Roberto Patarca-Montero, MD, PhD

Medical Etiology, Assessment, and Treatment of Chronic Fatigue and Malaise
Clinical Differentiation and Intervention

Pre-publication
REVIEW

"**D**r. Patarca-Montero is a concise and lucid author brimming with well-seasoned and equitable understanding of fatigue syndromes. Whether you are a patient, physician, or researcher, it will be impossible to open the book to any page without benefiting from his knowledgeable and balanced views. As in his previous books, there is an incredible and exhaustive bibliography that will be of incalculable benefit to any physician or researcher.

Dr. Patarca-Montero has the ability to focus on many of the areas of dispute surrounding CFS and give comprehensive clarifications and insights. It is a pleasure to read his unbiased, learned, and constructive views.

With the general failure of the majority of researchers and physicians to investigate the nature of the pathophysiology that is to be treated, patients with CFS and FS have turned in unprecedented numbers to alternative medicines, some useful, some dangerous, and some simply useless. The author discusses in considerable detail both conventional and alternative medications and herbals. His discussion is both informative and comprehensive.

It is impossible to read through the information packed into this book without believing that it will become the reference text for CFS for the next decade. This book is a marvel of information and I recommend any individuals with an interest in this complex and fascinating disease process to obtain a copy."

Byron Hyde, MD
Chairman,
Nightingale Research Foundation,
Ottawa, Ontario,
Canada

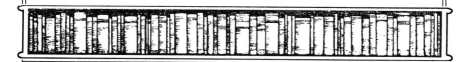

Medical Etiology, Assessment, and Treatment of Chronic Fatigue and Malaise

Clinical Differentiation and Intervention

THE HAWORTH MEDICAL PRESS®
Haworth Research Series
on Malaise, Fatigue, and Debilitation
Roberto Patarca-Montero, MD, PhD
Editor in Chief

Medical Etiology, Assessment, and Treatment of Chronic Fatigue and Malaise
Clinical Differentiation and Intervention

Roberto Patarca-Montero, MD, PhD

The Haworth Medical Press®
An Imprint of The Haworth Press, Inc.
New York • London • Oxford

Published by

The Haworth Medical Press ®, an imprint of The Haworth Press, Inc., 10 Alice Street, Binghamton, NY 13904-1580.

Publisher's Note

This book has been published solely for educational purposes and is not intended to substitute for the medical advice of a treating physician. Medicine is an ever-changing science. As new research and clinical experience broaden our knowledge, changes in treatment may be required. While many potential treatment options are made herein, some or all of the options may not be applicable to a particular individual. Therefore, the author, editor and publisher do not accept responsibility in the event of negative consequences incurred as a result of the information presented in this book. We do not claim that this information is necessarily accurate by the rigid scientific and regulatory standards applied for medical treatment. **No warranty, expressed or implied, is furnished with respect to the material contained in this book. The reader is urged to consult with his/her personal physician with respect to the treatment of any medical condition.**

Cover design by Marylouise E. Doyle.

Library of Congress Cataloging-in-Publication Data
Patarca-Montero, Roberto.
    Medical etiology, assessment, and treatment of chronic fatigue and malaise : clinical differentiation and intervention / Roberto Patarca-Montero.
        p. ; cm.
    Includes bibliographical references and index.
    ISBN 0-7890-2195-1 (case : alk. paper)—ISBN 0-7890-2196-X (soft : alk. paper)
    1. Fatigue—Etiology. 2. Fatigue—Diagnosis. 3. Fatigue—Treatment.
    [DNLM: 1. Fatigue—diagnosis. 2. Chronic Disease. 3. Diagnosis, Differential. 4. Fatigue—Etiology. 5. Fatigue—therapy. WB 146 P294m 2004] I. Title.
RB150.F37P383 2004
616'.0478—dc22
                                                                                        2003022502

CONTENTS

ABOUT THE AUTHOR

Roberto Patarca-Montero, MD, PhD, is Editor in Chief of The Haworth Medical Press. In his academic tenure, he has served as Assistant Professor of Medicine, Microbiology, and Immunology, and as Research Director of the E. M. Papper Laboratory of Clinical Immunology and Molecular Biology at the University of Miami School of Medicine. Previously, he was Assistant Professor of Pathology at the Dana-Farber Cancer Institute and Harvard Medical School in Boston.

Dr. Patarca served as Editor of *Critical Reviews in Oncogenesis* and of the *Journal of Chronic Fatigue Syndrome.* Dr. Patarca is also the author or co-author of more than 100 articles in journals or books, as well as *Chronic Fatigue Syndrome, Genes, and Infection: The Eta-1/Op Paradigm,* the *Concise Encyclopedia of Chronic Fatigue Syndrome,* and *Chronic Fatigue Syndrome: Advances in Epidemiologic, Clinical, and Basic Science Research.*

Dr. Patarca's research interests have focused on the pathophysiology and immunotherapy of AIDS and chronic fatigue syndrome; he was part of the American team that first characterized the AIDS virus and he also characterized several gene products that regulate its expression. Dr. Patarca was a member of the Board of Directors of the American Association for Chronic Fatigue Syndrome and the Acquired Non-HIV Immune Diseases Foundation and he is currently a member of the Chronic Fatigue Syndrome Coordinating Committee of the U.S. Department of Health and Human Services.

Chapter 1

Chronic Fatigue: Definition and History

DEFINITION OF CHRONIC FATIGUE

Fatigue is probably the most common symptom of illness affecting sufferers of most acute and chronic conditions. Fatigue is also a universal complaint that may sometimes be related to medical diagnoses or therapeutic treatments (Groopman, 1998; Ream and Richardson, 1996, 1997, 1999; Shapiro, 1998; Tiesinga, Dassen, and Halfens, 1996; White, 1997). In fact, Cox and colleagues (1987) reported that 20 percent of men and 30 percent of women always feel tired, and Shepherd and colleagues (1981) reported that 13 percent of men and 23 percent of women often get spells of complete exhaustion or fatigue. Therefore, confusion surrounds the definition and use of the term *fatigue*. As with many other medical concepts, it is a term frequently used in everyday language in the context of tiredness, weakness, exhaustion, decreased strength, decreased physical performance or endurance, sleepiness, lethargy, asthenia, difficulty concentrating, decreased memory, or lack of motivation, among others. Colloquial jargon to refer to fatigue states also changes, as exemplified by Ellis's statement (1984) that patients used to complain of not being "in the pink"; nowadays they are "bushed," "beat," or "washed out." Individuals also used to expect a simple diagnosis and treatment; now both are much more complex (Hurwitz, 1970). Other similarly nonspecific and less commonly used words in place of fatigue are the French terms malaise and lassitude. However, Glaus, Crow, and Hammond (1996a,b) found that the concept of malaise was neither identified nor understood as an expression of fatigue by the German-speaking population they studied.

Fatigue has been described for centuries in the medical literature. However, in 1921, Muscio (1921) concluded that the empirically vague term fatigue should be absolutely banished from scientific discussion, and consequently that attempts to obtain a fatigue test be abandoned. To this day, the term *fatigue* continues to elude precise definition or objective measurement in the research and clinical literature (Barofsky and Legro, 1991). The fact that the word *fatigue* is used to refer to many different physical and mental conditions, as well as personality disorders and traits, of diverse causes and characteristics adds to the confusion and, not uncommonly, also leads to stigmatization of the person labeled as "fatigued." In some instances, complaining of fatigue is perceived as a means of malingering and a reflection of laziness. Fatigue is often even considered, by both sufferers and the people who help them, as an inconvenience and a frustration that has to be dealt with for a limited time period. Some patients appear to gradually adjust and accommodate to the fatigue and are not really aware of the changes that take place over time (Hamilton et al., 2001).

The definitions of fatigue remain numerous, inconsistent, and varied according to the discipline of the author and the nature of the research (Richardson, 1998). Fatigue is a complex, nonspecific, and subjective phenomenon that has many causes and dimensions and for which no one definition is widely accepted and whose nature, intensity, and duration are influenced by the clinical, cultural, environmental, biochemical, personal, sociodemographic, and other variables of the context in which it manifests. The cause of fatigue may be physiological, psychological, pathological, or a combination thereof, and the variety of causes of fatigue determines the nature, frequency, and severity of its objective and subjective manifestations in particular individuals (Gall, 1996). The condition of fatigue therefore requires adequate assessments, innovative planning and interventions, and patient-centered evaluations by health care professionals. For instance, fatigue is often perceived as part of normal aging, yet for many active elderly, a complaint of generalized, nonspecific weakness should alert the physician to the existence of possible underlying pathology (Wolf-Klein et al., 1989).

Fatigue may be acute, episodic, or chronic, and it can be accompanied by a changing emotional or mental state. Not only is the recognition of fatigue as a symptom important to the diagnostic process, but fatigue, whether acute or chronic, needs to be recognized as a true and valid condition to be successful in its treatment and that of the illnesses it accompanies. Moreover, chronic fatigue and acute fatigue can be quite different conditions, requiring different approaches (Groopman, 1998; Ream and Richardson, 1996, 1997, 1999; Shapiro, 1998; Tiesinga, Dassen, and Halfens, 1996; White, 1997). The patterns and dimensions of fatigue have important implications in the care of individuals and patients, and further investigation in the area of fatigue is a critical aspect of quality-of-life improvement. Research into fatigue or other aspects of quality of life is curtailed by the fact that no animal protocols exist to individually study fatigue or other subjective symptoms such as depression, headache, or memory loss, and available tests lack sufficient specificity (Doull, 1996). Because of the lack of validated animal models of fatigue, it has generally been studied only as a self-reported phenomenon in humans.

In the clinical setting, as opposed to exercise physiology, fatigue is essentially a self-reported sensation that may have objectively measurable correlates which have yet to be identified and/or validated. In this respect, it is akin to the situation with nausea as opposed to vomiting. In animal models (e.g., in the ferret) the mechanical components (retching and vomiting) of the emetic response to anticancer therapies can be measured, but the subjective element of nausea cannot, although behavioral changes have been described that some consider to be correlates of the sensory experience (Morrow, Andrews, et al., 2002). Given the research tool limitations, fatigue is described as reduced capacity to sustain force or power output, reduced capacity to perform multiple tasks over time, and simply a subjective experience of feeling exhausted, tired, weak, or having lack of energy. Some authors think of fatigue as a subjective state of overwhelming, sustained exhaustion and decreased capacity for physical and mental work that may or may not be relieved by rest depending on whether fatigue is physiological or pathological. Therefore, for clinical and research purposes, fatigue is usually defined in the context that it manifests.

HISTORY OF CHRONIC FATIGUING ILLNESSES

Serious, disabling chronic fatigue is not a new, late-twentieth-century malaise. The history dates back several centuries, and with that history unfolds a complex, contradictory, and often controversial picture of puzzling illnesses with the cardinal symptom of chronic fatigue. The earlier models foreshadow the current conflicts among theoreticians, researchers, and clinicians about the nature of chronic fatiguing illnesses. As detailed in this section, the international historical trail that has led to the recognition of chronic fatiguing illnesses as disease entities is paved with terms that at different points have been used to refer to these unexplained symptom complexes of which fatigue is a prominent part.

In the sixteenth century, there is a reference to the "English sweats" of which Anne Boleyn was believed to be a sufferer (Cox, 2000). In the American Civil War there was an illness termed "soldiers' disease" for which the treatment was bed rest and hypernutrition for several months (Hyde, 1992a; Wessely, 1991). The term "fibrositis" was used in 1894 to refer to a chronic fatiguing illness; this term has now been replaced by fibromyalgia.

The 1982 publication of the resolution journal of Johann George Reinhold Forster included an account of an illness, termed "Tapanui flu," that was suffered by many of the sloop's crew, including Forster, after a period ashore at Queen Charlotte Sound, New Zealand. The symptoms of the illness were remarkably similar to those now clustered as the chronic fatigue syndrome (CFS) (St. George, 1996). In 1854, from the age thirty-five to sixty years, Florence Nightingale was reported as suffering from chest pain, headaches, rapid muscle fatigue, persistent upper back pain, and being unable to concentrate if more than one person was present in the room (Hyde, 1992a).

George Beard, an American neurologist, was responsible for publicizing the condition known as "neurasthenia" or "the disease of the century," beginning in 1869 (Beard, 1869; Friedberg and Jason, 1998). Neurasthenia dominated medical thinking on chronic fatiguing illnesses at the beginning of the twentieth century (Wessely, 1990, 1991). The syndrome was specified as having fatigue as its core symptom and was described as being brought on by mere thought of exertion or by the anticipation of any task. The signs were cited as worry, fatigue, and exhaustion (Wessely, 1990). It was most common among educated and professional classes. In 1880, Beard listed over seventy symptoms, with special attention being paid to specific areas: cardiac, gastrointestinal, temperature regulation, paresthesia, and pain syndromes (Wessely, 1991). Beard viewed this disabling condition as an entirely organic illness of profound fatigability of the body and mind beyond the reasonable results of mental or physical exertion and thereby partially or wholly incapacitating the suffering individual from his or her ordinary occupation or from the enjoyment of life (Hall, 1905). Neurasthenia was thought to derive from central exhaustion secondary to overwork, toxins, or metabolic or infective insults (Cox, 2000). "Organicists" such as Beard argued that affective changes were an understandable reaction to the illness (Wessely, 1991).

By the late 1800s, neurasthenia was one of the most frequently diagnosed illnesses. S. Weir Mitchell, a fellow neurologist of Beard and an American founder of neurology, proposed a "rest cure" that was later offered by private sanatoria and remained popular for about thirty years (Sabin and Dawson, 1993; Wessely, 1991). The rest cure prescription, in its extreme form, dictated total bed rest punctuated only by bathroom breaks. Patients were not permitted to read, write, think too hard, or even brush their teeth. Charlotte Perkins Gilman's (1993) famous short story "The Yellow Wallpaper" placed the rest cure in the cultural context of the late nineteenth century. The heroine of this tale was ordered to rest in an isolated room and was denied all visitors and reading materials. The story was a metaphor for the lives of middle-class women trapped in other people's expectations; the patient's Victorian physicians told her to rest until she wanted to pursue only "natural" womanly activities rather than the "unwomanly" intellectual activities that she craved. She eventually went mad, the only way she could become "free." An excellent discussion of the rest treatment approach for neurasthenia may be found in Ehrenreich and English's (1989) book *For Her Own Good: 150 Years of Experts' Advice to Women.*

By 1914, the observation that neurasthenia frequently followed an infection (influenza) was widely acknowledged (Wessely, 1991). However, by the end of World War I, the diagnosis of neurasthenia had almost disappeared. According to Wessely (1990), this change occurred as increasing medical skepticism and psychiatric sophistication led to the view that neurasthenia was a psychiatric rather than a neurological condition. In addition, the illness was increasingly perceived as an affliction of the lower social classes. In fact, prior to 1906, neurasthenia was viewed as a disease only of the upper classes. By 1906, it was viewed mainly as a disease of the lower social classes, and the term "mild melancholia" was also used. Diagnosis was made, according to Wessely (1991), for the comfort of the relatives and peace of mind of the patient.

It is not clear what influences led to these changing perceptions. Perhaps the upper classes rejected illnesses that had psychiatric implications, whereas those with fewer resources and limited access to needed care might have been more likely to be stigmatized with psychiatric labels. By 1926 there had been a move from neuroses to psychoneuroses. The diagnosis of neurasthenia was eventually discredited and became shameful for patients to confess. By the 1930s physicians generally used descriptive labels, such as chronic nervous exhaustion, tired, weak, or toxic, the main emphasis still being on psychological mechanisms (Wessely, 1990, 1991). In due course the diagnosis of neurasthenia was replaced by new psychiatric diagnoses of anxiety and depression (Wessely, 1990, 1991).

Chronic fatiguing illnesses were less frequently reported from World War I to the early 1980s. Friedberg and Jason (1998) posit that one or more of the following possibilities may have accounted for this decline: (1) the illness was, in fact, less prevalent; (2) physicians were less likely to diagnose it; (3) patients were less inclined to bring their complaints to physicians, who tended to perceive those complaints in psychiatric terms. It is unclear which one or combination of the three possible explanations accounts for the decrease in chronic fatiguing illness reporting. However, Friedberg and Jason (1998) believe that explanations (2) and (3) are more plausible. In an age when so many disorders had been traced to biological malfunctions, it was not difficult for physicians to conclude that an illness without consistent markers, such as neurasthenia, was an expression of a psychiatric condition. Once the leading physicians began to devalue neurasthenia as a psychiatric disorder, these patients may have been less likely to seek out medical services.

During this period, unexplained fatiguing illnesses also occurred in clustered outbreaks. As summarized in Cox (2000), notable epidemic outbreaks of chronic fatiguing illness occurred in the following locations:

1934, Los Angeles, California (198 hospital staff and community members)

1936, Fond-du-Lac, Wisconsin (thirty-five convent candidates and novices)

1937, Erstfeld, Switzerland (130 soldiers), and Frohburg, Switzerland (twenty-eight patients and staff)

1939, Harefield, England (seven hospital staff members), and Degersheim, Switzerland (seventy-three soldiers)

1945, Pennsylvania (university hospital)

1948-1949, Iceland (1,090 community members)

1949-1951, Adelaide, Australia (800 community members)

1950, Louisville, Kentucky (thirty-seven nursing students), and Upper New York State (nineteen community members)

1952, Middlesex Hospital, England (fourteen nursing students), Copenhangen, Denmark (more than seventy community members), and Lakeland, Florida (twenty-seven community members)

1953, Coventry, England (thirteen hospital staff and community members), and Rockville, Maryland (fifty nursing students and community members)

1954, Tallahassee, Florida (450 community members), Seward, Alaska (175 community members), and Berlin, Germany (seven in barracks group)

1954-1955, Johannesburg, South Africa (fourteen community members)

1955, Dalston, Columbia, England (community), Royal Free Hospital, England (300 hospital staff members), Perth, Australia (community), Gilfach Goch, Wales (community), East Ham, London, England (community), and Durban, South Africa (140 hospital staff and community members)

1955-1956, Segbwema, Sierra Leone (community members)

1956, Ridgefield, Connecticut (seventy community members), Punta Gorda, Florida (124 community members), and Pittsfield, Massachusetts (seven community members)

1956-1957, Coventry, England (seven community members)

1958, Athens, Greece (twenty-seven nursing students)

1959, Newcastle-upon-Tyne, England (community)

1961-1962, New York State (convent)

1964-1965, Galveston County, Texas (community)

1969, New York State (university medical center)

1970-1971, Great Ormond Street Hospital, London, England (hospital staff members)

1975, Sacramento, California (200 hospital staff members)

1976, South West, Ireland (community)

1979, Southampton, England (ten community members)

1980-1981, Ayrshire, Scotland (rural practice)

1980-1983, Helensburgh, Scotland (general practitioner practice)

1983-1984, West Otago, New Zealand (more than twenty community members)

1984, Lake Tahoe, Nevada (teachers and pupils)

1985, Lyndonville, New York (community)

Two epidemics that attracted considerable attention occurred in 1934 at the Los Angeles County Hospital and in 1955 at the Royal Free Hospital in Great Britain. Both outbreaks involved the medical staffs rather than the patients. The reported motor and sensory symptoms received diagnoses such as atypical poliomyelitis, neuromysthenia, or myalgic encephalomyelitis. Although most cases resolved within a few months, some of the affected individuals remained chronically ill with fluctuating symptoms and significant functional impairments (Briggs and Levine, 1994). Research studies were launched to better understand these outbreaks; however, physicians and researchers could not explain what had occurred. Because these outbreaks of acute illness affected relatively few people, they have become footnotes in medical history (Friedberg and Jason, 1998).

In the 1934 Los Angeles County Hospital epidemic all doctors and nurses were affected with an illness that was termed "atypical poliomyelitis" (Gilliam, 1992; Hyde et al., 1992b). In an attempt to treat their symptoms they were injected with immune prophylactic globulin (Cox, 2000). Their symptoms were described as follows: relapsing muscle weakness, inability to work, unusual pain syndromes, personality changes, memory loss, hysterical episodes, vertigo, major temperature fluctuations, pain in limbs, nausea, and aphasia. The disease was termed atypical poliomyelitis because the infective trigger was thought to be poliomyelitis. Other terms used were acute anterior poliomyelitis (1934) and abortive poliomyelitis (1937).

There appeared to be two forms of onset: acute and gradual. A greater predominance was noted in females. The sufferers were often later labeled as "malingerers" or as having "compensationitis." In 1968, when discussing the events of 1934, Marinacci stated that this attitude often produced a conflict between the patient and the attending medical staff, and the patients were transferred from clinic to clinic and from department to department (Hyde, 1992b). Fourteen to eighteen years later, twenty-one of those originally affected were examined. Their main complaints were recurring fatigue, pain, some muscle spasms (cervical and lumbosacral), persistence of symptoms, and impaired memory. Many were paralyzed and in wheelchairs (Hyde, 1992b).

In 1955, at the Royal Free Hospital in London (Compston, 1978), 200 cases of an unknown illness were identified with the following range of symptoms: headache, sore throat, malaise, lymphadenopathy, lassitude, vertigo, pain in limbs, nausea, dizziness, stiff neck, pain in back/chest, depression, abdominal pain, vomiting, diplopia, tinnitus, and diarrhea. The duration of hospital inpatient treatment varied from less than one month (114 individuals) to more than three months (14 individuals). Two years following the episode only four patients still had marked physical disability. The Royal Free Hospital epidemic was thought to be a manifestation of mass hysteria (Compston, 1978).

When comparing the 1934 and 1955 outbreaks, Parish (1978) found that the triggers in both appeared to be a virus. Both appeared to be a systemic illness, distinguished in many patients by a prolonged convalescence and portrayed by mental changes, particularly depression, autonomic disturbances, a profound tendency to fatigue easily, and relapses of the original features of the illness. In 1959, Donald Acheson described the symptoms of the illness as headache, low or absent fever, myalgia, and paresis with symptoms or signs suggestive of damage to the brain, in essence, mental symptoms. He also noticed a higher frequency in women, a predominantly normal cerebrospinal fluid, and that sufferers were prone to relapses.

A number of labels were being given to chronic fatiguing illnesses in this time period, such as epidemic neuromyasthenia (1950), neuritis vegetativa epidemica (1952), myalgic encephalomyelitis (1955), and Iceland or Akureyri disease. Chronic fatiguing illnesses were observed to be a frequent occurrence among young female nurses in hospital epidemics while patients remained unaffected, which writers at the time found surprising (Acheson, 1992).

In 1959, Acheson listed the common symptoms as generalized severe headache; stiffness in neck and back; and pain in the muscles of the neck, shoulders, and limbs that varied in intensity and was aggravated by exertion. The pain was often agonizing and unresponsive to opioids. When the pain was severe, exquisite muscle tenderness, tender nerve trunks, and skin sensitivity accompanied it. He also noted muscular twitching, cramps, low fever, and localized muscular weakness, which were variable in site and intensity. It was observed that full neurological examinations were rarely performed.

Many variations were seen between the numerous outbreaks that were reported and summarized (Cox, 2000). However, all were acute in duration with a range of four to twelve weeks. The acute symptoms often required hospitalization. Some people suffered relapses, although most recovered six months after onset. In some, relapses occurred with the menstrual cycle. Cyclical recurrences were seen in many of the epidemic patients two-and-a-half years after initial illness. The triggers appeared to be overexertion and cold, damp weather (Acheson, 1992).

It was noted in thirty-nine patients with Iceland/Akureyri disease (Sigurdsson and Gudmundsson, 1956) that six years after onset residual symptoms remained, although most had returned to work. Overall, there was a tendency toward slow improvement on a fluctuating course. The common symptoms remaining were nervousness, depression, fatigue, loss of memory, muscular pains, localized weakness, and poor concentration. Headache and joint pain were also common, with occasional upper respiratory or gastrointestinal disturbances and paresis. Lindal and colleagues (1997) noted that Iceland/Akureyri disease characterized by prolonged chronic fatigue resulted in anxiety disorders following infection. However, the more serious psychiatric disorders (agoraphobia with panic attacks, agoraphobia without panic attacks, social phobia, simple phobia, schizophrenia, and alcohol dependence) did not seem to play a role in the long run.

During the 1960s and 1970s, chronic brucellosis was often cited as the cause of chronic fatigue, but patients with this diagnosis were typically viewed as having psychiatric conditions, usually depression. During this time period, sporadic cases of chronic fatiguing illness were also noted (Parish, 1978). The predominant symptoms described were earache, headache, tinnitus, giddiness, muscular twitching, lassitude, cramps, low pyrexia, tremors, paresthesia, lymphadenopathy, muscle tenderness, stiffness of neck, and paresis.

In the acute stage, people described terrifying dreams, panic states, and hypersomnia. Later in the convalescent stage they described impairment of memory, difficulty in concentration, and depression. Acheson (1992) drew the conclusion that this was a disorder of an infection spread by personal contact (Parish, 1978). There appeared to be predominance in the medical and nursing professions, often with complete recovery within three months.

By 1960, U.S. reports linked chronic fatigue with the Epstein-Barr virus (Wessely, 1991). There was thought to be central nervous system involvement because of the common cognitive symptoms of diplopia, paresthesia, unsteadiness, vertigo, blurring of vision, emotional lability, impairment of memory and concentration, terrifying nightmares, and overelaborated recital of symptoms. Beginning in the mid-1980s, the term chronic Epstein-Barr virus (EBV) syndrome was used to explain chronic fatigue as a persistent viral illness caused by the same pathogen responsible for acute mononucleosis; however, this link was later discredited (Jones, 1991).

In 1984, in the Lake Tahoe region of Nevada, an epidemic of a mysterious disease occurred that was first termed "Lake Tahoe disease" and subsequently labeled chronic fatigue syndrome by infectious disease physicians at the Centers for Disease Control and Prevention (CDC) (Holmes et al., 1988). Some people prefer the term chronic fatigue immune dysfunction syndrome. Chronic fatigue syndrome includes cases of long-standing (six months or longer) fatigue that are not explained by an existing medical or psychiatric diagnosis, are not substantially alleviated by rest, and cause considerable disabilities in professional, social, and/or personal functioning (at least 50 percent reduction in baseline level). Secondary criteria for chronic fatigue syndrome include sore throat, fever, painful swollen lymph nodes (adenopathy, particularly cervical or axillary), muscle pain (myalgia), headaches (of a new type, pattern, or severity), multiple joint pain without joint swelling or redness, sleep disorders, and neuropsychological symptoms, such as self-reported persistent or recurrent impairment in short-term memory or concentration severe enough to cause substantial reductions in previous levels of occupational, educational, social, or personal activities. Although several studies have validated the use of these criteria (combinations of the primary and four secondary ones), much controversy persists and attempts at formulating new criteria based on laboratory parameters are being undertaken (Patarca, 2000; Riem, 1999; Wessely, 2001).

Chronic Fatiguing Illnesses and Infectious Diseases

The late twentieth century and the beginning of the twenty-first century witnessed the rise of the antiviral revolution era, which flourished from the knowledge provided by the molecular biological characterization of the genetic makeup of viruses. One of the corollaries of this revolution is that the realm of diseases is not only viral but also bacterial; microbial etiologies in general have also been expanded to include pathological processes such as atherosclerosis, autoimmune disease, and chronic fatiguing illnesses that would not have been previously recognized as secondary to infectious processes. A variety of viral and bacterial infections have been associated with chronic fatiguing illnesses. In addition to the terms cited previously, postviral fatigue syndrome, Coxsackie B virus infection, and yuppie flu (1986) have also been used as labels for chronic fatiguing illnesses.

Postpolio syndrome, another chronic fatiguing illness, affects more than 1.8 million North American polio survivors. A possible common pathophysiology and treatment for postpolio fatigue and chronic fatigue syndrome has been proposed (Bruno et al., 1996; Bruno, Creange, and Frick, 1998; Nollet et al., 1996; Thorsteinsson, 1997) based on the clinically significant fatigue, deficits on neuropsychologic tests of attention, histopathologic and neuroradiologic evidence of brain lesions, impaired activation of the hypo-thalamic-pituitary-adrenal (HPA) axis, increased prolactin secretion, elec-troencephalogram (EEG) slow-wave activity, and the influence of psycho-logical factors seen in both conditions (Bruno, 1998; Bruno, Creange, and Frick, 1998; Bruno et al., 1996, 1998; Schanke, 1997). However, persistent enteroviral infection has not been consistently demonstrated in CFS pa-tients.

Despite antibiotic treatment, a sequel of Lyme disease may be a post-Lyme disease syndrome, which is characterized by persistent fatigue, arthralgia, and neurocognitive impairment (Bujak, Weinstein, and Dorn-bush, 1996; Diamantis, 1996; Ellenbogen, 1997; Ravdin et al., 1996). An-other postinfection syndrome, the post-Q fever fatigue syndrome, is charac-terized by inappropriate fatigue, myalgia and arthralgia, night sweats, and changes in mood and sleep patterns following about 20 percent of labora-tory-proven cases of acute primary Q fever, a condition caused by *Coxiella burnetii* (Ayres et al., 1998; Bennett et al., 1998; Penttila et al., 1998) that can be transmitted through ticks, droplets, or raw milk from infected ani-mals.

A prospective cohort study (White et al., 1998) of 250 primary care pa-tients in England revealed a higher incidence and longer duration of an acute fatigue syndrome, and a higher prevalence of chronic fatigue syn-drome, after glandular fever versus an ordinary upper respiratory tract in-fection. The authors estimated that glandular fever accounts for 3,113 (95 percent) new cases of chronic fatigue syndrome per annum in England and Wales. New episodes of major depressive disorder were triggered by infec-tion, especially the Epstein-Barr virus, but lasted a median of only three weeks. No psychiatric disorder was significantly more prevalent six months after onset than before. A second study (White, Dash, and Thomas, 1998) by the same group found that the ability to process information after glan-dular fever or an ordinary upper respiratory tract infection is related to esti-mates of premorbid IQ, whereas poor concentration is related independ-ently to both psychiatric morbidity and a fatigue state, but not the particular infection itself.

Chronic Fatiguing Illnesses Associated with Defined Illnesses

The experience accumulated with the syndromes mentioned in the previ-ous section has been extended to conceptualize, define, and study fatigue in the context of cancer, as a complex syndrome termed *cancer-related fatigue* or *cancer-related fatigue syndrome* (Sadler et al., 2002; Winningham, 2001). Such a conceptual framework, reached by consensus from the clinical and research perspectives, facilitates the appreciation of the physical, affective, and cognitive manifestations of cancer-related fatigue. In 1999, cancer-related fatigue was accepted as a diagnosis in the *International Classification of Diseases*, Tenth Revision, Clinical Modification (ICD-10-CM) (Portenoy and Itri, 1999). Cancer-related fatigue is multifactorial and can be brought on by cancer treatment.

Postdialysis fatigue, another chronic fatiguing illness brought to its proper light in the late twentieth century and secondary to medical treatment, has been ascribed to excessive ultrafiltration and decline in osmolality during hemodialysis. As in chronic fatigue syndrome and other fatiguing illnesses, somnogenic cytokines such as tumor necrosis factor (TNF)-alpha, in this case induced by the hemodialysis process, play a role (Colton, 1988; Dreisbach et al., 1998; Herbelin et al., 1990; Patarca et al., 1992; Zaoui, Green, and Hakim, 1991). Patients undergoing chronic hemodialysis may also develop complications such as fever, hypotension, increased catabolism, acute-phase protein synthesis, beta2-microglobulin production, and cellular immune defects (Colton, 1988; Smetana et al., 1991).

Chronic Fatiguing Illnesses and the Environment

Progress in environmental and occupational medicine also evinced the role of toxins and other environmental agents as causes of chronic fatiguing illnesses. For instance, chronic ciguatera is a chronic fatiguing illness that may present in 20 percent of cases of ciguatera, a distressing form of fish poisoning caused by the ingestion of one or more of a series of ciguatoxins (Pearn, 1996, 1997). These poisons, some of the most potent mammalian neurotoxins known, are manufactured in reef-dwelling dinoflagellates and concentrated up the piscine food chain. Eating certain bottom-dwelling fish species poisons humans. The acute intoxication is clinically dramatic, resulting in paresthesias, dysesthesias, prostration, myalgia, and arthralgia. In approximately 20 percent of cases, symptoms of fatigue, reduced exercise tolerance, and nonspecific headaches and pains persist for months and, in a small percentage of cases, for years. Occasionally patients are encountered who have been diagnosed with chronic fatigue syndrome because of lack of awareness of the ciguatera syndrome, but in whom in retrospect the episode of acute fish poisoning can be established (Pearn, 1996, 1997).

A study (Iowa Persian Gulf Study Group, 1997) of 3,695 military personnel found that those who participated in the Persian Gulf War had a higher self-reported prevalence of medical and psychiatric conditions than contemporary military personnel who were not deployed to the Persian Gulf. Compared with non-Persian Gulf War military personnel, Persian Gulf War military personnel reported a significantly higher prevalence of symptoms of depression, post-traumatic stress disorder (PTSD), chronic fatigue, cognitive dysfunction, bronchitis, asthma, fibromyalgia, alcohol abuse, anxiety, and sexual discomfort. Assessment of health-related quality of life demonstrated diminished mental and physical functioning scores for Persian Gulf War military personnel. The New Jersey Center for Environmental Hazards Research (Fiedler, Kipen, Natelson, and Ottenweller, 1996) found that more than half of the Persian Gulf Registry veterans reported illness characterized by severe fatigue and symptoms consistent with chemical sensitivities. Human challenge testing procedures have been used unsuccessfully to test theories of causal relationships of airborne allergens and chemicals with allergic sensitization potential and the causal relationship of chemical exposure and the Persian Gulf War syndrome (Coker, 1996; Hyams, 1998; Nicolson, Bruton, and Nicholson, 1996; Selner, 1996). As will be discussed in Chapter 3, one report (Rook and Zumla, 1997) suggests that the symptoms of Persian Gulf War syndrome are compatible with the hypothesis that the immune system of affected individuals is biased toward a Th2 (humoral immunity-oriented) cytokine pattern. A factor that could lead to this pattern shift among Gulf War veterans includes exposure to multiple vaccinations. Some authors contend that because Armed Forces Reserve members, especially combat support units, were rapidly mobilized during Operation Desert Shield/Desert Storm, they were at higher risk for anxiety and stress-related disorders that may have contributed to the development of later symptoms (Malone et al., 1996).

Multiple chemical sensitivity (MCS) syndrome is part of the chemical sensitivity syndromes, which include the sick building syndrome and the Persian Gulf War syndrome, all related to chronic fatigue syndrome (Bell, Baldwin, and Schwartz, 1998; Weiss, 1998). Except for chronic fatigue syndrome, toxic chemical exposures are accorded a significant role in their etiologies. The connections are ambiguous because of the variety of chemical agents cited and, for the most part, the relatively low levels at which exposures occur. Conventional clinical signs are also typically lacking. Explanatory mechanisms include psychiatric diagnoses such as somatization, behavioral mechanisms such as conditioning and generalization, neuropharmacological mechanisms such as sensitization (including an olfactory-limbic neural sensitization model [Bell, Baldwin, and Schwartz, 1998] for intolerance to low-level chemicals in the environment), and psychoneuro-immunological mechanisms such as those involving the HPA axis. Laboratory animal experimentation and controlled clinical trials, especially with inhaled material, provide the means for exploring the proffered explanations.

A study (Fiedler, Kipen, DeLuca, et al., 1996) of twenty-three patients whose sensitivities to multiple low-level chemical exposures began with a defined exposure (MCS), thirteen patients with sensitivities to multiple chemicals without a clear date of onset chemical sensitivity (CS), and eighteen patients meeting CDC criteria for chronic fatigue syndrome found that subjects with sensitivities to chemicals (MCS and CS) reported significantly more lifestyle changes secondary to chemical sensitivities and significantly more chemical substances that made them ill compared with chronic fatigue syndrome and controls. MCS, CS, and CFS patients had significantly higher rates of current psychiatric disorders than controls and reported significantly more physical symptoms with no medical explanation. Seventy-four percent of MCS and 61 percent of chronic fatigue syndrome did not qualify for any current Axis I psychiatric diagnosis. Chemically sensitive subjects without a defined date of onset (CS) had the highest rate of Axis I psychiatric disorders (69 percent). In the Minnesota Multiphasic Personality Inventory (MMPI-2), 44 percent of MCS, 42 percent of CS, 53 percent of CFS, and none of the controls achieved clinically significant elevations on scales associated with somatoform disorders. With the exception of one complex test of visual memory, no significant differences were noted among the groups on tests of neuropsychological function. Standardized measures of psychiatric and neuropsychological function did not differentiate subjects with sensitivities to chemicals from those with chronic fatigue syndrome. Subjects with sensitivities to chemicals and no clear date of onset had the highest rate of psychiatric morbidity. Standardized neuropsychological tests did not substantiate the cognitive impairment reported symptomatically. Cognitive deficits may become apparent under controlled exposure conditions.

A study (Lohmann, Prohl, and Schwarz, 1996) of 320 cases with chronic neurotoxic health impairments, of which 136 showed signs of MCS, revealed that neurotoxic substances which were used as indoor wood preservatives (mainly Pentachlorophenol and/or Lindane) were the causative agents in 63 percent of the cases with neurotoxic health impairments and MCS. Other important neurotoxic substances to which the patients were mainly exposed were organic solvents (25 percent), formaldehyde (15 percent), dental materials (15 percent), pyrethroides (13 percent), and other biocides (19 percent) (multiple exposures were possible). The time of exposure was calculated as being more than or equal to ten years for 55 percent of the patients with MCS and for 50 percent of the group with neurotoxic health impairments, but without MCS. Out of the 184 cases with neurotoxic health impairments, but without MCS, there were 22 percent and, out of the

136 cases with MCS, 39 percent showed all symptoms of chronic fatigue syndrome. Fifty-three percent of the cases with MCS had an allergic disposition compared to only 20 percent of the cases without MCS. In a study (Gibson, Cheavens, and Warren, 1998) on social support, fatigue level, being in a romantic relationship, contact with a support group on a monthly or more frequent basis, chemical avoidance in the home, gender, and an improved course of illness predicted 19 percent of the variance for perceived social support among MCS patients.

Another chronic fatiguing illness of environmental etiology is sick building syndrome (SBS). Although a link has been proposed between chronic fatigue syndrome and sick building syndrome, the evidence indicates that they are distinctive entities. Sick building syndrome is an excess of work-related irritations of the skin and mucous membranes, and of symptoms such as headache (primary symptom), dry eyes, and fatigue in those working in modern air-conditioned buildings, with women reporting more symptoms than men (Citterio et al., 1998; Mendell et al., 1996). One study (Chester and Levine, 1997) of twenty-three individuals concluded that the fatigue related to sick building syndrome, including chronic fatigue syndrome (fifteen out of twenty-three cases), is significantly more likely to improve than fatigue identified in sporadic cases of chronic fatigue syndrome. Chronic fatigue syndrome has no clear etiology while, besides ventilation-related problems (Maehara et al., 1998), sick building syndrome has been linked to other etiologies. For instance, in an investigation (Sudakin, 1998) of health complaints among employees of a water-damaged office building, the environment showed evidence of high-level fungal contamination with the isolation of *Stachybotrys chartarum, Penicillium, Aspergillus versicolor,* and bacteria in bulk and surface samples. A health survey of building occupants revealed a high prevalence of multiple symptoms with the predominance of neurobehavioral and upper respiratory tract complaints. The majority of symptoms were significantly less prevalent after relocation from the water-damaged environment. Exposure to toxigenic fungi may therefore be responsible for the high prevalence of reported symptoms in this group. The gap between chronic fatigue syndrome and sick building syndrome is further delineated in a case-control study (Shefer et al., 1997) of over 3,300 current employees in two state office buildings in northern California and employees in a comparable "control" building. This study concluded that, despite the substantial number of employees with fatiguing illness in the two state office buildings, the prevalence was not significantly different than that of the comparable control building. Previously unidentified risk factors for fatigue of at least one month and at least six months identified in this population included Hispanic ethnicity, not completing college, and income below $50,000.

Chronic Fatiguing Illnesses and Rheumatology

Fibromyalgia is a form of nonarticular, or soft tissue, rheumatism characterized by spontaneous widespread musculoskeletal aching, tenderness on palpation with multiple tender points (at least eleven out of eighteen in defined locations) (hyperalgesia), decreased pain threshold (allodynia), fatigue, poor sleep, mood disturbances, and other symptoms (Ang and Wilke, 1999; Bennett, 1998; Briggs, 1997; Celiker et al., 1997; Clauw, 1995; Coward, 1999; "Fibromyalgia," 2000; Fordyce, 2000; Gerster, 1999; Gordon and Morrison, 1998; Hadler, 1996a,b; Healey, 1996; Krsnich-Shriwise, 1997; Leslie, 1999; Lilleaas, 1997; Littlejohn, 1996; MacFarlane et al., 1996; Mailis, 1996; Neeck, Riedel, and Vaitl, 1997; Nishikai, 1999; Parziale and Chen, 1996; Pasero, 1998; Proceedings of the International Fibromyalgia Conference, 1998; Rankin, 1999; Raspe and Croft, 1995; Reiffenberger and Amundson, 1996; Reveille, 1997; Reynolds, 1996; Romano, 1998; Siegmeth, 1999; Simms, 1996; Slavkin, 1997; Tabeeva, Korotkova, and Vein, 2000; Unger, 1996; Van Santen-Hoeufft, 1996; Wallace, 1997, 1999; Wallace, Shapiro, and Panush, 1999; Winfield, 1997; Wootton, 2000; Xie and Ye, 1997). The concept and diagnosis of fibromyalgia became popular, especially in North America, in the 1970s. It is noticeable that there does not appear to be an early case report, as there is, for instance, for gout, rheumatoid arthritis, or certain vasculitides. Operational definitions and classification criteria were given in 1990, with the endorsement of the American College of Rheumatology, and are now the most widely used.

Although nearly all rheumatologists now accept fibromyalgia as a distinct diagnostic entity, and it is also recognized by the World Health Organization (WHO), the validity of fibromyalgia as a distinct clinical entity has been challenged for several reasons: the subjective nature of chronic pain; the subjectivity of the tender point examination; the failure to agree on the importance and biological nature of tenderness itself; the lack of a gold standard laboratory test; the absence of a clear pathogenic mechanism; the use of a syndromic description without a unifying concept; the relative nature of the pain-distress relationship in the rheumatology clinic; the apparently continuous relationship between tender points and somatic distress across a variety of clinical disorders; the failure to distinguish a clinical feature from a disease process; legal defenses of insurance carriers motivated by economic concerns; psychiatric dogma; uninformed posturing; suspicion of malingering; ignorance of nociceptive physiology; and, occasionally, honest misunderstanding (Buskila, Neumann, et al., 1997; Cathebras, Lauwers, and Rousset, 1998; Cathebras, 2000; Cohen, 1999; Finestone, 1997; Fitzcharles, 1999; Gamaz-Nava et al., 1998; Goldenberg, 1999; Gordon, 1997; Hadler, 1996a,b, 1997a,b; Hamilton, 1998; Handler, 1998;

Hantzschel and Boche, 1999; Helliwell, 1995; Hellsstrom, 1995; Hilden, 1996; Holoweiko, 1996; Hudson, 1998; Hunt, Starkebaum, and Thompson, 1998; Hyams, 1998; Jones, 1996; Kaden and Bubenzer, 1999; Katz et al., 1997; Kissel and Mahnig, 1998; Laser, 1998; Leonhardt, 2000; Lindberg and Lindberg, 2000; Makela, 1999; Marlowe, 1998; Matsumoto, 1999; Neeck, 1998; Neerinckx et al., 2000; Peloso, 1998; Quintner and Cohen, 1997, 1999; Raspe, 1996; Rau and Russell, 2000; Rekola et al., 1997; Romano, 1998; Russell, 1999; Safran, 1998; Shojania, 2000; Smith MD, 1998; Smith WA, 1998; Solomon and Liang, 1997; Thorson, 1998; Wessely and Hotopf, 1999; White and Harth, 1998; Wigley, 1999; Wilke, 1996a,b; Wolfe, 1997; Wolfe et al., 1997). In the United States, fibromyalgia is the third or fourth most common reason for rheumatology referral (Celiker et al., 1997; Gamez-Nava et al., 1998; Wallace, 1997), and several Web sites are dedicated to this condition (Armstrong, 2000; Jahn and Klenke, 1999). Fibromyalgia is predominant in middle-aged women but has also been reported in men, elderly individuals, and the pediatric population (Borenstein, 1996; Buskila, 1999; Cathebras, Lauwers, and Rousset, 1998; Holland and Gonzalez, 1998).

According to the American College of Rheumatology, the diagnosis of fibromyalgia is based on criteria consisting entirely of clinical signs and symptoms (Alarcon, 1997; Barth, 1997; Bassetti, 1996; Brown, 1997; Garfin, 1995; Hart, 1998; Jacobsen, 2000; Kavanaugh, 1996; Kjaergaard, 1998; Maier, 1998; MedLetter Associates, 1998; Pongratz and Sievers, 2000; Reinhold-Keller, 1997; Weber, 1998; Xie and Ye, 1997; Zborovskii and Babaeva, 1998). The American College of Rheumatology criteria, established in 1990, provide the primary care provider with definitive subjective and objective findings that have shown to be 88 percent accurate in their ability to diagnose patients with the syndrome (Smith MD, 1998; Smith WA, 1998). In the majority of fibromyalgia patients generalized pain is preceded by localized or regional pain, usually in the musculoskeletal system. In many fibromyalgia patients there are findings compatible with tissue injury pain, with pain mechanisms involving both the primary afferent neuron and the nociceptive system in the central nervous system (Henriksson, 1999; Olin and Lidbeck, 1996). The distinction between fibromyalgia (tender points) and myofascial pain syndrome (trigger points) is essential (Klineberg et al., 1998; Uppgaard, 2000). Also, macrophagic fasciitis, a recently identified inflammatory myopathy that can be detected by deltoid muscle biopsy and is manifested mainly in the lower limbs, can be differentiated from fibromyalgia and sarcoidosis by gallium-67 scintigraphy (Cherin et al., 2000). Fitzcharles and Esdaile (1997) reported that eleven women with spondyloarthritis had been incorrectly diagnosed as having fibromyalgia. Internal and neurological disorders as a primary cause of fibromyalgia have to be excluded (Olin and Lidbeck, 1996).

The etiology and pathogenesis of fibromyalgia still remain uncertain, and some reports suggest a genetic component (Bennett, 1998; Gelfand, 1998; Kelly, 1997; Kenner, 1998; Monroe, 1998; Shelkovnikov and Krivoruchko, 1997). Fibromyalgia symptoms last, on average, at least fifteen years after illness onset (De Jesus, 2000; Kennedy and Felson, 1996). However, most patients experience some improvement in symptoms before that time (Kennedy and Felson, 1996). Patients with fibromyalgia report greater difficulty in performing activities of daily living (ADL) as well as increased pain, fatigue, and weakness compared with healthy controls (Bennett, 1998; Celiker et al., 1997; Hadler, 1996a,b; Kennedy and Felson, 1996; MacFarlane et al., 1996; Slavkin, 1997). Associated disorders are restless leg syndrome (RLS), irritable bowel syndrome (IBS), irritable bladder syndrome, interstitial cystitis, headaches, ocular and vestibular complaints, cognitive dysfunction, cold intolerance, multiple sensitivities, and dizziness (Asencio-Marchante and Terriza-García, 1998; Bennett, 1998; Maurizio and Rogers, 1997; Siegmeth, 1999). Some muscle abnormalities have been reported (Park et al., 1998); the myopathological patterns in fibromyalgia are nonspecific: type II fiber atrophy, an increase in lipid droplets, a slight proliferation of mitochondria, and a slightly elevated incidence of ragged red fibers (Pongrantz and Sievers, 2000). However, most studies agree on an absence of inflammatory or structural musculoskeletal abnormalities (Masumoto, 1999), and, therefore, the original term "fibrositis" was replaced with fibromyalgia (Simms, 1998).

There is clinical, and in many cases demographic, overlap between fibromyalgia, chronic fatigue syndrome, Persian Gulf War syndrome, silicone implant-associated syndrome, sick building syndrome, multiple chemical sensitivity, and syndromes including neurally mediated hypotension, abnormalities of the growth hormone-insulin-like growth factor-1 axis, chemical intolerance, altered functioning of the stress-response system, and the presence of autoantibodies (Baschetti, 1999b; Bazelmans, Vercoulen, et al., 1997; Bennett, 1998; Buchwald, 1996; Buskila, 1999, 2000; Chambers, 1997; Csef, 1999; Goldenberg, 1997; Granzow, 1999; Hoffmann et al., 1996; Kelly, 1997; Kenner, 1998; Klimas, 1998; Pocinki, 1997; Robertson, 1999; Sabal, 1997; Slavkin, 1997; Vree, 1997; Wallace, 1997; Wessely and Hotopf, 1999). However, there are differences among the latter syndromes (Matsumoto, 1999). Fibromyalgia may also be affected by psychosocial, cultural, psychological, and environmental factors (Affleck et al., 1998; Ben-Zion, Shieber, and Buskila, 1996; Cathebras, 1997; Hadler, 1996a,b; Hausotter, 1998; Kissel and Mahnig, 1998; Kuhn, 2000; Kurtze, Gundersen, and Svebak, 1998; Reid, Lang, and McGrath, 1997; Schaefer,

1997; Schuck, Chappel, and Kindness, 1997; Turk et al., 1996). On the other hand, fibromyalgia may complicate other syndromes (Kelemen and Muller, 1998; Potter, 1997), as is the case in some patients with hyperlaxity syndromes, such as benign joint hypermobility syndrome (Grahame, 2000).

Fibromyalgia patients journey along a continuum from experiencing symptoms, through seeking a diagnosis, to coping with the illness. Experiencing symptoms usually entails pain, a precipitating event, associated symptoms, and modulating factors. Seeking a diagnosis is associated with frustration and social isolation. Confirmation of diagnosis brings relief but also anxiety about the future. After diagnosis, several steps lead to creation of adaptive coping strategies (Mannerkorpi, Kroksmark, and Ekdahl, 1999; Raymond and Brown, 2000; Thorson, 1999). Treatment of patients with fibromyalgia and chronic fatigue syndrome continues to be of limited success, although the role of multidisciplinary group intervention appears promising (Bennett, 1998; Celiker et al., 1997; Goldenberg, 1996, 1997; Hadler, 1996a,b; MacFarlane et al., 1996; Slavkin, 1997) and several strategies have proven useful (Keitel, 1997; Maidannik, 1996; Moldofsky et al., 1996; Reiffenberger and Amundson, 1996; Scharf et al., 1998; Stoll, 2000; Wilke, 1996a,b). The conventional medical model fails to address the complex experience of fibromyalgia, and adopting a patient-centered approach is important for helping patients cope with this disease (Cunningham, 1996; Fitzcharles, 1999; Hellstrom et al., 1998; Leslie, 1999; Raymond and Brown, 2000; Romano, 1999; Smith MD, 1998; Smith WA, 1998).

DEFINITION OF CHRONIC FATIGUE SYNDROME AND CANCER-RELATED FATIGUE

Chronic fatigue syndrome and cancer-related fatigue are among the most studied chronic fatiguing illnesses, and this book will focus on these two syndromes because they illustrate the range of chronic fatiguing illnesses mentioned previously and in the rest of the book, and the concepts discussed are broadly pertinent. One, chronic fatigue syndrome, is of unknown proven cause and association with known pathologies, and the other, cancer-related fatigue, although multifactorial, is associated with a known pathology, namely, cancer. Fibromyalgia and other chronic fatiguing illnesses will also be included in the following discussions whenever appropriate.

Chronic Fatigue Syndrome

As stated previously, the diagnosis of chronic fatigue syndrome is based on clinical criteria and is largely dependent upon ruling out other organic and psychological causes of fatigue (Baschetti, 1997a; Bertolin and Calvo, 1997; Buchwald, Umali, et al., 1996; Butler and Rollnick, 1996; Caplan, 1998; Chalder, Powell, and Wessely, 1996; Chester, 1997a; Cook and Boore, 1997; De Loos, 1997; Delbanco, Daley, and Hartman, 1998; DeLuca et al., 1997; Dickinson, 1997; Dyck et al., 1996; Fuller and Morrison, 1998; Gompels and Spickett, 1996; Goshorn, 1998; Hadler, 1997a; Hakimi, 1996; Harrigan, 1998; Hartz, Kuhn, and Levine, 1998; Hausotter, 1996; Heyll et al., 1997; Hickie, Hadzi-Pavlovic, and Ricci, 1997; Hickie et al., 1996; Houde and Kampfe-Leacher, 1997; Joyce, Rabe-Hesketh, and Wessely, 1998; Kenner, 1998; Komaroff, 1997; Komaroff and Buchwald, 1998; Layzer, 1998; Lapp and Hyman, 1997; Lee, 1998; Levine, 1998; Lieb et al., 1996; Lipkin, Papernik, and Kaan, 1997; MacDonald et al., 1996; Massey, 1996; McCluskey, 1998; Mellergard, 1997; Miro et al., 1997; Mulube, 1996; Nisenbaum et al., 1998; Plioplys, Plioplys, and Davis, 1997; Ross, 1996; Salit, 1996, 1997; Sibbald, 1998; Simpson, Bennett, and Holland, 1997; Streeten, 1998; Suarez-Lozano, 1996; Teran Diaz, 1996; Tuck and Human, 1998; Van der Meer et al., 1997; Van Waveren, 1996; Wessely, 1996, 1997, 1998). Chronic fatigue syndrome is defined by primary and secondary criteria that are, however, largely subjective. Although several studies have validated these criteria, much controversy persists, and attempts at formulating new criteria based on laboratory parameters are being undertaken. The working case definition of chronic fatigue syndrome in 1988 was an attempt to establish a uniform basis for the previously heterogeneous approaches to research of this severe and inexplicable state of fatigue. At the same time, researchers wished to narrow down a pathogenetically founded disease entity a priori by specifying precise disease criteria. The case definition has also been used to establish prevalence estimates using physician-based surveillance and random digit dial telephone surveys. Although the original 1988 definition was revised in 1994, the empirical data gathered in accordance with the chronic fatigue syndrome definition have failed to confirm the assumption that the disease entity is pathogenetically uniform.

The onset of chronic fatigue syndrome may be associated with preceding stressful events and multiple other precipitants. A study that divided CFS patients into two groups based on whether onset was sudden or gradual found that the rate of concurrent psychiatric disease was significantly greater in the CFS-gradual group relative to the CFS-sudden group. Although both groups showed a significant reduction in information processing ability relative to controls, impairment in memory was more severe in the CFS-sudden group. Some authors also make a distinction between an acute phase (up to one month after the first consultation), a subacute phase (until six months after the onset of the complaints and disabilities), and a chronic phase (from six months after the onset of the complaints and disabilities) of the disease. Chronic fatigue syndrome evolves toward chronicity in an important number of cases.

Somatic pathogenetic hypotheses for chronic fatigue syndrome include persisting infections, intoxications, metabolic or immunologic disturbances, nervous system diseases, endocrine pathology, and psychosomatic influences. An infectious illness is not uniformly present at the onset, and no single infectious agent has been found. Various components of the central nervous system appear to be involved in chronic fatigue syndrome, including the hypothalamic pituitary axes, pain-processing pathways, sleep-wake cycle, and autonomic nervous system. Many studies have provided evidence for abnormalities in immunological markers among individuals diagnosed with chronic fatigue syndrome. Nonetheless, a clear picture has not been achieved in any area of research because of the noticeable variability in the nature and magnitude of the findings reported by different groups. Moreover, little support has been garnered for an association between the laboratory abnormalities and the diverse physical and health status changes in the CFS population. For instance, some authors think that although a subset of chronic fatigue syndrome patients with immune system activation can be identified, serum markers of inflammation and immune activation are of limited diagnostic usefulness in the evaluation of patients with chronic fatigue syndrome and chronic fatigue because changes in their values may reflect an intercurrent, transient, common condition such as an upper respiratory infection, or may be the result of an ongoing illness-associated process. On the other hand, other authors have found that CFS patients can be categorized based on immunological findings or that when patients are classified according to whether the disease started suddenly or gradually, immunological changes are apparent. It is also worth noting that although the degree of overlap between distributions of soluble immune mediators in chronic fatigue syndrome and controls has fueled criticism on validity or clinical significance of immune abnormalities in chronic fatigue syndrome, the degree of overlap is not unique to chronic fatigue syndrome and is also present, for instance, in sepsis syndrome and HIV-1-associated disease, clinical entities in which studies of immune abnormalities are providing insight into pathophysiology. This observation also applies to nonimmunological parameters in chronic fatigue syndrome.

Based on the discrepancies described, some authors argue that the conceptual model of chronic fatigue syndrome needs to be changed from one determined by a single cause/agent to one in which dysfunction is the end stage of a multifactorial process. A study of author bias in literature citation in chronic fatigue syndrome reviews revealed that citation of literature is influenced by the author's discipline and nationality, a finding which is compatible with the lack of consensus and integrated efforts among professionals from different disciplines who are working on chronic fatigue syndrome.

In light of current knowledge limitations, treatment plans for chronic fatigue syndrome are interdisciplinary and holistic, and most patients include alternative therapies. Empathy and compassion are essential components of providing care for CFS patients. Chronic fatigue syndrome patients need the support and reassurance of their physicians to help them cope with their symptoms and resume normal, productive lives. The first and most important task for the health care professional is to develop mutual trust and collaboration with the patient. The second is to complete an adequate assessment, the aim of which is either to make a diagnosis of chronic fatigue syndrome or to identify an alternative cause for the patient's symptoms. The history is most important and should include a detailed account of the symptoms, the associated disability, the choice of coping strategies, and, most important, the patient's own understanding of his or her illness. The assessment of possible comorbid psychiatric disorders, such as depression or anxiety, is mandatory. When the physician is satisfied that no alternative physical or psychiatric disorder can be found to explain symptoms, a diagnosis of chronic fatigue syndrome can be made. The treatment of chronic fatigue syndrome requires that patients be given a positive explanation of the cause of their symptoms, emphasizing the distinction among factors that may have predisposed them to develop the illness (lifestyle, work stress, personality), triggered the illness (viral infection, life events), and perpetuated the illness (cerebral dysfunction, sleep disorder, depression, inconsistent activity, and misunderstanding of the illness and fear of making it worse). Interventions are then aimed at overcoming these illness-perpetuating factors.

Epidemiological studies of chronic fatigue syndrome have been hampered by the absence of a specific diagnostic test, but with increasing interest in this disorder there has been a greater understanding of the risk factors, illness patterns, and other aspects of this multisystem disorder. Working case definitions have been developed for research purposes, but they have continued to change over time and have not always been utilized precisely by various investigators. This had been a major factor in the widely varying estimates of prevalence rates (Sutton, 1996), but two different studies using the same working definition and including a medical workup have estimated the prevalence to be approximately 200 cases per 100,000 individuals in the United States (Fukuda et al., 1997). A study of the epidemiology of chronic debilitating fatigue based on questionnaires completed by members of the Irish College of General Practitioners yielded an estimated 2.1 cases per practice and an incidence of one per 1,000 in the general population (Fitzgibbon et al., 1997). In a study of 214 primary care patients in England (Wessely et al., 1997), the point prevalence of chronic fatigue was 11.3 percent, falling to 4.1 percent if comorbid psychological disorders were excluded. The point prevalence of chronic fatigue syndrome was 2.6 percent, falling to 0.5 percent if comorbid psychological disorders were excluded. The prevalence of chronic fatigue syndrome based on a study of 601 patients in four family practices in Leyden was estimated to be at least 1.1 per 1,000 patients (Versluis et al., 1997). Extrapolation of the results from a study (Bazelmans, Vercoulen, et al., 1997) based on questionnaires filled out by general practitioners indicates that there are at least 17,000 CFS patients in the Netherlands. The prevalence of chronic fatigue syndrome in teenagers is 10 to 20 per 100,000 inhabitants in the Netherlands (De Jong, Prins, et al., 1997). A nationwide survey (Minowa and Jiamo, 1996) conduced using the Japanese version of the CDC criteria for chronic fatigue syndrome in all clinical departments of internal medicine, pediatrics, psychiatry, and neurology at university hospitals and at ordinary hospitals with 200 or more beds yielded a period prevalence adjusted for a response rate of 0.85 (0.63 for males and 1.02 for females) per 100,000 population and a response adjusted incidence estimate of 0.46 per 100,000 person-years.

Clusters of chronic fatigue syndrome cases, which appear to be related to earlier reports of "epidemic neuromyathenia," have attracted considerable attention and appear to be well documented, although investigated with varying methodology and often with dissimilar case definitions (Fukuda et al., 1997; Minowa and Jiamo, 1996). Risk factors for cases occurring in clusters and sporadically appear to be similar, the most consistent ones being female gender and the coexistence of some form of stress, either physical or psychological (Fukuda et al., 1997). In a study (Levine et al., 1997) of a 1984 outbreak of an illness characterized by prolonged unexplained fatigue reported in West Otago, New Zealand, twenty-three of the twenty-eight patients in the original report were contacted and ten (48 percent) of the twenty-one patients with satisfactory interviews appeared to meet the current CDC case definition of chronic fatigue syndrome, while eleven were classified as having prolonged or idiopathic fatigue. Not all cluster cases have been confirmed. For instance, data (Levine, 1997) collected from 1,698 households in four rural Michigan communities did not confirm a reported cluster of cases resembling chronic fatigue syndrome. The prevalence of households containing at least one fatigued person was similar between communities thought to harbor the cluster and communities selected for comparison.

In terms of possible infectious or environmental etiologies of chronic fatigue syndrome, a prospective cohort study (White et al., 1998) of 250 primary care patients revealed a higher incidence and longer duration of an acute fatigue syndrome, and a higher prevalence of chronic fatigue syndrome, after glandular fever versus an ordinary upper respiratory tract infection. A conservative estimate is that glandular fever accounts for 3,113 new cases of chronic fatigue syndrome per annum in England and Wales. In another study (Jason et al., 1998) based on data collected on two samples of nurses recruited through mailed questionnaires, a physician review team estimated the prevalence of chronic fatigue syndrome to be 1,088 per 100,000 among these health care professionals. These findings suggest that nurses might represent a high-risk group for this illness, possibly secondary to occupational stressors (exposure to viruses, shift schedules, and other stressors). Other studies disagree with this conclusion.

Although the prognosis of chronic fatigue syndrome is difficult to predict, cases occurring as part of clusters appear to have a better prognosis as a group than sporadic cases, and those with an acute onset have a better prognosis than those with gradual onset (Fukuda et al., 1997). One report (Joyce, Hotopf, and Wessely, 1997) documented that, of 26 studies on patients with chronic fatigue syndrome or chronic fatigue, four studied fatigue in children and found that 54 to 94 percent of children recovered over follow-up periods. Another five studies operationally defined chronic fatigue syndrome in adults and found that less than 10 percent of subjects return to premorbid levels of functioning, and the majority remain significantly impaired. The remaining studies used less stringent criteria to define their cohorts. Among patients in primary care with fatigue lasting less than six months, at least 40 percent of patients improved. As the definition becomes more stringent the prognosis appears to worsen. Consistently reported risk factors for poor prognosis are older age, more chronic illness, having a comorbid psychiatric disorder, and holding a belief that the illness is secondary to physical causes. These findings were confirmed in other studies (Aylward, 1996; Vercoulen, Swanink, Fennis, et al., 1996), one of which found that the improvement rate in CFS patients with a relatively long duration of complaints is small (among 246 patients, 3 percent reported complete recovery and 17 percent reported improvement) and influenced by psychological and cognitive factors (Vercoulen, Swanink, Fennis, et al., 1996).

Cancer-Related Fatigue

The other chronic fatiguing illness emphasized in this book is cancer-related fatigue. Fatigue is the most frequently reported symptom, occurring in 60 to more than 90 percent, of patients with cancer, as the result of a combination of physical and psychological causes that may be related directly or indirectly to the cancer itself or to its treatment (Aistars, 1987; Allard, 2000; Barnes and Bruera, 2002; Barnish, 1994; Bazzi and Kellogg, 1991; Blesch et al., 1991; Boxer et al., 1978; Bruera and MacDonald, 1988; Cella et al., 1998; Clarke and Lacasse, 1998; Cleeland, 2001; Coackley et al., 2002; Curt, 2000a,b, 2001a,b; Dean et al., 1995; Delaplace, 1997; Dilhuydy et al., 2001; Dodd, 2000; Eaton and Worrall, 1998; Escalante et al., 2001; Feyer, 2000; Foltz, Gaines, and Gullatte, 1996; Fulton and Knowles, 2000; Gall, 1996; Glaus, 1998a,b, 2001; Graydon et al., 1998; Gutstein, 2001; Harpham, 1999; Holland, 1973; Irvine et al., 1991; Krishnasamy, 2000; Llewelyn, 1996; Magnusson et al., 1999; Moore, 1998; Nail et al., 1991; Okuyama, Akechi, Kugaya, Okamura, Imoto, et al., 2000; Okuyama et al., 2001; Patenaude et al., 2002; Pearce and Richardson, 1994, 1996; Piper, Lindsey, and Dodd, 1987; Portenoy, 2000; Potter, 1998; Ream and Richardson, 1996, 1997, 1999; Richardson, 1995; Richardson and Ream, 1996; Sadler and Jacobsen, 2001; Smets et al., 1993; Sobrero et al., 2001; Stone, 2002; Stone, Hardy, et al., 2000; Stone, Richards, and Hardy, 1998; Stone, Richards, et al., 2000; Stone, Richardson, et al., 2000; Stone et al., 1999; Trabacchi, 1997; Valdres, Escalante, and Manzullo, 2001; Valentine and Meyers, 2001; Valdini, 1985).

A large number of studies classify fatigue as the most distressing phenomenon among cancer patients, and fatigue has a significant impact in the quality of life and functionality not only of cancer patients but also of their caregivers, family, or others (Bernhard and Ganz, 1991; Bernhard et al., 1996; Cella et al., 1998; Cleeland et al., 2000; Delaplace, 1997; Escalante et al., 2001; Feyer, 2000; Graydon et al., 1998; Greifzu, 1998; Haylock and Hart, 1979; Held, 1994; Hilton, Fitch, and Deane, 1998; Hollen et al., 1994; Howell, 1998; Hurny et al., 1993; Jensen and Given, 1991; Lutz et al., 1997, 2001; Manzullo and Escalante, 2002; Mast, 1998; Mings, 1998a-d; Mock, 2001a,b; Morris, 1986; Nail and King, 1987; Nail et al., 1991; Oberst et al., 1991; Piper, 1993; Potempa, 1993; Poulson, 1998, 2001; Rieger, 1988; Rubenstein, 1998; Smets et al., 1993; Trabacchi, 1997; Wells and Fedric, 2001; Winningham, 2001; Winningham et al., 1994; Witt and Murray-Edwards, 2002). In fact, fatigue affects more cancer patients and more persistently than any other symptom, and it is regarded by patients as being more distressing than pain, nausea, vomiting, or depression (Curt, 2001a,b; Stone et al., 2000).

The interest in cancer-related fatigue seems to be growing. Simon and Zittoun (1999) reported that a Medline search of the National Library of Medicine combining the key words "fatigue" and "cancer" yielded 248 entries in 1999 compared with 72 entries in 1989. There has also been increased diversification of the populations studied; for instance, the first report describing fatigue in children and adolescents with cancer was published in 1998.

Current literature suggests that fatigue is the most important under-diagnosed and undertreated symptom in cancer medicine. With almost 8 to 10 million Americans alive today who have been through the cancer experience, it is important to develop interventions to maintain quality of life, an important component of which is fatigue, following cancer diagnosis and treatment. Cancer-related fatigue has therefore gone from being an orphan topic to a global concern. For instance, Central Eastern European countries are involved in clinical trials of supportive care in cancer patients and, although not currently running, are interested in trials centered on cancer-related fatigue (Bosnjak, 2002).

In the cancer setting, fatigue is defined as a chronic whole-body experience of tiredness, which is perceived by the patient as being unusual, excessive, or abnormal, and absolutely disproportionate or unrelated to the amount of exercise or activity the patient has carried out and which is not alleviated or relieved by resting or sleeping (Anconi-Israel, Moore, and Jones, 2001; Tavio, Milan, and Tirelli, 2002). Morrow, Andrews, and colleagues (2002) point out that cancer-related fatigue differs from that induced by other causes, such as sleep disturbance and exertion- or exercise-induced fatigue, because the latter, non-cancer-related causes, are typically alleviated by a period of rest.

According to the tenth revision of the *International Classification of Diseases,* exhaustion and tiredness are subsumed under the diagnosis of cancer-related fatigue (Zahner, 2000; Zahner, Meran, and Karthaus, 2001). However, in contrast to cancer-related fatigue, which comprises physical, mental, and emotional dimensions, exhaustion and tiredness primarily refer to physical symptoms: Lacking resilience for activities of daily life, day sleepiness and nocturnal insomnia, as well as restricted power of concentration are the mainstays of exhaustion and tiredness. However, as illustrated in Figure 1.1, it should be noted that regarding lacking interests, diminished energy, and reduced mental capacity, exhaustion and fatigue partly overlap.

Fatigue and pain also have several components in common, such as being subjective, prevalent in most patients with cancer, and caused by multiple factors of both a physical and psychological nature (Kaasa et al., 1999). A study of 1,488 patients by Wolfe, Hawley, and Wilson (1996) documented that correlates of fatigue, such as pain, sleep disturbances, and disability, are generally similar across many fatiguing illnesses such as fibromyalgia, rheumatoid arthritis, and osteoarthritis. Fatigue in different contexts is also associated with all measures of distress and is a predictor of work dysfunction and overall health status.

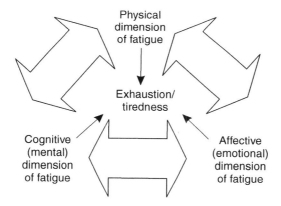

FIGURE 1.1. Contributions of fatigue dimensions to exhaustion/tiredness

In a qualitative study to explore the concept of cancer-related fatigue in twenty cancer patients and in twenty healthy individuals, Glaus, Crow, and Hammond (1996a,b, 1999a,b) found that physical signs of fatigue were more frequent than affective and cognitive signs in both groups. In the cancer patients, fatigue involved decreased physical performance, extreme and unusual tiredness, weakness, and an unusual need for rest that was distinctly different from healthy persons. Affective and cognitive distress was also more prominent in cancer patients (Glaus, Crow, and Hammond, 1996a,b, 1999a,b).

Holley (2000a,b) undertook a naturalistic inquiry to understand, from the patient's perspective, the differences between cancer-related fatigue and "typical" fatigue and to describe its impact on their lives. In a sample of seventeen adult patients with cancer, cancer-related fatigue was found to be more rapid in onset, more energy draining, more intense, longer lasting, more severe, and more unrelenting when compared with "typical" fatigue. Cancer-related fatigue caused distress in the physical, social, spiritual, psychological, and cognitive domains of the participants' lives. All participants agreed that cancer-related fatigue was different than the typical fatigue of everyday life (Holley, 2000a,b). Richardson and Ream (1996) also reported that cancer patients made a distinction between fatigue and tiredness. The following list summarizes the salient distinguishing features of cancer-related fatigue as compared to fatigue in healthy individuals.

- More rapid onset
- More energy draining (extreme and unusual tiredness)

- More intense
- Longer lasting
- More severe
- More unrelenting
- More affective and cognitive distress
- More unusual need for rest
- Similarly present in all age groups

Servaes and colleagues (2001) documented that 19 percent of the eighty-five adult disease-free (off treatment for at least six months) cancer patients they studied were severely fatigued. Their fatigue experience was comparable to that of patients with chronic fatigue syndrome. Severe fatigue was associated with problems of concentration and motivation, reduced physical activity, emotional health problems, and pain. In a later study, Servaes and colleagues (2002) concentrated on breast cancer survivors and documented that, in comparison to severely fatigued disease-free breast cancer patients, chronic fatigue syndrome patients score more problematic with regard to the level of fatigue, functional impairment, physical activity, pain, and self-efficacy. However, a subgroup of severely fatigued disease-free breast cancer patients reported the same number of problems as chronic fatigue syndrome patients with regard to psychological well-being, sleep, and concentration. Moreover, chronic fatigue syndrome patients and severely fatigued breast cancer patients score equal on measures of social support (Servaes et al., 2002).

Cancer-related fatigue is a subjective experience that has a clear detrimental effect on a cancer patient's quality of life and ability to sustain the usual personal, professional, and social relationships. The intensity of cancer-related fatigue varies with tumor site. For instance, patients with advanced pancreatic cancer experience significantly greater fatigue and general psychological disturbance than patients with another type of advanced abdominal neoplasm (Holland et al., 1986). Cancer-related fatigue has a temporal variation. Richardson, Ream, and Wilson-Barnett (1998) reported that fatigue in patients receiving chemotherapy varied throughout the day, more frequently occurring in the afternoon and early evening. Although Aapro, Cella, and Zagari (2002) found no correlation between cancer patient age and fatigue, among healthy individuals the cohort aged 65 or older reported more fatigue than did younger subjects. Cancer-related fatigue can be pervasive: cancer patients frequently report that fatigue begins with treatment, continues during the course of chemotherapy or radiation treatment, and declines somewhat—but frequently sustains at a higher-than-baseline rate—

after treatment is over. It may also persist for several years even in patients with no apparent disease (Morrow, Andrews, et al., 2002).

Ashbury and colleagues (1998) interviewed 913 cancer patients who received treatment within the previous two years and found that the most prevalent symptoms were fatigue and anxiety (78 and 77 percent, respectively), with fatigue being the most debilitating. Fatigue was most likely to be self-rated as moderate to severe and was most likely to interfere in normal daily activities. Respondents who experienced fatigue reported a more frequent use of health care services (including complementary therapies) than those who did not experience fatigue. Half of the respondents reported trying to find information on fatigue, but only half of these said they had obtained information. The most helpful sources of information were nurses, specialists, and other cancer patients. Respondents were more likely to be dissatisfied with their treatments for their symptoms than for their cancer (Ashbury et al., 1998).

FACTORS THAT INFLUENCE THE DIAGNOSIS AND TREATMENT OF FATIGUE AND CHRONIC FATIGUING ILLNESSES

The following list summarizes several reasons for the deficiencies in the diagnosis and treatment of fatigue and chronic fatiguing illnesses, and the following subsections discuss them in detail and point out how they are being addressed.

1. Definition of fatigue and chronic fatiguing illnesses
2. Illness beliefs/attributions
   Patient
   Health care professional
   Caregiver
3. Sociodemographic factors
   Age
   Gender
   Geocultural setting
4. Measurement of fatigue perception and severity

The previous section addressed the definition of fatigue and chronic fatiguing illnesses. The following subsection addresses the influence of the different perspectives (illness beliefs or attributions) of the patients, health care providers, and family and caregivers on the diagnosis and treatment of fatigue.

Illness Beliefs/Attributions

Attribution is an individual's perception of fact, and belief is what a person feels is real and true, something on which an individual bases his or her trust and confidence. The literature on the role of illness beliefs/attributions on the part of both patients and health care professionals is widely divided, and some have gone as far as suggesting that fatigue is merely a question of belief or attribution (Lloyd, 1998; Fry and Martin, 1996b; Bleijenberg, 1997). In this extreme, Barsky and Borus (1999), among other authors (Ford, 1997; Masi, 1998; Robbins, Kirmayer, and Hemami, 1997; Walker, Katon, et al., 1997), have applied the term "functional somatic syndromes" to several related syndromes characterized more by symptoms such as fatigue, suffering, and disability than by consistently demonstrable tissue abnormality. These syndromes include multiple chemical sensitivity, sick building syndrome, repetition stress injury, the side effects of silicone breast implants, Persian Gulf War syndrome, chronic whiplash, chronic fatigue syndrome, irritable bowel syndrome, and fibromyalgia. Barsky and Borus (1999) purport that although discrete pathophysiologic causes may ultimately be found in some patients with functional somatic syndromes, the suffering of these patients is exacerbated by a self-perpetuating, self-validating cycle in which common, endemic, somatic symptoms are incorrectly attributed to serious abnormality, reinforcing the patient's belief that he or she has a serious disease. Ford (1997) considers these syndromes a "fashionable" way to hide the diagnosis of hysteria.

The arguments described are not applicable to the context of a clear underlying pathology, as is the case in the syndrome of cancer-related fatigue. However, as discussed in the following subsections, illness beliefs and attributions, not only on the part of patients, but also of health care professionals, caregivers, and family, play important roles in the recognition and treatment of fatigue, and on bidirectional patient-health care system, patient-family, and patient-society interactions.

Patients' Illness Beliefs/Attributions

Some studies emphasize the individual's beliefs of fatigue as the cause for symptomatology. Patients' perceptions and coping styles also determine quality of life (Soderberg, Lundman, and Norberg, 1997). For instance, a study (Stewart, Abbey, et al., 1998) of 153 women from the Toronto area who were attending a women's health symposium yielded an overwhelming endorsement of social determinants as the cause of their persistent fatigue. Although depression and anxiety had the most robust associations with persistent fatigue in primary care and community studies, women in this sample ranked these factors in seventh place in their attributions. Similarly, although physicians often presuppose physical causes for fatigue, women, based on their own attributions, gave a low ranking for physical health as a cause for their fatigue.

The reality of a cancer diagnosis or its treatment fosters a set of beliefs and attributions of fatigue among cancer patients that stands in sharp contrast to those of women in the general population described earlier. For instance, a study to explore twelve patients' perceptions of fatigue in response to biochemotherapy treatment for metastatic melanoma found that all patients reported that the most direct causes of their fatigue were metastatic melanoma and biochemotherapy treatment (Fu et al., 2002).

Although cancer patients may more uniformly perceive their fatigue as caused by the cancer or its treatment, their report and perception of fatigue are colored by several factors. In this respect, fatigue report among cancer patients is influenced by tumor site, treatment stage, and patients' expectations, among other factors (Llewellyn-Thomas et al., 1992). For instance, men with Hodgkin's disease report more generalized symptoms: fatigue, energy loss, and work impairment, as compared to men with testicular cancer who report more focused and site-specific symptoms: less sexual enjoyment and poor health habits (Bloom et al., 1993).

Patients do not necessarily share doctors' priorities in decision making or place the same emphasis on different types of morbidity, and on many occasions patients consider fatigue as more important than other symptoms. Turner and colleagues (1996) interviewed 165 adult patients with Hodgkin's disease following treatment to examine their perceptions of actual and desired involvement and provision of information in the treatment decision-making process. Patients who felt satisfied with the adequacy of information given were significantly more likely to feel happy with their level of participation in the overall process of decision making. The observation was independent of the degree to which patients felt they had been involved in the decision-making process and of the outcome of their particular treatment. As part of a strategy investigating patients' priorities, patients were asked to rank a series of possible acute and late treatment-related morbidities. Contrary to expectations, the majority of long-term survivors felt early short-term side effects were more or equally important as late morbidity with respect to influencing choice of therapy. Unpredictably from doctors' perceptions, importance was placed by patients on side effects such as weight gain and fatigue in relation to other complications such as infertility and risk of relapse (Turner et al., 1996).

Fatigue is an important determinant of quality of life, and as such it has become increasingly important as the number of newly diagnosed patients with cancer increases and survival improves. In 1983, Coates and colleagues reported a survey of patient perceptions of the side effects of cancer chemotherapy and showed the importance of including patient feedback for the accurate assessment of quality of life. More recently, Carelle and colleagues (2002) carried out a similar survey in 100 patients (sixty-five women and thirty-five men) with cancer. In the survey, patients identified all side effects associated with their treatment using a set of forty-five cards that named physical side effects (group A) and a set of twenty-seven cards that named nonphysical side effects (group B), and the patients ranked these side effects according to severity. The top five cards from each group were then combined, and the resulting ten cards were rated again by severity, regardless of group. Patients rated "affects my family or partner" as the most severe side effect, alopecia as second, and fatigue as the third most severe. Effects on work or home responsibilities, effects on social activities, and loss of interest in sex were ranked fourth, fifth, and sixth, respectively.

The summarized results contrast with those of the early survey by Coates and colleagues (1983), in which "affects my family or partner" was ranked tenth, and fatigue was ranked eighth. Therefore, patient perceptions of the side effects of cancer chemotherapy have changed markedly. In the more recent study by Carelle and colleagues (2002), fatigue and psychosocial quality-of-life concerns predominated, compared with nausea, vomiting, and negative reactions to the treatment visit in the original survey. The more recent findings are consistent with the progress that has been made in reducing certain chemotherapy-associated toxicities. Fatigue, however, remains a major concern. The following list summarizes the factors that influence patients' attributions of cancer-related fatigue.

- Tumor site
- Treatment stage
- Cancer treatment type
- Effectiveness of controlling treatment side effects
- Patient's expectations
- Patient's health priorities

What the patient perceives as the underlying cause of fatigue plays a role in the cancer patient's quality of life and the level of disability associated with the fatigue. Experience with other fatiguing illnesses is informative in this respect. For instance, among patients with chronic fatigue syndrome, physical illness attributions and the presence of an emotional disorder have been shown to be associated with disability (Sharpe et al., 1992). Wilson and colleagues (Wilson, Hickie, Lloyd, Hadzi-Pavlovic, et al., 1994; Wilson, Hickie, Lloyd, and Wakefield, 1994) arrived at a similar conclusion, namely, that the belief of the illness as a physical one was predictive of poor outcome. It has also been postulated that individual differences in beliefs about chronic fatigue syndrome may influence the limits and boundaries that patients with this disorder set in their level of functioning (Petrie, Moss-Morris, and Weinman, 1995). In particular, catastrophic thinking may be an important factor in determining disability associated with chronic fatigue syndrome (Petrie, Moss-Morris, and Weinman, 1995). Likewise, Broeckel and colleagues (1998) found that more severe fatigue among breast cancer patients was associated with greater use of catastrophizing as a coping strategy.

In the presence of any long-term illness, it can be very difficult to retain a positive outlook in the face of prolonged disability, restriction of everyday life, and absence of a ready cure. The feelings, such as frustration, anger, irritability, anxiety, demoralization, and profound change in mood, could therefore impair recovery from any chronic fatiguing illness (Surawy et al., 1995). For instance, a study by Clements and colleagues (1997) reported that most patients with chronic fatigue syndrome believed that they could control their symptoms to some degree but could not alter the course of the underlying disease process. The coping methods they described were resting, avoiding activity, and reducing activity. Personal experience of feeling worse after activity was a major factor in the adoption of rest and activity avoidance (Clements et al., 1997; Ray, Jefferies, and Weir, 1995). This is also true for cancer-related fatigue. Upon investigation of why some individuals with lung or colorectal cancer develop fatigue whereas others do not, Olson and colleagues (2002) found that an adaptive behavioral mode labeled gliding characterized those who reported little or no fatigue, even when hemoglobin levels were low, while three other nonadaptive behavioral modes (inertia, disorganization, and overexertion) characterized those who reported fatigue. Therefore, interventions that either discourage avoidance or excess of activity or enhance perceived control could benefit the course of the illness (Ray, Jefferies, and Weir, 1997).

Neerinckx and colleagues (2000) found that the majority of patients with chronic fatigue syndrome and fibromyalgia reported a great diversity of attributions ("a chemical imbalance in my body," "a virus," "stress," and "emotional confusion") open to a preferably personalized cognitive-behavioral approach. Neerinckx and colleagues (2000) recommend paying special attention to patients with symptoms existing for more than one year and to those who had previous contact with a self-help group because they particularly show external, stable, and global attributions that may compromise feelings of self-efficacy in dealing with the illness.

Barsevick, Whitmer, and Walker (2001) conducted a small study of eight cancer patients known to be experiencing fatigue to describe cancer-related fatigue from the perspective of individuals experiencing it and to examine the fit of their descriptions with the concepts from the Common Sense Model of Illness Representation. All statements describing cancer-related fatigue could be classified using the major constructs of the Common Sense Model of Illness Representation: representation, coping, and appraisal. The majority of statements were classified as representations of fatigue (67 percent), with smaller proportions classified as coping (26 percent) and appraisal (7 percent). This study also provides evidence to support the validity of the Common Sense Model of Illness Representation constructs as an organizing framework in the conduct of research (Barsevick, Whitmer, and Walker, 2001).

As described in this subsection, patients' attributions are important in the diagnosis and management of cancer-related fatigue. Attributions or illness beliefs are amenable to modification through cognitive-behavioral therapy, a topic addressed in Chapter 4.

Health Care Professionals' Beliefs/Attributions

Several studies have emphasized the role of the physician in fatigue perpetuation, underdiagnosis, and undertreatment. For instance, Curt and colleagues (2000) reported that 40 percent of the 379 cancer patients they interviewed were not offered any fatigue treatment recommendations, despite the fact that physicians were the health care professionals most commonly consulted (79 percent) to discuss fatigue. A significant communication gap exists between patients and physicians regarding fatigue and nonspecific physician responses to patient reports (Curt, 2000a,b). This finding suggests that patients may benefit from physician initiation of discussion of the causes and treatments of fatigue and from physician education regarding available treatment modalities. Physician education is also important to minimize stigmatization of the patient with fatigue. In this respect, a study of adolescent cancer survivors who pursued postsecondary education revealed a stigmatization of patients with cancer by professional health workers. This observation underscores the need to confront the value that health professionals place on the stigmatized population with fatigue and health professionals' contribution to the broader societal posture (Griffith and Hart, 2000).

Stigmatization percolates to all chronic fatiguing illnesses, and even the diagnostic labels may contribute to this phenomenon. Several studies reviewed by Jason, Eisele, and Taylor (2001) highlight the effect of diagnostic labeling and the salience of similar types of brief communications used to describe illnesses such as chronic fatigue syndrome. They suggest that the name given to a syndrome can influence public attributions about those with the syndrome. For instance, two studies reviewed whether different names for chronic fatigue syndrome indeed prompt different attributions regarding its cause, nature, severity, contagion, and prognosis among samples of medical trainees and university undergraduates (Jason, Eisele, and Taylor, 2001). In these studies, three different diagnostic labels (chronic fatigue syndrome, Florence Nightingale disease, and myalgic encephalopathy) were tested to determine their effects on the attributions of medical trainees and college undergraduates regarding this syndrome. Participants were randomly assigned to one of three groups, with the only difference between groups being in the type of diagnostic label given as the diagnosis for the same case study of a patient with prototypic symptoms of chronic fatigue syndrome.

Results of these studies suggested that participants' attributions about chronic fatigue syndrome change based on the different diagnostic labels used to characterize it. The myalgic encephalopathy label was associated with the poorest prognosis, and this term was more likely to attribute a physiological cause to the illness and less likely to consider the patient in the case study as a potential candidate for organ donation. Results of a third investigation (Taylor, Jason, et al., 2001) indicated that physician recommendation for treatment of chronic fatigue syndrome can also influence subsequent attributions about the illness among health care practitioners. When a medically based treatment (antiviral drug) was recommended, the practitioners were significantly more likely to believe that the patient was significantly more disabled than those prompted with recommendation for a psychologically based treatment (cognitive-behavioral therapy with graded activity). These findings highlight distinctions in attributions that can result from recommending a medically based orientation toward chronic fatigue syndrome treatment versus one based heavily on minimizing medical factors and emphasizing psychiatric factors (Jason, Eisele, and Taylor, 2001).

Communication problems between patient and doctor easily arise because of different attributions of the fatigue complaints; these problems affect the nature and effectiveness of medical consultations. A study (De Rijk, Schreurs, and Bensing, 1998) of 2,097 individuals in the Netherlands found that more psychosocially attributed fatigue correlated with medical consultations characterized by less physical examination; more diagnostic procedures to reassure; fewer diagnostic procedures to discover underlying pathology; more counseling; less medical treatment; less prescription; and a longer duration than consultations with more somatically attributed fatigue. The study concluded that general practitioners do not discriminate between social groups when attributing fatigue to either somatic or psychosocial causes. The presence and character of other complaints and underlying diseases/problems, rather, relate to the general practitioners' somatic psychosocial attributions, which are then associated with particular aspects of the consultation.

For patients and oncologists, improving the quality of life of cancer patients requires a heightened awareness of fatigue, a better understanding of its impact, and improved communication and familiarity with interventions that can reduce its debilitating effects (Vogelzang et al., 1997). Vogelzang and colleagues (1997) conducted a study of patient, caregiver, and oncologist perceptions of cancer-related fatigue by using a three-part assessment survey of 419 cancer patients recruited from 100,000 randomly selected households nationwide. Patients provided access to 200 primary caregivers (usually family members), who were also interviewed by telephone. In a separate mail survey, 197 of 600 randomly sampled oncologists (unrelated to the patients) responded to a questionnaire that assessed perceptions and attitudes concerning fatigue in cancer patients who had received chemotherapy or radiotherapy and their caregivers.

In the study by Vogelzang and colleagues (1997), the median patient age was sixty-five years, and the primary cancer diagnoses were breast (females) and genitourinary (males). Thirty-five percent of the patients had received chemotherapy alone, 39 percent radiation therapy alone, and 24 percent both; 20 percent of patients received their last treatment within six weeks, 31 percent within seven weeks to one year, and 49 percent more than one year ago. More than three-quarters of patients (78 percent) experienced fatigue (defined as a general feeling of debilitating tiredness or loss of energy) during the course of their disease and treatment. Thirty-two percent experienced fatigue daily, and 32 percent reported that fatigue significantly affected their daily routines. Caregivers reported observing fatigue in 86 percent of the index patients, and oncologists perceived that 76 percent of their patients experienced fatigue.

Although oncologists believed that pain adversely affected their patients to a greater degree than fatigue (61 versus 37 percent), patients felt that fatigue adversely affected their daily lives more than pain (61 versus 19 percent). Most oncologists (80 percent) believed fatigue is overlooked or undertreated, and most patients (74 percent) considered fatigue a symptom to be endured. Fifty percent of patients did not discuss treatment options with their oncologists, and only 27 percent reported that their oncologists recommended any treatment for fatigue. When used, patients and caregivers generally perceived treatments for fatigue as successful. These data confirm the high prevalence and adverse impact of cancer-related fatigue, although it is seldom discussed and infrequently treated.

The limitations in physician-patient communication were also highlighted by a study in which Osse and colleagues (2002) reported a comprehensive overview of the problems that patients experience in a palliative phase of cancer. They used a two-step qualitative method: in-depth interviews with nine patients and seven relatives, followed by interviews with thirty-one patients and fifteen relatives using a checklist to confirm and complete the picture. Patients experienced problems in all quality-of-life and quality-of-palliative-care domains, although individual patients may have experienced only a few problems. Fatigue, feelings of futility, reluctance to accept help, fear of suffering, and the fear that help would not be available if needed were common problems. Communication problems arose when a grudge against a general practitioner had remained, or because one family member tried to spare the other a confrontation with his or her feelings of fear or grief (Osse et al., 2002).

Despite increasing recognition of the importance of maintaining patients' health-related quality of life as a goal of palliative treatment, the amount of patient-physician communication devoted to such issues remains limited and appears to make only a modest contribution, at least in an explicit sense, to the evaluation of treatment efficacy in daily clinical practice (Detmar et al., 2001). Detmar and colleagues (2001) assessed patient-physician communication in a population of ten oncologists and 240 of their patients who had incurable cancer and were receiving outpatient palliative chemotherapy. Physicians devoted 64 percent of their conversation to medical/technical issues and 23 percent to health-related quality-of-life issues. Patients' communication behavior was divided more equally between medical/technical issues (41 percent) and health-related quality-of-life topics (48 percent). Of the independent variables investigated, patients' self-reported health-related quality of life was the most powerful predictor of discussing health-related quality-of-life issues. Nevertheless, in 20 to 54 percent of the consultations in which patients were experiencing serious problems with health-related quality of life, no time was devoted to discussion of those problems. In particular, these patients' emotional functioning and fatigue were unapprised 54 and 48 percent of the time, respectively. However, discussion of health-related quality-of-life issues was not more frequent in consultations in which tumor response was evaluated.

The evaluation process of a fatigue complaint is complicated by the presence of multiple associated disorders, the prevalence of the complaint, and cost/benefit issues facing the primary care physician (Groopman, 1998; Llewelyn, 1996; Ream and Richardson, 1996, 1997, 1999; Shapiro, 1998;

Tiesinga et al., 1996; White, 1997). In a review of 425 medical charts, Ward and colleagues (1996) found that the workup for chronic fatigue is often incomplete or lacks documentation. This oversight is likely secondary to the problem that focus is not being directed at the chronic fatigue complaints.

Litwin and colleagues (1998) analyzed information on 2,252 patients with early-stage or advanced prostate cancer and found significant differences between physician and patient assessment of clinical domains, such as physical, sexual, urinary, and bowel function, fatigue, and bone pain. In all domains urologists underestimated patient symptoms, causing health-related quality-of-life impairment. A study of sixty-three patients with newly diagnosed M1 prostate cancer also found that physicians' ratings may not accurately reflect the functional health and symptom experience of their patients (Da Silva et al., 1996). In fact, an earlier trial by Da Silva (1993a,b) revealed that many clinicians exhibit considerable reluctance to perform quality-of-life research, partly because of feasibility problems and partly because of doctors' doubts about the value of such efforts. However, among patients, psychological distress, fatigue, issues of social and family life, and pain were found to be the most important concerns on a subjective basis, and this finding was confirmed by objective parameters (Da Silva et al., 1993). Although oncologists' perceptions may not accurately reflect their patients' reported physical and psychosocial experiences (Alberts et al., 1997; Hockenberry-Eaton et al., 1998; Labots and Puhlmann, 1997; Le Grand, 2002; Newell et al., 1998; Raber, 2001; Schneider, 1998a,b; Stein et al., 1998; Vastag and Bleider, 1998; Yarbro, 1996), doctors are able to influence these attributions actively in a favorable direction. The following list summarizes the items that complicate the diagnosis, evaluation, and treatment of fatigue.

- High prevalence of fatigue complaints
- Presence of multiple associated disorders
- Fatigue considered less prioritary by health care providers
- Cost/benefit dilemmas facing the health care provider
- Limits on time for patient-health care provider interaction

Nurses also play a very significant role in the diagnosis and management of fatigue (Fitch, Bakker, and Conlon, 1999; MacAvoy and Moritz, 1992; Robinson and Posner, 1992; Taplin, Blanke, and Baughman, 1997). To evaluate Swedish nurses' estimation of fatigue as a symptom in cancer patients and the strategies they used in its management, a questionnaire was mailed to 442 registered nurses in the autumn of 1995. The response rate was 49 percent. The responses showed that these nurses regarded fatigue as the most common symptom in cancer patients, but there were few established nursing interventions. Also, nurses wanted further education and tools for evaluation of fatigue, its causes, and treatment (Magnusson et al., 1997). Knowles and colleagues (2000) arrived at a similar conclusion after conducting a survey that evaluated how eighty-four nurses in a cancer center in Edinburgh define and assess fatigue. The results demonstrated that although the problems associated with fatigue were acknowledged, assessment tools were not widely used and the majority of nurses reported that they would benefit from further education on the subject to assist in the care of patients. From the responses of 249 oncology nurses in Canada, the following items were ranked as the top ten problems in clinical practice: anxiety, coping/stress management, bereavement/death, fatigue, metastatic disease, comfort, pain control and management, quality of life, recurrence of primary cancer, and nurse burnout. Overwhelming fatigue hinders patients in taking physical care of themselves and may be overlooked by the nurse since the patients' motor capabilities seem intact (Persson and Hallberg, 1995; Persson, Hallberg, and Ohlsson, 1997).

As in the case of doctors, nurses' perceptions may also differ from those of their patients. Parsaie, Golchin, and Asvadi (2000) compared the perceptions of chemotherapy treatment stressors among twenty-one nurses and fifty-seven patients. The greatest physical stressor mentioned by the patients was fatigue (66 percent), and by nurses, hair loss (alopecia) (62 percent). Nurses' perceptions of psychosocial items causing the greatest stress included fear of disease recurrence (90.5 percent), fear of death (90.5 percent), economic problems (90.5 percent), and appearance changes (90.5 percent). In contrast, patients perceived dependency (80 percent), economic problems (70 percent), and loss of social activity (66 percent) as the greatest stressors. The study also revealed disagreement between the two groups on intensity of physical and psychosocial stressors. The results from this study increased awareness among the nurses involved of important stress factors in chemotherapy treatment. Identification of the situations perceived to be more stressful than others helped clinical nurses to modify their care and provide for their patients in a way that removes or reduces the stressors (Parsaie, Golchin, and Asvadi, 2000).

The health care professional's role in combating fatigue extends beyond treatment side effects and spans the treatment continuum from prevention to research. This role includes patient assessment to identify those at high risk and to evaluate potential causes of fatigue, as well as the implementation of interventions to manage the fatigue, such as patient and family education, self-care activities, and treatment of specific problems (Butler, 1998; Yarbro, 1996). Participation of health care professionals in multidisciplinary community education programs on fatigue and its management provides a valuable service for patients, a rewarding experience for educators, and facilitated communication between patient and health care providers (Grant et al., 2000; Reh, 1998).

Change in clinical practice is occurring, albeit slowly. Dean and Stahl (2002) reported that one major change which occurred in their cancer center as an effort to change clinical practice of fatigue assessment and management was the inclusion of a fatigue question in the daily patient care record. This inclusion signified a commitment by the institution to address the deficient report and treatment of fatigue. Many cancer centers have incorporated tertiary clinics that focus on fatigue and its management, and a number of resources have become available for patients with cancer-related fatigue (Whitmer and Barsevick, 2001). For instance, the Fatigue Coalition, a multidisciplinary group of medical practitioners, researchers, and patient advocates, developed a series of educational and research initiatives designed to help patients and physicians better understand chemotherapy-related fatigue and provide successful interventions (Wolfe, 2000).

Multisite research and personal or computerized education projects have also been implemented (Nail et al., 1998; Skalla and Lacasse, 1992; Stacey, 1998; Sweeney, 2000; Wydra, 2001). Literacy is an important factor in materials development. The efficacy of computer-assisted learning, audio and video programs, and telephone interventions are also supported in a variety of patient groups. Wilkie and colleagues (2001) evaluated the feasibility of an innovative computerized symptom assessment tool, SymptomReport, and a computerized, tailored education tool, SymptomConsult, in a sample of forty-one outpatients with cancer. The study found that patients required less than forty minutes on average to complete SymptomReport. The mean acceptability score was high. The twelve patients who completed SymptomConsult did so in an average of twenty minutes. The majority of participants indicated that the computer programs were easy, enjoyable, and informative tools.

Education projects and a greater awareness of the importance of correctly informing patients on their conditions are helping to address deficiencies documented earlier. For instance, in 1995, Sarna and Ganley (1995) examined the readability and content of educational materials developed specifically for lung cancer patients and identified in a survey of fifty-four cancer organizations and institutions and a literature review. Only five educational resources specifically developed to address the needs of lung cancer patients were identified. Only two addressed fatigue, shortness of breath (dyspnea), loss of appetite, pain, risk of recurrence, sexuality, smoking cessation, rehabilitation, or palliation. None addressed reduced functional abilities resulting from disease or treatment. All of the materials reviewed were written at a reading level of tenth grade or higher. The authors concluded that lung cancer patient-education materials were inadequate and required advanced reading skills.

Presenting clear, concise, and well-timed communication to patients regarding fatigue management is an important role for health care providers (Jakel, 2002). Whelan and colleagues (1997) reported that patients with newly diagnosed cancer commonly report symptoms related to fatigue, pain, and psychological distress. Other frequently reported items relate to the need for information and social concerns regarding the patients' ability to take care of their home and maintain family and other relationships. Awareness of these issues is important for planning supportive care interventions for newly diagnosed cancer patients. Fatigue is very distressing to patients, who often view it as an indication that their disease is progressing or that treatment is ineffective. Patients with a cancer diagnosis frequently have psychological distress. Communication and information help patients cope with the diagnosis of cancer and with the management of side effects.

Based on an extensive review of the literature, Chelf and colleagues (2001) concluded that cancer patients want and benefit from information, especially when making treatment decisions. Education helps patients manage side effects and improves adherence (Crang, 1999). Appropriate information on fatigue is also important for conducting clinical research in cancer and cancer-related fatigue. In a study of expectations of cancer patients participating in clinical trials, Yoder and colleagues (1997) found that patients expected symptoms such as fatigue, nausea and vomiting, and weight loss to improve during therapy, but their expectations were not met. One theme that emerged from the data was hope/optimism. Yoder and colleagues (1997) recommend that health care professionals, particularly oncology nurses, must allow cancer patients who are undergoing investigational therapy to maintain a level of hope, while realistically counseling them about their progress during clinical trial participation.

Better awareness of fatigue also helps to better manage other associated symptoms of cancer, such as pain, that affect quality of life and disability level. The experience with the positive effects of increased awareness on cancer-related fatigue should be extended to other patient populations. For example, current published data also indicate barriers and deficiencies in health care for women with physical disabilities. A survey of 170 women with physical disabilities in metropolitan Philadelphia revealed that the respondents experienced on average twelve secondary complications in the past year that moderately impaired their functioning (Coyle and Santiago, 2002). Although many of these complications (fatigue, spasticity, deconditioning, joint pain, depression, social isolation) are preventable, only about half of the women had seen a rehabilitative service provider (e.g., physical therapist, mental health worker) in the past six months, despite most (96 percent) of them having seen a general care provider. However, women who saw their general health care provider most frequently were more likely to also be receiving services from a rehabilitative service provider (Coyle and Santiago, 2002).

Family and Caregivers

Besides health care providers, family members and caregivers can enhance problems with the diagnosis and management of fatigue. Several studies have addressed the reliability of caregivers' perceptions on the levels of fatigue experienced by cancer patients. In a study of 103 pairs of patients, with either recently diagnosed or recurrent brain cancer, and their primary caregivers (75 percent spouses, 22 percent relatives, and 3 percent friends), Sneeuw and colleagues (1997) found that approximately 60 percent of the patient and proxy scores were in exact agreement, with more than 90 percent of scores being within one response category of each other. For most health-related quality-of-life dimensions assessed, moderate to good agreement was found. Statistically significant differences in mean scores were noted for several dimensions, with proxies tending to rate the patients as having a lower quality of life than the patients themselves. With the exception of fatigue ratings, this response bias was of a limited magnitude. Less agreement and a more pronounced response bias was observed for the more impaired patients, and particularly for patients exhibiting mental confusion.

The finding was confirmed by longitudinal analyses that indicated lower levels of patient-proxy agreement at follow-up for those patients whose physical or neurological condition had deteriorated over time (Sneeuw et al., 1997). In a study of 172 patients and eighty-three spouses/partners who completed quality-of-life questionnaires in a prostate cancer health education lecture series, Kornblith and colleagues (1994) reported that spouses reported significantly greater psychological distress than did patients. The authors recommend a two-stage clinical evaluation, in which quality-of-life questionnaires would initially be used to identify patients and spouses experiencing problems in adaptation for further evaluation by a mental health professional to receive appropriate treatment or assistance.

Caregiver perception of fatigue is also influenced by caregiver gender. Kurtz and colleagues (1996) reported that in a sample of 216 patients and their family caregivers, the rate of symptom report agreement between patient and caregiver was highest for fatigue and lowest for insomnia, whether the entire sample, male or female caregivers, was considered. However, female caregivers had a higher percentage of agreement with their patients and a higher level of association between patient and caregiver responses than male caregivers, uniformly for all symptoms.

Kurtz and colleagues (1996) further stress that health care professionals must recognize that reports of patient symptoms from the patient and the caregiver may not always be in agreement, and that awareness of variables which may cloud family caregivers' observations is needed, so that accurate symptom reporting occurs and appropriate management can be initiated to enhance quality of life for the patient as much as possible. It is also important for health care professionals to educate family caregivers about the nuances of symptom distress presentation and to teach caregivers techniques to elicit accurate information so that timely, appropriate management can be initiated.

Harden and colleagues (2002) conducted a descriptive, qualitative study that explored the experiences of couples living with prostate cancer, the impact of the illness on their quality of life, their ability to manage symptoms, and their suggestions for interventions that would help them to improve their daily experiences. Six focus groups were used to obtain the data; two were patient-only groups, two were spouse-caregiver groups, and two were dyad groups. The study included a total of forty-two participants: twenty-two men with prostate cancer and twenty spouse-caregivers. Four major themes emerged from the data: enduring uncertainty, living with treatment effects, coping with changes, and needing help. Participants had a need for information and support. Both men and spouse-caregivers felt unprepared to manage treatment effects. Symptoms had a broad effect on couples, not just men. Positive effects of the illness, as well as negative effects, emerged from the themes. Harden and colleagues (2002) concluded that attention needs to be given to methods of providing information and support to couples coping with prostate cancer. Both patients and partners need to be included in discussions about the effect of the illness and treatments so that both can feel more prepared to manage them.

Wong and colleagues (2002) set out to determine the content and format most suitable for educational events targeting advanced cancer patients and their caregivers. One hundred forty-four respondents completed the Advanced Cancer Information Needs survey. The participants identified the management of pain, fatigue, and home palliative care resources as the areas in which information was most needed. Caregivers displayed greater interest, and the range of topics in which they continue to seek additional information is wider. Thirty-one percent of respondents said they would participate in an educational event. A one-on-one interview approach and short written materials were the preferred sources of information (Wong et al., 2002).

A women's study (Libbus, 1996) showed that some women were able to identify specific ways in which the family and important others could help them to decrease or prevent their fatigue. However, many expressed the belief that significant others were unconcerned and unwilling to assist them in any substantive way. In contrast to the latter perception, a study by Hamilton and colleagues (2001) of twenty-two lung cancer patients and fourteen family members six weeks postcompletion of radiation therapy revealed that over half of the family members felt more of the impact of fatigue than did their loved ones afflicted by cancer. Family members subtly assumed or took over responsibilities and activities that the patient could no longer perform.

It should be pointed out that fatigue has a significant impact in the quality of life and functionality not only of cancer patients but also of their caregivers, family or otherwise. Therefore, the assessment and treatment of fatigue in the latter group are also of paramount importance (Bernhard et al., 1996; Escalante et al., 2001; Greifzu, 1998; Hollen et al., 1994; Hurny et al., 1993; Jensen and Given, 1991; Lutz et al., 2001; Mings, 1998c; Mock, 2001a,b; Rieger, 1988; Wells and Fedric, 2001; Winningham, 2001; Winningham et al., 1994). The experience in this respect with other fatiguing illness is revealing. Neumann and Buskila (1997) reported that the quality of life and physical functioning of the relatives of fibromyalgia patients were impaired, especially for female relatives and those with undiagnosed fibromyalgia, a finding that may be attributed to the psychological distress in families of fibromyalgia patients and to the high prevalence (25 percent) of undiagnosed fibromyalgia among relatives. Similarly, studies have evinced that difficulties in relieving fatigue and strain in relatives curtail home care of patients with terminal cancer (Hinton, 1994, 1996).

Fatigue is a complex symptom prevalent in informal caregiving, and when role demands exceed caregiver resources, fatigue ensues and caregiving can be compromised. Teel and Press (1999) compared perceptions of fatigue among ninety-two older adults caring for spouses with Alzheimer's disease, Parkinson's disease, or cancer with a control group of thirty-three older adults whose spouses required no extra care. Caregiving elders reported more fatigue, less energy, and more sleep difficulty than did control participants. All caregiving groups reported similar levels of fatigue, energy, sleep, and self-reported health even though there were marked differences regarding spousal status. Health care providers can support older caregivers in monitoring their own health and in recognizing the need for services that support the caregiving role (Teel and Press, 1999). At the other age extreme, Wolfe and colleagues (2000) interviewed the parents of 103 children who had died of cancer. The authors reported that, according to the parents, 89 percent of the children suffered "a lot" or "a great deal" from at least one symptom in their last month of life, most commonly pain, fatigue, or shortness of breath. On the basis of a review of the medical records, parents were significantly more likely than physicians to report that their child had fatigue, poor appetite, constipation, and diarrhea.

Family members require assistance for their distress as patient status deteriorates. In a study of Chinese immigrant and North American Caucasian families, Leavitt and colleagues (1999) reported that all families complained of emotional and physical fatigue and the need to adapt to a tentative future with their child. A study by Jason and colleagues (1997) revealed that families of patients undergoing high-dose multiple daily fractionated radiotherapy for malignant astrocytomas showed slightly less "conflict" and slightly more "cohesion" than the norm; this was especially true when patients had a greater cognitive deficit. Emotional state of spouses was variable, with increased fatigue or reduced activity most commonly reported, followed by depression and anxiety. Mostly this improved with time or remained stable (Jason et al., 1997). In a study of 208 cancer patients in treatment and their caregivers, Kurtz and colleagues (1994) revealed significant differences by survival groups for caregiver depression, caregiver reactions, and patient assistance.

Describing what happens to individuals and their families as a result of fatigue and identifying what individuals do to manage or reduce the impact of fatigue are essential elements in determining multidimensional health care interventions. Curt and colleagues (2000) reported that 65 percent of 379 cancer patients they interviewed indicated that their fatigue resulted in their caregivers taking at least one day (average of 4.5 days) off work in a typical month. Patients also reported that fatigue interferes with both their own and their caregivers' careers and economic status (Curt, 2000a,b). As mentioned earlier, there is a growing awareness that oncology health care professionals should care for both patients and their caregivers. However, although some transplant programs provide services to support lay caregivers, studies indicate that these individuals continue to feel stressed by their situation. Rexilius and colleagues (2002) proposed that massage therapy might be one intervention which can be used by nurses to decrease feelings of stress in patients' caregivers.

Sociodemographic Factors

Race and sex disparities in health outcomes have been extensively documented (Alexander and Sehgal, 1998; Ayanian et al., 1999; Bierman and Clancy, 2001; Cooper, Hill, and Powe, 2002; Fiscella et al., 2000; Keppel, Pearcy, and Wagener, 2000; Lynch et al., 2000; Sehgal, 2003; Williams and

Rucker, 2000), and the influence of several sociodemographic factors on chronic fatiguing illnesses has been studied in different combinations. For instance, results from a study of 455 ambulatory cancer patients suggested that gender, education, employment status, household size, performance status, and depressive mood were all associated with fatigue (Akechi et al., 1999). The following subsections address some of the factors that have been better studied. Other factors, such as ethnicity and socioeconomic status, remain to be studied more rigorously.

Age

Aapro, Cella, and Zagari (2002) found no correlation between cancer patient age and fatigue, while in controls the cohort aged sixty-five or older reported more fatigue than did younger subjects. A descriptive study of twelve adult ovarian cancer patients who were receiving chemotherapy and twelve apparently healthy adult women also failed to reveal a relationship between fatigue and age. In contrast to the latter observations, Pater and colleagues (1997) reported that the oldest cancer patients they studied had less fatigue. Furthermore, in a sample of 263 cancer patients who were undergoing chemotherapy, older age was associated with better quality of life and less fatigue, insomnia, anxiety, and depression (Redeker, Lev, and Ruggiero, 2000).

Although most studies suggest that among cancer patients the manifestation of fatigue appears to be independent of age, it is worth understanding the special features of recognizing and managing fatigue in different age groups. This understanding is particularly important because the population is aging and the prevalence of cancer is increasing. In fact, the incidence of cancer increases from 500 in 100,000 to 2,000 to 4,000 in 100,000 as women or men age from fifty to eighty years. Moreover, the five-year survival rate for many cancer sites exceeds 50 percent, an observation which suggests that these patients are living longer and may be considered to have a chronic illness (Gerber, 2001).

Many conditions that would not be considered normal in a younger population are routinely accepted in older people as a part of so-called normal aging. Fatigue is one among many other such chronic and debilitating conditions, which include chronic pain, insomnia, weakness, and anemia (Aapro, Cella, and Zagari, 2002). However, the latter chronic conditions are not normal in an aging population: all patients with chronic conditions should be adequately treated and counseled for their conditions (Aapro, Cella, and Zagari, 2002; Sheehan and Forman, 1997). Older women with breast cancer, as compared to a control group, are more vulnerable to fatigue-related losses in their cognitive capacity to direct attention, an essential capacity for self-care and independent functioning. This reduced performance in a cognitive function persists over an extended interval (Cimprich and Ronis, 2001).

Cleary and Carbone (1997) point out that many older patients are treated within community hospitals, in which anticancer therapies are less likely to be given and in which the palliation of symptoms should be of primary importance. Elderly patients are less likely than younger patients to receive proper pain and fatigue management. Elderly patients also are less likely to take opioids for pain because of their attitudes and beliefs. Treatments for cancer are quite complex, and they are often delivered to elders who have a variety of medical problems and are receiving additional medications that may complicate overall patient management. Hence, these patients may have extremely complex functional problems. Cancer patients need comprehensive care designed to relieve symptoms of pain, fatigue, and weakness. They need education to help support their ability to reach functional independence and maintain quality of life (Gerber, 2001).

Aggressive treatment should not be withheld from older patients simply because of their age (Nerenz et al., 1986). In a study of 1,000 patients referred to a palliative medicine program, Walsh, Donnelly, and Rybicki (2000) found that although fatigue was among the ten most reported symptoms, younger age was associated with eleven symptoms: blackout, vomiting, pain, nausea, headache, sedation, bloating, sleep problems, anxiety, depression, and constipation. In a sample of 217 patients receiving initial chemotherapy treatment for breast cancer or lymphoma, Nerenz and colleagues (1986) found that elderly patients reported no more difficulty with treatment or emotional distress than did younger patients. This general pattern held across disease types, with some exceptions.

Langer (2002) points out that tremendous bias exists against treating the elderly cancer patients; therapeutic nihilism and constrained societal/financial resources conspire to maintain the status quo. For instance, although 60 percent of those diagnosed with non-small-cell lung cancer are sixty years of age or older, the elderly are often undertreated. Furthermore, those older than age seventy are underrepresented in clinical research trials and there is a prevailing notion that the elderly respond more poorly to treatment. Weighted survival analyses that deduct time spent with progressive disease or significant toxicity have reinforced this notion.

In advanced non-small-cell lung cancer, fit elderly patients who receive platinum-based regimens do as well, or nearly as well, as patients younger than age seventy, although the incidence of neutropenia and fatigue is often higher. Platinum doses above 75 mg/m^2 every three to four weeks are relatively more toxic in the elderly than are lower doses. Three separate studies from Italy have formally assessed the elderly. One study showed superiority for single-agent vinorelbine versus best supportive care regarding survival rates and quality of life. A second showed a marked survival advantage for combination vinorelbine and gemcitabine versus vinorelbine alone. However, a much larger, more credible study demonstrated no benefit for combination vinorelbine and gemcitabine versus the constituent single agents. To date, no elderly-specific trials have addressed the role of taxanes or platinum-based combination therapy versus nonplatinum monotherapy or doublets. Comprehensive evaluation of comorbidities and their influence on outcome have not been conducted, and there are virtually no data for patients older than age eighty (Langer, 2002).

Based on a study of 907 cancer patients aged sixty-five or older, Given and colleagues (2000) documented that elderly patients with cancer report levels of function similar to other chronic conditions. Although scores on physical function varied by site of cancer, the pattern of change was similar among sites. Age, comorbidity, treatment modalities, and fatigue and pain symptom reports each had an independent effect on loss of functioning. In a study of 208 cancer patients in treatment and their caregivers, Kurtz and colleagues (1994) showed that although symptoms varied significantly by survival status, age demonstrated no independent effect on patient variables, including symptom severity, patient depression, and activities of daily living or immobility.

The significant link between symptoms and loss of physical functioning has important implications for health care providers caring for patients with cancer as they deal with symptom management and quality-of-life issues. In a sample of 279 patients with cancer, Kurtz and colleagues (1993) studied the trajectories of symptoms and loss of physical functioning over time. Findings at the first assessment time point indicated that age and comorbidity were significantly correlated, and loss of physical functioning was associated primarily with symptoms and, to a lesser degree, with age. Loss-of-function scores varied significantly according to cancer site, with higher levels for patients with lung cancer and lower levels for patients with breast or colorectal/gastrointestinal cancer. The most frequently occurring symptoms were fatigue, insomnia, pain, and nausea. Average levels of symptoms and loss of physical functioning were lower six months later, indicative of a possible treatment-related effect (at this time point, a smaller percentage of patients had recently undergone treatment). Although comorbidity was only modestly correlated with symptoms and loss of function for the total sample, it was highly correlated with both symptoms and loss of physical functioning for the younger patients (those younger than sixty years of age).

In line with the previous study, Given and colleagues (Given, Given, Azzouz, and Stommel, 2001; Given, Given, Azzouz, Kozachik, and Stommel, 2001) studied physical functioning of 841 elderly (sixty-five years of age or older) patients with breast, colon, lung, or prostate cancer prior to diagnosis and following initial treatment. The authors found that site and stage of cancer prior to diagnosis do not affect functioning. Moreover, older cancer patients report higher functioning than their counterparts in the U.S. population; changes in functioning following diagnosis varied by cancer site; treatments were related to loss in functioning, but comorbidity was not; and fatigue, pain, and insomnia were significant and independent predictors of change in patient functioning. In the year following diagnosis, patients improved with respect to their reports of pain and/or fatigue; stage, more comorbidity, and lung cancer were related to both pain and fatigue; and chemotherapy was related to reports of fatigue but did not have an extended effect on fatigue.

Deconditioning, often caused by treatment-induced fatigue, along with impaired physical function, sensory-neurological deficits, and use of multiple medications, are among the risk factors for falls in cancer patients (Holley, 2002c). A major risk factor is aging; because people often are diagnosed with cancer at an older age or are living longer with cancer, many are at risk for falls. Of all types of accidents, falls pose the most serious threat to the elderly. Fall injuries in the elderly population can have serious consequences related to reduced physical functioning and quality of life (Holley, 2002c). It is therefore important to evaluate, diagnose, and treat fatigue and other symptoms that affect the quality of life of elderly patients with cancer. The following list summarizes the factors that may limit such endeavors and that should be overcome.

- More likely to be treated in less-specialized centers
- More coexisting medical problems
- Patient on more medications
- Patient less likely to take certain medications because of beliefs
- Constrained societal/financial resources
- Underrepresentation in clinical trials
- Erroneous notions that fatigue is normal part of aging

At the other end of the age spectrum, Hinds and Hockenberry-Eaton (2001) have pointed out that although fatigue may be a universal experience for children and adolescents who are being treated for a malignancy, it may also be the most unrecognized, and thus untreated, symptom experienced by this population (Clarke-Steffen, 2001; Clarke-Steffen et al., 2001; Hockenberry-Eaton and Hinds, 2000). Fatigue can occur in children who receive chemotherapy, radiotherapy, and biotherapy, and in children who are treated with bone marrow transplantation (White, 2001). Education of the patient and family regarding the potential for fatigue is helpful in preparing them for the cancer experience. Factors that contribute to and alleviate fatigue can be identified for each patient, taking into consideration age, developmental level, and cultural background. Parents and patients, especially adolescent patients, may have different opinions about what fatigue is and what may be helpful.

Fatigue in pediatric patients exists within a greater context of illness, treatment, and child and family development. Any effort to define, measure, and intervene with fatigue needs to take into consideration the major components of these children and adolescents' treatment context. A study by Hinds and colleagues (Hinds, Hockenberry-Eaton, Gilger, et al., 1999; Hinds, Hockenberry-Eaton, Quargnenti, et al., 1999) revealed that children, adolescents, parents, and staff define patient fatigue differently. The conceptual definition from the child data emphasizes the physical sensation of the fatigue; alternating and at times merging physical and mental tiredness are emphasized in the adolescents' definition (Hinds, Quargnenti, and Wentz, 1992). Staff perceive fatigue to be a debilitating symptom for these children. When attempting to determine the presence or absence of fatigue, health care staff members primarily compare a child's current state with his or her previous state rather than that of other children. Parents and staff view themselves as responsible for causing and alleviating patient fatigue; patients viewed rest and distraction as their primary sources of improving fatigue (Hinds, Quargnenti, and Wentz, 1992; Hinds, Hockenberry-Eaton, Gilger, et al., 1999; Hinds, Hockenberry-Eaton, Quargnenti, et al., 1999).

Davies and colleagues (2002) performed a typology study of fatigue in twenty children with cancer and eighteen parents and found that energy, as an overriding phenomenon, was a core concept in the descriptions of fatigue. Children with cancer may experience three subjectively distinct types of fatigue that represent different levels of energy: typical tiredness, treatment fatigue, and shutdown fatigue. The successful treatment for children with cancer has greatly increased the survival rates for these young people compared to children diagnosed with cancer in the 1970s. These new medical realities direct attention to the psychosocial consequences of successful treatment and subsequent survival. Zebrack and Chesler (2002) assessed quality of life in 176 childhood cancer survivors (aged sixteen through twenty-eight) using a survey instrument designed for cancer survivors. Survivors indicate that symptoms often associated with treatment are at a minimum but that other long-term effects such as fatigue, aches, and pain negatively impact quality of life.

Although chronic fatigue syndrome was originally thought to be mainly a disease of adults, pediatric chronic fatigue syndrome is a significant problem and also the subject of much controversy (Bell et al., 1999; Carter et al., 1996; Cohen, 1997; De Jong, Prins, et al., 1997; Dowsett and Colby, 1997; Hume, 1997; Jacobs, 1997; Marcovitch, 1997; Plioplys, 1997b; Stein, First, and Friedman, 1998). A study encompassing chart review and telephone follow-up revealed that although the clinical features associated with chronic fatigue in children and adolescents are similar to those described in adults, they present earlier in the course of the illness and the prognosis is better (Gibbons et al., 1998). Proposed criteria for the diagnosis of chronic fatigue syndrome in adolescence are absence of a physical explanation for the complaints, a disabling fatigue for at least six months and prolonged school absenteeism, or severe motor and social disabilities. Exclusion criterion should be a psychiatric disorder (Arzomand, 1998). Analysis of data on severely disabled juvenile chronic fatigue syndrome patients in the United Kingdom shows a modal age of onset of eleven to fifteen years and a tendency to deterioration in patients' cognitive and functional stati between onset and recruitment (Wright and Beverly, 1998). Certain psychological factors can discriminate chronic fatigue from depressive symptomatology as well as normal functioning in children and adolescents (Krilov et al., 1998). Although an equal prevalence of chronic fatigue syndrome was found among boys and girls in two schools in England, the number of chronic fatigue syndrome cases was higher in the inner-London borough-like school as compared to the more greenbelt borough (Jordan et al., 1998).

The frequency of chronic pain syndromes in pediatric rheumatology has increased over the past twenty-five years. Diagnosis is complex: underlying organic illness, somatization, and growing pains are all possibilities (Cassidy, 1998). Fibromyalgia has also been recognized in children and adolescents as juvenile fibromyalgia (Buskila, 1996; Clark et al., 1998; Kulig, 1991; Sherry, 1997; Tayag-Kier et al., 2000). Juvenile rheumatoid arthritis and juvenile fibromyalgia can coexist (Schikler, 2000). For the patients with the initial diagnosis of either juvenile rheumatoid arthritis or juvenile fibromyalgia whose clinical response to therapy is not in keeping with expectations or physical examination findings or whose clinical course worsens without explanation, reevaluation to determine if juvenile fibromyalgia in the juvenile rheumatoid arthritis patient has developed or juvenile rheumatoid arthritis in the juvenile fibromyalgia patient has emerged is warranted.

The clinical spectrum of fibromyalgia in children (diffuse aching, headaches, sleep disturbances, and, less commonly, stiffness, subjective joint swelling, fatigue, abdominal pain, joint hypermobility, dizziness, and depression) is similar to that of adults but with better outcomes (Gedalia et al., 2000; Mikkelsson, Salminen, and Kautiainen, 1997; Mikkelsson et al., 1997; Mikkelsson, 1999; Rusy, Harvey, and Beste, 1999; Sieb et al., 1997;

Siegel, Janeway, and Baum, 1998). Tayag-Kier and colleagues (2000) also demonstrated, in sixteen children and adolescents with juvenile fibromyalgia, abnormalities in sleep architecture, including periodic limb movement in sleep, similar to those seen in adult fibromyalgia patients. However, Breau, McGrath, and Lu (1999) suggest that fibromyalgia and chronic fatigue syndrome may be related in children and may not be duplicates of the adult disorders; that psychological and psychosocial factors are unlikely contributors to the etiology of these disorders; and that the evidence is increasingly pointing to a role for genetic factors in their etiology. Roizenblatt and colleagues (1997) reported a significant concordance of fibromyalgia diagnosis and significant correlations between polysomnographic indexes, sleep anomalies, and pain manifestations in children and their mothers.

Gedalia and colleagues (2000) reported that active exercise programs seem to correlate with better outcomes in juvenile fibromyalgia. However, Kujala, Taimela, and Viljanen (1999) point out that, in addition to its likely long-term health benefits, vigorous physical activity causes musculoskeletal pains during adolescence, which should be considered as a confounder in epidemiological studies on fibromyalgia and related issues. In terms of other factors that affect juvenile fibromyalgia symptomatology, Schanberg and colleagues (1998) found that family environment and parental pain history may be related to how children cope with juvenile fibromyalgia. Behavioral interventions targeting the family may improve the long-term functional status of children with juvenile fibromyalgia (Haavet and Grunfeld, 1997; Schanberg et al., 1996). In this respect, Reid, Lang, and McGrath (1997) point out that disability among children with fibromyalgia or juvenile rheumatoid arthritis is a function of the children's psychological adjustment and physical state, and of the parents' physical state and method of coping with pain.

Gender

Pater and colleagues (1997) reported that female gender is associated with greater fatigue severity. In a sample of 263 cancer patients who were undergoing chemotherapy, women had more anxiety and fatigue and poorer quality of life than did men (Redeker, Lev, and Ruggiero, 2000). Similarly, a study to explore patients' perceptions of fatigue in response to biochemotherapy treatment for metastatic melanoma found that female patients' total fatigue scores were higher than those of male patients (Fu et al., 2002). Based on a study of 907 cancer patients aged sixty-five or older, Given and colleagues (2000) reported that men scored ten points higher on physical function than women at all observation points, and surgery, female gender, and number of symptoms reliably predicted change in function. Taking gender into account for the appropriate diagnosis and management of cancer and cancer-related fatigue is therefore important (Millner and Widerman, 1994).

In a study of 109 cancer patients post-bone marrow transplantation, Heinonen and colleagues (2001) reported that independent of the time post-transplantation, perceived physical well-being, age at transplantation, and education, females reported worse emotional well-being and more fatigue than males. Females also indicated more tiredness and less quality sleep. Males were found to experience less satisfaction with social support regardless of marital status. On the other hand, married males were more satisfied with their sexual life, more interested in sexual relationships, and more sexually active compared to married females. However, no significant differences between males and females were found in terms of overall physical, functional, and social well-being (Heinonen et al., 2001).

Knobel and colleagues (2000) also reported that fatigue was highly prevalent among thirty-three lymphoma patients treated with high-dose therapy supported by autologous bone marrow transplantation, and females reported significantly more fatigue and impaired health-related quality of life compared to males and the normal population. Gonadal dysfunction was found in the majority of the patients, but no statistically significant endocrinological or immunological associations with fatigue could be demonstrated. The high level of fatigue among female long-term survivors after autologous bone marrow transplantation may be related to the gonadal dysfunction, but further studies are necessary.

The prevalence of comorbid conditions with cancer-related fatigue may also vary by gender. For instance, in a study of 1,000 patients referred to a palliative medicine program, Walsh, Donnelly, and Rybicki (2000) found that while fatigue was among the ten most frequently reported symptoms, comorbid symptoms had a different gender distribution. Males had more dysphagia, hoarseness, greater than 10 percent of weight loss, and sleep problems, while females had more early satiety, nausea, vomiting, and anxiety.

Similar to cancer-related fatigue, several studies have documented female gender predominance for other fatiguing illnesses and in the incidence of chronic fatigue in the general population. For instance, a survey of 3,500 Norwegians, aged eighteen to ninety, revealed that women were more fatigued than men (Loge, Ekeberg, and Kaasa, 1998). A study (Fitzgibbon et al., 1997) of 118 questionnaires completed by members of the Irish College of General Practitioners yielded a male-to-female ratio of 1:2 with all social classes represented, while a male-to-female ratio of 1:5 was found in a study (Versluis et al., 1997) of 601 patients in four practices in Leyden.

Moreover, a cross-sectional telephone screening survey, followed by interviews of 8,004 households (16,970 residents) in San Francisco revealed that chronic fatigue illnesses were most prevalent among women. In a study of 1,108 Japanese female full-time workers, Araki, Muto, and Asakura (1999) found high rates of complaints of fatigue (44.1 percent), eye discomfort (53.6 percent), headache (43 percent), and menstrual pain (32.5 percent) in association with irritability or depression. Amount of overtime work, marital status in the thirty to forty-four age group, and the presence of children were found to be important factors in determining health status.

In contrast to the studies described previously, the findings of one group (Van Mens-Verhulst and Bensing, 1997, 1998) disagree with the female predominance of fatigue: Diaries kept by Dutch citizens over a twenty-one-day period showed that the majority of those with persistent fatigue complaints were male, middle-aged, less educated, and unemployed, and they had more psychological and psychosocial problems than the incidental fatigue sufferers. Moreover, a study (Versluis et al., 1997) of primary care patients in England found that rates of chronic fatigue and chronic fatigue syndrome did not vary by social class and that, after adjustment for psychological disorders, being female was modestly associated with chronic fatigue.

The findings described could be reconciled by a study (Levine et al., 1997) on the natural history of a 1984 outbreak of an illness characterized by prolonged unexplained fatigue in West Otago, New Zealand. The outbreak resembled other reported outbreaks of epidemic neuromyasthenia in that affected individuals presented with a spectrum of complaints ranging from transient diarrhea and upper respiratory disorders to chronic fatigue syndrome. The study revealed a female predominance among patients meeting the CDC case definition for chronic fatigue syndrome, whereas males predominated among patients diagnosed as having prolonged or idiopathic fatigue. The findings are in line with those of another study in which Euga and colleagues (1996) compared subjects fulfilling criteria for chronic fatigue syndrome and identified as part of a prospective cohort study in primary care, to adults fulfilling the same criteria referred for treatment to a specialist chronic fatigue syndrome clinic. The study showed that although women were overrepresented in both primary care and hospital groups, the high rates of psychiatric morbidity and female excess that characterize chronic fatigue syndrome in specialist settings are not secondary to selection bias.

The prevalence rates of the most common causes of arthralgia and arthritis, osteoarthritis, and rheumatoid arthritis, and the prevalence rates of less common diseases that cause arthralgia and fatigue, including systemic lupus erythematosus, systemic sclerosis, and fibromyalgia, are between two and ten times higher in women (Buckwalter and Lappin, 2000; Burckhardt and Bjelle, 1996; Schaefer, 1997). The heterogeneous group of diseases that causes chronic arthralgia and arthritis, along with fatigue, is also the most common cause of activity limitation and disability among middle-aged and older women (Holtedahl, 1999; Stormorken and Brosstad, 1999). For reasons that remain poorly understood, this group of diseases affects women substantially more frequently than men (Belilos and Carsons, 1998; Forseth, Forre, and Gran, 1999; Meisler, 1999). Forseth, Gran, and Husby (1997) estimated an annual incidence of fibromyalgia in women of 583 per 100,000.

A study by Buskila and colleagues (2000), comparing forty men and forty women with fibromyalgia, concluded that although fibromyalgia is uncommon in men, its health outcome is worse than in women (more severe symptoms, decreased physical function, and lower quality of life in men despite similar mean tender point counts). In contrast, Yunus and colleagues (2000), in a comparative study of sixty-seven men and 469 women with fibromyalgia, found that male fibromyalgia patients had fewer symptoms and fewer tender points and less common "hurt all over" complaints, fatigue, morning fatigue, and irritable bowel syndrome, compared with female patients. Further studies of gender comparisons in cancer-related fatigue and other fatiguing illnesses are needed.

Geocultural Setting

In a study in Switzerland, Glaus, Crow, and Hammond (1996a,b) found that linguistic differences in the description of fatigue/tiredness between healthy and ill individuals revealed different perceptions of the phenomenon. Winstead-Fry (1998) also noted differences between rural and urban persons experiencing cancer that may make the experience of fatigue more difficult for rural cancer patients. The goal of the Rural Cancer Care Project is to assist patients and families residing in rural areas to receive the highest-quality cancer care in their own communities (White, Given, and Devoss, 1996). In the rural setting, knowledge deficit proved to be one of the most frequently identified problems (in 78 percent of the 170 patients evaluated), although the patient and family had often received care at a community oncology center with specialist health care professionals. Teaching was a major nursing intervention employed in patient care to address patient problems and needs as presented (e.g., chronic pain, fatigue). Patients had more knowledge needs in the later stages of disease when they had cancers in all sites but the breast, where patients with stage I and II disease had the greater learning needs (White, Given, and Devoss, 1996).

A comparison of caregiving for children with cancer by Chinese immigrant and North American Caucasian families revealed that cultural differences and immigrant status contributed to lower verbal expression of distress, more isolation, and lower attention to emotional distress for the Chinese. Caregiving emphases were dietary for the Chinese and emotional for the Caucasians (Leavitt et al., 1999). Chan and Molassiotis (2001) studied the impact of fatigue on Chinese cancer patients in Hong Kong (twenty-two chemotherapy patients and fifteen radiotherapy patients) by the end of the second week after commencement of their treatment. Six themes emerged that illustrated the impact of fatigue on patients' lives within the Chinese cultural context: work and role functioning, daily routines, social life, mental ability, emotional status, and appetite and oral intake.

MEASUREMENT OF FATIGUE PERCEPTION AND SEVERITY

Several instruments, some with both scales and subscales (for instance, physical, emotional, cognitive, and/or temporal) have been developed and validated in particular populations to assess fatigue and other quality-of-life parameters among patients with cancer, chronic fatiguing illnesses, other diseases, and in the general population (Aaronson et al., 1993; Ahsberg and Furst, 2001; Belza et al., 1993; Chalder et al., 1993; Cleeland et al., 2000; Collins et al., 2000; De Haes, van Knippenberg, and Neijt, 1990; Fisk et al., 1994; Furst and Ahsberg, 2001; Hann et al., 1998; Hann, Denniston, and Baker, 2000; Holley, 2000b; Ishihara et al., 1995a,b; Kirsh et al., 2001; Krupp et al., 1989; Lee, Hicks, and Nino-Murcia, 1991; Levine et al., 1988; McNair, Lorr, and Droppleman, 1992; Meek et al., 2000; Mendoza et al., 1999; Okuyama, Akechi, Kugaya, Okamura, Imoto, et al., 2000; Okuyama, Akechi, Kugaya, Okamura, Shima, et al., 2000; Okuyama et al., 2001; Padilla, 1992; Piper, 1990; Piper, Lindsey, et al., 1989; Piper, Rieger, et al., 1989; Piper et al., 1998; Ray et al., 1992; Rhoten, 1982; Schneider, 1998a,b, 1999; Schwartz AL, 1998b; Schwartz AH, 2002; Schwartz, Jandorf, and Krupp, 1993; Schwartz and Meek, 1999; Sigurdardottir et al., 1993; Smets et al., 1995, 1996; Stein et al., 1998; Varni et al., 2002; Ware and Sherbourne, 1992; Whitmer, Jakubek, and Barsevick, 1998; Winstead-Fry, 1998; Wu and McSweeney, 2001; Yellen et al., 1997). These instruments include the Piper Fatigue Scale; Fatigue Scale; Energy/Fatigue Scale; Visual Analogue Scale for Fatigue (VAS-F); Rhoten Fatigue Scale; Fatigue Symptom Checklist; Rotterdam Symptom Checklist; Fatigue Symptom Inventory; Fatigue Severity Scale; Schwartz Cancer Fatigue Scale; Bidimensional Fatigue Scale; Fatigue Assessment Instrument; Multidimensional Assessment of Fatigue; Fatigue Impact Scale; Multidimensional Fatigue Inventory; Swedish Occupational Fatigue Inventory; Brief Fatigue Inventory; Fatigue Symptom Inventory; Pearson Byars Fatigue Feeling Checklist; Functional Assessment of Cancer Therapy (FACT) General and Fatigue subscales (FACT-G and FACT-F, respectively); Cancer-Related Fatigue Distress Scale; Profile of Fatigue-Related States; and Profile of Mood States (POMS).

However, the instruments available to measure fatigue have numerous limitations: many have been generated from investigators' observations, not actual experiences described by patients; others operationalize different definitions of fatigue or differ in dimensionality, which leads to limited reliability and validity testing (Wu and McSweeney, 2001). Initially, instruments were developed for use with healthy populations, such as airmen and workers engaged in manual and clerical work (Richardson, 1998). In the more recent instruments, fatigue is often found as a single item or scale in self-report measures of symptoms, mood, and functional status reflecting the effect of fatigue and the interaction of fatigue with other symptoms or concepts related to quality of life.

As reviewed by Friedberg and Jason (1998), instruments to measure fatigue have one of three response formats: visual analog, verbal rating, and numerical rating scales with item numbers ranging from one to sixty-two. The visual analog scale is rarely used and presents some difficulties exemplified in the next paragraph regarding the Piper Fatigue Scale. A verbal rating scale is a list of adjectives that describe different levels of fatigue intensity, such as mild and moderate. The verbal rating scale is easy to administer and score, easy for the respondent to comprehend, and shows good compliance. Alternatively, the numerical rating scale instructs the patient to provide a single rating of his or her fatigue-related problem on a 0-to-10 or 0-to-100 scale. The 0 point indicates no fatigue-related problem and the 10 or 100 point indicates a fatigue-related problem as bad as it could be. The number chosen by the patient signifies the severity of the fatigue-related problem for the patient. Numerical rating scales of fatigue are extremely easy to administer and score and have shown sensitivity to treatment effects.

The Piper Fatigue Scale (Piper, Lindsey, et al., 1989; Piper, Rieger, et al., 1989) is a forty-two-item visual analog scale designed to evaluate seven dimensions of fatigue, including a temporal dimension (i.e., duration), an intensity/severity dimension, an affective dimension, and a sensory dimension. The Piper Fatigue Scale is the first modern scale to subdivide the experience of fatigue into several distinct dimensions. These dimensions may be useful in developing a more sophisticated conceptualization of this complex subjective state. The initial validation of the Piper Fatigue Scale

(Piper, Lindsey, et al., 1989; Piper, Rieger, et al., 1989) was conducted on fifty cancer patients starting their first week of outpatient radiation therapy. Twenty-four percent of these patients reported difficulties in responding to the visual analog scale format. Eight patients were dropped from the study because of unanswered questions on the Piper Fatigue Scale. Internal consistency for the entire measurement was high. However, the length of the Piper Fatigue Scale combined with some participants' difficulties in using a visual analog scale suggests that the Piper Fatigue Scale is impractical for quick assessment in clinical and research settings. Moreover, Gledhill and colleagues (2002) pointed out serious limitations in a study intended to validate the French version of the Piper Fatigue Scale. Other more recent scales, such as the Schwartz Cancer Fatigue Scale with its four subscales (physical, emotional, cognitive, and temporal), have been developed specifically for the cancer patient (Schwartz, Jandorf, and Krupp, 1993; Schwartz and Meek, 1999).

For all assessment domains, regardless of the instrument used, the type and extent of the fatigue evaluation is dependent on the clinical setting or research project. For instance, Leddy (1997) found no significant differences in healthiness, fatigue, and symptom experience in women with and without breast cancer, while many other studies disagree with that conclusion. Unfortunately, there is no gold standard of fatigue intensity to confirm the adequacy of any particular scale. Rather, the construct of fatigue intensity is often validated against other fatigue measures or functional impairment measures. Selecting a fatigue intensity scale may become a matter of the practical issues of patient comprehension and ease of administration and scoring. In fact, measuring the effect of fatigue on function is considered by some researchers to be more informative about specific fatigue-related dysfunction than is a fatigue intensity measure or a generic functional status measure. Some instruments focus on the effect of fatigue on affect.

Fatigue assessment instruments also have to allow detection of temporal changes in fatigue status. For instance, to aid interpretation of fatigue scale scores and planning studies using these measures, Schwartz and colleagues (2002) determined the minimally important clinical difference (MICD) in fatigue as measured by the Profile of Mood States, Schwartz Cancer Fatigue Scale, General Fatigue Scale, and a ten-point single-item fatigue measure. The MICD is the smallest amount of change in a symptom (e.g., fatigue) measure that signifies an important change in that symptom. Subjects rated the degree of change in their fatigue over two days on a global rating scale. One hundred three patients were enrolled on this multisite, prospective, repeated measures design. MICD was determined following established procedures at two time points. Statistically significant changes were observed for moderate and large changes in fatigue, but not for small changes. The scales were sensitive to increases in fatigue over time (Schwartz et al., 2002).

Most useful studies use a variety of fatigue rating scales and other instruments that rate other symptoms and quality of life. Among these instruments, one can mention the Memorial Symptom Assessment Scale-Short Form; the Depression Scale; the Cancer-Related Fatigue Distress Scale; the Center for Epidemiological Studies Depression Questionnaire; the Hamilton Depression Inventory; the Functional Living Index-Cancer (FLIC); the European Organization for Research and Treatment of Cancer 30-item Quality of Life Questionnaire (EORTC QLQ-C30); Lung Cancer Symptom Scale; Quality of Life Index-Cancer version; the Karnofsky Performance scale; M.D. Anderson Symptom Inventory; the Hospital Anxiety and Depression Scale (HADS); and the Eysenck Personality Inventory (EPI); among others.

For instance, the European Organization for Research and Treatment of Cancer Quality of Life Core Questionnaire (EORTC QLQ-C30) incorporates nine multi-item scales: five functional scales (physical, role, cognitive, emotional, and social); three symptom scales (fatigue, pain, and nausea and vomiting); and a global health and quality-of-life scale (Bjordal and Kaasa, 1992; Du, Shi, and Zhang, 1997; Flechtner et al., 1998; Fossa, Aaronson, Newling, et al., 1990; McLachlan, Devins, and Goodwin, 1999; Niezgoda and Pater, 1993; Osoba et al., 1994; Schaafsma and Osoba, 1994). Several single-item symptom measures that assess both symptoms and economic consequences of the disease are also included. The EORTC QLQ-C30 seems to yield high test/retest reliability in patients with various cancer diagnoses whose condition is not expected to change during the time of measurement (Hjermstad et al., 1995). In an evaluation of the QLQ-C30, Aaronson and colleagues (1993) reported that while all interscale correlations were statistically significant, the correlation was moderate, indicating that the scales were assessing distinct components of the quality-of-life construct. Most of the functional and symptom measures discriminated clearly between patients differing in clinical status as defined by the Eastern Cooperative Oncology Group performance status scale, weight loss, and treatment toxicity. There were statistically significant changes in the expected direction, physical and role functioning, global quality of life, fatigue, and nausea and vomiting for patients whose performance status had improved or worsened during treatment. The reliability and validity of the questionnaire were highly consistent across the three language/cultural groups studied: patients from English-speaking countries, Northern Europe, and Southern Europe.

Isaka and colleagues (1993) and Kobayashi and colleagues (1998) validated the EORTC QLQ-C30 in Japanese patients with prostate cancer and lung cancer, respectively. Kyriaki and colleagues (2001) validated the EORTC QLQ-C30 among Greek cancer patients. Brunelli and colleagues (2000) validated the QLQ-C30 instrument for the evaluation of quality of life among patients with malignant dysphagia. Blazeby and colleagues (Blazeby, Brookes, and Alderson, 2000; Blazeby et al., 1995) also validated the QLQ-C30 among patients with esophageal cancer but stated limitations in terms of its usefulness with respect to certain cancer-specific symptoms such as dysphagia (difficulty swallowing). However, Bye, Ose, and Kaasa (1995) pointed out that when measuring specific phenomena such as diarrhea in a clinical trial, the EORTC QLQ-C30 questionnaire does not seem to be as sensitive as specific trial-related instruments. Moreover, in a study of fifty-four cancer patients, Hendricks, van Beijsterveldt, and Schouten (1998) concluded that although the EORTC QLQ-C30 may be helpful to analyze overall quality of life after bone marrow transplantation, it provides no information on individual effects on quality of life.

Ishihara and colleagues (1996) developed and validated a questionnaire on quality of life of patients with chemotherapy-induced vomiting. The questionnaire consisted of fifteen items which included descriptive questions on appetite, feeling, sleep, mental fatigue, anxiety, pain, sputum, respiratory distress, nausea, vomiting, abdominal condition, daily life in a hospital, and relationship with family, a linear analog scale representing influence of nausea and vomiting on patient's life during twenty-four hours, and a face scale as the global scale. Based on a comparison of the Functional Living Index and the QLQ-C30 questionnaires, King, Dobson, and Harnett (1996) concluded that the choice of quality-of-life instrument for use in a particular trial affects both the results and conclusions. It is important, therefore, to consider carefully which instrument is most likely to detect important differences relevant to the patients' lives in that setting.

Bagust, Barraza-Llorens, and Philips (2001) derived and validated a new compound quality-of-life measure from the EORTC QLQ-C30/LC13 instrument which maximizes the use of the information collected and can serve as a proxy utility measure for economic evaluation. This approach yields relative weightings and rankings for the main issues affecting quality-of-life ratings in lung cancer patients, most importantly fatigue, breathlessness, poor concentration, and disruption to family and social life. A study comparing EORTC QLQ-C30, the Medical Outcome Study Quality of Life Questionnaire Short Form 36 (SF-36), and the Functional Living Index-Cancer questionnaire showed that overall health subscales of these three questionnaires cannot be equated, while most specific subscales provide valid results (Kuenstner et al., 2002).

Zachrisson and colleagues (Zachrisson, Regland, Jahreskog, Kron, and Gottfries, 2002) constructed an observer's rating scale, the FibroFatigue scale, that seems to be a reliable and valid measuring instrument with capacity to monitor symptom severity and change during treatment of patients with fibromyalgia and chronic fatigue syndrome. The FibroFatigue scale rates twelve items measuring pain, muscular tension, fatigue, concentration difficulties, failing memory, irritability, sadness, sleep disturbances, and autonomic disturbances (items derived from the Comprehensive Psychopathological Rating Scale) and irritable bowel, headache, and subjective experience of infection (new items).

Fatigue was among the eight symptoms endorsed by more than 20 percent of ninety-five hepatobiliary cancer experts for inclusion in the Functional Assessment of Cancer Therapy-Hepatobiliary Symptom Index-8 (FHSI-8). Among fifty-one hepatobiliary cancer patients, the FHSI-8 showed good internal consistency, test-retest reliability, a strong association with mood, patient differentiation by performance status rating, and treatment status. Symptom scaling in diseases such as hepatobiliary cancer is therefore feasible and may provide an efficient, clinically relevant end point for following groups over time (Yount et al., 2002). It is probably the combined use of fatigue rating scales, symptom distress scales, and psychometric evaluation of patients that is yielding the most information while a better approach to the study of fatigue and other cancer-related symptoms is deciphered. Chapter 2 describes the interrelatedness of fatigue and other cancer- and chronic fatiguing illnesses-associated symptoms.

Chapter 2

Relevance of Fatigue to Other Symptoms, and to Diagnosis, Predisposition, and Treatment of Illnesses Such As Cancer

RELEVANCE OF FATIGUE TO SYMPTOM DISTRESS AND QUALITY OF LIFE

Experience of cancer-related fatigue by cancer patients, regardless of their diagnosis, disease stage, treatment regimen, or age, influences all aspects of quality of life and aggravates the experience of other distressing symptoms such as pain, nausea, and shortness of breath (Cassetta, 1995; Constantini et al., 2000; Nail, 2001; Nail and King, 1987; Nail et al., 1991; Vordermark et al., 2002; Vroegop and Burghouts, 1989; Walker et al., 1996). In fact, the burden of distressing symptoms and the side effects of cancer treatments may be so great for some patients that they make a decision not to continue with treatment (Redmond, 1996).

Drawing from the experience of other fatiguing illnesses, quality of life is significantly affected in patients with rheumatic diseases, such as fibromyalgia, rheumatoid arthritis, and Sjögren's syndrome (Buskila, Zaks, et al., 1997; Ruiz Moral et al., 1997; Strombeck et al., 2000). Comorbid conditions such as anxiety and depression further affect quality of life (Kurtze, Gundersen, and Svebak, 1999). Schlenk and colleagues (1998) found that fibromyalgia patients had comparable quality-of-life scores to patients with chronic obstructive pulmonary disease (COPD), AIDS, or urinary incontinence, and worse scores than patients with prostate cancer or hyperlipidemia. Wolfe and Hawley (1997) found that fibromyalgia patients have lower quality-of-life scores compared to patients with rheumatoid arthritis or osteoarthritis.

Fatigue affects more cancer patients for more of the time than any other symptom, and patients regard fatigue as being more important than pain, nausea, vomiting, or depression (Curt, 2001a,b; Stone, Hardy, et al., 2000; Stone, Richards, et al., 2000). However, in a study of 1,307 cancer patients, Stone, Richards, and colleagues (2000) found that fatigue had never been reported to the hospital doctor by 52 percent of patients with this symptom, and only 14 percent had received treatment or advice about the management of their fatigue. Fatigue was reported to be not well managed by 33 percent of patients with this symptom, while the comparable figures for pain and nausea/vomiting were 9 percent and 7 percent, respectively. Determining the prevalence of fatigue among cancer patients is also complicated by the high prevalence of fatigue symptoms in the general population (Cella et al., 2002; Rieger, 2001). More accurate prevalence estimates of cancer-related fatigue may result in its improved diagnosis and management (Cella et al., 2001).

In a prospective six-month randomized-control trial with forty-eight subjects newly diagnosed with advanced lung cancer, predominantly non-small cell, Sarna (1998) randomly assigned subjects to structured assessment of symptom distress or usual care. The authors found that, as documented in a previous study (Sarna and Brecht, 1997), fatigue was the most common severely distressing symptom. Systematic use of structured symptom assessment forestalled increased symptom distress over time. Chemotherapy lessened symptom distress, but the impact diminished with time. Subjects with more depression and greater functional limitations had greater symptom distress (Sarna, 1998).

A study by Schumacher and colleagues (2002) underscored that fatigue is an important aspect of quality of life in patients with acute myeloid leukemia. The study consisted of twelve sequential time-point evaluations of 101 patients with acute myeloid leukemia undergoing intensive and prolonged treatment. For the thirty-seven patients who completed the course of inpatient treatment, quality of life improved from the beginning of chemotherapy to the end of inpatient treatment. Patients who subsequently went off protocol did not differ significantly in their self-assessed quality of life when compared with patients who completed therapy. Fatigue was more closely related to quality of life than nausea/vomiting or appetite loss but did not correlate with hemoglobin levels. Fatigue, pain, worry, anxiety, mood disorder, and depression are the main symptoms reported by patients with head and neck cancer (De Boer et al., 1999).

Pain, fatigue, and psychological distress were the most prevalent symptoms among 151 ovarian cancer patients studied by Portenoy and colleagues (1994). Pain, easy fatigue, and anorexia were consistently among the ten most prevalent symptoms at all seventeen primary sites in a study of 1,000 patients with advanced cancer (Donnelly and Walsh, 1995; Donnelly, Walsh, and Rybicki, 1995). When pain, anorexia, weakness, anxiety, lack of energy, easy fatigue, early satiety, constipation, and shortness of breath were present, 60 to 80 percent of patients rated them as moderate or severe, i.e., of clinical importance. The most common symptoms also were the most severe (Donnelly and Walsh, 1995; Donnelly, Walsh, and Rybicki, 1995). Fatigue, pain, and depression were the most common symptoms in chemotherapy-treated breast cancer patients and were all significantly correlated to one another and to total health status (Gaston-Johansson et al., 1999).

In a set of 2,000 cancer patients and 1,000 controls, cancer patients experienced significantly more fatigue compared with controls (Aapro, Cella, and Zagari, 2002). Stone, Richards, and colleagues (2000) reported that severe fatigue (defined as a score on the Fatigue Severity Scale in excess of the ninety-fifth percentile of the control group with no cancer) is a common problem among cancer patients, particularly those with advanced disease. In the population of 227 cancer patients studied, the prevalence of severe fatigue was 15 percent among patients with recently diagnosed breast cancer, 16 percent among patients with recently diagnosed prostate cancer, 50 percent among patients with inoperable non-small-cell lung cancer, and 78 percent among patients receiving specialist inpatient palliative care. Fatigue was significantly associated with the severity of psychological symptoms (anxiety and depression) and with the severity of pain and shortness of breath (Stone, Richards, et al., 2000). In another study (Pater et al., 1997), factors associated with greater fatigue severity included female gender, presence of metastatic disease, and poorer performance status. In addition, the oldest patients were found to have less fatigue, as were patients with breast cancer, while patients with ovarian and lung cancer experienced greater fatigue.

A study of 180 cancer patients at a veterans administration medical center found that increased fatigue levels were associated with greater symptom distress and decreased quality of life and that fatigue severity predicted survival. The Karnofsky Performance Scale score, stage of disease, and number of symptoms independently predicted survival in cancer patients with fatigue (Hwang et al., 2002). A study of 171 patients with advanced lung cancer documented that fatigue and shortness of breath interfered with at least one daily life activity in more than 50 percent of patients, while pain did so in about 40 percent. Fatigue and shortness of breath predominantly interfered with physical activities, such as walking and work, whereas pain interfered with all activities almost equally (Tanaka et al., 2002). In a study of 130 advanced cancer patients, lung involvement, anxiety, fatigue/tiredness, and vital capacity were significantly correlated with the intensity of shortness of breath (Bruera et al., 2000).

Fifty percent of a sample of 228 patients being treated for leukemia and non-Hodgkin's lymphoma reported severe fatigue (Wang et al., 2002); more patients with acute leukemia (61 percent) reported severe fatigue compared with those with chronic leukemia (47 percent) and non-Hodgkin's lymphoma (46 percent). Increased fatigue severity significantly compromised patients' general activity, work, life enjoyment, mood, walking, and relationships with others. Fatigue severity was strongly associated with performance status, use of opioids, blood transfusions, gastrointestinal symptoms, and sleep disturbance items, as well as with low serum hemoglobin and albumin levels. Nausea was the significant clinical predictor of severe fatigue, and low serum albumin was the significant laboratory value predictor. These results support better control of gastrointestinal symptoms for fatigue management in this patient population and also suggest a possible nutritional factor for fatigue in hematological malignancies (Wang et al., 2002).

Jacobsen and colleagues (1999) reported that breast cancer patients experienced worse fatigue than women with no cancer history. These differences were evident before and after patients started chemotherapy. In addition, fatigue worsened among patients after treatment started. More severe fatigue before treatment was associated with poorer performance status and the presence of fatigue-related symptoms (e.g., sleep problems and muscle weakness). Increases in fatigue after chemotherapy started were associated with continued fatigue-related symptoms and the development of chemotherapy side effects (e.g., nausea and mouth sores). These findings demonstrate the clinical significance of fatigue in breast cancer patients before and during adjuvant chemotherapy treatment. Jacobsen and colleagues (1999) concluded that results suggest that aggressive management of common side effects, such as nausea and pain, may be useful in relieving chemotherapy-related fatigue.

Cimprich (1999) showed a discernible pattern of symptom distress before any treatment in a study of seventy-four women newly diagnosed with breast cancer, indicating a need for early intervention to promote the initial process of adjustment. Higher levels of distress were related to a triad of symptoms, namely, insomnia, fatigue, and loss of concentration. Also, lowered effectiveness in cognitive function and significant disturbances in mood state were observed. Women younger than fifty-five years of age reported significantly greater overall symptom distress than older women did.

Dow and colleagues (1996) evaluated the quality of life of 294 breast cancer survivors, and found that

1. fatigue, aches and pains, and sleep problems were persistent after treatment ended;
2. psychological distress from cancer diagnosis and treatment, and fear of recurrent, metastatic, and recurrent disease were problematic over time;
3. family distress, sexuality, and family burden issues were of greatest social concern; and
4. uncertainty over the future plagued breast cancer survivors long term.

In a study of eighty-six breast cancer patients who survived two to five years following initiation of adjuvant cytotoxic and/or hormonal therapy, Lindley and colleagues (1998) found that the reported frequency of moderate to severe symptoms was generally low (less than 15 percent), with fatigue (almost 32 percent), insomnia (23.3 percent), and local numbness at the site of surgery (22.1 percent) occurring with greatest frequency. A study of the effect of perioperative chemotherapy on the quality of life of patients with early breast cancer revealed that although the treated group reported more fatigue and considered hair loss a severe side effect, no differences were found in overall physical and physiological well-being, perceived social interaction, and activity level at two months as compared to a group that did not receive perioperative chemotherapy. One year after surgery no differences were found between the two groups (Kiebert et al., 1990).

Fatigue was among four variables identified by Peng, Manz, and Keck (2001) as effective predictors of pain reporting by cancer patients during chemotherapy; the other variables were depression, severity of colds or viral infections, and insomnia. Conversely, other cancer-related symptoms can also affect the intensity of fatigue. For instance, Blesch and colleagues (1991) reported that level of pain was a significant correlate of fatigue in breast and lung cancer patients.

Burrows, Dibble, and Miaskowski (1998) reported that cancer patients with somatic and visceral pain had significantly higher fatigue scores than pain-free cancer patients. In addition, patients with somatic and visceral pain had significantly lower physical well-being, nutrition, and total quality-of-life scores and more symptom distress than pain-free patients. In a veterans affairs medical center study, Chang and colleagues (2000) reported that patients with moderately intense pain or fatigue also were more likely to experience nausea, shortness of breath, and lack of appetite. Among women with breast cancer, Graydon (1994) reported that those who experienced the most fatigue had the most symptoms and the poorest level of functioning.

Spiegel, Sands, and Koopman (1994) found that the prevalence of depressive disorders of all types was significantly higher in a high-pain than in a low-pain group of cancer patients. Furthermore, a significantly higher history of major depression was present in the low-pain group as compared to the high-pain group. Also, in comparison with patients in the low-pain group, patients in the high-pain group were significantly more anxious and emotionally distressed. Pain intensity correlated significantly with fatigue, vigor, and total mood disturbance, and pain frequency correlated significantly with fatigue, vigor, and depression (Spiegel, Sands, and Koopman, 1994).

Lilleby and colleagues (1999) stress that clinicians should be aware that general quality-of-life dimensions (physical function, emotional function, fatigue) are as a rule of greater significance for quality of life than sexuality and lower-urinary-tract symptoms. Kunkel and colleagues (Kunkel, Bakker, et al., 2000; Kunkel, Myers, et al., 2000) also emphasize that fatigue, urinary incontinence, and sexual dysfunction are major emotional and physical stressors for prostate cancer patients, and therefore point out that consultation-liaison psychiatrists and physicians need to be aware of the psychosocial sequels of both prostate cancer and treatment-related side effects.

Ample evidence suggests that quality-of-life parameters are also important prognostic factors for cancer patients (Wisloff and Hjorth, 1997). For instance, worse fatigue, appetite loss, and constipation scores were significantly associated with shorter survival in esophageal cancer patients (Blazeby, Brookes, and Alderson, 2000). Fatigue was also among the significant survival prognostic factors recognized in a study of advanced breast cancer patients by Kramer and colleagues (2000). Other factors included multiple sites of visceral disease, pain, and global quality of life. For treatment response, fatigue, along with age, shortness of breath, and global quality of life, was a significant predictive factor. Likewise, fatigue, splenomegaly, hepatomegaly, and anemia are associated with poor survival among patients with chronic lymphocytic leukemia (Chen et al., 1997). Fatigue was one of six factors, out of sixteen analyzed prospectively in 395 metastatic cancer patients seen in a dedicated palliative radiotherapy clinic, that had a statistically significant impact on survival (Chow et al., 2002). However, a study of 206 patients with advanced non-small-cell lung carcinoma showed that although fatigue was among the predictors of poor survival, after adjustment for significant clinical factors, a patient-provided pain report had the greatest prognostic importance (Herndon et al., 1999).

In a study of 434 newly diagnosed ambulatory cancer patients, eighty-two of whom had lung cancer, Degner and Sloan (1995) reported that the single measure of symptom distress was a significant predictor of survival in lung cancer patients, with the exception of three patients who had substantial postthoracotomy symptoms. The most problematic symptoms for patients were fatigue and insomnia, with 40 and 30 percent having moderate or high scores on these symptoms, respectively. Patients with advanced disease reported more distress than those with early-stage disease; women reported more distress than men; older patients had less distress than younger patients; distress was highest in lung cancer patients and lowest in men with genitourinary cancers.

Van Andel, Kurth, and de Haes (1997) reported that global health status and quality of life were independent factors for progression in untreated patients with lymph node–positive prostate cancer. Moreover, an increase in prostate-specific antigen in hormonally treated patients indicated not only hormonal escape but also a decrease in quality of life. Fatigue, lower-urinary-tract symptoms, and prostate-specific antigen levels were also found to be independent predictive factors for global quality of life after initial treatment in patients with prostate cancer in other studies (Fossa, 1996; Fossa, Paus, et al., 1992; Fossa et al., 1997). To develop a predictive model for survival from the time of presentation in an outpatient palliative radiotherapy clinic, Chow and colleagues (2002) prospectively analyzed sixteen factors in 395 patients. Fatigue was among the six prognostic factors that had a statistically significant impact on survival, the others being primary cancer site, site of metastases, Karnofsky Performance Score, appetite, and shortness of breath scores from the modified Edmonton Symptom Assessment Scale. If validated in an independent series of patients, this and other models that include fatigue can be used to guide clinical decisions, plan supportive services, and allocate resource use.

Based on the results of four randomized clinical trials conducted over six years in a total of 501 patients, Maisey and colleagues (2002) reported that baseline quality of life, including fatigue scales, predicts survival in patients with advanced colorectal cancer. Pretreatment health-related quality-of-life scores also appear to have value in predicting which patients will experience chemotherapy-induced vomiting. In a study of the effect of postchemotherapy nausea and vomiting on health-related quality of life, Osoba and colleagues (Osoba, Zee, Warr, et al., 1997) reported that the group with both nausea and vomiting postchemotherapy showed statistically significantly worse physical, cognitive, and social functioning, global quality of life, fatigue, anorexia, insomnia, and shortness of breath as compared to the group with neither nausea nor vomiting. Patients with nausea but no vomiting tended to have less worsening in functioning and symptoms as compared to those having both nausea and vomiting. Increased severity of vomiting (more than two episodes) was associated with worsening of only global quality of life and anorexia as compared with one to two episodes of vomiting (Osoba, Zee, Pater, et al., 1997).

In a related study, Osoba and colleagues (Osoba, Zee, Pater, et al., 1997) found that a history of low alcohol use was also associated with postchemotherapy vomiting, whereas increased fatigue and lower performance status were associated with postchemotherapy nausea. Moreover, an earlier study had shown that in patients who did not vomit, the pretreatment fatigue and anorexia scores were better than in patients who did vomit (Osoba et al., 1996). In the week following chemotherapy, health-related quality-of-life-change scores from prechemotherapy values for cognitive function, global quality of life, fatigue, anorexia, insomnia, and shortness of breath were significantly worse in the group experiencing vomiting than in the group who remained completely free of vomiting. No differences in physical, role, emotional, and social function were attributable to chemotherapy-induced vomiting (Osoba et al., 1996).

In a prospective longitudinal study, Molassiotis and colleagues (2002) assessed the pretreatment factors predicting the development of postchemotherapy nausea and vomiting in seventy-one Chinese breast cancer patients. Regression analyses revealed that nonpharmacological factors explained part of the variance of nausea/vomiting, the most common predictors being a history of labyrinthitis, expectation of developing nausea/vomiting after chemotherapy, younger age, stage of disease, and state anxiety, but not fatigue. The results indicate that consideration of the role of nonpharmacological factors in the development of nausea/vomiting could lead to more effective management of this complication induced by chemotherapy.

Despite the findings described, and as pointed out in Chapter 1, fatigue and other symptoms have not received adequate attention in part because of the lack of their conceptual definitions and of methods to accurately measure them. The latter deficiencies are particularly evident for cancer-related fatigue. Moreover, some studies on fatigue have failed to include a control group, have not controlled for possible confounding variables, and have restricted measurement to unidimensional scales with limited reliability and validity, deficiencies which have also shed inconsistency on correlations with weight loss, anemia, psychological distress, or other variables (Chiu, Hu, and Chen, 2000; Irvine et al., 1991).

A major reason for inadequate symptom relief in cancer patients is lack of effective symptom assessment. Accurate assessment of fatigue and other cancer-related symptoms is necessary before any treatment can be undertaken, and to this end several instruments have been developed and validated in particular patient populations (Burge, 1993; Butow et al., 1991; Cassetta, 1995; Cella and Webster, 1997; Cella et al., 1996; Chang et al., 2000; Chapman, Elstein, et al., 1999; Chapman and Nelson, 1994; Cleeland, 2000; Cohen, Kahn, and Steeves, 1998; Collins et al., 2000; Costantini et al., 2000; Esper and Redman, 1999; Fairclough et al., 1999; Faithfull, 1998; Fiedler et al., 1997; Fiedler, Neef, and Rosendahl, 1999; Fossa, 1996; Fossa et al., 1989; Fossa, Aaronson, de Voogt, and da Silva, 1990; Fossa, Aaronson, Newling, et al., 1990; Furst, 1996; Gaston-Johansson et al., 1990; Genre et al., 2002; Glaus, 1993a,b, 1994; Gledhill and Bacon, 2001; Grant et al., 1998; Groopman and Itri, 1999; Hann et al., 1997, 1999; Hann, Winter, and Jacobsen, 1999; Held-Warmkessel, Volpe, and Waldman, 1998; Hogan, 1998; Jakobsson, Hallberg, and Loven, 1997; Kaasa et al., 1998; Kasai, 1994; Kato et al., 1990; Kurihara et al., 1990; Kuriya et al., 1996; Lakusta et al., 2001; Lindley and Hirsch, 1992; McMillan, 1996; Naughton and Homsi, 2002; Wang, 2002; Murphy, 1999; Nail and Winningham, 1995; Norum and Wist, 1996; Osoba, 2000; Osoba et al., 1994, 1996, 2000;

Osoba, Aaronson, et al., 1997; Osoba, Zee, Pater, et al., 1997; Osoba, Zee, Warr, et al., 1997; Padilla, 1990; Passik et al., 2002; Rhodes, Watson, and Hanson, 1998; Rhodes et al., 2000; Samarel et al., 1996; Sanchez-Ortiz et al., 2000; Schumacher et al., 1998; Stein et al., 2000; Strohl, 1988; Tamburini et al., 1996; Thomas, 1998b; Tishelman, Denger, and Mueller, 2000; Van Basten et al., 1997; Velikova et al., 1999, 2001; Wenzel et al., 1992; Whynes and Neilson, 1993; Williams et al., 2001).

Hakamies-Blomqvist and colleagues (2001) point out that timing of assessments of cancer-related symptoms and quality of life is also important. In fact, incorrect timing of quality-of-life assessments in oncological trials jeopardizes both the reliability of the quality-of-life findings within treatment and the validity of quality-of-life outcome comparisons between treatments. This item should be emphasized in the planning of both the study design and clinical routines. For instance, Hanson Frost and colleagues (2000) examined the differences in the physical and social well-being of women during the following breast cancer states: newly diagnosed, adjuvant therapy, stable disease, and recurrent disease (thirty-five, fifty-two, eighty-four, and sixty-four individuals, respectively). Differences were found across phases of disease on various subscales, including those representing perceived health states, overall impact, medical interactions, physical function, role function, fatigue, pain, social function and satisfaction with health, somatization, global psychosocial measures, and sexual and marital relations. While individuals with recurrent disease often experienced more difficulties with their well-being than women in the other groups, women newly diagnosed and in the adjuvant group experienced more difficulties in select areas of well-being when compared with women in the stable group. Health care professionals need to recognize differences between groups to better meet the needs of patients with a breast cancer diagnosis (Hanson Frost et al., 2000).

Quality-of-life studies available demonstrate that approximately 10 percent of testicular cancer patients will suffer from enduring long-term problems, namely, fatigue, anxiety, depression, and disrupted intimate relationships (Heidenreich and Hofmann, 1999). Since the different therapeutic strategies in clinical stage I testicular cancer result in the same high cure rates but may encounter various levels of psychosocial distress, quality of life appears to represent the most important end point of different treatment modalities in the clinical setting, and quality-of-life documentation must be integrated in all clinical study protocols (Heidenreich and Hofmann, 1999).

Patients' fears and expectations also influence fatigue and other quality-of-life parameters. In this respect, Passik and colleagues (2001) investigated patients' anticipatory fears about chemotherapy. Hair loss, vomiting, infection, nausea, and weight loss were ranked as the most feared side effects of cancer treatment for the group as they began treatment. Patients beginning chemotherapy endorsed frequent or intense levels of fatigue, worrying about the future, pain, and sleep problems. No differences were found in the reporting of symptoms based on gender, age, or educational level. Although changes in symptom distress over the study period were unremarkable, changes in fears about chemotherapy were of interest. The most feared symptoms were reordered following the treatment experience. The rankings of nausea and vomiting, hair loss, and loss of appetite decreased significantly. Thirty-five percent fewer chemotherapy patients reported vomiting as one of their most feared side effects; 45 percent fewer patients who received antiemetics reported vomiting as one of their most feared side effects. Effective treatments, such as those that have been developed to treat acute chemotherapy-related vomiting, can relieve the fears of patients on treatment. Passik and colleagues (2001) concluded that patients' fears about treatment are fluid, malleable, and change in response to the provision of adequate management.

Questions of meaning and challenge by illness, i.e., the spiritual dimension of quality of life, traditionally played an important role in anthroposophically oriented medicine and have gained importance in palliative medicine and supportive care (Van Wegberg et al., 1998). However, in a study of eighty-nine patients with advanced breast and gastrointestinal cancer, no association was found between spiritual quality of life and any EORTC QLQ-C30 subscales, including that assessing fatigue (Van Wegberg et al., 1998), an observation which suggests that this dimension should be assessed separately.

Chronic fatigue syndrome is associated with considerable personal and occupational disability and high rates of unemployment (Bombardier and Buchwald, 1996; Versluis et al., 1997). The potentially large economic burden of this disorder underscores the need for accurate estimates of direct and indirect costs, the relative contribution of individual factors to disability, and the need to develop targeted rehabilitation programs. The Medical Outcomes Study Short-Form General Health Survey (SF-36) is useful in assessing functional status in patients with fatiguing illnesses. In one study (Buchwald, Pearlman, et al., 1996), patients with chronic fatigue syndrome and chronic fatigue (lowest scores) were differentiated from those with major depression and acute infectious mononucleosis (intermediate scores), and from controls (highest scores); however, the SF-36 did not discriminate between chronic fatigue and chronic fatigue syndrome patients. A large study (Komaroff, Fagioli, Doolittle, et al., 1996) showed that CFS patients had marked impairment in comparison with the general population and disease comparison groups with hypertension, congestive heart failure, type II diabetes mellitus, acute myocardial infarction, multiple sclerosis, and depression. Moreover, the degree and pattern of impairment was different from that seen in patients with depression; CFS patients scored significantly lower on all SF-36 scales except for those measuring mental health and role disability secondary to emotional problems, on which they scored significantly higher. The relationship between cognitive impairment and functional disability in chronic fatigue syndrome cannot be explained entirely on the basis of psychiatric factors (Christodoulou, DeLuca, et al., 1998).

In medicine, response shift refers to a change—as a result of an event such as a therapy—in the meaning of one's self-evaluation of quality of life. Response shift can be viewed as a change in internal standard. Because of response shift, estimates of side effects of radiotherapy may be attenuated if patients adapt to treatment toxicities. If patients experience extreme fatigue during treatment, they may judge the level of fatigue following this experience differently from how they would have judged it before. In fact, Visser and colleagues (2000) explored whether a response shift might have occurred in 199 patients receiving radiotherapy and found that patients retrospectively minimized their pretreatment level of fatigue.

Jansen and colleagues (2000) assessed to what extent two components of response shift, scale recalibration, and changes in values occur in early-stage breast cancer patients undergoing radiotherapy and examined what the implications would be for treatment evaluation. Significant scale-recalibration effects were observed in the areas of fatigue and overall quality of life. When the groups were divided according to their subjective transition scores, significant scale-recalibration effects were found in worsened quality of life for fatigue and overall quality of life, and improved quality of life for fatigue and psychological well-being. The effects of scale recalibration observed would have significantly affected quality-of-life evaluations, in that the impact of radiotherapy on fatigue and overall quality of life would have been underestimated (Jansen et al., 2000).

Sprangers and colleagues (1999) examined whether response shift resulting from changes in internal standards occurred in ninety-nine newly diagnosed cancer patients undergoing radiotherapy. The pattern of mean scores indicative of response-shift effects was found in two distinct subgroups: patients experiencing diminishing levels of fatigue and patients facing early stages of adaptation to increased levels of fatigue. Because response shift may adversely affect the results of self-reported outcomes in clinical trials or other longitudinal research, further research is needed (Sprangers et al., 1999).

A study by Janda and colleagues (2000) revealed that after radiotherapy for prostate carcinoma, patients experience a temporary deterioration of fatigue and role functioning. Despite physical deterioration, the authors observed an improvement in emotional functioning scores with both questionnaires. This may have been secondary to psychological adaptation and coping (Janda et al., 2000). In a study of sixty-three patients with newly diagnosed M1 prostate cancer who completed a pretreatment questionnaire, Da Silva and colleagues (1996) found that before treatment, fatigue, pain, and decreased social role and sexual functioning were the problems most frequently reported by patients. Correlation analysis in an earlier trial by Da Silva (1993a,b) showed that reduced social life, impaired sexual potency, and fatigue played important roles in overall psychological well-being. Herr and O'Sullivan (2000) evaluated a cohort of 144 men with locally advanced prostate cancer or prostate-specific antigen relapse after local therapy and found that men who received androgen suppression had more fatigue, loss of energy, emotional distress, and a lower overall quality of life than men who deferred hormone therapy. Combined androgen blockade had a greater adverse effect on quality of life than monotherapy.

Understanding the underlying mechanisms for cancer-related fatigue and fatigue in general can lead toward more effective and innovative programs, which in turn will translate into improvement in functioning and quality of life for cancer patients at all stages of disease and may constitute valuable adjuncts to standard therapies that are also applicable to other medical conditions (Winningham, 2001). For instance, peripheral neuropathy is a troublesome symptom that frequently occurs in patients with cancer and is associated with certain neurotoxic chemotherapeutic agents. Ultimately, peripheral neuropathy can be recognized as a significant symptom, such as pain or fatigue. Therefore, monitoring for such symptoms is of importance to the recognition and timely management of this complication (Sweeney, 2002).

This conclusion is further underscored by studies of visual disturbances in advanced cancer patients, a complication that is very rarely signaled, evaluated, or adequately treated (Saita, Polastri, and De Conno, 1999). The main causes of sight disturbances are primary eye tumors, ocular metastases, and some paraneoplastic syndromes. Sight alteration can also be associated with fatigue, asthenia, anemia, and hypovitaminosis. These symptoms can be monocular or binocular, and their gravity and evolution can vary. Based on a survey of 156 patients, Saita, Polastri, and De Conno (1999) estimated the prevalence of visual disturbances to be 12 percent in advanced cancer patients.

The National Institutes of Health Consensus Development Panel (2001) concluded that quality of life needs to be evaluated in selected randomized clinical trials to examine the impact of the major acute and long-term side effects of adjuvant treatments, particularly fatigue, premature menopause, weight gain, and mild memory loss. In terms of the best way to follow up quality of life, a randomized controlled trial in which 296 women with breast cancer in remission received routine follow-up either in hospital or in general practice revealed that general practice follow-up is not associated with increase in time to diagnosis, increase in anxiety, or deterioration in health-related quality of life (Grunfeld et al., 1996). Women detect most recurrences as interval events and present to the general practitioner, regardless of continuing hospital follow-up.

Servaes and colleagues (2001) documented that 19 percent of the eighty-five adult disease-free (off treatment for at least six months) cancer patients they studied were severely fatigued. Their fatigue experience was comparable to that of patients with chronic fatigue syndrome. Severe fatigue was associated with problems of concentration and motivation, reduced physical activity, emotional health problems, and pain. Furthermore, a relationship was found between fatigue and depression and anxiety, while no relationship was found between fatigue and type of cancer, former treatment modalities, duration of treatment, and time since treatment ended (Servaes et al., 2001). In a later study, Servaes and colleagues (2002) concentrated on breast cancer survivors and documented that, in comparison to severely fatigued disease-free breast cancer patients, CFS patients score more problematic with regard to the level of fatigue, functional impairment, physical activity, pain, and self-efficacy. However, a subgroup of severely fatigued disease-free breast cancer patients reported the same amount of problems as CFS patients with regard to psychological well-being, sleep, and concentration, and CFS patients and severely fatigued breast cancer patients scored equal on measures of social support (Servaes et al., 2002).

A survey of 298 breast cancer survivors by Ferrell and colleagues (1998) revealed continued physical demands of breast cancer, including fatigue and pain, as well as psychological burdens related to fear of breast cancer recurrence and anxiety, living with uncertainty, and maintaining hope. Breast cancer survivors also reported positive aspects and life changes after successfully facing breast cancer (Ferrell et al., 1996, 1998). In a study of sixty-one women with breast cancer, Broeckel and colleagues' (1998) former adjuvant chemotherapy patients reported more severe fatigue and worse quality of life because of fatigue as compared to women without cancer. More severe fatigue among patients was significantly related to poorer sleep quality, more menopausal symptoms, greater use of catastrophizing as a coping strategy, and current presence of a psychiatric disorder. Bower and colleagues (2000) reported that the level of fatigue reported by the 1,957 breast cancer survivors they surveyed was comparable to that of age-matched women in the general population, although the breast cancer survivors were somewhat more fatigued than a more demographically similar reference group. Approximately one-third of the breast cancer survivors assessed reported more severe fatigue, which was associated with significantly higher levels of depression, pain, and sleep disturbance. In addition, fatigued women were more bothered by menopausal symptoms and were somewhat more likely to have received chemotherapy (with or without radiation therapy) than nonfatigued women. Depression and pain emerged as the strongest predictors of fatigue.

In a study of 134 disease-free breast cancer patients who had undergone successful surgical treatment, Okuyama and colleagues (Okuyama, Akechi, Kugaya, Okamura, Imoto, et al., 2000; Okuyama et al., 2001) found that fatigue was significantly correlated with shortness of breath, insufficient sleep, and depression, and these three variables accounted for a total of 46 percent of variance in fatigue. Factors concerned with the cancer and treatment, such as disease stage, lymph node metastasis, number of days since operation, past intravenous chemotherapy, radiotherapy, current use of fluoropyrimidine compounds, and current use of tamoxifen citrate were not correlated with fatigue. The results suggest that fatigue in this population is determined by current physical and psychological distress rather than by the cancer itself and prior cancer treatments, and that the management of shortness of breath, insomnia, and depression might be important in reducing fatigue in this population (Okuyama, Akechi, Kugaya, Okamura, Imoto, et al., 2000). The observations described for breast cancer patients apply to other malignancies. For instance, regardless of tumor cell type (small- versus non-small-cell), depression is common and persistent in lung cancer patients, especially those with more severe fatigue and functional impairment (Hopwood and Stephens, 2000).

An evaluation of 100 long-term survivors of Hodgkin's disease in Calvados, France, revealed that, compared with controls, Hodgkin's disease patients reported more physical, role, and cognitive functioning impairments, as well as shortness of breath and chronic fatigue, despite there being no apparent statistical difference in global health status between the two groups (Joly et al., 1996). Loge and colleagues (1999, 2000) also reported increased prevalence of fatigue among Hodgkin's disease survivors as compared to the general population in Norway. Kornblith and colleagues (1998) reported greater fatigue among Hodgkin's disease as compared to acute leukemia survivors. Knobel and colleagues (2001) reported that survivors of Hodgkin's disease with pulmonary dysfunction suffered more fatigue than those with normal pulmonary function. Gas transfer impairment was the most prevalent pulmonary dysfunction, and three times as many patients with gas transfer impairment reported chronic fatigue (duration, six months or longer), compared with patients without pulmonary dysfunction. No associations were found between cardiac sequels or hypothyroidism and fatigue in this patient population.

Crom and colleagues (1999) assessed 220 individuals who had survived a pediatric solid tumor fifteen years or longer and found that health status and health-related quality of life were better in survivors treated with low-intensity therapy. One hundred thirty respondents (59.1 percent) reported at least one serious toxicity. Shortness of breath and fatigue were commonly reported in survivors of Hodgkin's disease. Correlational analyses showed that predictors of health status included socioeconomic status, marital status, and the presence of comorbid factors. One-third of survivors reported that their history of cancer had an adverse impact on their current financial status. Consistent predictors of health-related quality-of-life outcomes among three models included health status, presence of shortness of breath or pain, marital status, and socioeconomic status (Crom et al., 1999).

Although technological advances and insights into the mechanisms of cancer and cancer treatments have resulted in hope of increased survival and even cure in many cancer populations, parallel efforts to promote quality of life through a commitment to fatigue management, rehabilitation, and aggressive palliation have lagged (Curt, 1999; Esper and Redman, 1999). Outcome in palliative care can be defined as patients' quality of life, quality of death, and satisfaction with care (Miccinesi et al., 1999; Sahlberg-Blom, Ternestedt, and Johansson, 2001; Sebastian et al., 1993). A number of symptoms, including fatigue, cause physical or mental distress and suffering in the terminal and dying patient (Sheehan and Forman, 1997). Fatigue, along with pain, cachexia, nausea, vomiting, constipation, delirium, and shortness of breath, is among the most common symptoms in the terminal stages of an illness such as cancer or acquired immunodeficiency syndrome (AIDS) (Ross and Alexander, 2001). In fact, fatigue is the most common symptom at the end of life, but little is known about its pathophysiology and specific treatment (Ross and Alexander, 2001; Sahlberg-Blom, Ternestedt, and Johansson, 2001).

In a prospective study of 117 patients (96 percent with a cancer diagnosis) in a Danish hospice, all symptoms causing distress were assessed daily in three degrees of severity (Henriksen et al., 1997). The ten most frequently recorded symptoms were fatigue, pain, weakness, shortness of breath, immobility/paresis, anorexia, general malaise, nausea/vomiting, edema, and amnesia. Fatigue was registered on 60.9 percent of the admission days, pain on 27.3 percent, shortness of breath on 19.2 percent, and nausea/vomiting on 8.5 percent. The prevalence of pain, shortness of breath, nausea/vomiting, thirst, and anxiety did not increase during the last seven days of life (Henriksen et al., 1997). Balducci and Extermann (2000) point out that although the frail person with advanced cancer is not a candidate for aggressive life-prolonging antineoplastic treatment, he or she is a candidate for aggressive palliation of symptoms, including fatigue. Moreover, when cancer progresses despite treatment, goals change from cure to prolongation of life with the best possible quality for the patient.

Fatigue and other symptoms, such as nausea and vomiting, nutrition, and hydration, need to be controlled in the terminally ill (Anderson, 1994). Medical staff need to understand and utilize management strategies for common symptoms from which terminally ill cancer patients suffer (fatigue, cancer pain, anorexia, shortness of breath, nausea/vomiting, constipation, hypercalcemia, and psychological symptoms) (Ikenaga and Tsuneto, 2000). Fatigue was among the most intense symptoms of cancer patients seen by a palliative care consult team in a tertiary referral hospital (Jenkins et al., 2000).

In a self-assessment study of cancer patients referred to palliative care, Stromgren and colleagues (2002) reported that almost all ninety-one participating patients suffered from impaired role function and physical function and had high levels of pain, fatigue, and other symptoms. Forty-seven percent of patients suffered from depression. Outpatients had better scores than both inpatients and patients in palliative home care for physical function, role function, cognitive function, depression, and inactivity.

In the palliative care population a high level of fatigue and pain was reported zero to one month before death (Kaasa et al., 1999). To explore the relationship between fatigue and pain, Kaasa and colleagues (1999) used data from five studies: two random samples from the Norwegian population (2,323 and 1,965 individuals, respectively), 459 Hodgkin's disease survivors, 434 palliative care patients, and ninety-four patients with bone metastases. The level of fatigue was much higher in the two palliative care populations as compared to the normal population samples. Patients with bone metastases had significantly more pain than the patients in the palliative care trial and norms. In the two palliative care and bone metastases populations fatigue was almost unchanged over time, while pain was reduced.

A request for euthanasia in the terminally ill raises concerns that physical and/or mental suffering have not been addressed and thus mandates a critical appraisal of the physical and psychosocial aspects of the individual concerned. Among 490 patients referred to a palliative care service, six requests for euthanasia (1.6 percent) were recorded (Virik and Glare, 2002). Four of these patients had a cancer diagnosis (all had metastatic disease) and the contributing factors identified were uncontrolled symptoms (2/6—severe constipation in both), depression (1/6), issues of burden/dependency (6/6), lack of autonomy/control (4/6), sense of hopelessness (3/6), and social isolation (4/6). The patient-rated main problems were physical symptoms (5/6), specifically pain (2/6), shortness of breath (2/6), fatigue (1/6) and nausea (1/6), and psychosocial issues (4/6). Thus assessment and management of fatigue and related symptoms are also critical in terminally ill patients (Virik and Glare, 2002).

RELEVANCE OF FATIGUE IN THE DIAGNOSIS OF OTHER DISEASES SUCH AS CANCER

The recognition of fatigue as an important manifestation of cancer helps in the diagnosis of cancer itself. In fact, fatigue can be an ominous sign of an undiagnosed malignancy (Abasiyanik et al., 1996; Abe et al., 1994; Ako et al., 2000; Alderson and Delalle, 2002; Aozasa et al., 1982; Archer, Kourlas, and Mazzaferri, 1998; Asari et al., 1987; Bachle et al., 2001; Baddley, Daberkow, and Hilton, 1998; Bakhshandeh et al., 2000; Banno et al., 1989, 1993; Barwich and Rohl, 1974; Benz et al., 1999; Berent et al., 1998; Berge et al., 1999; Berndt, 1992; Bierens de Haan and Chapuis, 1972; Biesiada and Kalinowska-Nowak, 1999; Billeter, Streit, and Deuel, 1991; Bjernulf et al., 1970; Black and Zervas, 1997; Blade, Kyle, and Greipp, 1996; Blade, Lust, and Kyle, 1994; Blegvad et al., 1990; Blevins et al., 1992; Bohgaki et al., 1999, 2000; Bohle et al., 1997; Boxer et al., 1978; Bozbora et al., 2000; Burski et al., 2002; Canver et al., 1990; Carlin et al., 1986; Castellano et al., 1981; Chen, Nakazawa, and Hori, 1993; Chow et al., 1998; Ciccarelli, Welch, and Kent, 1987; Cicogna and Visioli, 1988; Colovic et al., 2000; Craig et al., 1996; Crombleholme et al., 1993; D'Amato et al., 1998; De Gramont, 1990; Dencker, 1972; Dhodapkar, Li, et al., 1994; Diamond and Matthay, 1988; Dickson and Franks, 1988; Eadington, 1988; Eskelinen et al., 1992; Esrig et al., 1992; Falk, Krishnan, and Meis, 1993; Flandrin and Daniel, 1974; Frangoul et al., 2000; Frankel, Shapiro, and Weidner, 2000; Fujisawa et al., 1992; Fujiyama et al., 1990; Fujiwara et al., 1992; Funabashi et al., 1989; Furuya et al., 1992; Galton et al., 1974; Gates et al., 1995; Gelston and Sheldon, 1981; Gentiloni et al., 1997; Ghobrial et al., 2002; Gilcrease et al., 1998; Gohji et al., 1989; Gotoh et al., 1995; Graham et al., 1996; Grantham et al., 1998; Grimmond and Spencer, 1986; Grundmann and Wolff, 2000; Hamilton, Daly, and Furlong, 2002; Hansen, Vogt, et al., 1998; Hara et al., 1999; Harada et al., 1975; Hasegawa et al., 2002; Hayashi et al., 1983; Helgesen and Fuglsig, 2000; Hellsten, Berge, and Wehlin, 1981; Herrmann et al., 1992; Hettich et al., 1990; Hill et al., 1991; Hippo et al., 1997; Hirai et al., 1999; Hollerbach et al., 1995; Hoogendoorn et al., 1997; Horny et al., 1988; Huntrakoon, Callaway, and Vergara, 1987; Hurd, 1983; Ichiba, Nishizaki, and Tanizaki, 1992; Ichihara and Mori, 1969; Iida et al., 1991, 1994; Imai et al., 1981, 1982, 1986, 1991; Inaba et al., 1996; Invernizzi et al., 1991; Ishikawa et al., 1995, 1997; Izban et al., 2001; John et al., 2001; Juman et al., 1994; Kamiya et al., 1985;

Kamiyama et al., 1990; Kanou et al., 1986; Katayama et al., 1989; Kawabata et al., 1999; Kawanishi et al., 2001; Kazumori et al., 1998; Klima et al., 1993; Koike et al., 1992; Kramer et al., 1993; Krumholz, 1988; Kukita et al., 1992; Kullavanijaya and Kulthanan, 1990; Kumita et al., 1989; Kurihara et al., 2000; Kuroda et al., 1992; Kyle, 1999; Kyle and Bayrd, 1975; Lands and Foust, 1996; Lauritzen et al., 1994; Lee et al., 1985; Leger-Ravet et al., 1996; Lind et al., 1990; Lumachi et al., 2000; Majumdar, Fletcher, and Evans, 1999; Mark et al., 1976; Marks et al., 1978; Masuda et al., 1998; Masutani et al., 1997: Mathiak et al., 1996: Matsuda et al., 1992; Matsumoto et al., 2001; Matsuoka et al., 1992; McClenathan, 1989; Mehregan, Su, and Kurtin, 1994; Metz-Kurschel and Wehr, 1989; Meyer et al., 1998; Micieta et al., 1972; Miller et al., 1972, 2000; Mimori et al., 1989; Misonou, Kanda, Miyake, et al., 1990; Misonou, Kanda, Shishido, et al., 1990; Mitsudo et al., 2000; Miyagawa et al., 1993; Mizusawa et al., 1995; Morishima et al., 1996; Morishita et al., 1988; Motohashi et al., 1990; Mraz et al., 1995; Muraoka et al., 1990; Murthy et al., 1976; Nagai et al., 1993; Nakajima et al., 1995; Nakashima et al., 2000; Nanjo et al., 1996; Natori et al., 1990; Needleman et al., 1981; Newman and Ravin, 1980; Newton et al., 1973; Nishida et al., 1992; Nishiyama, Kinoshita, et al., 1996; Notermans et al., 1998; Notsu et al., 1994; O'Quinn, 2001; Oberg, 1994; Ogasawara et al., 1984; Ogata et al., 1996; Ogawa et al., 1989, 1991, 1995; Ohsaki et al., 2000; Ohshima et al., 1991; Ojeda, Mech, and Hicken, 1998; Olson et al., 1982; Orii et al., 1997; Osterwalder et al., 1998; Otani et al., 2001; Otsuji et al., 1994; Otsuka et al., 1996; Ozawa et al., 1997; Paal et al., 2001; Paelinck et al., 1995; Pedersen-Bjergaard, Worm, and Hainau, 1977; Peters et al., 1974; Picus and Schultz, 1999; Povoa et al., 1991; Prian, Scott, and Robinson, 1978; Raizner and Heck, 1995; Ramot et al., 1996; Rector et al., 1993; Rettmar et al., 1993; Rivoire, 1992; Rostoker et al., 1986; Rundles and Moore, 1978; Ryan et al., 1988; Saeki et al., 1990; Sakai et al., 1984, 1990, 2000; Sanders et al., 1996; Sane and Roggli, 1995; Sato et al., 1995; Savage, Szydlo, and Goldman, 1997; Sawada et al., 1986; Scamps, O'Neill, and Purser, 1971; Scherrer et al., 1980; Schleef et al., 1999; Schloss et al., 1975; Seo, 2002; Sexauer, Kass, and Schnitzer, 1974; Shaheen, Ghanghroo, and Malik, 1999; Shimooki et al., 1995; Solves et al., 1999; Sone et al., 1989; Stancu et al., 2002; Stanley-Brown and Dargeon, 1966; Stein, First, and Friedman, 2001; Stimpel et al., 1985; Strum, 1987; Studer, Staub, and Wyss, 1971; Sugie et al., 1992; Sugita et al., 1996; Suzuki et al., 1987; Tada et al., 1989; Takechi et al., 1991; Tamura et al., 1994; Tanaka et al., 1990; Tokunaga et al., 2000; Torii et al., 1989; Tsuji et al., 2001; Tsutsumi et al., 2001; Tucker, Bardales, and Miranda, 1999; Uchita et al., 1998; Uemura, Okano, and Sato, 1992; Uetsuji et al., 1990; Van de Wal et al., 1988; Van der Meer and Elving, 1997; Van Dijk et al.,

1985; Van Ert, Foss, and Barlow, 1981; Vanel et al., 1983; Walger et al., 1992; Watanabe, 2001; Watanabe et al., 1997; Wataya et al., 1998; Werner, 1974; Werner et al., 1985; Wilson et al., 1995; Yahchouchi and Cherqui, 2000; Yamaguchi et al., 1993; Yamamoto et al., 1998; Yamamoto, Masu-yama, and Hori, 1999; Yata et al., 1999; Yoshida et al., 1997; Yoshioka et al., 1994; Yu, Zhang, and Shi, 1997; Zhu, 1988; Zutic, 1999).

Children ultimately diagnosed with malignancy are referred to pediatric rheumatology clinics with provisional rheumatic diagnoses because of overlapping nonspecific symptoms such as fatigue. Cabral and Tucker (1999) performed a retrospective review of the case records of twenty-nine children with malignancy who were referred to two pediatric rheumatology centers between 1983 and 1997. The suspected diagnoses on referral were juvenile rheumatoid arthritis (twelve), nonspecific connective tissue disease (four), discitis (three), spondyloarthropathy (three), systemic lupus erythematosus (two), Kawasaki disease (two), Lyme disease (one), mixed connective tissue disease (one), and dermatomyositis (one). The final diagnoses were leukemia (thirteen), neuroblastoma (six), lymphoma (three), Ewing's sarcoma (three), ependymoma (one), thalamic glioma (one), epithelioma (one), and sarcoma (one). Patients had features typical of many rheumatic disorders including musculoskeletal pains (82 percent), fever (54 percent), fatigue (50 percent), weight loss (42 percent), hepatomegaly (29 percent), and arthritis (25 percent).

Features that were suggestive of malignancy in the study included non-articular "bone" pain (68 percent), back pain as a major presenting feature (32 percent), bone tenderness (29 percent), severe constitutional symptoms (32 percent), clinical features "atypical" of most rheumatic disease (48 percent), and abnormal initial investigations (68 percent). The atypical features included night sweats (14 percent), ecchymoses and bruising (14 percent), abnormal neurological signs (10 percent), abnormal masses (7 percent), and ptosis (3 percent). Initial investigations with abnormal findings included complete blood count/smear (31 percent), discordant erythrocyte sedimentation rate and platelet count (28 percent), elevated lactate dehydrogenase level (24 percent), plain skeletal X-ray films (28 percent), bone scan (21 percent), and abdominal ultrasonography (17 percent). Findings of investigations done before referral to the rheumatology clinic were not recognized as abnormal in eleven patients (40 percent) (Cabral and Tucker, 1999).

These findings underscore the fact that patients with a diverse group of malignancies, other than leukemia, may present to the pediatric rheumatologist and not the oncologist. Therefore, rheumatic diagnoses should be reevaluated in the presence of any atypical or discordant clinical features. Likewise, at the other end of the age spectrum, primary-care physicians often provide care to elderly patients presenting with nonspecific general complaints. These may include anorexia, weight loss, and fatigue associated with laboratory test results consistent with an inflammatory process (increased erythrocyte sedimentation rate, increased C-reactive protein, anemia of inflammatory origin). In elderly patients, inflammatory diseases of unknown origin are most often related to an infectious illness (particularly bacterial endocarditis or tuberculosis), a systemic autoimmune disorder (temporal arteritis, polymyalgia rheumatica, or vasculitis), or a neoplastic process (Cogan, 2000).

Several case reports illustrate this point. Gray, Bridges, and McNeill (1992) reported a case of a forty-year-old man who suffered eight years of vague but disabling symptoms, initially thought to be related to postviral fatigue syndrome but ameliorated by the removal of a large atrial myxoma. Chudgar and colleagues (1991) reported that weakness and fatigue were the most common presenting symptoms (66 percent of cases studied) of hairy cell leukemia. Kanazawa and colleagues (1998) reported on a case of rapidly progressing small-cell lung cancer incidentally found during the course of renal failure in a sixty-five-year-old man. The patient had a medical history of hypertension, diabetes mellitus, and cardiovascular disease. Hemodialysis was introduced following renal failure, but pneumonia resulted in a transient exacerbation and his complaint of general fatigue did not improve. Examination for the fatigue revealed no apparent abnormalities. Three months later, he died of small-cell lung cancer.

Smith and Anderson (1985) documented that, contrary to clinical impressions, most early-stage ovarian cancers produced symptoms and were more likely than late-stage ovarian cancers to cause fatigue and urination problems; however, only irregular menstrual cycles were more likely to convince patients with early-stage ovarian cancers to seek a diagnosis. Fatigue was also among the presenting features of epidermodysplasia verruciformis in a sentinel case tied to fourteen members of a pedigree with an intriguing squamous cell carcinoma transformation (Sehgal, Luthra, and Bajaj, 2002). Ueno and colleagues (2002) reported on an adenosquamous cell carcinoma of the papilla major case in a forty-seven-year-old man who was admitted to hospital with complaint of general fatigue. A mixed-type thymoma with pure red cell aplasia was diagnosed in a seventy-one-year-old man who was admitted to the hospital because of general fatigue (Adachi et al., 2001).

Tumors may produce abnormal quantities or particular molecules, or homologues thereof, such as hormones, which in turn cause physiological derangements termed paraneoplastic syndromes. Some paraneoplastic syndromes can also manifest as fatigue preceding the diagnosis of the cancer (Andersson and Lindholm, 1967; Asanuma et al., 2002; Bajorunas, 1990;

Base, Navratilova, and Cap, 1993; Cavestro et al., 2002; Chigot, Menegaux, and Achrafi, 1995; Mischis-Troussard et al., 2000; Nishimura et al., 1994; Palmer, 1983; Ralston et al., 1990; Schaefer et al., 1986; Schneider et al., 2001; Sivula and Ronni-Sivula, 1984; Tezelman et al., 1993, 1995; Von Petrykowski et al., 1983; Wada et al., 1999; Zaloga, Gil, and Medbery, 1985).

In the case of Lambert-Eaton myasthenic syndrome that is usually associated with small-cell lung cancer, the clinical presentation is characterized by fatigue, weakness of the proximal muscles of the pelvis, thighs, shoulders, and arms, and a weakening or absence of deep tendon reflexes. The latter are manifestations of an abnormality at the neuromuscular junction that may precede the diagnosis of lung cancer (Bergmans, De Meirsman, and Rosselle, 1975; Courau et al., 1998; Harada et al., 1992; Ishikawa et al., 2000; Ozata et al., 1997; Perel'man et al., 1979, 1984; Struthers, 1994). A significant clinical overlap has also been noted between chronic fatigue disorders and the paraneoplastic syndrome of serum inappropriate antidiuretic hormone (SIADH). SIADH is characterized by lethargy and mental confusion, induction or exacerbation by viral illnesses, physical exertion, emotional stress and/or hypotension, and response to treatment with salt loading and glucocorticoids (Peroutka, 1998). For instance, Asada and colleagues (1996) reported on a sixty-one-year-old woman who was admitted to the hospital complaining of fatigue and was diagnosed with a ganglioneuroblastoma of the thymus and the syndrome of inappropriate secretion of antidiuretic hormone.

Bauer, Muha, and Pytel (1976) provided another illustration of the use of fatigue or fatigability as an aid in the diagnosis of cancer. These authors designed a facial fatigability test to detect "latent" facial motor lesions by fatigability. The test revealed pathological fatigability in eight cases: two intrameatal and four large acoustic neuromas, and two inflammatory processes in the internal auditory meatus. However, the test failed in one case of intrameatal acoustic neuroma.

RELEVANCE OF FATIGUE AND CHRONIC FATIGUING ILLNESSES IN PREDISPOSITION TO DISEASES SUCH AS CANCER

Another facet of the association between cancer and fatigue has been suggested by some authors who have put forth the hypothesis that not only is fatigue the consequence of cancer but also that cancer may be the outcome of fatiguing illnesses, in particular those associated with immune dysregulation. In this respect, a series of studies at the University of Pittsburgh Cancer Center focused on an apparent outbreak of a fatiguing illness involving members of a symphony orchestra in North Carolina (Grufferman et al., 1988; Eby et al., 1989). The studies documented four cases of cancer (B-cell non-Hodgkin's lymphoma, glioblastoma multiforme, parotid acinar carcinoma, and breast cancer) among the orchestra members and close contacts. The cancer cases had lower levels, as compared to controls, of activity of natural killer cells, a set of white blood cells that can directly kill cancer cells.

The findings of the studies described are also consistent with those of another study of natural killer cell activity in a family with members who had developed a fatiguing illness, namely chronic fatigue syndrome, as adults. Low natural killer cell activity was present in six out of eight cases of fatiguing illness, and in four out of twelve unaffected family members. Two of the offspring of the fatiguing illness cases had pediatric malignancies. Based on these observations, the authors suggested that the low natural killer cell activity in this family may be a result of a genetically determined immunological abnormality predisposing to cancer and the fatiguing illness (George, Evans, and Gunn, 1997; Levine, Whiteside, et al., 1998).

As an additional approach to investigating a possible link between cancer and fatiguing illnesses, another study reviewed data from the population-based Nevada Cancer Registry and focused on counties where an outbreak of fatiguing illness had been noted. Higher incidences of non-Hodgkin's lymphoma and primary brain tumors, but not of breast or lung cancer, were noted in two northern Nevada counties (Washoe and Lyon). In these counties, outbreaks of a fatiguing illness, including cases of chronic fatigue syndrome, had been documented, compared to a southern Nevada county (Clark), where no such illness was reported (Levine, Fears, et al., 1998). The study concluded that a link between neoplasia and the fatiguing illness was premature and required further study (Levine et al., 1994; Levine, Jacobson, et al., 1992; Levine, Fears, et al., 1998; Levine, Peterson, et al., 1992; Levine, Whiteside, et al., 1998).

In a ten-year follow-up study, thirteen out of 123 patients with fatigue also reported a history of cancer (Strickland et al., 2001). Five of these stated their cancer occurred prior to the onset of fatigue, and eight reported malignancies occurring subsequent to the onset of fatigue. Two of the patients had two tumors subsequent to their acute illness (a transitional-cell carcinoma of the bladder and basal-cell carcinoma in one and a thyroid carcinoma and fatal brain tumor in the second). The other lesions identified in patients subsequent to the onset of fatigue included a B-cell lymphoma (stage IIIA), an adenocystic carcinoma of the breast, and a melanoma. Although the follow-up study did not have sufficient numbers of patients, the small study group had patients with non-Hodgkin's lymphoma and brain cancer, both noted to be in excess in the initial study (Strickland et al., 2001).

An association between Whipple's disease and Ki-1 anaplastic large-cell lymphoma to Gulf War syndrome has been suggested, and Cannova (1998) presented an unusual case of multiple giant cell tumors of the hand in a patient with documented Gulf War syndrome. This syndrome is another fatiguing illness whose most commonly reported symptoms include chronic fatigue, headache, and neurological disorders (Carver et al., 1994). Further studies are needed to substantiate a possible association between neoplasia and certain fatiguing illnesses. Also, research studies need to address whether, as suggested by associations between immune dysregulation and particular tumor types (Filipovich et al., 1992), the disordered immunity seen in some patients with fatiguing illness can also increase their risk of developing cancer. In this respect, studies on particular metabolic pathways in immune cells are providing intriguing clues. For instance, lymphocytes in a subset of patients with chronic fatigue syndrome display decreased apoptotic (programmed cell death) activity and increased cleavage of the tumor-suppressor gene *p53,* findings that could explain the increased propensity for lymphomas described earlier (De Meirleir et al., 2002).

Another intriguing relationship between chronic fatiguing illness and cancer predisposition has been put forth by studies of magnesium deficiency. Marginal magnesium deficiency is associated with the so-called latent tetany syndrome that is characterized by fatigue, muscle weakness and pain (aching and/or cramps with spasms or tetany), abnormal sleep patterns, and inner ear problems (Durlach, 1980, 1988). It has been postulated that the chronic fatiguing illness of latent tetany syndrome may also predispose to cancer. The latter proposal is based on several observations (Seelig, 1998): magnesium deficiency is associated with lower natural killer cell activity (Flynn and Yen, 1981); magnesium-deficient rats have lower natural killer cell activity and have a higher frequency of thymic lymphomas and leukemias (Bois, 1968; Bois and Beaulnes, 1966); immunosurveillance against neoplastic cells seems to be diminished by magnesium deficiency (Hass et al., 1981); and higher frequencies of lymphomas and both lympho-leukemias and granuloleukemias of cattle and humans have been associated with areas in Poland with mineral (e.g., magnesium) deficiencies (Aleksandrowicz and Skotnicki, 1982). The following list summarizes the links discussed in this section. Again, further research is warranted in this area.

- Low natural killer cell syndrome
- Chronic fatigue syndrome
- Gulf War syndrome
- Latent tetany syndrome

RELEVANCE OF FATIGUE IN THE TREATMENT
OF OTHER DISEASES SUCH AS CANCER

General cancer-treatment-related disorders may include fatigue, nausea, and physical disability secondary to surgery, sexual dysfunction, neurological and musculoskeletal disorders, hearing loss, and cognitive impairment. Cancer patients in general typically experience fatigue while undergoing treatment for their diseases (Hishikawa et al., 1983; Yasko and Greene, 1987). In fact, fatigue is regarded as the universal, most common, most distressing, and unavoidable side effect of cancer therapy (De Jong et al., 2002; Kobashi-Schoot et al., 1985; Morrow, Andrews, et al., 2002; Schwartz, Mori, et al., 2001; Schwartz, Ilson, et al., 2001). For instance, fatigue was the most problematic side effect over time among women under treatment for breast cancer, and fatigue burden was associated negatively with quality of life at different evaluation time points (Longman, Braden, and Mishel, 1996, 1997, 1999).

Although some cancer treatments may not differ in their antitumor effectiveness, they may be associated with differential incidence of fatigue and alteration of quality of life, a feature that in turn influences choice of therapy. For instance, Silberfarb and colleagues (1983) found that among seventy-seven patients with small-cell lung carcinoma who were assigned randomly to two chemotherapy regimens, one regimen produced less depression and fatigue than the other, despite the absence of differences in tumor response. Therefore, fatigue and other quality-of-life variables are increasingly included as end points in cancer therapy trials, thereby supplementing such traditional end points as survival time in the evaluation of the effects of cancer treatments (Moinpour, 1994).

Fatigue may also interfere with cancer therapy compliance and even limit the amount and frequency of treatment that a patient receives (Yarbro, 1996). For instance, a study by Genre and colleagues (2002), although limited by a small patient cohort of forty-seven nonmetastatic breast cancer patients, showed that shortening cycles of doxorubicin plus cyclophosphamide to increase dose intensity had relatively few consequences on adverse treatment effects but a highly negative impact on patients' quality of life, including fatigue. Moreover, in a study of tamoxifen in thirty-six patients with advanced breast cancer, therapy had to be stopped in two patients because of fatigue (Haarstad et al., 1992).

Women with breast cancer are at high risk for fatigue as a side effect of treatment with surgery, radiation, and chemotherapy. The fatigue experience includes a physical component of decreased functional status, an affective component of emotional distress, and a cognitive component of difficulty concentrating (Becque and Blok, 1997; Beisecker et al., 1997;

Gallagher and Buchsel, 1998; Mock, 1998; Sadler and Jacobsen, 2001). The latter variables have different weights in different patients, and fatigue and its contributing factors in breast cancer survivors vary by type of cancer therapy (Woo et al., 1998). In a study of posttreatment fatigue in eighty-eight breast cancer survivors, Andrykowski, Curran, and Lightner (1998) found that survivors reported more fatigue, more weakness, and less vitality relative to a group of eighty-eight women with benign breast problems. However, no relationship was found in the breast cancer group between fatigue and extent of treatment or time since treatment completion.

Fatigue, breast soreness, sensation, and skin changes are common symptoms with breast irradiation that resolve over time. Nausea, vomiting, fatigue, hair loss, menopausal symptoms, and weight gain are predictable chemotherapy-related side effects and are reported as mild to moderately distressful by the majority of patients. Consistency of information, support, collaboration, coordination of care, and communication among patients and health care providers are essential to meet the challenge of successful treatment and rehabilitation (Knobf, 1986, 1990).

Other complications associated with fatigue may also develop during cancer treatment. For instance, in a study by Warner and colleagues (1997) of eight women with no previous rheumatic history, four developed polyarthritis (one seropositive), three fibromyalgia, and one spondylosis after the diagnosis and during or after treatment of breast cancer. Of fifteen women with breast cancer who had previous rheumatic symptoms, twelve developed worse and/or new symptoms after chemotherapy. In both groups, the symptoms had a significant negative impact on functional status, and in some cases resolution was only partial even after many years of follow-up. Warner and colleagues (1997) suggest that prospective studies are needed to determine the incidence, risk factors, and optimal management of fibromyalgia or nondestructive polyarthropathy in women who receive systemic adjuvant therapy for breast cancer. Some chemotherapeutic agents, such as tamoxifen, may help relieve fibromyalgia symptoms (Simonson, 1996).

Schwartz and colleagues (2000) reported that chemotherapy-related fatigue peaks in the days after chemotherapy, whereas radiation therapy-related fatigue gradually accumulates over the course of treatment. The fatigue associated with both forms of treatment gradually declines over time. Fatigue may persist even decades after cancer treatment: Hodgkin's disease survivors are one example (Brice, 2002; Kaasa et al., 1998; Loge et al., 1999, 2000).

Irvine and colleagues (1994) found no differences in the mean pretreatment levels of fatigue among fifty-four patients receiving treatment with radiotherapy and forty-seven on chemotherapy as compared to that in fifty-three apparently healthy auxiliary staff working at three cancer treatment facilities. However, cancer patients experienced a significant increase in fatigue over a five- or six-week course of radiotherapy and fourteen days after treatment with chemotherapy, and these increases were significantly greater than the fatigue reported by healthy control subjects. The prevalence of fatigue among patients after undergoing cancer treatment was determined to be 61 percent. The results of this study were confirmed in another study of seventy-six women with breast cancer receiving external radiation therapy (Irvine et al., 1998). Fatigue significantly increased over the course of treatment, was highest at the last week of treatment, and returned to pretreatment levels by three months after treatment. Fatigue was not influenced by the patient's age, stage of disease, time since surgery, weight, and length of time since diagnosis.

Chan and Molassiotis (2001) reported that by the end of the second week after commencement of their treatment, chemotherapy patients reported greater severity of fatigue than did radiotherapy patients. In contrast, in a study of 448 breast cancer patients free from recurrence two to ten years after primary surgical therapy, Berglund and colleagues (1991) found that those who had received adjuvant chemotherapy scored their overall quality of life higher than those patients who had received postoperative radiotherapy. The radiotherapy patients had significantly greater problems with decreased stamina, symptoms related to the operation scar, and anxiety. The chemotherapy patients had significantly more problems with smell aversion. Activity level inside and outside the home, anxiousness, and depressive symptoms were similar in both groups (Berglund et al., 1991).

Use of the Schwartz Cancer Fatigue Scale, with its physical, emotional, cognitive, and temporal subscales, has also evinced differences in fatigue between those people who are currently receiving treatment and those who have completed treatment (Schwartz, 1998a,b; Schwartz and Meek, 1999). In fact, in a sizable number of people, fatigue persists well beyond active treatment. This feature is illustrated by the study of 379 individuals who had been treated with chemotherapy, either alone or in combination with radiation therapy. Among these patients 37 percent had at least two weeks of fatigue in the previous month. Moreover, of the respondents who had received their last treatment more than five years ago, 33 percent still reported at least a two-week period of fatigue in the month before the interview (Cella et al., 2001).

In a cross-sectional study of 235 gynecological cancer patients, the levels of functioning and symptomatology were also time dependent (Carlsson, Strang, and Bjurstrom, 2000). Patients with short treatment-free intervals reported more problems than the other patients. Patients previously treated with chemotherapy had poorer role and cognitive functioning and more problems with fatigue, nausea, vomiting, shortness of breath, constipation, and finances, compared with those not treated with chemotherapy. Those patients who had been treated with external radiotherapy and/or brachytherapy had significantly more problems with flatulence and diarrhea (Carlsson, Strang, and Bjurstrom, et al., 2000).

De Jong and colleagues (2002) pointed out that high and fluctuating prevalence rates of fatigue have been found not only during but also after adjuvant cancer chemotherapy. The intensity of fatigue seems to be stable throughout the treatment cycles, despite the common perception that more chemotherapy treatments lead to greater fatigue. The first two days after a chemotherapy treatment seem to be the worst period. Payne (2002) also reported that subjective fatigue was experienced by the majority of seventeen adult patients studied with either early-stage breast or ovarian cancer receiving chemotherapy for the first time. The course of fatigue was irregular over time, intensified at three months, and continued six months after treatment ended. Likewise, the majority of patients in a descriptive-correlational, cross-sectional study of twelve adult patients between the ages of twenty-eight and seventy who received at least one cycle of biochemotherapy treatment for metastatic melanoma (stages III and IV) reported severe or moderate fatigue. Fatigue duration varied from hours to months, with a maximum duration of twelve months after biochemotherapy treatment (Fu et al., 2002).

Chemotherapy

Based on a twenty-five-minute telephone interview of 379 cancer patients having a prior history of chemotherapy, Curt and colleagues (2000) reported that 76 percent of patients experienced fatigue at least a few days each month during their most recent chemotherapy; 30 percent experienced fatigue on a daily basis. Ninety-one percent of those who experienced fatigue reported that it prevented a "normal" life, and 88 percent indicated that fatigue caused an alteration in their daily routine. Fatigue made it more difficult to participate in social activities and perform typical cognitive tasks. Of the 177 patients who were employed, 75 percent changed their employment status as a result of fatigue. Physicians were the health care professionals most commonly consulted (79 percent) to discuss fatigue. Bed rest/relaxation was the most common treatment recommendation (37 percent); 40 percent of patients were not offered any recommendations. Given the impact of fatigue documented in their study, Curt and colleagues (2000) recommended that treatment options should be routinely considered in the care of patients with cancer (Curt et al., 2000).

A descriptive study of twelve adult ovarian cancer patients who were receiving chemotherapy and twelve apparently healthy adult women revealed that while there was no significant relationship between fatigue and age, stage of disease, course of treatment, or depression, fatigue was related to levels of the cancer marker CA 125. The fatigue trajectory peaked at day seven and slowly declined during the remainder of the twenty-eight-day treatment course (Pickard-Holley, 1991). Fatigue was also a frequent acute complication during administration of methyl-glyoxal bis-guanylhydrazone (NSC 3296) in advanced ovarian cancer (Vogl, Pagano, and Horton, 1984), but not with administration of docetaxel-carboplatin as first-line chemotherapy for epithelial ovarian cancer (Vasey et al., 2001). Fatigue was common in a phase II study of weekly docetaxel in thirty-seven patients with metastatic breast cancer (Aihara, Kim, and Takatsuka, 2002). Fatigue was also a severe toxicity in 9.9 percent of seventy-two patients with advanced or recurrent breast cancer who received docetaxel in a late phase II clinical trial (Adachi et al., 1996). Moreover, fatigue became more common with repetitive dosing in a phase II study of weekly docetaxel and trastuzumab for thirty patients with HER-2-overexpressing metastatic breast cancer (Esteva et al., 2002). Fatigue was seen in 58 percent of thirty-six patients undergoing a phase II study of docetaxel for advanced malignant melanoma (Aamdal et al., 1994).

Fatigue was a common toxicity associated with daily perillyl alcohol use in patients with advanced ovarian cancer who had received prior platinum-based therapy and had residual or recurrent disease (Bailey et al., 2002). Only one patient developed significant fatigue as toxicity in a phase II study of low-dose infusional 5-fluorouracil and paclitaxel (Taxol) given every two weeks in twenty-one patients with recurrent or metastatic breast cancer, a treatment that did not prove effective (Collichio et al., 2002). Fatigue was a dose-limiting toxicity at higher doses of the farnesyl transferase inhibitor SCH66336 in a phase I trial that demonstrated clinical activity in twenty-nine patients with solid tumors (Adjei et al., 2000).

Fatigue, frequently associated with flulike symptoms, was reported by 39 percent of sixty-one patients with advanced and/or recurrent squamous-cell carcinoma of the head and neck and treated with the pyrimidine antimetabolite gemcitabine (Catimel et al., 1994). However, a phase I trial of weekly gemcitabine and concurrent radiotherapy in fifteen patients with locally advanced pancreatic cancer revealed that a significant number of patients did not develop fatigue as a toxicity (Ikeda et al., 2002). Fatigue is a toxicity, but not among the clinically significant ones, in patients with squamous cell carcinoma of the head and neck receiving oral uracil and ftorafur with leucovorin (Colevas et al., 2001). Fatigue is also one of the toxicities associated with administration of the potent inhibitor of topoisomerase I, topotecan, as shown in a study of twenty-six patients with refractory solid tumors (small- and non-small-cell lung cancer, ovarian cancer, melanoma, and cervical cancer) (Kakolyris, Kouroussis, Souglakos, Mavroudis, et al., 2001) where topotecan had some antitumor effect. A phase I clinical and pharmacological study of chronic oral administration of the farnesyl protein transferase inhibitor R115777 in 28 patients with advanced cancer revealed that fatigue was a common toxicity (Crul, De Klerk, et al., 2002). Fatigue was among the most prominent toxicities in a phase II evaluation of docetaxel plus one-day oral estramustine phosphate in the treatment of forty patients with androgen-independent prostate carcinoma (Sinibaldi et al., 2002).

In another study, only one of thirty-nine patients with advanced non-small-cell lung cancer treated with gemcitabine and vinorelbine experienced fatigue and stopped the treatment. However, despite the fact that the combination of gemcitabine and vinorelbine was relatively well tolerated and was associated with prolonged one-year survival and improvement in cancer-related symptoms, it showed a low objective response rate in this trial (Pectasides, Kalofonos, et al., 2001). Only one patient developed significant fatigue in a phase II trial of topotecan and gemcitabine in thirty-five patients with previously treated, advanced non-small-cell lung carcinoma (Rinaldi et al., 2002). Fatigue occurred in ten of thirty patients with chemotherapy-naive, advanced non-small-cell lung carcinoma and who were undergoing a phase II trial of gemcitabine and docetaxel (Popa et al., 2002).

Gemcitabine use in breast cancer is also associated with mild fatigue toxicity (Tripathy, 2002). A phase II trial of treatment of advanced breast cancer with docetaxel and gemcitabine with and without human granulocyte colony-stimulating factor in fifty-one patients concluded that the combination is well tolerated and effective (Kornek et al., 2002). In a study of eighteen patients, Wolff and colleagues (2001) concluded that although gemcitabine is a clinically relevant radiosensitizer in patients with pancreatic adenocarcinoma, the toxic effects are significant, prominent among which is fatigue, and suggest that until dose and scheduling issues are explored further, concomitant administration of gemcitabine and radiation therapy should still be considered investigational.

Ten percent of the fifty patients studied in a phase II trial of weekly chemotherapy with carboplatin, docetaxel, and irinotecan in advanced previously untreated non-small-cell lung cancer developed fatigue (Pectasides et al., 2002). Fourteen percent of patients with extensive-stage small-cell lung cancer exhibited fatigue after treatment with cisplatin, etoposide, and paclitaxel (Taxol) with granulocyte colony-stimulating factor (Kelly et al., 2001). Mavroudis and colleagues (2001) concluded in a separate study that the combination of cisplatin, etoposide, and paclitaxel is not more effective despite being significantly more toxic than cisplatin-etoposide, and these authors do not recommend its use. Seventy-eight percent of patients receiving paclitaxel/carboplatin for advanced non-small-cell lung cancer experienced fatigue and neuropathy that was cumulative and progressive over successive cycles of treatment (Langer, Leighton, Comis, et al., 1995; Langer, Leighton, McAleer, et al., 1995).

Joss and colleagues (1995) reported that whereas small-cell lung cancer patients achieve better subjective adjustment and less fatigue with early alternating chemotherapy, late alternating chemotherapy allows for higher received dose intensities of cisplatin, adriamycin, and etoposide, and a significantly longer median survival of patients with extensive disease. On the other hand, 6-hydroxymethylacylfulvene (MGI-114, irofulven) was toxic and ineffective in patients with advanced non-small-cell cancer previously treated with chemotherapy (Dowell et al., 2001). Fatigue or malaise was a common toxicity in a phase I clinical and pharmacological trial of intravenous estramustine phosphate in thirty-one patients with hormone-refractory prostate cancer. Dose-limiting fatigue and hypotension occurred at 3,000 mg/m^2, and cumulative fatigue developed after multiple cycles at 2,500 mg/m^2 (Hudes et al., 2002).

Current research reports provide many more examples of fatigue as a toxicity in chemotherapeutic trials for a diversity of cancers (Al-Karim et al., 2002; Albain et al., 1990; Alberto et al., 1986; Alberts et al., 1998, 2001; Ali et al., 1998; Anthoney and Twelves, 2001; Aoki et al., 2002; Aoyama et al., 1994; Ardizzoni et al., 1997; Asai and Fukuoka, 1999; Athanasiadis et al., 1995; Atkins et al., 1985, 1994; Bafaloukos et al., 1996; Bailey et al., 1992; Baldini et al., 2001; Barzacchi et al., 1994; Bashey et al., 2001; Bedikian et al., 1997, 1999; Belanger et al., 1993; Belani et al., 1996; Benedetti et al., 1997; Beran et al., 1997; Berg, 1998; Berlin et al., 1997, 1998-1999; Bhargava et al., 2001; Bissett et al., 2001; Blum, 1999; Blum et al., 1999; Boccardo, 2000; Boccardo et al., 1992; Bok and Small, 1999; Bokemeyer et al., 1996, 2000; Bolla et al., 2002; Bonfil, 2001; Borner et al., 1992; Brand, Capadano, and Tempero, 1997; Brandes et al., 1994; Braybrooke et al., 1997; Breuer, Diehl, and Ruffer, 2000; Briasoulis et al., 1999; Britten et al., 2001; Brogden and Nevidjon, 1995; Brophy and Sharp, 1991; Brunetti et al., 1994; Buchwalter, Miller, and Jenison, 2001; Buckingham, Fitt, and Sitzia, 1997; Buckner et al., 1998; Budman et al., 1994, 1999; Burris et al., 1994; Burstein et al., 2000; Buzaid, Murren, and Durivage, 1991; Buzdar, 2000; Buzdar et al., 1994; Calvo et al., 2001; Caponigro, 2002; Cardoso et al., 2001; Carducci et al., 2001; Carenza et al., 1986; Carpano et al., 1999; Carriere and Cummins-Mcmanus, 2001; Cascinu et al., 1996, 1999, 2001; Casper et al., 1993, 1997; Catimel et al., 1995; Chakravarthy et al., 2000; Chang and Garrow, 1995; Chang et al., 1995,

1998, 1999, 2001; Chapman et al., 1981; Chapman, Einhorn, et al., 1999; Cheeseman et al., 2000; Chen et al., 1998, 2000; Chi et al., 2001; Childs et al., 2000; Christodoulou, Ferry, et al., 1998; Chun, Leyland-Jones, and Cheson, 1991; Chung-Faye et al., 2001; Clemett and Lamb, 2000; Cohen et al., 1995, 2002; Coiffier et al., 1999; Colevas and Posner, 1998; Colevas et al., 2000; Collichio and Pandya, 1998; Comella and Southern Italy Cooperative Oncology Group, 2001; Conley et al., 1993, 1998, 2000; Conroy, 2002; Cooper et al., 1986; Creagan et al., 1986; Creaven et al., 1987; Creaven, Pendyala, and Petrelli, 1993; Creemers et al., 1996; Croghan, Booth, and Meyskens, 1988; Crul, Rosing, et al., 2002; Culine et al., 1999; Cyjon et al., 2001; Dahut et al., 1996; Davidson et al., 1996, 1999; De Jong, Mulder, et al., 1997; De Jongh et al., 2002; De Marinis et al., 1999; De Wit et al., 1997; Del Mastro et al., 1995, 2002; Delord et al., 2000; Demetri, von Mehren, et al., 2002; Dhingra et al., 1991; Dhodapkar, Richardson, et al., 1994; Dhodapkar et al., 1997; Dieras et al., 1996; Dijkman et al., 1997; Dikken and Sitzia, 1988; Dillman et al., 2000; Dimaggio et al., 1990; DiSaia and Gillette, 1991; Dombernowsky et al., 1998; Domenge et al., 2000; Dooley and Goa, 1999; Douillard et al., 2000; Dreyfuss et al., 1996; Durie et al., 1986; Dutcher et al., 2000; Eckhardt et al., 1998, 2000; Edmonson et al., 1988; Eifel et al., 2001; Einzig, Neuberg, et al., 1996; Einzig, Schuchter, et al., 1996; Eisenberger et al., 1993, 1995; Elling et al., 2000; Enzinger et al., 1999; Epstein et al., 2002; Eskens et al., 2000; Falcone et al., 1993, 1995, 1996, 1999; Falkson and Falkson, 1996; Falkson, Raats, and Falkson, 1992; Feliu et al., 2001; Feng, Xu, and Jiang, 1999; Feun et al., 1991, 1993, 1994, 1995, 2000; Flanigan et al., 1994; Fletcher et al., 1993; Forastiere et al., 1987, 1988; Fossa et al., 1986, 2001; Fossa, Martinelli, et al., 1992; Fountzilas et al., 1991, 2000; Fountzilas, Papadimitriou, et al., 2001; Fountzilas, Tsavdaridri, et al., 2001; Francis et al., 1996a,b; Frasci et al., 1993, 1999, 2001; Frasci, Iaffaioli, et al., 1994; Frasci, Tortoriello, et al., 1994; Fukuoka et al., 1997; Furuse, 1998; Furuse et al., 2001; Furuse, Kinuwaki, et al., 1994; Furuse, Ohta, et al, 1994; Fyfe et al., 2001; Ganju, Edmonson, and Buckner, 1994; Gause et al., 1998; Gelmon, 1995; Gelmon, Eisenhauer, et al., 1999; Gelmon, Tolcher, et al., 1999; Georgoulias, Kourousis, Androulakis, et al., 1997; Georgoulias, Kourousis, Kakolyris, et al., 1997; Georgoulias et al., 1998, 2001; Gerard et al., 1998; Gerrits et al., 1997; Gerrits, Burris, Schellens, Eckardt, et al., 1998; Gerrits, Burris, Schellens, Planting, et al., 1998; Giaccone et al., 1998; Giannakakis et al., 2000; Gianni et al., 1991; Gianola et al., 1986; Gilbert et al., 2001; Giles et al., 2002; Gill et al., 1992, 1995; Glisson et al., 1999; Goel et al., 2002; Goldberg, Kaufmann, et al., 2002; Goldhirsch et al., 1980; Gore et al., 1997, 2001; Goss, 1999; Goss et al., 1995, 1997, 1999; Grant et al., 1998; Greco, 1999; Greco et al., 2000; Greenberg et al., 1988;

Greenblatt et al., 1995; Greene et al., 1994; Grem et al., 1993, 1997, 2000, 2001; Gridelli, 2001; Gridelli et al., 2000; Grosh et al., 1983; Gulbrandsen et al., 2001; Gunthert et al., 1999; Haas et al., 2001; Hagemeijer, Prins, and Courtens, 1997; Hainsworth, Burris, and Greco, 1999; Hainsworth, Calvert, and Greco, 2002; Hainsworth et al., 1989, 1998, 1999, 2000, 2001; Hakamies-Blomqvist et al., 2000; Hallum et al., 1995; Hamm et al., 1991; Hart et al., 1982; Hartlapp et al., 1985, 1986; Hartmann et al., 1999; Havsteen et al., 1996; Heath et al., 2001; Hegarty et al., 1990; Heilmann et al., 2001; Herben et al., 1998; Herben, Panday, et al., 1999; Herben, van Gijn, et al., 1999; Herbst et al., 2001; Hesketh et al., 1999; Hill et al., 1997; Hocepied, Falkson, and Falkson, 1996; Hoffman et al., 1996; Hofstra et al., 2001; Homesley et al., 2001; Honkoop et al., 1996; Hood and Finley, 1991; Horti et al., 1988; Hortobagyi et al., 1986; Hovstadius et al., 2000; Hudes et al., 1989, 1995, 1997, 1999, 2000; Huizing et al., 1997; Humerickhouse et al., 1999; Ibrahim et al., 1999, 2000, 2001, 2002; Ikeda et al., 1998; Ilson et al., 1995, 2000; Inuyama et al., 1999; Ishii et al., 1988, 1996; Israel et al., 1995; Jacobs et al., 2000; John et al., 1993; Johnson, Paul, and Hande, 1997; Johnston et al., 1998; Kakolyris et al., 2000; Kakolyris, Kouroussis, Souglakos, Agelaki, et al., 2001; Karp, 2001; Katsumata et al., 1997; Kaur et al., 2002; Kayitalire et al., 1992; Keizer et al., 1995; Kelly et al., 1995, 2000: Kelsen, Chapman, et al., 1982; Kelsen, Yagoda, et al., 1982; Kemeny, Israel, and O'Hehir, 1990; Keren-Rosenberg and Muggia, 1997; Khayat et al., 1992; Khuri et al., 1998; Kidera et al., 1982; Kim et al., 1999, 2001; Kim, Zhi, et al., 1998; Kim, Kim, Cho, et al., 2002; Kim, Kim, Choi, et al., 2002; Kim, Roscoe, and Morrow, 2002; Kimura, 1984; Kimura, Yamada, and Yoshida, 1986; Kimura et al., 1986; Knuth et al., 1992; Koda et al., 1999; Kolitz et al., 1988; Kollmannsberger et al., 1999; Komaki et al., 2000; Koshizuka et al., 2001; Kosmas et al., 2000, 2002; Kouroussis et al., 2000, 2001; Kouroussis, Androulakis, et al., 1998; Kouroussis, Kakolyris, et al., 1998; Kreis and Budman, 1999; Kreis et al., 1999; Kriegmair, Oberneder, and Hofstetter, 1995; Kroep et al., 1999; Kuhn, 2002; Kunikane et al., 2001; Kurata et al., 2000; Kurie et al., 1996; Kurita et al., 1993; Kuroi et al., 2001; Kuzel et al., 2002; Labianca et al., 1992; Lamb and Adkins, 1998; Langer et al., 1998; Langer, Leighton, Comis, et al., 1995; Langer, Leighton, McAleer, et al., 1995; Lawrence et al., 1991; Leiby, Unverfurth, and Neidhart, 1986; Leonard et al., 2000; Lewis et al., 2002; Lilenbaum et al., 2001; Lin et al., 2001; Lippman et al., 1992; Liu et al., 2002; Lopez et al., 2000; Loprinzi et al., 1998; Ludwig et al., 1991; Lynch, 2001; Lynch et al., 1985, 2002; Mai et al., 1999; Macquart-Moulin et al., 1999, 2000; Madden et al., 2000; Malviya et al., 1996; Mandanas et al., 1993; Mani et al., 1998-1999, 1999, 2001; Marshall, Richmond, and DeLap, 1996; Marshall et al., 2002; Masuda et al., 2000; Mattioli et al., 1993; McDonald et al., 1998;

McGuire et al., 2000; McLaughlin et al., 1993; Meadows, Walther, and Ozer, 1991; Meden et al., 2001; Meropol et al., 1996; Meyerowitz, Sparks, and Spears, 1979; Meyers et al., 1998-1999; Michaelson, Kemeny, and Young, 1982; Minsky et al., 1992; Mitsuyama et al., 1999; Mittelman et al., 1999; Miyauchi et al., 2001; Mohiuddin, Cheu, and Ahmad, 1996; Moore et al., 1993; Moore, Pazdur, et al., 1995; Moore, Kaizer, et al., 1995; Morant et al., 2000; Morimoto, Abe, and Kinoshita, 1998; Mortimer et al., 1990; Mross et al., 1998; Murad et al., 2001; Murren et al., 1997, 2000, 2002; Muscato et al., 1995; Muss et al., 1985, 1990; Nagel, Wander, and Blossey, 1982; Naglieri et al., 1999; Neidhart et al., 1986, 1990; Neidhart, Gagen, et al., 1984; Neidhart, Gochnour, et al., 1984; Nicaise et al., 1983, 1986; Niimoto et al., 1985, 1986; Niitani et al., 1994; Nishiyama, Takahashi, et al., 1996; Noda et al., 1994, 1998; Nogue, Saigi, and Segui, 1995; Nole et al., 2001; Nomura et al., 1988, 1993; Novick and Warrell, 2000; Obrist et al., 1979; O'Dwyer et al., 1985, 1996; O'Reilly and Gelmon, 1995; Oevermann et al., 2000; Oh et al., 2001; Ohe et al., 2001; Oka et al., 2002; Okada et al., 1999; Olencki et al., 2001; Ormrod and Spencer, 1999; Osoba et al., 2001; Osterlund et al., 2001; Oura et al., 1999; Paciucci et al., 2002; Pajkos et al., 1998; Palmeri, Gebbia, and Rausa, 1990; Paoletti et al., 1980; Papakostas et al., 2001; Paredes Espinoza et al., 1994; Paridaens et al., 2000; Parra et al., 2001; Patnaik et al., 2002; Patt et al., 1996, 2001; Paz-Ares et al., 1998; Pazdur, 1997; Pazdur et al., 1993, 1995, 1999; Pazdur, Ajani, Abbruzzese, et al., 1992; Pazdur, Ajani, Winn, et al., 1992; Pazdur, Bready, et al., 1994; Pazdur, Lassere, et al., 1994, 1997; Pazdur, Moore, et al., 1994; Pazdur, Diaz-Canton, et al., 1997; Pectasides, Dimopoulos, et al., 2001; Perez et al., 1998; Perez-Soler et al., 1996; Petit et al., 1999; Pipas et al., 2001; Pisters et al., 1996; Pizzorno et al., 1998; Plummer et al., 2002; Poggi et al., 2002; Posner et al., 1990, 1992; Propper et al., 1998, 2001; Punt et al., 1997, 2001; Pyrhonen, Hahka-Kemppinen, and Muhonen, 1992; Quan and Mitchell, 1993; Quan, Dean, et al., 1994; Quan, Madajewicz, et al., 1994; Quan et al., 1996; Raats, Falkson, and Falkson, 1992; Rapoport et al., 1993; Ratain et al., 1997; Ratanatharathorn et al., 1998; Ravdin et al., 1991; Recchia et al., 2001; Reese, Corry, and Small, 2000; Reyno et al., 1995; Richner et al., 1992; Rinaldi et al., 1993, 1995, 1999; Rini et al., 2000; Ripple et al., 1998; Rischin et al., 2000; Roberts et al., 2000; Robins et al., 2002; Rogers, 1993; Rosen et al., 1996, 2001; Rosenthal and Oratz, 1998; Rosing et al., 2000; Rosso et al., 1992; Roth, Morant, and Alberto, 1999; Roth et al., 2000; Rothenberg et al., 2001; Rougier and Bugat, 1996; Rougier et al., 1997; Royce et al., 1999, 2001; Rozencweig et al., 1983; Ryan et al., 2002; Saeki et al., 1989; Sakuda et al., 1980; Sakuma et al., 1999; Salimen, Nikkanen, and Lindholm, 1997; Salminen et al., 1999; Saltz et al., 1993, 1994; Sandler et al., 1998; Sato et al., 2001;

Savarese et al., 2001; Scheulen et al., 2000; Schilsky et al., 1993, 1998, 2000; Schmid et al., 1997; Schoffski, Hagedorn, et al., 2000; Schoffski, Seeland, et al., 2000; Schomburg et al., 1993; Schornagel et al., 1989; Schuchter et al., 1992; Scott and Wiseman, 1999; Semb et al., 1998; Sertoli, Bernengo, et al., 1989; Sertoli, Brunetti, et al., 1989; Sessa et al., 1988, 1994, 1999, 2002; Seymour et al., 1999; Shade et al., 1998-1999; Shamdas et al., 1994; Shapiro et al., 1996, 1998, 1999; Sharma et al., 2002; Shimizu et al., 1984; Shimoyama et al., 1992; Shin et al., 1998, 2000; Shin, Glisson, Khuri, Clifford, et al., 2002; Shin, Glisson, Khuri, Lippman, et al., 2002; Shin, Khuri, Glisson, et al., 2001; Shin, Khuri, Murphy, et al., 2001; Shinoda et al., 1997; Sinibaldi et al., 1999; Sinnige et al., 1993; Sitzia, Hughes, and Sobrido, 1995; Sitzia et al., 1997; Sitzia and Huggins, 1998; Siu et al., 2002; Sjostrom et al., 1999; Sklarin et al., 1997; Slabber et al., 1996; Small et al., 2000; Smith et al., 1996, 2000; Smith, O'Brien, et al., 2001; Solal-Celigny et al., 1993; Sommer et al., 2001; Soni et al., 1997; Soori et al., 1999, 2000, 2002; Sorbe et al., 1994; Sordillo, Magill, and Welt, 1985; Sparano et al., 1993, 1996; Stadler et al., 1998, 1999; Stevenson et al., 1999, 2001; Stewart et al., 1996, 1999; Stopeck et al., 2002; Stoter et al., 1989, 1991; Stupp et al., 2001; Subramanyan et al., 1999; Sulkes et al., 1994; Sulkes, Benner, and Canetta, 1998; Suzuki, 1986; Szarka et al., 2001; Taguchi, 1987, 1994; Taguchi et al., 1996; Taguchi, Furue, et al., 1994; Taguchi, Hirata, et al., 1994; Taguchi, Mori, et al., 1994; Taguchi, Morimoto, et al., 1998; Taguchi, Sakata, et al., 1998; Takada et al., 1998; Talpaz et al., 2001; Tamura et al., 1989; Tan et al., 2002; Taylor, Modiano, et al., 1992; Taylor, Dorr, et al., 2001; Taylor, Jason, et al., 2001; Tefferi et al., 1994; Terao, 2002; Thodtmann, Depenbrock, Blatter, et al., 1999; Thodtmann, Depenbrock, Dumez, et al. 1999; Thomas, Arzoomanian, et al., 2001; Thomas, Dahut, et al., 2001; Thomson et al., 1993; Tolcher and Gelmon, 1995; Toma et al., 1994; Tominaga et al., 1992, 1993; Tominaga, Nomura, Adachi, Aoyama, et al., 1994; Tominaga, Nomura, Adachi, Takashima, et al., 1994; Touroutoglou et al., 1998; Treat et al., 1998; Triozzi et al., 1996; Trudeau et al., 1993, 1995; Trump et al., 1990; Tsavaris et al., 1993, 1995, 1996, 1997, 2000, 2001; Tsukagoshi, 1995; Tulpule et al., 1998, 2001; Twelves et al., 1994; Valero et al., 1999; Van Dam et al., 1980; Van der Lely, Brownell, and Lamberts, 1991; Van Groeningen et al., 1986; Van Herpen et al., 2000; Van Poznak et al., 2001; Varterasian et al., 1998, 2000; Varveris et al., 2003; Vasey et al., 1995; Verdi et al., 1992; Verschraegen et al., 1997, 2001; Vest, Bork, and Hansen, 1988; Vitale et al., 2000; Vokes et al., 2001; Von der Maase et al., 2000; Von Mehren et al., 1995; Von Pawel et al., 1999; Voravud et al., 1993; Wadler and Wiernik, 1990; Wadler et al., 1988, 1990, 1991, 1996, 1998, 2002; Walters et al., 1998; Wander et al., 1986; Wang et al., 1988; Warrell, Coonley, and Burchenal, 1983; Weiss et al., 1982, 1983, 1988, 1995, 1998; Westermann et al., 2000; White et al., 2000; Whitehead et al., 1997, 2001, 2002; Wiseman and Spencer, 1997; Wisloff et al., 1996; Woolley et al., 1996; Wymenga et al., 1999; Yamaguchi et al., 1999; Yang et al., 1999; Yap et al., 1981; Yoshida et al., 1994; Yoshimoto, Nasu, et al., 1985; Zamagni et al., 1998; Zarogoulidis et al., 1996; Zelefsky et al., 2000; Zujewski et al., 2000).

The fatigue toxicity of several new chemotherapeutic compounds currently under development remains to be determined (Zhai et al., 2002). For instance, only one patient, among twenty-seven patients with previously tamoxifen-treated metastatic breast cancer, experienced fatigue while on hormonal therapy with the new nonsteroidal aromatase inhibitor anastrozole in a trial that showed limited effectiveness (Lavrenkov et al., 2002). In a phase I trial of BCL-2 antisense oligonucleotide (G3139) administered by continuous intravenous infusion in thirty-five patients with advanced cancer, fatigue and transient reversible elevations of serum transaminases (grades 2-3) became apparent after seven days of treatment at the highest dose level examined (6.9 mg/kg/day) (Morris et al., 2002). Fatigue was among the toxicities in a phase I and pharmacokinetic study of E7070, a novel chloroindolyl sulfonamide cell-cycle inhibitor, administered as a one-hour infusion every three weeks in forty patients with advanced cancer (Raymond et al., 2002). Fatigue in three patients was among the dose-limiting toxicities in a phase I trial of the histone deacetylase inhibitor depsipeptide (FR901228, NSC 630176) in thirty-seven patients with advanced or refractory neoplasms (Sandor et al., 2002).

In some instances, fatigue, along with limited or no effectiveness of the agents tested, has disfavored use of a particular agent or combination of chemotherapeutic agents. For instance, Schwartz, Ilson, and colleagues (2001) reported that 93 percent of patients with advanced gastric carcinoma experienced fatigue after administration of the cyclin-dependent kinase inhibitor flavopiridol, and the researchers concluded that this agent was an ineffective treatment for this condition. Piroxantrone yielded similar results for metastatic gastric adenocarcinoma (Pazdur, Bready, et al., 1994). The combination of cytarabine and cisplatin was found to be of no clinical value as salvage therapy in patients with advanced colorectal cancer who failed 5-fluorouracil and folinic acid. The combination had significant toxicity (50 percent of patients experienced fatigue, vomiting, and severe hematological toxicity) and lacked efficiency (Adenis et al., 1995). Fatigue was a major toxicity in phase II studies of CPT-11 plus cisplatin and of irinotecan and cisplatin in patients with advanced, untreated gastric or gastroesophageal junction adenocarcinoma (Ajani et al., 2001, 2002). Fourteen percent of patients developed fatigue in a phase II trial that provided inconclusive evidence for the use of docetaxel chemotherapy in twenty-two patients with incurable metastatic or locally extensive adenocarcinoma of the esophagus (Heath et al., 2002). The topoisomerase-1 irinotecan is also associated with significant toxicity, including fatigue, and poor antitumor response in patients with advanced hepatocellular carcinoma (O'Reilley et al., 2001).

Treatment with all-*trans*-retinoic acid of patients with metastatic non-small-cell lung cancer was associated with fatigue in 36 percent of cases despite limited antitumor activity (Treat et al., 1994). A phase I trial showed no antitumor effectiveness but did cause fatigue as a side effect of administration of the polyamine biosynthesis inhibitors alpha-difluoromethyl ornithine and methylglyoxal bis (guanylhydrazone) in patients with advanced prostatic cancer (Herr, Warrel, and Burchenal, 1986). Abraham and colleagues (2002) conducted a phase II trial of continuous-infusion doxorubicin, vincristine, and etoposide with daily mitotane as a P-glycoprotein antagonist for the treatment of metastatic adrenocortical carcinoma. Daily mitotane made treatment difficult because it was associated with grade 1/2 nausea, diarrhea, fatigue, and neuropsychiatric changes in thirty-one of thirty-six patients (Abraham et al., 2002). Fatigue was also evident as a toxicity in 50 percent of eighteen patients in a phase II trial of JM-216, an orally bioavailable platinum compound that proved to have limited effectiveness in the treatment of advanced/recurrent squamous cervical cancer (Trudeau et al., 2002). A clinical trial showed that although time to progression in 371 metastatic breast cancer patients treated with epirubicin is not improved by the addition of either cisplatin or lonidamine (Berruti et al., 2002), the addition of lonidamine produced more myalgias and fatigue.

Stealth liposomal doxorubicin, although associated with little fatigue toxicity, lacks antitumor activity in the treatment of patients with anthracycline-resistant breast cancer (Rivera, Valero, et al., 2002). In contrast, a phase I evaluation of polymer-bound doxorubicin in twenty-five patients with primary or six with metastatic liver cancer evinced its induction of severe fatigue at the maximum tolerated dose (Seymour et al., 2002). Fatigue was among the most frequent toxicities in an initial clinical trial of oral TAC-101, a novel retinoic acid receptor-alpha selective retinoid, in twenty-nine patients with advanced cancer (Rizvi et al., 2002). Fatigue was among the most common toxicities (17 percent) in a multicenter phase II study of a twenty-eight-day regimen of orally administered eniluracil, a potent inactivator of dihydropyrimidine dehydrogenase, and fluorouracil. The latter combination proved to have modest activity in the treatment of eighty-four patients with anthracycline- and taxane-resistant advanced breast cancer (Rivera, Sutton, et al., 2002).

In contrast to the cases described, some chemotherapeutic treatments are effective without inducing fatigue in a significant number of patients. For instance, preoperative chemoradiation using oral capecitabine (Xeloda), a new orally administered fluoropyrimidine carbamate that was rationally designed to exert its effect by tumor-selective activation, is safe, well tolerated, and effective for locally advanced rectal cancer, and only four percent of patients complained of fatigue (Kim, Kim, Cho, et al., 2002). Another example is provided by the use of ketoconazole and hydrocortisone in the treatment of prostate cancer. High-dose (400 mg) oral ketoconazole three times daily with replacement doses of hydrocortisone has become a standard treatment option for patients with advanced prostate cancer that progresses after androgen deprivation. However, toxicity, including fatigue, can hinder the ability to deliver treatment, and the cost of the regimen can be substantial. Harris and colleagues (2002) conducted a prospective phase II study to assess the efficacy and safety of a regimen of low-dose (200 mg) oral ketoconazole three times daily with replacement doses of hydrocortisone (20 mg every morning and 10 mg at bedtime) in twenty-eight men with androgen-independent prostate cancer. The regimen of low-dose ketoconazole with replacement doses of hydrocortisone was well tolerated (fourteen percent of patients complained of fatigue) and had moderate activity in patients with progressive androgen-independent prostate cancer.

In a phase II study of induction chemotherapy with paclitaxel, ifosfamide, and carboplatin for fifty patients with locally advanced squamous cell carcinoma of the head and neck, fatigue developed in only 7 percent of them (Shin, Glisson, Khuri, Lippman, et al., 2002). Fatigue was among the lesser toxicities in a phase I clinical and pharmacokinetic study of protein kinase C-alpha antisense oligonucleotide ISIS 3521 administered in combination with 5-fluorouracil and leucovorin in fifteen patients with advanced cancer (Rudin et al., 2001). Fatigue was not a toxicity in a phase I study of the granulocyte-monocyte colony-stimulating factor (GM-CSF) antagonist E21R, whose administration proved to be safe in patients (eighteen males and four females) with solid tumors known to express GM-CSF receptors (two breast, four prostate, ten colon, and three lung cancer, and three melanoma cases) (Olver et al., 2002).

In a study of women with progressive human epidermal growth factor receptor (HER)-2-overexpressing metastatic breast cancer who may or may not have had prior chemotherapy, there was mild worsening of physical and role functioning and of fatigue throughout the duration of chemotherapy treatment. On the other hand, a similar comparison of those receiving chemotherapy with trastuzumab revealed mild worsening of role functioning at weeks eight and twenty and of fatigue only at week eight. These results suggest that trastuzumab may be associated with an amelioration of the deleterious effects of chemotherapy alone (Osoba and Burchmore, 1999).

The influence of factors such as pain, impaired quality of sleep, and depression are highly consistent across several studies, although it is often not clear whether it is the symptoms that cause the fatigue or vice versa. The outcomes of several studies indicate that many symptoms are interrelated in a network. For instance, based on two studies of patients receiving chemotherapy or radiotherapy, Irvine and colleagues (1994, 1998) reported that fatigue in cancer patients was found to covary with weight, symptom distress, mood disturbance, and alterations in usual functional activities. The best predictors of fatigue in the patient sample were their symptom distress and mood disturbance. Symptom distress and fatigue were significant predictors of impairment in functional activities related to illness (Irvine et al., 1994, 1998).

Based on a prospective, longitudinal study of ninety-three cancer patients, Dodd, Miaskowski, and Paul (2001) underscore the relevance of the possible synergistic adverse effects of the symptom cluster of pain, fatigue, and sleep insufficiency on functional status of patients after three cycles of chemotherapy. Quality-of-life findings from lung cancer clinical trials indicate a prevalence of symptom distress, fatigue, and decline in functional status, although patients also experience symptom management problems without treatment (Benedict, 1989). A summary of quality-of-life findings for two vinorelbine (Navelbine) trials (randomized and single-arm) in patients with non-small-cell lung cancer showed that symptom status was as good or better for patients receiving vinorelbine compared with those receiving 5-fluorouracil/leucovorin in the randomized study (Moinpour, 1994). A phase I/pilot study of sequential doxorubicin/vinorelbine concluded that the combination is feasible and associated with activation of *p53* and the repression of microtubule-associated protein 4, changes that lead to increased sensitivity to chemotherapy (Bash-Babula et al., 2002).

Immunotherapy

Interferon-Alpha

Alpha-interferons are biological response modifiers that regulate immune function, slow cell proliferation, and inhibit viral replication (Balmer, 1985). Interferon-alpha-2 was the first pure human protein found to be effective in the treatment of cancer, and it has served as a prototype for the clinical development of other immunomodulators such as interleukin-2 and several growth-regulating cytokines (Tsukagoshi, 1987). Interferon-alpha is a polypeptide cytokine that may be useful for single-agent or combined treatment of selected hematological malignancies, including cutaneous lymphomas, and of solid tumors such as renal cell carcinoma, among others (Bukowski et al., 2002; Bunn, Idhe, and Foon, 1987; Chimenti et al., 1995;

Connors and Silver, 1984; Connors et al., 1985; Cortes et al., 1996; De Palo et al., 1984, 1985; De Kernion et al., 1983; Di Bartolomeo et al., 1993; Doberauer et al., 1991; Edelstein et al., 1983; Edmonson et al., 1987; Eggermont et al., 1985, 1986; Einhorn et al., 1988; Elsasser-Beile et al., 1987; Finter et al., 1991; Grander and Einhorn, 1998; Grunberg et al., 1985; Gutterman et al., 1980, 1982; Horning et al., 1982, 1983, 1985; Iaffaioli et al., 1991; Ichimaru et al., 1988; Kamihira et al., 1983; Kankuri et al., 2001; Kanno et al., 1993; Kasamatsu et al., 1985; Kempf et al., 1986; Kobayashi et al., 1987, 1989; Lai et al., 1993; Marschalko et al., 2001; Marschner et al., 1991; Matsuyama et al., 1997; Moertel, Rubin, and Kvols, 1989; Morales et al., 1997; Motzer et al., 2001; Neefe et al., 1990; Neidhart, Gagen, et al., 1984; Niederle, Kurschel, and Schmidt, 1984; Niiranen et al., 1990; Niloff et al., 1985; Obbens et al., 1985; Oberg, 1992; Oberg and Eriksson, 1991a,b; Olesen et al., 1987; Olsen et al., 1989; Padmanabhan et al., 1985; Pizzocaro et al., 1993; Quesada, Swanson, and Gutterman, 1985; Sarna and Figlin, 1985; Sherwin et al., 1982; Taguchi, 1984, 1985; Urba and Longo, 1986; Van Zandwijk et al., 1990; Vugrin, Hood, and Laszlo, 1986; Wagstaff et al., 1984; Watanabe et al., 1994; Yasumoto et al., 1992; Yoshimoto, Tsushima, et al., 1985).

Hairy cell leukemia is the tumor most sensitive to interferon-alpha (Golomb et al., 1986, 1988; Niederle et al., 1987; Quesada, Hersh, et al., 1986; Smalley et al., 1991; Thompson, Rubin, and Fefer, 1987). Interferon-alpha-2 has been used to treat chronic myelogenous leukemia and other myeloproliferative disorders, such as multiple myeloma, with limited success (Blade et al., 1998; Foon, Bottino, et al., 1985; Foon, Roth, and Bunn, 1987; Freund et al., 1989; Gutterman et al., 1980; Koyama et al., 1988; Nagler et al., 1994; Ozer et al., 1983; Quesada, Alexanian, et al., 1986; Rozman et al., 1988; Suzuki, Iwase, et al., 1991; Takeuchi et al., 1995; Werter et al., 1988; Westin et al., 1995; Yoshida, 2001). There are at least fifteen different molecular species of interferon-alpha. Interferon-alpha-2a (Roferon-A/Roche) and interferon-alpha-2b (Intron A/Schering) are approved in the United States for treating hairy cell leukemia and AIDS-related Kaposi's sarcoma (Baumann et al., 1991; Borden, 1992a,b; Evans et al., 1991; Fischl et al., 1996; Hansen and Borden, 1992; Rios et al., 1985; Sawayama et al., 1996; Tur and Brenner, 1998). Deichmann and colleagues (1998) showed that interferon-alpha is also effective in the treatment of non-AIDS-associated Kaposi's sarcoma.

Despite its biological activities, administration of interferon is associated with toxicity. The acute syndrome of toxicity of interferon administration consists of fever, chills, myalgias, arthralgias, and headache, with some variation according to type of interferon, route of administration, schedule, and dose (Creagan et al., 1988; Crockett et al., 1987; Furue, 1985, 1986;

Gauci, 1987; Giles et al., 1991; Grion et al., 1994; Jones and Itri, 1986; Mittelman et al., 1990; Oh et al., 2002; Quesada, Talpaz, et al., 1986; Silver, Connors, and Salinas, 1985; Zimmerman et al., 1994). Fatigue is the most prevalent nonacute symptom. Hematological toxicity consists mainly of leukopenia, but anemia and thrombocytopenia occur in some patients. Nausea, vomiting, and diarrhea are the main gastrointestinal symptoms. Elevation of serum transaminases seems to reflect liver toxicity. Renal function is well preserved, except for rare instances of acute renal failure. Cardiac toxicity remains questionable, although heart failure and arrhythmias have been associated with the administration of interferons.

Most if not all of these effects, which can also contribute to fatigue, are reversible or can be ameliorated. With interferon-alpha, doses of 1 million to 9 million units (MU) are generally well tolerated, but doses greater than or equal to 18 MU yield moderate to severe toxicity. Doses greater than or equal to 36 MU can induce severe toxicity and significantly alter the performance status of the patient (Quesada, Talpaz, et al., 1986). Newer formulations of interferon-alpha with longer half-lives, such as pegylated interferon-alpha, are being used more frequently and share similar toxicity spectra as regular interferon-alpha (Bukowski et al., 2002).

A study revealed that interferon-alpha/beta is at least partially responsible for the early fatigue induced by polydI:dC, a double-stranded RNA interferon inducer that mimics the effects of viral infections, during prolonged treadmill running in mice (Davis, Weaver, et al., 1998). Poly dI:dC is somnogenic and pyrogenic; it induces a flulike syndrome in humans and has antiviral and possibly antitumoral activity (Carter and De Clercq, 1974; Droller, 1987; Freeman et al., 1977; Muller, Ushijima, and Schroder, 1994; Stevenson et al., 1985; Witt et al., 1996). Ampligen, a mismatched double-stranded RNA molecule, can also induce fatigue and somnolence (Brodsky et al., 1985).

Kirkwood and colleagues (2002) reviewed the toxicity profile of high-dose interferon-alpha therapy by examining data from U.S. cooperative group trials. The high-dose regimen is associated with acute constitutional symptoms, chronic fatigue, myelosuppression, elevated liver enzyme levels, and neurological symptoms. The majority of patients tolerate one year of therapy with an understanding of the anticipated toxicities in conjunction with appropriate dose modifications and supportive care. Many of the toxicities associated with interferon-alpha seem to be the result of endogenous cytokines and their effects on the neuroendocrine system. An increased understanding of the mechanisms of interferon-alpha-associated toxicity will lead to more rational and effective supportive care and improved quality of life.

In a study of thirty patients with malignant melanoma receiving interferon-alpha, Dean and colleagues (1995) found a consistent pattern of fatigue, with the most extreme fatigue scores in the affective domain, followed by the sensory, temporal, total fatigue, and fatigue severity scores (Symptom Distress Scale and Piper Fatigue Scale). Studies by Creagan and colleagues (Creagan, Ahmann, Green, Long, Frytak, et al., 1984; Creagan, Ahmann, Green, Long, Rubin, et al., 1984), Kirkwood and colleagues (1985), Legha and colleagues (1987), Maral and colleagues (1987), Neefe and colleagues (1990), and Sertoli and colleagues (Sertoli, Bernengo, et al., 1989; Sertoli, Brunetti, et al., 1989) indicated that recombinant interferon-alpha has some antitumor activity in patients with disseminated malignant melanoma. However, other studies stress that interferon-alpha-2b is ineffective in the treatment of malignant melanoma (Coates et al., 1986; Hersey et al., 1985).

Fatigue, reversible on discontinuation of treatment, was frequently a dose-limiting toxicity in patients with metastatic breast cancer, nodular poorly differentiated lymphocytic lymphoma, or multiple myeloma receiving 36 million units of leukocyte interferon (Quesada et al., 1984). However, leukocyte alpha-interferon is not an active agent in the treatment of advanced, refractory breast cancer when used at a maximum tolerated dose; all of the nineteen patients studied required dose reductions, most often for reasons of fatigue (Sherwin et al., 1983). A preliminary study of interferon-alpha use in breast cancer by Borden and colleagues (1982) was inconclusive as to efficacy.

High-dose interferon-alpha-2 was found to be ineffective in the treatment of metastatic colorectal cancer and also associated with substantial fatigue (Figlin, Callaghan, and Sarna, 1983; Furue, 1985, 1986; Silgals et al., 1984). From a small study of seventeen patients, Basser and colleagues (1991) concluded that although interferon-alpha-2b has activity against carcinoid tumors, its benefits are short-lived and toxicity, including fatigue, limits its use with increasing dose. Concomitant alpha-interferon and chemotherapy also appears ineffective in advanced squamous cell carcinoma of the head and neck (Benasso et al., 1993). Fatigue was also the most common toxicity associated with human lymphoblastoid interferon treatment of patients with advanced epithelial ovarian malignancies (Abdulhay et al., 1985). Addition of lymphoblastoid interferon-alpha-N1 to the combination of doxorubicin, cyclophosphamide, and cisplatin in the treatment of advanced epithelial ovarian malignancies resulted in severe fatigue and malaise, which was considered unacceptable (Di Saia and Gillette, 1991).

Chronic fatigue in twenty out of twenty-two patients was evident in a phase II trial of intracerebrospinal fluid interferon-alpha. The latter intervention proved to be of modest activity for the treatment of neoplastic meningitis, a metastatic complication of both primary central nervous system and systemic cancer that occurs in 1 to 5 percent of patients with known cancer (Chamberlain, 2002). The toxicity calls the treatment into question. The results of a study by Ardizzoni and colleagues (1994) indicate only marginal activity of interferon-alpha in the treatment of diffuse malignant pleural mesothelioma, with four out of thirteen patients assessed experiencing fatigue as a toxicity. Benedetti Panici and colleagues (1989) reported that systemic interferon-alpha had comparable efficacy to diathermoregulation in the treatment of primary multiple and widespread anogenital condyloma; fatigue was the most common chronic side effect.

A pilot study conducted by Dillman and colleagues (1995) concluded that although interferon-alpha-2a and external beam radiotherapy can be safely coadministered with tolerable fatigue toxicity in patients with gliomas, a randomized trial would be needed to establish clinical benefit. However, the need to add interferon is questioned by results of a phase III trial (Kiebert et al., 1998) that showed safety and efficacy of radiotherapy alone for treatment of patients with gliomas. Nemoto and colleagues (1997) also showed benefit of radiotherapy in the treatment of low-grade astrocytoma. The combination of interleukin-2 and interferon-alpha has been tested with limited success for the same indication (Merchant et al., 1992).

Combinations of interferon-alpha with other medications have proven useful in the treatment of certain neoplasias. For instance, only two patients developed mild fatigue in a phase I trial of interferon-alpha-2b and liposome-encapsulated all-*trans*-retinoic acid in the treatment of twelve patients with advanced renal cell carcinoma (Goldberg, Vargas, et al., 2002). *Trans*-retinoic acid is purported to augment the antitumor effects of interferon-alpha-2b. Moreover, although fatigue remains as a limiting toxicity, evidence exists that the toxicity of alpha-interferon can be ameliorated by coadministration of dexamethasone without compromise of therapeutic efficacy (Amato et al., 1995). Although the treatment was discontinued after six weeks because of increasing fatigue and anorexia, Ankerst and colleagues (1984) reported a six-month-long complete remission in a patient with acute myelogenous leukemia treated with leukocyte alpha-interferon and cimetidine. Steiner, Wolf, and Pehamberger (1987) arrived at a similar conclusion in a study on malignant melanoma. However, Creagan and colleagues (1986) found no benefit of adding cimetidine to interferon-alpha in the treatment of disseminated malignant melanoma. Similarly, histamine did not appear to add efficacy with respect to response in a low-dose schedule of interleukin-2 and interferon-alpha (Donskov et al., 2002).

Oberg (1996) combined interferon-alpha and octreotide treatment in twenty-four patients with malignant carcinoid tumors who did not respond biochemically to high-dose octreotide alone. Although biochemical re-

sponse occurred in 77 percent, no significant antitumor effect was noted besides disease stabilization in four cases. The combination therapy had an effect on clinical symptoms rather than tumor mass. However, interferon was
better tolerated when in the combination.

Kantarjian and colleagues (1999) evaluated the efficacy of the combination of interferon-alpha and daily low-dose cytarabine in the treatment of
patients with early chronic-phase chronic myelogenous leukemia (within
one year of diagnosis). The authors concluded that the combination seems
to be promising for this indication based on the observation of high rates of
remissions and cytogenetic response. Combination therapy with dacarbazine and interferon-alpha-2a has some therapeutic activity in the management of advanced malignant melanoma (Bajetta et al., 1990). Human
fibroblast interferon is effective and also associated with fatigue in cervical
and vulvar intraepithelial neoplasia associated with papillomaviral cytopathic effects (De Palo et al., 1984, 1985). Mild to moderate fatigue was
also evident in approximately one-third of patients with advanced squamous cell cancer of the skin undergoing treatment with alpha-interferon,
retinoic acid, and cisplatin (Shin, Glisson, Khuri, Clifford, et al., 2002). Although a phase I trial of interferon-alpha and pentostatin, an inhibitor of
adenosine deaminase, showed potential benefit in hematological malignancies, further studies are necessary (Bernard et al., 1991).

Fatigue was the most common toxicity associated with interferon-alpha,
leucovorin, and 5-fluorouracil treatment, which was partially effective in
some cases of advanced non-small-cell lung cancer and colon cancer (Quan,
Madajewicz, et al., 1994). In this case, higher doses of interferon-alpha also
resulted in higher prevalence and intensity of fatigue. Interferon-alpha-2a
and fluorouracil is also an active regimen that leads to fatigue in the treatment of patients with advanced esophageal cancer (Kelsen et al., 1992).
Eighty percent of forty-three patients receiving human leukocyte alpha-
interferon in a clinical trial for the treatment of renal cell carcinoma experienced fatigue, which was the most common side effect along with fever
(De Kernion et al., 1983). Fatigue was among the most common side effects
upon administration of combined interferon-alpha-2a and vinblastine treatment in patients with either advanced melanoma or renal cell cancer
(Kellokumpu-Lehtinen and Nordman, 1988, 1990; Kellokumpu-Lehtinen,
Nordman, and Toivanen, 1989).

Mattson and colleagues (1985) reported that although human leukocyte
interferon has a growth-delaying effect on small-cell lung cancer and potentiates the effects of radiation, fatigue, memory and psychomotor dysfunction, and anorexia are dose limiting with interferon therapy regardless of
dose or duration. Fatigue was also a toxicity in 31 percent of advanced non-
small-cell lung cancer patients treated with a combination chemotherapy

(cyclophosphamide, epidoxorubicin, and cisplatin) and interferon-alpha-2b (Ardizzoni et al., 1991). Fatigue was a toxicity during simultaneous homoharringtonine and interferon-alpha in the treatment of forty-seven patients with chronic-phase chronic myelogenous leukemia (O'Brien et al., 2002).

As detailed previously, fatigue occurs in more than 70 percent of patients treated with interferon-alpha, and interferon-alpha-associated fatigue is often the dominant dose-limiting side effect, worsening with continued therapy and accompanied by significant depression. Several hypotheses have been put forth to explain interferon-alpha-induced fatigue.

At high doses, interferons are neurotoxic, and the abnormalities seen by electroencephalography resemble those in diffuse encephalitis. Interferon-related neurotoxicity includes somnolence and confusion, fatigue, lethargy, psychiatric symptoms, conceptual disorganization, neurological deficits, cortical blindness, coma, and, rarely, death. The neurological syndromes seem to be more common in elderly patients, following intramuscular or intravenous administration, at higher doses of frequent injections of interferon-alpha and in primary renal cell carcinoma. The duration of the treatment is not strongly related to neurotoxicity. Computed tomography findings are nonspecific and include atrophy or periventricular lucencies. Electroencephalograph studies demonstrate a generalized increase in slow-wave activity that returns to normal after cessation of treatment (Merimsky and Chaitchik, 1992).

Adams, Quesada, and Gutterman (1984) suggested that the intense fatigue experienced by metastatic renal cell carcinoma patients on interferon-alpha therapy may be a manifestation of a complex neurotoxicity, most suggestive of frontal lobe changes, and resulting in neurasthenia syndrome with reversible impairment of some higher mental functions. Caraceni and colleagues (1998) reported that neurological dysfunction associated with low-dose adjuvant interferon-alpha therapy in patients with malignant melanoma metastatic to regional lymph nodes after radical surgery was mild and consisted mainly of action tremor. Psychiatric symptoms and neuropsychological impairment were not found. Levels of fatigue and anxiety were increased in the interferon-alpha group but without a sizable impact on quality-of-life measures.

Capuron and colleagues (2002) conducted a study of forty patients with malignant melanoma eligible for interferon-alpha treatment who were randomly assigned to receive either paroxetine or placebo in a double-blind design. The authors documented that neurovegetative and somatic symptoms including anorexia, fatigue, and pain appeared within two weeks of interferon-alpha therapy in a large proportion of patients. In contrast, symptoms of depressed mood, anxiety, and cognitive dysfunction appeared later during interferon-alpha treatment and more specifically in patients meeting diagnostic criteria for major depression. Symptoms of depression, anxiety, cognitive dysfunction, and pain were more responsive, whereas symptoms of fatigue and anorexia were less responsive to paroxetine treatment. These data demonstrate distinct phenomenology and treatment responsiveness of symptom dimensions induced by interferon-alpha and suggest that different mechanisms mediate the various behavioral manifestations of cytokine-induced "sickness behavior" (Capuron et al., 2002).

The induction of proinflammatory cytokines observed in patients treated with interferon-alpha is also consistent with a possible mechanism of neuromuscular pathology that could manifest as fatigue. In this respect, neuromuscular fatigue in interferon-alpha-induced fatigue is similar to that observed in patients with post-polio fatigue syndrome. Post-polio fatigue syndrome, which affects more than 1.8 million North American polio survivors, is characterized by clinically significant fatigue, weakness, and pain, decades after paralytic poliomyelitis. The syndrome also includes other overlapping features with chronic fatigue syndrome and fibromyalgia such as deficits on neuropsychological tests of attention, histopathologic and neuroradiologic evidence of brain lesions, impaired activation of the hypothalamic-pituitary-adrenal axis, increased prolactin secretion, and EEG slow-wave activity (Bruno, 1998; Bruno, Creange, and Frick, 1998; Bruno et al., 1996, 1998; Nollet et al., 1996; Schanke, 1997; Thorsteinsson, 1997; Trojan and Cashman, 1995).

Interferon-alpha-induced fatigue may also be associated with the development of immune-mediated endocrine diseases, in particular hypothyroidism and hypothalamic-pituitary-adrenal axis-related hormonal deficiencies (Dalakas, Mock, and Hawkins, 1998; Jones, Wadler, and Hupart, 1998). Thyroid dysfunction, associated with the development of auto-antibodies, is seen in 8 to 20 percent of patients receiving interferon-alpha (Malik, Makower, and Wadler, 2001).

Clinical management of interferon-mediated fatigue is challenging because the syndrome is variable in onset and severity and the pathophysiology is poorly understood. Current management typically centers on dose reduction, but ancillary nonpharmacologic measures may help improve symptoms. Other strategies include antidepressant or anxiolytic therapy and treatment of coexisting hypothyroidism (Malik, Makower, and Wadler, 2001).

Interferon-Beta

Interferon-beta in a dose-intensive regimen has antineoplastic activity in patients with low- and high-grade astrocytomas and brainstem gliomas

(Allen et al., 1991; Bogdahn et al., 1985). Fatigue is a prominent toxicity of interferon-beta (Bukowski et al., 1991; Hawkins et al., 1984; Mani, Todd, and Poo, 1996; Quesada, Gutterman, and Hersh, 1982; Wisloff and Gulbrandsen, 2000) and further studies are needed for the indication mentioned here or others. In this respect, interferon-beta proved ineffective in the treatment of metastatic breast cancer (Barreras et al., 1988), advanced sarcomas (Borden et al., 1992), and gynecological tumors (Kanazawa et al., 1984).

Preclinical data have demonstrated synergy between interleukin-2 and beta-interferon in stimulating natural killer cell activity and in increasing expression of interleukin-2 receptors (Krigel et al., 1988, 1990). Phase I trials also showed that in some the latter combination is tolerable and has some biological activity in the treatment of renal cell carcinoma (Krigel et al., 1988, 1990).

Interferon-beta-serine is a muteine, recombinant interferon that is tolerated at a dose fivefold to tenfold higher than interferon-alpha and interacts with the same cell membrane receptor as interferon-alpha. A study by Kinney and colleagues (1990) demonstrated that interferon-beta-serine given in high doses exhibits significant antitumor activity in renal cell carcinoma; however, the objective response rate is 20 percent, and interferon-beta-serine is therefore not associated with a greater response than interferon-alpha. Sarna, Figlin, and Pertcheck (1987) showed limited activity of interferon-beta-serine in the treatment of advanced malignant melanoma.

Interferon-Gamma

Interferon-gamma also has antitumor activity (Bonnem and Oldham, 1987; Silver et al., 1990). Heavy fatigue with somnolence or lethargy, which was reversible upon drug cessation, was among the main toxicities associated with administration of human recombinant interferon-gamma in patients with various advanced cancers (Adachi et al., 1985; Digel et al., 1991; Foon, Sherwin, et al., 1985; Kawai et al., 1990; Kobayashi and Urabe, 1988; Kurzrock et al., 1985; Machida et al., 1987; Mahmoud et al., 1992; Mahrle and Schulze, 1990; Mani and Poo, 1996; Marth et al., 1989; Ogawa et al., 1987; Sherwin et al., 1984; Sriskandan et al., 1986; Vadhan-Raj et al., 1986; Van der Burg et al., 1985). There is only minimal activity of recombinant interferon-gamma as a single agent in neoplasms of B-cell origin (Quesada et al., 1988). Although interferon-gamma alone is effective in Philadelphia chromosome-positive chronic myelogenous leukemia (Silver et al., 1990), side effects can substantially limit the dosage and duration of treatment (Russo et al., 1989). Quesada and colleagues (1987) reported that interferon-gamma also has minimal activity against renal cell cancer.

Phase II clinical trials of vinblastine and interferon-gamma combination with and without 13-*cis* retinoic acid for twenty-nine and forty patients with advanced renal cell carcinoma in each trial, respectively, showed no benefit of addition of vinblastine and no increased fatigue (Bacoyiannis et al., 2002). Interferon-gamma did not prove effective in the treatment of malignant melanoma even though the side effects were manageable (Creagan et al., 1987; Ernstoff et al., 1987). Combinations of interferon-alpha and interferon-gamma demonstrate synergistic antiviral and antiproliferative activity in vitro (Kurzrock et al., 1986). However, although subjective improvement was demonstrated in six out of twelve patients studied, combined alpha- and gamma-interferon therapy lacked antitumoral effects for malignant midgut carcinoid tumors (Janson, Kauppinen, and Oberg, 1993). Limited efficacy was also seen for the latter combination in the treatment of renal cell carcinoma (Kawai et al., 1990; Naito et al., 1995). A combination of interferon-gamma and interleukin-2 did not prove to be effective for the treatment of advanced cancer (Reddy et al., 1997). Combination of interferon-beta and -gamma is not effective for the treatment of malignant melanoma (Schiller et al., 1988; Smith et al., 1991) or other cancers (Schiller et al., 1987) because the doses that are necessary to achieve therapeutic activity are highly toxic (Schiller et al., 1990).

Interleukin-2

Interleukin-2 was the first cytokine to be discovered and characterized, and it remains the most therapeutically useful of the interleukins studied (see Chapter 3 for more details on cytokines). The physiology of interleukin-2 has been well studied. Upon binding of an antigen to receptors on an individual T cell, the antigen stimulates the T cell to secrete interleukin-2 and to make interleukin-2 receptors. The interleukin-2 receptor acts as an on-off switch, and activated T cells undergo complex changes in morphology, metabolism, expression of surface receptors, and production of cytokines. The activated T cell starts to synthesize DNA and divides, producing two T cells that can now be activated by antigen. In addition to its role as an inducer of T-cell proliferation, interleukin-2 stimulates the proliferation and differentiation of B cells, helping them to secrete antibodies. Killer T cells, which appear to be in a constant state of activation, also respond to interleukin-2 (Meropol et al., 1998). The maturation and differentiation of lymphocytes in the thymus and bone marrow may also be influenced by interleukin-2 (Gelfand, 1990; Hamilton, 1993; Smith, 1990a,b).

Recombinant interleukin-2 use in metastatic renal cell carcinoma or malignant melanoma is associated with fatigue as a toxicity (Figlin et al., 1992;

Mier et al., 1988; Mittelman et al., 1991; Von der Maase et al., 1991). High-dose intravenous interleukin-2, with or without lymphokine-activated killer cells or interferon-alpha, has been reported to have activity in certain solid tumors. However, toxicity, including fatigue, has usually required hospitalization for its administration (Allison, Jones, and McGuffey, 1989; Creekmore et al., 1989; Hersh et al., 1989; Mier et al., 1988; Oldham et al., 1992; Sarna et al., 1989; Sawaki, 1990; Sharp, 1993; Sondel et al., 1988; Sznol et al., 1990; Taylor, Chase, et al., 1992; Tursz et al., 1991; Urba et al., 1993; Whitehead, Wolf, et al., 1995). Treatment with concomitant interleukin-2 and interferon-alpha-2a as outpatient therapy for patients with advanced malignancy also results in fatigue as treatment-limiting toxicity (Kroger et al., 1999; Kruit et al., 1991; Lipton et al., 1993; Nagler et al., 1994; Ratain et al., 1993; Ravaud et al., 1994; Schantz et al., 1992; Weiner et al., 1991). Patients with colon cancer metastatic to the liver tolerated the latter combined treatment less than patients with other tumors. Okuno and colleagues (1992) also showed feasibility of intrasplenic arterial infusion of interleukin-2 to patients with advanced cancer.

Combined interleukin-2 and interferon-alpha treatment is ineffective for advanced non-small-cell lung cancer (Jansen et al., 1992). Several studies suggest that combined interleukin-2 and interferon-alpha treatment had significant activity against advanced renal cell cancer with less toxicity (Bergmann et al., 1993; Eton et al., 1996; Hirsh et al., 1990). However, other studies conclude or suggest that the combination is more toxic and ineffective (Clark et al., 1999; Jayson et al., 1998). Prolonged low-dose subcutaneous interleukin-2 administration may also be of use in treatment of advanced malignancies (Angevin et al., 1995; Farag et al., 2002; Gause et al., 1996; Huberman et al., 1991; Ikemoto et al., 1990; Kashani-Sabet et al., 1999; Whitehead et al., 1990; Vlasveld et al., 1992). Combination of subcutaneous interleukin-2 and interferon-alpha is effective in the treatment of metastatic renal cell carcinoma and melanoma and has less toxicity, including fatigue, than the intravenous intervention (Atzpodien et al., 1993; Dutcher et al., 1997; Karp, 1998; Vogelzang, Lipton, and Figlin, 1993; Vuoristo et al., 1994; Whitehead et al., 1993).

Since metastatic renal cell carcinoma has poor prognosis, and treatment strategies, including hormone therapy, chemotherapy, and immunotherapy, have little impact on the quality of life and global survival statistics, new interest has recently focused on the combination of immunochemotherapy using pyrimidine analogs, such as gemcitabine. A phase II trial of weekly intravenous gemcitabine administration with standard doses of interferon and low doses of interleukin-2 immunotherapy for metastatic renal cell cancer showed that, despite the small sample size of fifteen patients, this biotherapeutic combination is effective and well tolerated (Neri et al.,

2002). However, a phase II trial of intravenous gemcitabine and 5-fluor-ouracil with subcutaneous interleukin-2 and interferon-alpha in forty-one patients with metastatic renal cell carcinoma demonstrated that addition of gemcitabine and 5-fluorouracil did not improve the rate of response seen with interleukin-based therapy only (Ryan, Vogelzang, and Stadler, 2002). Toxicity was moderate to severe, with fatigue, fever, anorexia, or nausea experienced by 75 to 90 percent of patients.

Tumor Necrosis Factor

Administration of tumor necrosis factor (TNF) to AIDS patients with Kaposi's sarcoma, although ineffective as an antitumor or antiviral agent, results in fatigue (Aboulafia et al., 1989). A small study by Bartsch and colleagues (1989) suggested that a high concentration of recombinant TNF-alpha at the tumor site has the potential to induce local tumor regressions. Instillation of recombinant tumor necrosis factor appears to be an effective method that can be used for pleurodesis with relatively few side effects (Rauthe and Sistermanns, 1997, 1998). However, both local and systemic administrations of TNF-alpha are associated with fatigue as a side effect (Bartsch et al., 1988; Chang et al., 1986; Chapman et al., 1987; Creagan et al., 1998; Del Mastro et al., 1995; Eskander et al., 1997; Feinberg et al., 1988; Schiller et al., 1991; Schwartz et al., 1989; Sherman et al., 1988; Skillings et al., 1992; Spriggs et al., 1988; Taguchi, 1986; Wiedenmann et al., 1989).

Combinations of TNF-alpha and interferon-gamma demonstrate synergistic antiproliferative activity in vitro, and fatigue is also an associated toxicity evident in clinical trials of this combination (Kurzrock et al., 1989). A phase II trial demonstrated that recombinant TNF-alpha is inactive as a single agent in patients with previously treated metastatic breast cancer (Budd et al., 1991). Recombinant tumor necrosis factor did not demonstrate antitumor efficacy against adenocarcinomas of the stomach and the pancreas (Muggia et al., 1992). Tumor necrosis factor is also ineffective in patients with advanced cancer (Jakubowski et al., 1989).

Other Cytokines

Recombinant human granulocyte colony-stimulating factor alone or with other cytokines or chemotherapeutic agents also causes fatigue and asthenia (De Gast et al., 2000; Gozdasoglu et al., 1995; Hovgaard and Nissen, 1992; Milkovich et al., 2000; Osborne et al., 1994; Punt and Kingma, 1994; Rifkin, Hersh, and Salmon, 1988; Rini et al., 1998; Ryan et al., 2000; Simmons et al., 1999). However, granulocyte colony-stimulating factor is useful to speed recovery and minimize side effects from chemotherapeutic interventions. For instance, recombinant human granulocyte-macrophage colony-stimulating factor can be administered safely to patients with Hodgkin's disease and results in improved hematological recovery after chemotherapy. Full-dose subcutaneous administration proved to be at least as effective as continuous intravenous infusion and should be preferred (Hovgaard and Nissen, 1992).

In a review article, Kitamura (1993) points out that interleukin-1 has antitumor effects, especially on cutaneous lymphoma and brain tumors, and also functions as hematopoietic growth factor for very immature hematopoietic stem cells. The side effects of interleukin-1 are variable but tolerable and include fatigue, fever, and skin redness, among others. Fatigue was also a common toxicity in clinical evaluations of intravenous recombinant human interleukin-3, -4, -6, -11, or -12 in patients with advanced malignancies (Atkins et al., 1992, 1997; Bouffet, Philip, et al., 1997; Cornacoff et al., 1992; Gilleece et al., 1992; Gordon et al., 1996; Kudoh and Yamada, 1998; Kudoh et al., 1986; Lundin et al., 2001; Ohe et al., 1998; Rinehart et al., 1995, 1997; Robertson et al., 2002; Schuler et al., 1998; Sosman et al., 1997; Stadler, Rybak, and Vogelzang, 1995; Tate et al., 2001; Taylor et al., 2000; Tepler et al., 1994, 1996; Vadhan-Raj et al., 1994; Veldhuis et al., 1996; Vokes et al., 1998; Weber et al., 1993; Weisdorf et al., 1994; Whitehead, Friedman, et al., 1995; Whitehead et al., 1998; Yamamoto et al., 1999; Younes et al., 1996).

Radiation Therapy

Radiotherapy-induced fatigue is a common early and chronic side effect of irradiation, reported in up to 80 and 30 percent of patients during radiation therapy and at follow-up visits, respectively (Jereczek-Fossa, Marsiglia, and Orrecchia, 2001, 2002). Medical and nursing staff members frequently underestimate radiation-therapy-associated fatigue; only about 50 percent of patients discuss it with a physician; and in only one-fourth of cases is any intervention proposed to the patient. The patients rarely expect fatigue to be a side effect of treatment. The etiology of this common symptom, its correlates, and prevalence are poorly understood.

Fatigue is a significant problem for patients with breast or prostate cancer receiving radical radiotherapy, although its severity is relatively modest (Greenberg et al., 1992; Stone et al., 2001). Radiotherapy was associated with a decline in global quality of life, role, cognitive, and social functioning, and an increase in nausea/vomiting, pain, insomnia, diarrhea, and financial difficulty. Before radiotherapy, 39 percent of the variation in fatigue scores among patients could be explained by a combination of measures of their global quality of life and physical functioning. A combination of fatigue and anxiety scores at baseline was able to predict 54 percent of the variation in fatigue scores at the completion of radiotherapy (Stone et al., 2001). Teh and colleagues (2001) reported that adding a gene-therapy approach to radiotherapy intervention for prostate cancer did not increase toxicity, including fatigue.

In a prospective, descriptive study by Christman, Oakley, and Cronin (2001), at least 40 percent of forty-nine women undergoing external beam radiation and low-dose rate brachytherapy for cervical or uterine cancer reported difficulty sleeping, fatigue, diarrhea, anorexia, nausea, urinary frequency, dysuria, vaginal discharge, and perineal irritation. Incidence and timing of symptoms varied by operative status and brachytherapy timing.

Fatigue is also associated with preoperative hyperfractionated radiation therapy for locally advanced rectal cancers (Allal et al., 1999, 2002). A study by Mannaerts and colleagues (2002) of fifty-five patients with locally advanced primary and sixty-six patients with locally recurrent rectal cancer treated with high-dose preoperative external beam irradiation, followed by extended surgery and intraoperative radiotherapy, revealed fatigue in 44 percent, perineal pain in 42 percent, radiating pain in the leg(s) in 21 percent, walking difficulties in 36 percent, and voiding dysfunction in 42 percent of the patients as symptoms of ongoing morbidity.

Fatigue syndrome was evident in 49.2 percent of women and 28.3 percent of men as an immediate toxicity secondary to fractionated total-body irradiation prior to bone marrow transplantation (Buchali et al., 2000). Bjordal, Kaasa, and Mastekaasa (1994) found that long-term survivors of head and neck cancer reported a high level of disease and radiotherapy treatment-related symptoms. However, in certain circumstances radiotherapy may help both survival and fatigue management. Palliative versus more intensive radiotherapy for patients with inoperable non-small-cell lung cancer and good performance status is useful to improve fatigue and quality of life (Langendijk, Aaronson, et al., 2000; Langendijk, ten Velde, et al., 2000; Macbeth et al., 1996).

Although a prospective, observational study of forty-five adults with primary cancer of the lung receiving outpatient primary or adjuvant radiation therapy did not identify an increase in fatigue during radiation therapy (Beach et al., 2001), Langendijk and colleagues (2001) reported a poor quality-of-life response rate for fatigue (28 percent) in a prospective study on radical radiotherapy in non-small-cell lung cancer. In another study, Langendijk and colleagues (2002) also documented a significant, gradual increase over time in fatigue, shortness of breath, and appetite loss, together with a significant deterioration of role functioning, after curative radiotherapy in forty-six patients with medically inoperable stage I non-small-cell lung cancer. Possible explanations for the observations are preexisting, slowly progressive chronic obstructive pulmonary disease and radiation-induced pulmonary changes. Morever, Hickok and colleagues (1996) reported that fatigue developed in thirty-nine of the fifty patients (78 percent) receiving radiation therapy for histologically diagnosed lung cancer and was not strongly related to demographic or disease variables. Forty patients experienced pain (80 percent), but depression was noted in the records of only six patients (12 percent). Onset of fatigue closely followed development of pain in only eleven patients. Lower frequency of fatigue in patients with previous surgery or chemotherapy and the likelihood of a response shift suggest these were not significant causes of fatigue. Concurrent capecitabine and radiation therapy in thirty-two patients with gastrointestinal malignancies was well tolerated, and only one patient developed fatigue (Vaishampayan et al., 2002).

Langendijk and colleagues (2002) reported that after curative radiotherapy for stage I medically inoperable non-small-cell lung cancer, there is a gradual increase in fatigue, shortness of breath, and appetite loss, together with a significant deterioration of role functioning, possibly because of pre-existing, slowly progressive chronic obstructive pulmonary disease and radiation-induced pulmonary changes. Fatigue is also associated with shortness of breath before treatment in this patient population (Langendijk, Aaronson, et al., 2000). Van de Pol and colleagues (1997) reported that prophylactic cranial irradiation in patients with small-cell lung cancer was also associated with fatigue.

In numerous studies the level and time course of radiation-therapy-associated fatigue was demonstrated to depend on the site of tumor and the treatment modalities. For example, psychological mechanisms have been proposed to explain fatigue in women receiving irradiation for early breast cancer, whereas decline in neuromuscular efficiency rather than psychological reasons can lead to the fatigue observed in patients undergoing radiotherapy for prostate cancer. Radiation-therapy-associated fatigue can affect global quality of life more than pain, sexual dysfunction, and other cancer- or treatment-related symptoms (Jereczek-Fossa, Marsigha, and Orecchia, 2001, 2002).

In a prospective study of fatigue in thirty-six patients with localized prostate cancer undergoing radiotherapy, Monga and colleagues (1999) observed that fatigue scores (Piper Fatigue Scale) were significantly higher at completion of radiotherapy as compared with preradiotherapy values. Moreover, patients scoring higher on the Piper Fatigue Scale were more likely to report a poorer quality of physical well-being on the Functional Assessment of Cancer Therapy–Prostate (FACT-P). In contrast, no significant changes were noted in mean scores of hematocrit, body weight, Beck Depression Inventory, and Epworth Sleepiness Scale during the study period. These results suggest that fatigue may not be the result of depression or sleep disturbance, and the authors proposed that the physical expression of fatigue may be secondary to a decline in neuromuscular efficiency and enhanced muscle fatigue (Monga et al., 1999).

A previous small study on thirteen patients by the same research group provided evidence of transient decline in neuromuscular efficiency (as assessed by sustained isometric contraction of the tibialis anterior for sixty seconds on a force dynamometer) in prostate cancer patients at the completion of radiotherapy. The effect seemed to be specific for neuromuscular performance alone and independent of the cardiovascular (as assessed by treadmill stress testing with a modified Bruce protocol) or psychological (as assessed by the Piper Fatigue Scale, Beck Depression Inventory, and Epworth Sleepiness Scale) fatigue status of the patients (Monga et al., 1997).

Lovely (1998) reported that the main problems among brain tumor patients include memory loss, fatigue, and loss of concentration. In a study of sixty individuals, Lovely, Miaskowski, and Dodd (1999) reported that patients with glioblastoma multiformae experience increases in fatigue after radiation therapy. Increases in fatigue are associated with decreases in almost all aspects of patients' quality of life. Merchant and colleagues (2002) assessed sustained attention, impulsivity, and reaction time during radiotherapy for thirty-nine pediatric patients with localized primary brain tumors. Continuous performance test scores exhibited an increasing trend for errors of omission (inattentiveness), decreasing trend for errors of commission (impulsivity), and slower reaction times. However, none of the changes were statistically significant. Older patients (age greater than twelve years) were more attentive, less impulsive, and had faster reaction times at baseline than the younger patients. The reaction time was significantly reduced during treatment for the older patients and lengthened significantly for the younger patients. Taphoorn and colleagues (1994) reported no adverse effect on quality of life in patients with glioma treated with radiotherapy.

Ahsberg and Furst (2001) reported that although fatigue in cancer patients increased significantly at the end of radiotherapy, as compared to pretreatment, it decreased after treatment. The highest fatigue ratings concerned lack of energy, lack of motivation, and sleepiness (Ahsberg and Furst, 2001). Geinitz and colleagues (2001) studied forty-one patients who received adjuvant radiotherapy after breast-conserving surgery. Fatigue intensity increased until treatment week four and remained elevated until week five. Two months after radiotherapy, the values had fallen to the pretreatment levels.

De Graeff and colleagues (De Graeff, de Leeuw, Ros, Hordijk, Batter-mann, et al., 1999) reported that after radiotherapy for laryngeal cancer, a temporary deterioration of physical functioning and symptoms occurs, mostly caused by side effects of treatment. Despite physical deterioration, an improvement of emotional functioning and mood occurs after treatment, probably as a result of psychological adaptation and coping processes (De Graeff, de Leeuw, Ros, Hordijk, Battermann, et al., 1999).

Smets and colleagues (Smets, Visser, Garssen, et al., 1998; Smets, Visser, Willems-Groot, Garssen, Oldenburger, et al., 1998; Smets, Visser, Willems-Groot, Garssen, Schuster-Uitterhoeve, and de Haes, 1998) reported that fatigue in disease-free postradiotherapy cancer patients did not differ significantly from fatigue in the general population. However, for 34 percent of the patients, fatigue following treatment was worse than antici-pated, 39 percent listed fatigue as one of the three symptoms causing them the most distress, 26 percent of patients worried about their fatigue, and pa-tients' overall quality of life was negatively related to fatigue. The degree of fatigue, functional disability, and pain before radiotherapy were the best predictors of fatigue at nine-month follow-up. Postradiotherapy, fatigue in disease-free patients was significantly associated with gender, physical dis-tress, pain rating, sleep quality, functional disability, psychological distress, and depression, but not with medical (diagnosis, prognosis, comorbidity) or treatment-related (target area, total radiation dose, fractionation) variables (Smets, Visser, Garssen, et al., 1998; Smets, Visser, Willems-Groot, Gars-sen, Oldenburger, et al., 1998; Smets, Visser, Willems-Groot, Garssen, Schuster-Uitterhoeve, and de Haes, 1998). The significant associations be-tween fatigue and both psychological and physical variables once again un-derscore the complex etiology of this symptom in patients and point out the necessity of a multidisciplinary approach for its treatment.

The time course of fatigue after radiation therapy in cancer patients is also described in a study of fifteen women with stage I or II node-negative breast cancer, but who were otherwise healthy. Greenberg and colleagues (1992) noted that fatigue did not increase linearly with cumulative radiation dose over time; it dropped from the first to second week and rose in the third week. The cumulative effects reached a plateau in the fourth week (after an average of seventeen fractions), which was maintained during the remain-ing weeks of treatment. Within three weeks after treatment, fatigue had di-minished. No patient had sustained depressive symptoms, and cardio-pulmonary exercise capacity in five patients at six and twelve weeks did not change from just before radiation. Other markers, including reverse triiodo-thyronine and pulse change with orthostatic stress, did not correlate with ei-ther subjective fatigue or cumulative radiation in fifteen patients. The curve of the fatigue manifestation during treatment conforms to the adaptation of the organism to a continuing stress.

The level and timing of fatigue may also be dependent on the type or extent of radiation treatment. Based on a small study, Beard and colleagues (1997) reported that in the fatigue, energy, and vigor subscales, patients who received whole-pelvis treatment fared significantly worse than those receiving small-field or conformal radiation. However, Fieler (1997) reported that patients receiving high-dose rate brachytherapy experienced similar side effects to patients receiving external beam radiation to the same site.

Surgery

Surgery for cancer is also associated with fatigue (Watt-Watson and Graydon, 1995). Krupp and colleagues (1975) stressed that surgeons should strive to reduce morbidity, mortality, and operating time as well as surgical fatigue. There is also variability in the intensity of fatigue experienced after different surgical interventions for the same problem in cancer patients (Dutta et al., 2002).

Brandberg and colleagues (2000) reported that up to 75 percent of patients with uveal melanoma reported fatigue after either enucleation or radiotherapy. Fatigue is also reported in laryngectomized patients (Coelho and Sawada, 1999; Major et al., 2001; Muller et al., 2001; Pourel et al., 2002), in long-term survivors after curative transhiatal esophagectomy for esophageal carcinoma (Brooks et al., 2002; De Boer et al., 2000; O'Hanlon et al., 1995; Zieren et al., 1996), in postadrenalectomy patients (Telenius-Berg et al., 1989), in postpneumonectomy patients (Fiedler et al., 1997; Fiedler, Neef, and Rosendahl, 1999), in patients posttranssphenoidal microsurgery (Flitsch, Spitzner, and Ludecke, 2000), postorchiectomy (Nygard, Norum, and Due, 2001), and in patients postsurgery for colorectal and gastric cancer (Forsberg, Bjorvell, and Cedermark, 1996; Galloway and Graydon, 1996; Koch, 2002; Pringle and Swan, 2001; Schwenk, Bohm, and Muller, 1998; Wu et al., 2000).

Bone marrow transplantation is also associated with subsequent fatigue (Bellm et al., 2000; Bush et al., 1995, 2000; Hjermstad, Evensen, et al., 1999; Hjermstad, Loge, et al., 1999; Kopp et al., 1998; Lawrence, Gilbert, and Peters, 1996; McQuellon et al., 1996, 1998; Molassiotis, 1999; Molassiotis and Morris, 1999; Whedon, Stearns, and Mills, 1995; Zittoun, Achard, and Ruszniewski, 1999). During autologous stem cell rescue for breast cancer, women experience fatigue that is worse than what is "normally" experienced. This fatigue interferes with daily functioning and quality of life and is related to both medical (i.e., time since transplant) and psychosocial factors (Hann et al., 1997, 1999; Jacobsen and Stein, 1999; Winer et al., 1999).

In a study of 227 women, physical and treatment-related problems were reported frequently one month after breast cancer surgery and occurred with equal frequency in women receiving modified radical mastectomy or breast-conservation treatment (Shimozuma et al., 1999). No significant differences in problems were reported at one year by type of surgery; however, frequently reported problems included "numbness in the chest wall or axilla," "tightness, pulling, or stretching in the arm or axilla," "less energy or fatigue," "difficulty in sleeping," and "hot flashes." No relationship was found between the type of surgery and mood or quality of life. Poorer quality of life one year after surgery was significantly associated with greater mood disturbance and body-image discomfort one month after surgery, as well as positive lymph node involvement. Although the majority of patients experienced substantial disruptions in the physical and psychosocial dimensions of quality of life postoperatively, most women recovered during the year after surgery, with only a minority (less than 10 percent) significantly worsening during that time (Shimozuma et al., 1999).

Hoskins (1997) collected data at six time points: seven to ten days, one month, two months, three months, six months, and one year postsurgery in a sample of ninety-three women with breast cancer. Fatigue and emotional distress were persistent issues. Psychological distress and perceived health status improved with no significant differences between breast-conservation treatment and mastectomy groups. Significant differences existed between patients receiving chemotherapy versus no therapy between three and six months. Significant changes also existed in perceived health status and psychological distress in both the positive- and negative-node groups, with no differences between groups. The authors concluded that adjustment, a multidimensional and complex process, occurs over time (Hoskins, 1997). Wyatt and Friedman (1998) also stressed the need to address fatigue and other related symptoms postmastectomy or -lumpectomy.

Jones and colleagues (1992) assessed the quality of life of forty-eight patients treated surgically for head and neck cancer. Five groups of patients were considered: laryngectomy, pharyngolaryngoesophagectomy, craniofacial procedure, "other operations," and patients with disease recurrence. Laryngectomy and "other operation" patients reported relatively few problems, whereas patients with disease recurrence described difficulties in all of the domains examined. Symptoms of fatigue were common (Jones et al., 1992). In a study of 141 patients with brain tumors with cortical lesions caused by microsurgical tumor resection, Irle and colleagues (1994) found that patients with lesions of the ventral frontal cortex or the temporoparietal cortex reported postoperatively significantly worse mood states (anxiety/

depression, irritability/anger, fatigue) than did patients in the other lesion and control groups.

Quality-of-life parameters, including fatigue, after rectal cancer surgery change with time, being generally worst in the early postoperative period (Camilleri-Brennan and Steele, 2001). De Graeff and colleagues (De Graeff, de Leeuw, Ros, Hordijk, Blijham, and Winnubst, 1999) reported that surgical treatment for oral or oropharyngeal cancer results in significant deterioration of physical functioning and symptoms during the first year, especially when combined with radiotherapy. Despite this, an improvement of emotional functioning is noted after treatment, probably as a result of adaptation and coping processes.

In contrast to the outcomes associated with the surgical procedures mentioned previously, a study of 192 patients surviving pancreaticoduodenectomy revealed that they had near-normal quality-of-life scores. Although many patients reported weight loss and symptoms consistent with pancreatic exocrine and endocrine insufficiency, most patients had quality-of-life scores comparable to those of control patients and could function independently in daily activities (Huang et al., 2000).

Schroeder and Hill (1993) prospectively determined postoperative fatigue, as defined by a 10-point scale (1 = fit, 10 = fatigued), in eighty-four patients undergoing major surgery. The best predictor of postoperative fatigue was preoperative fatigue, with lesser correlations with diagnosis (especially cancer); preoperative weight, particularly total body protein; and weight loss, grip strength, and age. Postoperative fatigue was not correlated with preoperative anxiety, depression, or hostility, involuntary muscle function, gender, preoperative stress, or changes in total body protein or fat over the two postoperative weeks. Schroeder and Hill (1993) concluded that patients who present for surgery already fatigued are the ones most likely to suffer from prolonged postoperative fatigue, particularly if they are elderly, suffer from cancer, or have few extra reserves of body protein.

Other Treatment Modalities

A phase I trial of fourteen patients with a variety of neoplasms not responsive to standard forms of therapy as well as other related studies revealed that fatigue is a toxicity of whole-body hyperthermia (Bull et al., 1979; Cole et al., 1979). Whole-body hyperthermia is a potential adjuvant to chemotherapy or other forms of cancer therapy. Koltyn and colleagues (1992) demonstrated a statistically significant increase in fatigue associated with decreased vigor that returned to baseline values by seventy-two hours following whole-body hyperthermia. In contrast, a significant improvement in depression was evident through seventy-two hours following treatment.

The following study illustrates the use of this cancer treatment modality. Ostrow and colleagues (1981) treated seven patients with advanced cancer with whole-body hyperthermia using a nylon and vinyl mesh, water-perfused suit. Treatments were given at 41.8°C for four hours. Five patients received concomitant cyclophosphamide with hyperthermia. Compared to baseline (37°C) conditions, there was a significant rise in pulse rate, a fall in diastolic pressure, and an increase in respiratory rate. Toxic effects included fatigue, extremity edema, diarrhea, nausea and vomiting, and respiratory depression in a patient with cerebral metastases. Compared to baseline values, there was a significant increase in serum glucose and decreases in serum calcium and phosphorus. Significant elevations in serum lactate dehydrogenase and aspartate aminotransferase values occurred twenty-four hours following hyperthermia, suggesting hepatic sensitivity to heat. The physiologic alterations observed and the toxic effects documented indicate that careful monitoring of patients is necessary (Ostrow et al., 1981).

Alternative and complementary treatments of cancer, cancer-related fatigue, and chronic fatiguing illnesses are covered in Chapter 4.

Chapter 3

Possible Causative, Predisposing, and Perpetuating Factors of Chronic Fatiguing Illnesses

Although a number of researchers have speculated about the nature of chronic fatigue and chronic fatiguing illnesses, little systematic research has been conducted on their cause or treatment. In many aspects, our knowledge of the fatigue mechanisms in, for instance, cancer patients is at a similar stage to that reached in our understanding of anticancer therapy-induced nausea and vomiting in the 1980s (Morrow, Andrews, et al., 2002). Many factors (summarized in the following list) have been associated with the mediation, predisposition, and/or perpetuation of fatigue, and they will be discussed by body organ system in the following sections.

I. Body defenses (immunological)
   A. The soldiers of the immune army: immune cell phenotypic distributions and function
      1. T and B lymphocytes
      2. Natural killer (NK) cells
      3. Neutrophils, monocytes, and eosinophils
   B. Cytokines
      1. Cytokines and cancer-related fatigue
      2. Cytokines and chronic fatigue syndrome
      3. The Th1-type (cell-mediated immunity)/Th2-type (humoral immunity) cytokine imbalance paradigm in cancer and fatigue
         a. Th2-type predominance in several cancers
         b. Th2-type predominance in fatiguing illnesses
   C. Autoantibodies
   D. Major histocompatibility genes
   E. Macrophage activation (Neopterin)
   F. Viral reactivation and microbial attack
      1. Viruses
      2. Bacteria
      3. Fungi

G. Reaction to foreign substances: silicone breast implants
H. Environmental toxins
II. Endocrine
   A. Hypothalamic-pituitary-adrenal (HPA) stress system
III. Neurological
   A. Autonomic dysfunction
      1. The vagal afferent hypothesis
   B. Sleep and circadian rhythm
   C. Cognition
   D. Brain injury
   E. Ion channelopathy
IV. Psychological and psychiatric
   A. Behavior
   B. Personality
   C. Psychosocial adaptation
   D. Mood
V. Hematological
   A. Anemia
VI. Musculoskeletal
   A. Skeletal muscle wasting
      1. Low cysteine-glutathione syndrome
   B. Muscle physiology in chronic fatigue syndrome
VII. Nutritional
   A. Carnitine deficiency
   B. Phosphate deficiency
   C. Magnesium deficiency
   D. Low serum albumin levels
   E. High cerebrospinal fluid homocysteine levels
   F. Vitamins C and B-12 and folate
   G. Amino acids
   H. The adenosine triphosphate (ATP) hypothesis

It should be pointed out that some of the factors discussed have more weight for particular forms of cancer, cancer treatments, or chronic fatiguing illnesses, and these situations will be indicated. Moreover, although the material is presented by organ system, it should be kept in mind that the body and the mind function as a whole. Any partitioning of the contributions of bodily functions to fatigue is artificial and done in part because that is how knowledge is acquired in the different specialties and in part because of the limitations in said knowledge.

As we learn more about how the human body works, we realize the many links that underlie apparently unrelated phenomena and the picture becomes simpler. One unifying concept is that disorders of the neuroendocrineimmunological circuitry such as fatigue, related to the noxious stimulation of a cancerous or other processes, can lead to, or result from, neurological, endocrinological, immunological, psychiatric, nutritional, or multiorgan pathology. This link has encouraged a search for markers with functional or pathological correlates for fatigue. Although cancer or particular pathologies may underlie fatigue, they are never alone as a stimulus and many other intrinsic and extrinsic factors have a contribution.

The immune, nervous, and endocrine axes communicate with one another through a network of shared or system-unique molecules that collectively produce a coordinated response to internal and external challenges. Part of this adaptive phenomenon, which is necessary for the survival of the organism, is thought to involve the release of proteins called cytokines, which inform the brain about immune activation, from activated cells. The brain then organizes a series of neuroendocrine responses that participate in the regulation of the host response. The trigger for the adaptive response may also be neuroendocrine, which in turn leads to the local production of cytokines within the nervous system which then activates the rest of the response. Cytokines produce activation of the hypothalamic-pituitary-adrenal axis in response to various threats to homeostasis, the regulated balance of the bodily functions (Turnbull and Rivier, 1995a,b).

The extensive interactions between different cytokines, hormones, and neurotransmitters, the broad spectrum of pathophysiologies associated with increased production of these mediators, and the number of tissues/cells capable of either synthesizing or responding to these mediators suggest that multiple mechanisms mediate their influence. This interconnectivity between different bodily systems is critical to the understanding of fatigue and chronic fatiguing illnesses and renders insufficient the distinction of a particular origin for their manifestation as simply neurological, immunological, endocrinological, or nutritional. Environmental, sociodemographic, cultural, and emotional influences also need to be considered. The following sections address the different parts of the puzzle and whenever possible try to integrate them into a more coherent scene that is useful for intervention.

One useful integrative paradigm is provided by psychoneuroimmunology, the disciplinary scientific field concerned with interactions among behavior, the immune system, and the nervous system. Its clinical aspects are based on an understanding of the biological mechanisms underlying the influence of psychosocial factors on onset and course of immunologically induced psychiatric symptoms. Its bioregulatory aspects include understanding the complex interaction of neuroendocrine and immunologically generated networks in maintaining health and combating disease (Solomon, 1995).

Through the ages and across cultures, physicians have linked psychic and bodily well-being (Solomon, 1995). In 1680, the Transylvanian physician Papai Pariz Ferenc essentially reiterated Aristotle and anticipated psychoneuroimmunology when he said, "When the parts of the body and its humors are not in harmony, then the mind is unbalanced and melancholy ensues, but on the other hand, a quiet and happy mind makes the whole body healthy" (Solomon, 1995, pp. 1ff). In 1990, the Dalai Lama said that practices that promote enlightenment have "mundane benefits, such as good health." In 1992, the New Zealand immunologist Roger Booth in collaboration with Kevin Ashbridge of Switzerland stated:

> There is a need to reassess and perhaps redefine the concepts, symbols and languages of immunology and psychology in ways which allow the relationships between immunological and psychological processes to be expressed in terms of a coherent teleological perspective. . . . To make sense of psychoimmune relationships we must be open to modifying some of our preconceptions about the nature of our immune system and of our psyche. (Solomon, 1995, pp. 1ff)

We need be reminded, as the great humanistic psychologist Abraham Maslow explained in 1972, that science is a human creation. "Its laws, organization, and articulations rest not only on the nature of the reality that it discovers, but also on the nature of the human nature that does the discovering" (Solomon, 1995, pp. 1ff). Modern clinical medicine and its related basic sciences have evolved through a number of developmental phases, one of which, psychosomatic medicine, moved toward an integrative or holistic approach to at least some diseases. Solomon (1995) expressed that psychoneuroimmunology is a field of conceptual breakthrough which offers the opportunity, at last, to approach the body and its health and disorders from a new theoretical systems perspective.

As the philosophers David Letvin and George Freeman Solomon pointed out in 1990 (Solomon, 1995), the body itself is more than an evolutionary biological entity; it is a result of processes that communicatively interact with its biological nature, develop, and transform it. Human bodies are sociable from their beginning and biologically organized for communication processes, both via the senses and the immune system. Thus it is hard to draw a line between the body of nature and the body of experience. The history of medicine has presented many different, often conflicting, representations of the human body. The advancement of medicine depends now more than ever on breaking free of schemata that are incomplete and no longer work. The ancients placed what went on within the body in communication with natural and supernatural forces outside the body. However, medicine in the Middle Ages and the Renaissance went from abstraction to concreteness and interiority with the beginnings of dissection by Da Vinci and Vesalius. The body as a machine (for example, the central nervous system as analogous to a telephone switchboard in the late nineteenth century or to a computer in the mid-twentieth) led to linear concepts of causality of disease, the malfunctioning of the machine. Early-modern medicine was concerned with structures and how they worked. Late-modern medicine, with more complexity, has been concerned with functions and processes, finally to a commitment to understanding of systems.

Understanding of the endocrine system set the stage for a blurring of the distinction between the inner (homeostasis) and the outer (adaptation). Now we can come to the point of systemic integration, as exemplified by psychoneuroimmunology with its nervous, neuroendocrine, and immune components. The shift from the structural to the functional was useful but still mechanistic. Although the complexity of systems and processes has been recognized, Solomon (1995) urges that we need now to develop new, nonlinear, nonmechanistic understandings based on systems, chaos, and informational theories. Extremely linear mathematics points out that small perturbations can change sine waves to bimodal or trimodal waves and then chaotic fluctuations—and back. Some systems are so complex and so interrelated that the conditions of the whole are not predictable on the basis of their elements. The body is more than anatomy, physiology, biochemistry, or even psychosomatics and molecular biology. Disease may be more complex than even a multifactorial biopsychosocial model can adequately describe.

Psychoneuroimmunology increasingly is dissolving dualisms of mind-body, body-environment, and individual-population (Solomon, 1995). In realizing that states of the medical body are correlated with the individual's bodily experienced meanings, Levin and Solomon expressed the hope that patients themselves will begin to understand their bodies in new ways (Solomon, 1995). Each patient may begin to realize the extent to which the body that he or she presents to medicine for diagnosis and treatment is a body of meaningful experience, of significant intelligence, informed about itself and its environment, and influenced by internal sensitivity and embodied awareness. The degree to which the patient is skilled at sensing the body's diseases and its health are also conditions of meaning as integrated through interpretations of life experienced by the mind-brain-immune system (Solomon, 1995).

BODY DEFENSE FACTORS
(IMMUNOLOGICAL FACTORS)

The cells of the immune system circulate in the blood (white blood cells) or populate many tissues and mucous surfaces, and they predominate in certain organs (such as the spleen and bone marrow). Immune cells act as an army in charge of defending the body by attacking foreign invaders and cancer cells and disposing of the remains of dead cells (see Figure 3.1 for illustration). The immune system communicates across both short and long distances. It is the ability of the immune system to successfully communicate among its many parts that enables it to function properly, protecting us from potentially harmful organisms and molecules. Our health and well-being, therefore, depend on the communication from immune system cell to immune system cell, as well as from the immune system to other organ systems.

The Soldiers of the Immune Army: Immune Cell Phenotypic Distributions and Function

Macrophages (from the Greek word for "big eaters"; also called monocytes when they circulate in the blood) are immune cells that survey the

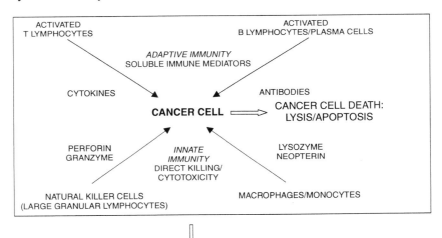

FIGURE 3.1. Immune cells and mediators associated with attack on cancer cells and fatigue

body for the presence of microbes or dead cells. Macrophages/monocytes engulf dead cells, digest them, and present the resulting pieces to the T cells (or T lymphocytes). The T cells (the "T" comes from the observation that they were originally found to predominate in the thymus), which can be considered the generals of the immune system army, then decide if the digested particle pieces are foreign to the body or abnormal.

If T cells are presented with a foreign or abnormal particle, they become activated. Activated T cells start to divide and secrete cytokines to stimulate other T cells, macrophages/monocytes, natural killer cells, or B cells. Natural killer cells are immune cells that are able to kill microbial infected or cancer cells by themselves, with or without orders from the generals. B cells (the "B" comes from the observation that they are the predominant cells in the bursa of birds; in humans their source is the bone marrow), upon activation, differentiate into plasma cells which act similar to cannons that fire the bullets known as immunoglobulins.

Analysis of the complex interactions underlying immune responses was greatly facilitated by the development of monoclonal antibodies to various surface proteins on lymphoid cells, which defined functionally distinct subsets (Cantor and Boyse, 1977; Reinherz and Schlossman, 1981; Romain and Schlossman, 1984). Such analysis has also demonstrated that each type of lymphoid cell is genetically programmed to carry out defined immunological functions that are predictable on the basis of surface phenotype (Romain and Schlossman, 1984).

Surface-marker phenotyping of peripheral blood lymphoid cells has also allowed insight into the cellular basis of immune dysfunction associated with pathologies of many organ systems with diverse causes, including viral, autoimmune, and genetic, among others (see for example Calabrese, Kling, and Gold, 1987; Fletcher et al., 1989; Griffin, 1991; Klimas et al., 1992; McAllister et al., 1989; Raziuddin and Elawad, 1990; Villemain et al., 1989). Several reports also documented alterations in the distribution of various lymphoid cell subsets among CFS patients. Certain discrepancies in the findings from different study groups can be attributed to group nonequivalences on diverse parameters such as demographic variables (gender, age, socioeconomic status), medical status variables predating onset of disease, medication use, concomitant substance abuse, nutritional status, and the effects of time of sample collection (diurnal or seasonal variations) (Fletcher et al., 1989; Herberman, 1991; Lahita, 1982; Malone et al., 1990; Martin, Muler, and Dionel, 1988; Patarca, Sandler, et al., 1995; Roberts et al., 1998; Schulte, 1991; Whiteside, 1994). Methodological flaws are also to blame because some studies used frozen cells in their assessments, and cryopreservation is known to affect the expression of many surface markers and cytokines.

T and B Lymphocytes

The immune army activation process is mediated by the group of T-cell generals known as T-helper cells, which derive their name from the fact that they "help" or "boost" the immune attack. Another group of T-cell generals, known as the T-suppressor cells, is in charge of halting the immune response and returning the army to its resting state. As in the army, where one can identify the rank and function of soldiers or officers by their uniform and insignia, the cells of the immune system carry particular surface markers that are associated with particular functions and have been given cluster designation or cluster differentiation (CD) numbers. All T cells carry the CD3 surface marker, also known as the T-cell receptor, the portal of presentation of particles to T cells by macrophages/monocytes and B cells, the so-called antigen-resenting cells. T-helper cells carry on their surface a molecule known as CD4, and T-suppressor cells carry CD8.

CD4+ T cells (helper/inducer cells) are the principal source of "help" for antibody production by B cells in response to T-cell-dependent antigenic stimulation, as well as inducers of cytotoxic and suppressor T-cell function (CD8+ cells; Reinherz and Schlossman, 1981). Discrepant results have been reported in reference to CD4+ and CD8+ T-cell counts in CFS patients. Straus and colleagues (1985) reported a statistically higher percentage of CD4+ lymphocytes with normal numbers of CD8+ cells and CD4/CD8 ratio; several groups found normal percentages of CD4+ and CD8+ cells as well as a normal CD4/CD8 ratio (Borysiewicz et al., 1986; Gupta and Vayuvegula, 1991; Jones, 1991; Jones and Straus, 1987; Jones et al., 1985; Landay et al., 1991; Lloyd et al., 1992; Tirelli et al., 1994); Lloyd and colleagues (1989) found decreased numbers of both CD4+ and CD8+ T cells; Buchwald and Komaroff (1991) found reduced numbers of CD8+ cells and higher-than-normal CD4/CD8 ratios; and Klimas and colleagues (1990) found that most CFS subjects studied had a normal number of CD4+ cells and an elevated number of CD8+ cells, which resulted in a decrease in the CD4/CD8 ratio. Decreased CD4/CD8 ratios in 20 to 100 percent of patients have been demonstrated by other investigators (Aoki, Usuda, and Miyakoshi, 1987; DuBois, 1986; Jones, 1991; Jones and Straus, 1987; Jones et al., 1985; Linde et al., 1992).

The conflicting results summarized here may be associated with the fluctuation in clinical manifestations of these patients or with other factors mentioned previously. In fact, several researchers have detected fluctuations in several immunological parameters and in the severity of symptoms in longitudinal follow-up investigations of CFS patients. Moreover, Mawle and colleagues (1997) found that although only marginal differences in cytokine responses and cell surface markers were apparent in the total CFS population they studied, when the patients were subgrouped by type of disease onset (gradual or sudden) or by how well they were feeling on the day of testing, more pronounced differences were seen. It is also worth noting that although Peakman and colleagues (1997) did not find significant differences in the percentage levels of total CD3+, CD4+, CD8+, and activated, naive, and memory T-cell subsets between CFS patients and controls, they cryopreserved the cells before flow cytometric analysis, and cryopreservation can differentially affect the representation of T-cell subsets.

A study by Sandman and colleagues (1992) found that elevated CD4+ and CD8+ cell counts in CFS patients were related to decreases in priming of memory and speed of memory scanning, and increases in errors on a memory fragility test. However, that study did not control for depression severity, and it is not clear whether the finding is related to comorbid depression or to chronic fatigue syndrome itself.

Klimas and colleagues (1990) found a decreased proportion of CD4+CD45RA+ cells, which are associated with suppressor/cytotoxic cell induction (Morimoto et al., 1985), but Natelson, LaManca, and colleagues (1998) found no significant change in the proportions of CD4+CD45RA+ and CD4+CD45RO+ cells in CFS patients. Franco and colleagues (1987) also described a decrease in the number of CD4+CD45RA+ lymphocytes in two patients with severe, chronic Epstein-Barr (EBV) virus infection; one of the two patients showed a persistent diminished number of cells despite clinical improvement with interleukin-2 treatment. Several publications have associated alterations in the latter subset of T cells with a number of clinical entities, particularly autoimmune diseases (Alpert et al., 1987; Emery et al., 1987; Klimas et al., 1992; Morimoto et al., 1985; Sato et al., 1987; Sobel et al., 1988). In a study of lymph node and peripheral blood lymphocytes, Fletcher and colleagues (2000) reported decreased proportion of naive T cells in both lymph node and peripheral blood. They also found that in CFS patients, as in normal controls, approximately 80 percent of lymph node lymphocytes are CD3+, of which over 65 percent are CD4+ (Black, Leong, and Crowed, 1980; Bryan et al., 1993; Kelly-Williams, Zmijewski, and Tomaszewski, 1989; Lindelman, Mellstedt, and Biverfeld, 1983; Tedla et al., 1999). The variance of CD8+ cell proportions among the different studies may be related to the specific location of the nodes studied, the status of nodal reactivity at the time of harvest, the technique used to make the lymphocyte suspensions, as well as the methods of staining and analysis (Tedla et al., 1999).

Increased numbers of T cells expressing the activation marker CD26, probably as a result of CD8+ activation, have also been reported in CFS patients (Klimas et al., 1990). In this respect, an increased proportion of CD8+ cells expressing the activation marker human leukocyte antigen (HLA)-DR

(Barker et al., 1994; Hassan et al., 1998; Klimas et al., 1990; Landay et al., 1991) have been reported in CFS patients, whereas normal proportions of CD4+ T cells coexpressing the HLA-DR marker or the interleukin-2 receptor (CD25) were found in one study (Landay et al., 1991), normal proportions of CD8+, CD38+, CD8+CD11b-, CD8+HLA-DR+, and CD8+CD28+ were found in another study (Natelson, LaManca, et al., 1998), and normal proportions of CD8+HLA-DR+ and CD8+CD38+ were found by Swanink and colleagues (1996). In contrast to some of the latter findings, Hassan and colleagues (1998) found significantly decreased expression of CD28 on CD8 cells, and Barker and colleagues (1994), Landay and colleagues (1991), and Swanink and colleagues (1996) found significantly decreased expression of CD11b on CD8 cells. Higher expression of CD38 on CD8 cells was found by Barker and colleagues (1994), Landay and colleagues (1991), and Peakman and colleagues (1997).

It is worth noting that relatively high proportions of HLA-DR+ T cells have been reported in a number of autoimmune disorders (Alviggi et al., 1984; Canonica et al., 1982; Jackson et al., 1984; Koide, 1985; Rabinowe et al., 1984), and that Hassan and colleagues (1998) found that chronic fatigue syndrome patients with increased HLA-DR expression had significantly lower Short Form-36 health questionnaire total scores, worse body pains, and poorer general health perception and physical functioning scores. The increased expression of class II antigens and the reduced expression of the costimulatory receptor CD28, which is a marker of terminally differentiated cells, lend further support to the concept of immunoactivation of T lymphocytes in chronic fatigue syndrome and may be consistent with the notion of a viral etiopathogenesis in the illness.

A study of the association between chronic fatigue syndrome physical symptoms, illness burden, and lymphocyte activation markers in twenty-seven newly diagnosed CFS patients (Helder et al., 1998) revealed that elevations in T-helper/inducer cells were associated with a greater frequency and severity of tender lymph nodes, greater severity of memory and concentration difficulties, and headaches. Greater numbers of activated T cells (CD2+CD3+CD26+) were associated with a greater frequency of tender lymph nodes and cognitive difficulties, and more activated cytotoxic/suppressor cells (CD8+CD38+HLA-DR+) were associated with greater severity of tender lymph nodes, fatigue, and sleep problems. Conversely, lower percentages of regulatory cells such as CD3+CD8+ were associated with a greater number of cognitive difficulties, greater Sickness Impact Profile (SIP) total, greater SIP physical impairment, and an increased frequency and severity of memory problems, increased frequency of headaches, and increased severity of fatigue. Thus among CFS patients the degree of cellular immune activation is associated with the severity of CFS physical symptoms, cognitive complaints, and perceived illness burden.

In terms of B-cell numbers, Gupta and Vayuvegula (1991), Klimas and colleagues (1990), Landay and colleagues (1991), Lloyd and colleagues (1992), and Barker and colleagues (1994) found normal levels of CD20+ resting B cells, whereas other teams reported both increased and decreased levels (Borysiewicz et al., 1986; Buchwald and Komaroff, 1991; Linde et al., 1992; Tirelli et al., 1994). The proportion of CD5-bearing B cells was found to be increased in two studies (Klimas et al., 1990; Tirelli et al., 1994), and decreased in one study (Landay et al., 1991). B cells bearing the cell marker CD5 have been associated with autoimmunity (Casali and Notkins, 1989).

Depressed responses to phytohemagglutinin (PHA) and pokeweed mitogen (PWM), an indication of dysfunction in cellular immunity, were found in the CFS patients studied by most teams (Aoki, Usuda, and Miyakoshi, 1987; Behan, Behan, and Bell, 1985; Borysiewicz et al., 1986; Hassan et al., 1998; Jones et al., 1985; Jones and Straus, 1987; Jones, 1991; Klimas et al., 1990; Lloyd et al., 1989, 1992; Straus et al., 1985; Tobi et al., 1982). Mawle and colleagues (1997) found no change. Gupta and Vayuvegula (1991) found that the lymphocyte DNA synthesis in response to PHA, PWM, and concanavalin A was normal in CFS patients, but the response to soluble antigens (mumps, *Escherichia coli*) was significantly reduced. Roberts and colleagues (1998) found that the degree of PWM-induced lymphoproliferative response is associated with Rh status among healthy controls but not among CFS patients and thus recommended controlling future studies for Rh status. In terms of the functional implications of decreased lymphoproliferative activities in chronic fatigue syndrome, Hassan and colleagues (1998) reported that PHA proliferative responses were lower in patients with poor emotional and mental health scores, and the anti-CD3/anti-CD28 response was low in those with low general health perception scores. T-cell dysfunction in CFS patients has been suggested to result from decreased surface expression of CD3, an important component of the T-cell receptor complex (Subira et al., 1989), and Barker and colleagues (1994) found no significant increase in the mean proliferation of peripheral blood cells when stimulated with the anti-CD3 antibody.

In terms of the impaired lymphocyte responses seen in CFS patients, Bounous and Molson (1999) pointed out that, as an antioxidant, glutathione (GSH) is essential for allowing the lymphocyte to express its full potential without being hampered by oxyradical accumulation. Hence, protracted challenge of the immunocytes may lead to cellular GSH depletion. Bounous and Molson (1999) hypothesized that because GSH is also essential to aerobic muscular contraction, an undesirable competition for GSH precursors between the immune and muscular systems may develop. It is conceivable that the priority of the immune system for the survival of the host has drawn the ever-diminishing GSH precursors to this vital area, thus depriving the skeletal muscle of adequate GSH precursors to sustain a normal aerobic metabolism, resulting in fatigue and eventually myalgia (Bounous and Molson, 1999).

In terms of B-cell function, spontaneous and mitogen-induced immunoglobulin synthesis are also affected. Despite these deficits in B-cell function, stimulation with allergens provides differential lymphocyte responsiveness. Greater in vitro lymphocyte responses to specific allergens, greater baseline levels of lymphocyte incorporation of tritiated thymidine, and an increased number of immunoglobulin E-bearing B and T lymphocytes have been reported (Olson, Kanaan, Gersuk, et al., 1986; Olson, Kanaan, Kelley, and Jones, 1986). Elevation in levels of certain cytokines, such as interleukin-4, -5, and -6, may underlie the latter effects. In a sample of sixty-five CFS patients, Lutgendorf and colleagues (Lutgendorf, Antoni, et al., 1995; Lutgendorf, Klimas, et al., 1995) observed that decreased lymphoproliferative responses to PHA and PWM were associated with increased cognitive difficulties and greater SIP physical illness burden.

Another area of research in chronic fatigue syndrome is that of apoptosis, the process of programmed cell death, which is regulated by several genes including *Bax* and *Bcl-2*. The Bcl-2 protein forms a heterodimer with Bax that inhibits apoptosis, whereas the Bax-Bax homodimer promotes it. A report by Hassan and colleagues (1998) found no association between surface and intracellular immunologic and apoptotic markers and functional lymphocyte assays after stimulation with anti-CD3/anti-CD28 antibodies or with apoptosis repressor ratio of Bcl-2/Bax in both CD4 and CD8. However, recent evidence indicates that induction of apoptosis might be mediated in a dysregulated immune system, such as that present in chronic fatigue syndrome, by the up-regulation of growth-inhibitory cytokines. In this respect, Vojdani and colleagues (1997) found an increased apoptotic cell population in CFS individuals as compared to healthy controls. The increased apoptotic subpopulations in CFS individuals was accompanied by an abnormal cell arrest in the S phase and the G2/M boundary of the cell cycle as compared to the control group. In addition, CFS individuals exhibited enhanced mRNA and protein levels of the interferon-induced protein kinase RNA (PKR) product as compared to healthy controls. In 50 percent of the CFS samples treated with 2-aminopurine (a potent inhibitor of PKR) the apoptotic population was reduced by more than 50 percent. PKR-mediated apoptosis may thus contribute to the pathogenesis and the fatigue symptomatology associated with chronic fatigue syndrome. See and colleagues (1998) found that the addition of a glyconutrient compound (dietary supplement that supplies the eight crucial monosaccharides required for synthesis of glycoproteins) to peripheral blood cells of CFS patients in vitro significantly decreased the percentage of apoptotic cells (all three parameters were deficient at baseline).

In contrast to the studies previously described, Swanink and colleagues (1996) found no obvious difference in apoptosis in leukocyte cultures from CFS patients.

Natural Killer Cells

Klimas and colleagues (1990), Morrison, Behan, and Behan (1991), Peakman and colleagues (1997), and Tirelli and colleagues (1994) found increased numbers of natural killer cells, whereas Barker and colleagues (1994), Landay and colleagues (1991), Lloyd and colleagues (1992), and Natelson, LaManca, and colleagues (1998) found normal numbers, and Masuda and colleagues (1994) and Gupta and colleagues (1997) found decreased numbers of natural killer cells. Despite the discrepancy in total numbers of natural killer cells measured by different groups, Caligiuri and colleagues (1987) and Morrison, Behan, and Behan (1991) found an increased proportion of CD56+CD3+ T cells, which may account for the decreased natural killer cell cytotoxic activity seen in several studies of CFS patients. Morrison, Behan, and Behan (1991) also found a decreased percentage of CD56+Fc gamma receptor+ natural killer cells, which suggests a reduced capacity for antibody-dependent cellular toxicity.

Several studies revealed impaired natural killer cell function in CFS patients as assessed by cytotoxic activity against K562 cells (Barker et al., 1994; Caligiuri et al., 1987; DuBois, 1986; Kibler et al., 1985; Klimas et al., 1990; Ojo-Amaise, Conley, and Peters, 1994; See et al., 1997; Straus et al., 1985; Whiteside and Friberg, 1998) and a decreased number of CD56+ CD3– lymphocytes (Caligiuri et al., 1987; Morrison, Behan, and Behan, 1991). A study by Levine, Whiteside, and colleagues (1998) on natural killer cell activity in a family with members who had developed chronic fatigue syndrome as adults, as compared who those had not, documented low NK cell activity in six out of eight cases and in four out of twelve unaffected family members. Two of the offspring of the CFS cases had pediatric malignancies. Based on these observations, the authors suggested that the low natural killer cell activity in this family may be a result of a genetically determined immunologic abnormality predisposing to chronic fatigue syndrome and cancer. Gold and colleagues (1990) were the only group to find elevated NK cell activity among the CFS patients they studied, whereas

Mawle and colleagues (1997) found no change in natural killer cell function.

The changes in natural killer cell cytotoxic activity found by most groups could be related to several findings:

1. CD56+CD3– cells are the lymphoid subset with highest natural killer cell activity, and a decrease in their representation is expected to lower the value for the natural killer cell activity per effector cells.
2. The reduction in CD4+CD45+ T cells described previously may also result in decreased induction of suppressor/cytotoxic T cells.
3. Reduced natural killer cell activity may be associated with deficiencies in the production of interleukin-2 and interferon-gamma by T cells or in the ability of natural killer cells to respond to these lymphokines.

Buchwald and Komaroff (1991) found that stimulation with interleukin-2 failed to result in improvement of cytolytic activity in many patients with chronic fatigue syndrome.

Poor natural killer cell function may also be related to the finding of an impaired ability of lymphocytes from CFS patients to produce interferon-gamma in response to mitogenic stimuli (Kibler et al., 1985; Klimas et al., 1990). Although one study reported elevated interferon-gamma production (Altman, Larratt, and Golubjatnikov, 1988) and another demonstrated normal production (Morte et al., 1988), the inability of lymphocytes from CFS patients to produce interferon-gamma found by Klimas and colleagues (1990), Kibler and colleagues (1985), and Visser and colleagues (1998) might represent a cellular exhaustion as a consequence of persistent viral stimulus. The postulate is supported by Morag and colleagues' (1982) and Straus and colleagues' (1985) findings of elevated levels of leukocyte 2'5'-oligoadenylate synthetase, an interferon-inducible enzyme, in lymphocytes of CFS patients. Furthermore, the lack of interferon-gamma production in CFS patients may be responsible for the impaired activation of immunoregulatory circuits, which in turn facilitates the reactivation and progression of viral infections. In this respect, Lusso and colleagues (1987) described the prevention of intercellular spread of Epstein-Barr virus mediated by the interferon released as a consequence of cellular response, and Borysiewicz and colleagues (1986) described normal natural killer cell activity but reduced EBV-specific cytotoxic T-cell activity in their CFS patients. Reactivation/replication of a latent virus (such as Epstein-Barr virus) secondary to decreased natural killer cell activity has also been proposed to modulate the immune system to induce chronic fatigue syndrome (Glaser and Kiecolt-Glase, 1998).

More recent research had provided alternative explanations for the decreased natural killer cell activity observed in chronic fatigue syndrome. A study by Ogawa and colleagues (1998) revealed a possible dysfunction in the nitric oxide (NO)-mediated natural killer cell activation in CFS patients based on the observations that twenty-four-hour treatment of natural killer cells with L-arginine, one of the essential amino acids, enhanced natural killer cell activity in controls but not in CFS patients. Although the expression of inducible nitric oxide synthase (the enzyme involved in the synthesis of nitric oxide from L-arginine) transcripts in peripheral blood mononuclear cells was not significantly different between healthy control subjects and CFS patients, incubation with S-nitro-N-acetylpenicillamine, a nitric oxide donor, stimulated natural killer cell activity in healthy control subjects but not in CFS patients. See and colleagues (1998) reported that in vitro addition of a glyconutrient compound (dietary supplement that supplies the eight crucial monosaccharides required for synthesis of glycoproteins) to peripheral blood cells from CFS patients significantly enhanced natural killer cell activity, increased the expression of the glycoproteins CD5, CD8, and CD11a, and decreased the percentage of apoptotic cells, parameters that were all deficient at baseline. The last observation would be consistent with a defect in glycoprotein synthesis.

See and Tilles (1996) treated thirty CFS patients with interferon-alpha-2a or placebo in a double-blind crossover study. Outcome was evaluated by natural killer cell function, lymphocyte proliferation to mitogens and soluble antigens, CD4/CD8 counts, and a ten-item quality-of-life survey. Although mean natural killer cell function increased after twelve weeks of interferon therapy, no significant change was seen in the other immunologic parameters or quality-of-life scores. When the twenty-six patients who completed the study were stratified according to their baseline natural killer cell function and lymphocyte proliferation, four groups were identified: three patients had normal natural killer cell function and lymphocyte proliferation when compared to normal, healthy controls; nine had isolated deficiency in lymphocyte proliferation; seven had diminished natural killer cell function only; and seven had abnormalities for both parameters. Quality-of-life scores were not significantly different for the four groups at baseline. After twelve weeks of interferon therapy, quality-of-life scores significantly improved in each of the seven patients with isolated natural killer cell dysfunction compared to baseline. In these patients the mean natural killer cell function increased. Significant improvement was not recorded for quality of life in the other three groups. Thus therapy with interferon-alpha has a significant effect on the quality of life of that subgroup of patients with chronic fatigue syndrome manifesting an isolated decrease in natural killer cell function.

Pursuing the hypothesis that the low-grade fever and fatigue in low natural killer cell syndrome—a condition resembling chronic fatigue syndrome in many but not all ways (Aoki et al., 1993; Aoki, Usuda, and Miyakoshi, 1987)—might be abrogated by interventions that normalize natural killer cell functioning, one group has tested the effects of immunopotentiators with patients diagnosed with low natural killer cell syndrome. They found in single-blind trials (contents of medication were not revealed to patients) that although the administration of antipyrectics, nonsteroidal anti-inflammatory drugs, or antibiotics had no detectable effects on fever, lentinan (a glucon extracted from Japanese mushrooms) improved clinical symptoms and increased natural killer cell cytotoxicity and antibody-dependent cellular cytotoxicity in patients with low natural killer cell syndrome (Miyakoshi, Aoki, and Mizukoshi, 1984). Although preliminary, this is one of the only studies to document parallel improvements in CFS-like clinical symptoms and natural killer cell cytotoxicity following an experimental manipulation. However, this study did not focus specifically on CDC-diagnosed CFS patients.

Neutrophils, Monocytes, and Eosinophils

Previously described relationships between basal circulating neutrophil numbers and plasma progesterone concentrations and between exercise-induced neutrophilia and urinary cortisol and plasma creatine kinase concentrations in healthy women were not observed in CFS women. Observations suggest that normal endocrine influences on the circulating neutrophil pool may be disrupted in CFS patients (Cannon et al., 1998).

Prieto and colleagues (1989) found significant monocyte dysfunction in patients with chronic fatigue syndrome, such as reduced display of vimentin, phagocytosis index, and surface expression of HLA-DR. These deficits responded to naloxone treatment, an observation which suggests that increased interaction of endogenous opioids with monocyte receptors might account for the monocyte dysfunction. Gupta and colleagues (1997) found that monocytes from CFS patients display an increased density of intercellular adhesion molecule (ICAM-I) and lymphocyte factor activation (LFA-1), but showed decreased enhancing response to recombinant interferon-gamma in vitro. In contrast to the latter studies, Barker and colleagues (1994) did not find abnormalities in superoxide anion production and phagocytosis in CFS patients. Moreover, lack of a consistent elevation of neopterin, a macrophage activation marker, suggests that monocytes do not appear to account for the imbalances in interleukin-1.

Conti and colleagues (1996) provided evidence for eosinophil activation in chronic fatigue syndrome by demonstrating elevated serum levels of eosinophil cationic protein (ECP). In the CFS population they studied, the prevalence of reaction allergen-specific testing (RAST) positivity to one or more allergens was 77 percent, and no control showed positive RAST. Twelve of the fourteen CFS patients with increased ECP serum levels were RAST positive. However, CFS, RAST-positive patients had no significantly higher ECP serum levels than CFS, RAST-negative patients did. It remains to be determined whether eosinophil activation has a pathogenetic role in chronic fatigue syndrome or a common immunologic background may exist for both atopy and chronic fatigue syndrome.

Although a higher prevalence of allergy (Steinberg, Pheley, and Peterson, 1996) and delayed-type hypersensitivity (Lloyd et al., 1989, 1992) can be detected in CFS patients, a trial with antihistamine treatment did not provide significant improvement (Steinberg et al., 1996). Other authors, such as Mawle and colleagues (1997), found no significant difference in the incidence of delayed-type hypersensitivity and allergic responses among CFS patients. Baraniuk and colleagues (Baraniuk, Clauw, and Gaumond, 1998; Baraniuk et al., 1998) found that 30 percent of CFS patients had positive skin tests, a feature that suggests the potential for allergic rhinitis complaints, and 46 percent had nonallergic rhinitis; they suggested that although atopy may coexist in some CFS subjects, it is unlikely that it plays a causal role in CFS pathogenesis. Borish and colleagues (1998) proposed that in at least a large subgroup of CFS subjects with allergies, the concomitant influences of immune activation brought on by allergic inflammation in an individual with the appropriate psychological profile may interact to produce the symptoms of chronic fatigue syndrome. Borok (1998) suggested that food intolerance, in a genetically predisposed group of people, causes symptoms akin to both the major and minor criteria of chronic fatigue syndrome, and it should be screened for to avoid confusion. On the other hand, some authors have associated chronic fatigue syndrome with nickel allergy (Marcusson, Lindh, and Evengard, 1999; Regland et al., 2000; Uter, 2000). Although the controversy of atopy and chronic fatigue syndrome continues, it may be possible that these two conditions share some common denominators that are worth pursuing, particularly in light of the proposed Th2-type cytokine predominant pattern discussed in the following section.

Cytokines

The immune system cells closely network with one another and with cells of other bodily systems through either direct interactions or a series of message conveyors known as cytokines (*cyto* stands for cell, and *kinein* for to move, i.e., messages that get cells going). Cytokines are endowed with the capacity to interact with different cell types and modulate their function. The immune system dictates which cells will respond to the cytokine signals by strictly controlling the expression of cytokine receptors, cell surface proteins that bind a specific cytokine and transmit a signal to the interior of the cell.

A cytokine and its receptor are complementary in shape in the regions where they interact, much like a key fitting into a lock. Only a particular cytokine receptor (or sometimes several of them) has the proper three-dimensional shape to interact with and hold onto its respective cytokine. Once a cytokine has bound to its receptor on the surface of a cell, the tail of the receptor molecule that extends into the cytoplasm of the cell initiates an intracellular biochemical cascade. The outcome of this cascade is the expression of new genes by the cell receiving the cytokine signal (known as the target cell), which in turn ultimately results in changes in the biologic activity of the target cell. The biologic effects of cytokines are extremely diverse, in part because a single cytokine may be pleiotropic, meaning that the same cytokine signal could have different effects on different types of target cells.

Some of the cytokines produced in the immunological battlefield travel into the protected environment of the central nervous system and warn the brain that the body is defending itself from a foreign invader or a cancer. One such cytokine is interleukin-1 (*inter* meaning between, and *leukin* referring to leukocyte or white blood cell, because cytokines were originally believed to be message conveyors only between white blood cells). Interleukin-1 travels to the region of the brain known as the hypothalamus, the body's thermostat. Interaction of interleukin-1 with hypothalamic cells leads to fever (microbes or cancer cells usually replicate less efficiently at higher body temperatures) and somnolence (sleep allows the body to conserve and focus energy on the battle against the invading microbe or cancer). Other cytokines, such as tumor necrosis factor (TNF), are also fever inducers, the so-called pyrogens.

Every cytokine has natural endogenous antagonists that quench their activity and allow the control of the extent of the battle led by the immune system defense mechanisms. Cytokines can be synergistic or antagonistic, either complementing or inhibiting each other's signals. These properties give rise to a highly complex cytokine network where signals are delivered, sometimes in cooperation and sometimes in opposition with one another, to target cells throughout the immune system. The process keeps immune cells and those of other bodily systems functioning in response to pathogenic or toxic challenges (Heilig et al., 1993; Kalinkovich et al., 1993; Patarca, Klimas, Lutgendorf, et al., 1994; Patarca, Klimas, Walling, et al., 1995; Prince et al., 1990).

Activation of the immune system by cancer cells, pathogens, or pathogen-infected cells may evoke feelings of fatigue, which are also mediated by proinflammatory cytokines and other soluble immune mediators (Pui, 1989). For instance, the majority of patients with inoperable non-small-cell lung cancer have evidence of a systemic inflammatory response, whose magnitude is associated with more fatigue, greater weight loss, poorer performance status, and poorer survival (Scott et al., 2002). Osterlund and colleagues (2002) reported that raltitrexed treatment promotes systemic inflammatory reaction in colorectal carcinoma patients, with 94 percent of the 52 patients they studied reporting fatigue.

Bower and colleagues (2002) studied forty breast cancer survivors (twenty fatigued, twenty nonfatigued) and found that fatigued breast cancer survivors showed elevations in serum markers associated with proinflammatory cytokine activity an average of five years after diagnosis. Fatigued breast cancer survivors had significantly higher serum levels of several markers associated with proinflammatory cytokine activity than nonfatigued survivors, including interleukin-1 receptor antagonist, soluble tumor necrosis factor receptor type II, and neopterin. They were also more likely to report behavioral problems that co-occur with fatigue in the context of immune activation. Fatigued cancer survivors had significantly lower serum levels of cortisol than the nonfatigued group as well as differences in two lymphocyte populations, observations that may account for the enduring immune activation (Bower et al., 2002).

Cytokines and Cancer-Related Fatigue

The immune, endocrine, and nervous systems respond to external and internal challenges, including cancer, and communicate and regulate one another by means of shared or system-unique hormones, growth factors, neurotransmitters, and neuromodulators. Therefore, the nervous, endocrine, and immune systems are major adaptive systems of the body, a feature that is important to maintain homeostasis or balanced physiological function (Crofford, 1998a,b; Morand et al., 1996; Pellegrini, Berghella, Di Loreto, et al., 1996). Many types of cancer cells have the capacity to produce the factors that the immune and nervous system use to communicate and maintain a balanced functioning of the body. This process leads to imbalance and several cancer-related manifestations of disease, many of which contribute to fatigue, such as anemia, weight loss, fever, pain, and infection.

In cancer patients, many pathological manifestations are influenced by a frequently disrupted balance between endogenous cytokine levels and their natural antagonists (Kurzrock, 2001). Indeed, cancer cells and the immune system appear to overexpress a range of cytokines in patients with malignancies that are associated with cancer-related manifestations, such as anemia, cachexia, fever, night sweats, and pain, among others (see Table 3.1). In fact, during acute febrile illness, septic shock, and some tumors, cytokines initiate an acute-phase response, which is characterized by fatigue, fever, inactivity, anorexia, and catabolism (Akira, Taga, and Kishimoto, 1993; Calabrese, Kling, and Gold, 1987). Profound neuroendocrine and metabolic changes also take place: the liver produces acute-phase proteins; bone marrow function and the metabolic activity of leukocytes are greatly increased; and specific immune reactivity is suppressed.

Some cytokines act as autocrine or paracrine growth factors for the neoplastic tissue while simultaneously causing secondary symptoms related to fatigue (Akiyama et al., 1994; Chopra, Dinh, and Hannigan, 1998; Emilie et al., 1992; Fischer et al., 1994; Patarca and Fletcher, 1997; Pawelec, Zeuthen, and Kiessling, 1997; Samaniego et al., 1995). For instance, tumors such as atrial myxoma, plasmacytoma, and Lennert's T-cell lymphoma secrete interleukin-6. The resulting elevated circulating interleukin-6 levels correlate in many cases with disease severity as seen in other fatigue-associated pathologies, such as endotoxemia, systemic inflammatory response syndrome, systemic lupus erythematosus, familial hemophagocytic lymphohistiocytosis, and rheumatoid arthritis (Akira et al., 1990; Akira, Taga, and Kishimoto, 1993; Casey, Balk, and Bone, 1993; Henter et al., 1991; Hirano et al., 1988; Maini, Elliott, Brennan, and Feldman, 1995; Maini, Elliott, Brennan, Williams, et al., 1995; Rosenbloom et al., 1995; Spronk et al., 1992).

TABLE 3.1. Cytokines associated with cancer-related manifestations and fatigue

	Anemia	Cachexia	Fever and Night Sweats
Interleukin-1	X		X
Interleukin-6	X		
Tumor necrosis factor	X	X	X
Interferon-gamma		X	
Leukemia inhibitory factor		X	

High serum levels of interleukin-1, interleukin-6, and TNF-alpha have been found in cancer patients, and the levels of these cytokines correlate in many cases with tumor progression (Moldawer, Gelin, and Schersten, 1987; Moldawer, Andersson, and Galin, 1988; Moldawer et al., 1992; Strassman, Fong, et al., 1992). In this respect, progression of cervical cancer has also been associated with elevated levels of circulating cytokines (Chopra, Dinh, and Hannigan, et al., 1998). However, it should be pointed out that although interleukin-6, along with interleukin-1 and oncostatin M, is also a growth factor for Kaposi's sarcoma (Brown et al., 1991; Chandran Nair et al., 1992), its elevated serum levels in AIDS patients with Kaposi's sarcoma are unrelated to disease extent (De Wit et al., 1991; Hamilton et al., 1994; Louie et al., 1995; Sinkovics, 1991). In other cases, such as that illustrated by prostate cancer, several studies have identified cytokines not specific to the disease, the levels of which correlate with prognosis (Thompson, 1990).

Several ongoing studies are trying to elucidate the role of particular cytokines in fatigue per se and in other cancer-associated symptoms that can lead to fatigue. For instance, cancer-associated anemia may be secondary to a blunted erythropoietin response and/or cytokines (interleukin-1, interleukin-6, and TNF-alpha) that suppress erythropoiesis.

Similarly, fever and night sweats are influenced by pyrogenic cytokines such as interleukin-1 and tumor necrosis factor (Kurzrock, 2001). One should note that although these cytokines are the most well known pyrogens, other cytokines may be involved in the manifestation of fever and night sweats. For instance, although interleukin-1 can be identified in Reed-Sternberg cells, granulocytes, and small to medium cells of undetermined origin in about half the cases of Hodgkin's disease, demonstration of interleukin-1-positive cells does not correlate with the presence of fever, weight loss, and night sweats (Ree, Crowley, and Dinarello, 1987).

The characteristic picture of anorexia—tissue wasting, the loss of body weight accompanied by a decrease in muscular mass (protein reserves) and adipose tissue (energy reserves), and the poor performance status preceding death—so often found in advanced-stage cancer patients is termed cancer-related anorexia/cachexia syndrome (CACS) (Baracos, 2001; Brennan, 1997; Bruera, 1992; Finley, 2000; Glaus, 1998b; Heber, Byerley, and Chi, 1986; Nelson and Walsh, 1991; Ockenga et al., 2002; Puccio and Nathanson, 1997).

Cancerous cachexia, a wasting syndrome and a hallmark of cancer, can be attributed to loss of appetite or enhanced energy expenditure leading to fatigue (Glaus, 1998b; Tait and Aisner, 1989). St. Pierre, Kasper, and Lindsey (1992) proposed that one physiologic mechanism of cancer-related fatigue involves changes in skeletal muscle protein stores or metabolite concentration. A reduction in skeletal muscle protein stores may result from endogenous tumor necrosis factor or from tumor necrosis factor administered as antineoplastic therapy. TNF-alpha has also been implicated in HIV-related wasting (Abrams, 1996; Fauci, 1993).

Cancerous cachexia may result from circulating factors produced by the host or by the tumor itself. A number of cytokines, including interleukin-1 and interleukin-6, as well as tumor necrosis factor, interferon-gamma, and leukemia inhibitory factor, have been proposed as mediators of the cachectic process and they act as cachectins in animal models. Moreover, the chronic administration of these factors in humans, either alone or in combination, is capable of reproducing the different features of CACS (Busbridge, Dacombe, and Hopkins, 1989; Gelin, Moldawer, and Lonnroth, 1991; Ilyin and Plata-Salaman, 1996a,b; McLaughlin, Rogan, and Ton, 1992; Moldawer, Rogy, and Lowry, 1992; Patarca and Fletcher, 1998; Strassmann, Fong, et al., 1992; Strassmann, Jacob, et al., 1992).

The nonsteroidal anti-inflammatory drug zaltoprofen improves the decrease in body weight in rodent sickness behavior models (Okamoto, 2002). However, the results of numerous clinical and laboratory studies suggest that the action of cytokines alone is unable to explain the complex mechanism of CACS (Espat, Copeland, and Moldawer, 1994; Mantovani et al., 1998; McNamara, Alexander, and Norton, 1992; Noguchi et al., 1996; Tisdale, 1997a,b). More direct evidence of a cytokine involvement in CACS is provided by the observations that cachexia in experimental animal models (Matthys and Billiau, 1997; Noguchi et al., 1996; Sherry, Gelin, and Fong, 1991) can be relieved by administration of specific cytokine antagonists. These studies also revealed that cachexia can rarely be attributed to any one single or specific cytokine but rather to a set of cytokines that work in concert. The same cytokines seem to play a role in cachexia-related inflammation and in the acute-phase response (Moldawer and Copeland, 1997).

Coats (2002) points out that in many underlying conditions associated with cachexia, the patient also suffers an often-unexplained severe shortness of breath along with weakness, asthenia, and exhaustion. There appear to be marked similarities in the cause of shortness of breath and fatigue between different cachectic conditions. For instance, in cardiac cachexia, evidence exists for a linkage between skeletal muscle reflex inputs to ventilatory control and exaggerated chemoreflex responses as candidates for the heightened perception of shortness of breath which cannot be explained by heart or lung dysfunction in many patients. Similar processes may occur in other cachexias, especially those complicating cancer, AIDS, chronic liver disease, and chronic lung disease (Coats, 2002).

Cytokines may underlie the development of depression among cancer patients. Depression is also a common side effect of biotherapy of cancer with cytokines. However, great differences exist in the prevalence of the development of depressive symptoms across studies of interferon-alpha or interleukin-2 administration (Wichers and Maes, 2002). Differences in doses and duration of therapy may be sources of variation as well as individual differences of patients, such as a history of psychiatric illness. In addition, sensitization effects may contribute to differential responses of patients to the administration of cytokines.

In animals, administration of proinflammatory cytokines induces a pattern of behavioral alterations called "sickness behavior" that resembles the vegetative symptoms of depression in humans. Changes in serotonin receptors and in levels of serotonin and its precursor tryptophan in depressed people support a role for serotonin in the development of depression. In addition, evidence exists for a dysregulation of the noradrenergic system and a hyperactive hypothalamic-pituitary-adrenal axis in depression. Some mechanisms exist that make it possible for cytokines to cross the blood-brain barrier.

Proinflammatory cytokines such as interleukin-1beta, interferon-alpha, interferon-gamma, and TNF-alpha affect serotonin metabolism directly and/or indirectly by stimulating the enzyme indoleamine 2,3-dioxygenase which leads to a peripheral depletion of tryptophan. Interleukin-1, interleukin-2, and TNF-alpha influence noradrenergic activity, and interleukin-1, interleukin-6, and TNF-alpha are found to be potent stimulators of the HPA axis. Altogether, administration of cytokines may induce alterations in the brain resembling those found in depressed patients, which leads to the hypothesis that cytokines induce depression by their influence on the serotonin, noradrenergic, and hypothalamic-pituitary-adrenal axis systems (Wichers and Maes, 2002).

Changes in serum cytokine levels may also be one of the mechanisms by which radiation therapy triggers fatigue. In a study of fifteen men undergoing external beam radiation for prostate cancer, Greenberg and colleagues (1993) reported that ranked weekly mean fatigue scores for each subject increased at week 4 then reached a plateau and rose in weeks 6 and 7. In week 6, the last week of full-volume radiation, subjects slept most compared to all other weeks, including week 7 when treatment was coned down. Ranked serum interleukin-1 tended to rise between weeks 1 and 4, as fatigue scores rose. The authors suggest that localized radiation treatment is associated with increased fatigue and sleep requirement independent of depressive symptoms. Relative serum interleukin-1 changes may be one signal for the systemic reaction and subjective fatigue associated with the acute effects of radiation (Greenberg et al., 1993). However, in another study, no evidence was found that serum levels of interleukin-1beta, interleukin-6, TNF-alpha, declining hemoglobin levels, anxiety, or depression were responsible for fatigue induced by adjuvant radiotherapy after breast-conserving surgery in patients with breast cancer (Geinitz et al., 2001).

Cytokines and Chronic Fatigue Syndrome

Interleukin-1 and soluble interleukin-1 receptors. Interleukin-1 is the term for two distinct cytokines—interleukin-1alpha and interleukin-1beta— that share the same cell-surface receptors and biological activities (Dinarello, 1991; Platanias and Vogelzang, 1990). One study of CFS patients (Patarca, Lugtendorf, et al., 1994) found elevated levels of serum interleukin-1alpha but not of plasma interleukin-1beta in 17 percent of patients studied. When the cohort was examined as to severity of symptoms, the top quartile in terms of disability had the highest level of interleukin-1. Curiously, use of reverse transcriptase-coupled polymerase chain reaction (RT-PCR) revealed interleukin-1beta, but not interleukin-1alpha messenger RNA (mRNA) in peripheral blood mononuclear cells (PBMCs) of several CFS patients with highly elevated levels of interleukin-1alpha. RT-PCR of fractionated cell populations showed that lymphocytes accounted for the interleukin-1beta mRNA detected in PBMCs. The fact that interleukin-1alpha mRNA was not detectable by RT-PCR in either PBMCs or granulocytes suggests that serum interleukin-1alpha in CFS patients is probably derived from a source other than peripheral blood cells. Other potential sources are tissue macrophages, endothelial cells, lymph node cells, fibroblasts, central nervous system microglia, astrocytes, and dermal dendritic cells (Dinarello, 1991).

Linde and colleagues (1992) found significantly higher levels of interleukin-1alpha in chronic fatigue syndrome and mononucleosis patients, but Lloyd and colleagues (1992), Peakman and colleagues (1997), and Rasmussen and colleagues (1994) found no difference. Five studies, in addition to the one previously described by Patarca, Lutgendorf, and colleagues (1994), found no difference in the levels of interleukin-1beta in CFS patients (Linde et al., 1992; Morte et al., 1989; Peakman et al., 1997; Rasmussen et al., 1994; Straus et al., 1989).

The signs and symptoms of chronic fatigue syndrome, which include fatigue, myalgia, and low-grade fever, are similar to those experienced by patients infused with cytokines such as interleukin-1. Elevated serum levels of interleukin-1alpha found in a significant number of CFS patients could underlie several of the clinical symptoms. Interleukin-1 can gain access to the brain through the preoptic nucleus of the hypothalamus, where it induces fever and the release of adrenocorticotropin hormone (ACTH)-releasing factor (Arnason, 1991; Berkenbosch et al., 1987; Besedovsky et al., 1986;

Sapolsky et al., 1987), which in turn would lead to release of ACTH and cortisol. The observation that cortisol levels tend to be low in CFS patients regardless of interleukin-1alpha levels suggests a role of a defective hypothalamic feedback loop in the pathogenesis of chronic fatigue syndrome. The presence of such a defect has been documented in Lewis rats, which are particularly susceptible to the induction of a variety of inflammatory and autoimmune diseases and exhibit reduced levels of ACTH-releasing hormone, ACTH, and cortisol in response to interleukin-1.

Besides its effects on the hypothalamic-pituitary-adrenal axis, interleukin-1 has other effects on the pituitary; it has been shown to augment release of prolactin and growth hormone and to inhibit release of thyrotropin and luteinizing hormone (Bernton et al., 1987; Rettori et al., 1991). The growth hormone deficiency state associated with chronic fatigue syndrome may also be a reflection of the defect in the hypothalamic feedback loop that renders it inadequately responsive to interleukin-1.

Interleukin-1 and tumor necrosis factor provoke slow-wave sleep when placed in the lateral ventricles of experimental animals (Shoham et al., 1987). The inordinate fatigue, lassitude, and excessive sleepiness associated with chronic fatigue syndrome (Holmes et al., 1988; Moldofsky, 1989a) could well be a consequence of the direct action of these cytokines on neurons. Neurotoxic effects secondary to chronic overexpression of interleukin-1alpha and/or beta of S100—a small (10 kDa), soluble calcium-binding protein that is synthesized and released by astroglia (Van Eldik and Zimmer, 1987)—has been proposed to underlie progressive neurological degeneration in Alzheimer's disease (Griffin et al., 1989).

Interleukin-1 induces prostaglandin (PGE_2, PGI_2) synthesis by endothelial and smooth muscle cells (Dejana et al., 1987). These substances are potent vasodilators, and interleukin-1 administration in animals and humans produces significant hypotension. Interleukin-1 has a natriuretic effect (Caverzasio, Rizzoli, and Dayer, 1987) and may affect plasma volume.

Chronic fatigue syndrome, as well as other chronic fatiguing illnesses, affects women in disproportionate numbers and is often exacerbated in the premenstrual period and following physical exertion. Cannon and colleagues (1997) found that isolated peripheral blood mononuclear cells from healthy women, but not from CFS patients, exhibited significant menstrual cycle-related differences in interleukin-1beta secretion that were related to estradiol and progesterone levels. Interleukin-1 receptor antagonist secretion for CFS patients was twofold higher than controls during the follicular phase, but luteal phase levels were similar between groups. In both phases of the menstrual cycle, interleukin-1 soluble receptor type II release was significantly higher for CFS patients compared to controls. The only changes that might be attributable to exertion occurred during the follicular phase in the control subjects, who exhibited an increase in interleukin-1beta secretion forty-eight hours after the stress. These results suggest that an abnormality exists in interleukin-1beta secretion in CFS patients that may be related to altered sensitivity to estradiol and progesterone. Furthermore, the increased release of interleukin-1 receptor antagonist and soluble interleukin-1 receptor type II by cells from CFS patients is consistent with the hypothesis that chronic fatigue syndrome is associated with chronic, low-level activation of the immune system.

In contrast to the studies mentioned previously, Swanink and colleagues (1996) found no obvious difference in the levels of circulating cytokines, and ex vivo production of interleukin-1alpha and interleukin-1 receptor antagonist. Although endotoxin-stimulated ex vivo production of TNF-alpha and interleukin-1beta was significantly lower in chronic fatigue syndrome, none of the immunologic test results correlated with fatigue severity or psychological well-being scores. Swanink and colleagues (1996) concluded that these immunologic tests cannot be used as diagnostic tools in individual CFS patients.

Tumor necrosis factor and soluble tumor necrosis factor receptors. Tumor necrosis factor-alpha and -beta are cytokines produced on lymphoid cell activation (Beutler and Cerami, 1988). Twenty-eight percent of CFS patients studied by Patarca, Lutgendorf, and colleagues (1994) had elevations in serum levels of TNF-alpha and -beta, usually with elevation in serum levels of interleukin-1 or soluble interleukin-2 receptor. Tumor necrosis factor-alpha expression in CFS patients is also evident at the mRNA level, an observation that suggests de novo synthesis rather than release of a preformed inducible surface TNF-alpha protein upon activation of monocytes and CD4+ T cells (Kriegler et al., 1988). The levels of spontaneously (unstimulated) produced TNF-alpha by nonadherent lymphocytes were also significantly increased as compared to matched controls simultaneously studied by Gupta and colleagues (1997). Moss, Mercandetti, and Vojdani (1999) also found elevated levels of TNF-alpha in CFS patients compared to non-CFS controls. Tumor necrosis factor-alpha may be associated with central nervous system pathology because it has been associated with demyelination and may also lead to loss of appetite (Beutler and Cerami, 1988; Wilt et al., 1995). A study by Dreisbach and colleagues (1998) suggests that TNF-alpha may be involved in the pathogenesis of postdialysis fatigue. In contrast to the studies previously discussed, Lloyd and colleagues (1992) found no difference in the levels of TNF-alpha and -beta in CFS patients, and Rasmussen and colleagues (1994) and Peakman and colleagues (1997) found no differences in the levels of TNF-alpha and -beta, respectively. The latter discrepancies are likely secondary to the fact that TNF levels decrease precipitously if the serum or plasma is not frozen within thirty minutes from collection (Patarca, Sandler, et al., 1995).

Tumor necrosis factor-alpha's proinflammatory effects may be mediated by induction of gene expression for neutrophil activating protein-1 and macrophage inflammatory proteins, resulting in neutrophil migration and degranulation (Dinarello, 1992). Thus it is reasonable that TNF elevations may also be associated with markers of macrophage activation such as serum neopterin. In fact, among CFS patients studied at the University of Miami, illness-burden scores were significantly positively correlated with elevated TNF-alpha serum levels.

Chronic fatigue syndrome patients have higher serum levels of soluble tumor necrosis factor receptor type I (sCD120a) and soluble tumor necrosis factor receptor type II (sCD120b) (Patarca, Klimas, Sandler, et al., 1995). Higher levels of soluble TNF receptors are negatively correlated with natural killer cell cytotoxic and lymphoproliferative activities in chronic fatigue syndrome, an observation that is consistent with the activities of these soluble mediators.

Interleukin-2 and soluble interleukin-2 receptor. As mentioned in Chapter 2, interleukin-2, formerly termed "T-cell growth factor," is a glycosylated protein produced by T lymphocytes after mitogenic or antigenic stimulation (Watson and Mochizuki, 1980). Interleukin-2 acts as a growth factor (Fletcher and Goldstein, 1987) and promotes proliferation of T cells (Morgan, Ruscetti, and Gallo, 1976) and, under particular conditions, B cells and macrophages (Malkovsky et al., 1987; Tsudo, Ichiyama, and Uchino, 1984). Although serum interleukin-2 levels were found to be elevated in CFS patients compared with control individuals in one study (Cheney, Dorman, and Bell, 1989), decreased levels were reported in two other studies (Gold et al., 1990; Kibler et al., 1985), and no difference was reported in three studies (Linde et al., 1992; Patarca, Lutgendorf, et al., 1994; Straus et al., 1989). Rasmussen and colleagues (1994) reported a higher production of interleukin-2 by stimulated peripheral blood cells from CFS patients as compared to controls. Cheney, Dorman, and Bell (1989) found no obvious relationship between interleukin-2 serum levels and severity or duration of illness in chronic fatigue syndrome.

Elevated levels of soluble interleukin-2 receptor, a marker of lymphoid cell activation, have been found in a number of pathological conditions, including viral infections, autoimmune diseases, and lymphoproliferative and hematological malignancies (Cohen, Stempel, and Colombe, 1990; Pui, 1989). Twelve percent of CFS patients studied by Patarca, Lutgendorf, and colleagues (1994) had elevated levels of soluble interleukin-2 receptor. This observation is consistent with the increased proportion of activated T cells and the reduced levels of interleukin-2 or decreased natural killer cell cytotoxic activity found in several studies of CFS patients previously discussed. However, Linde and colleagues (1992) found no elevation in soluble interleukin-2 receptor levels in CFS patients.

Interferons. The interferons comprise a multigenic family with pleiotropic properties and diverse cellular origin. Data from six studies indicate that circulating interferons are present in three percent or less of patients studied (Aoki, Usuda, and Miyakoshi, 1987; Borysiewicz et al., 1986; Buchwald and Komaroff, 1991; Ho-Yen, Carrington, and Armstrong, 1988; Jones et al., 1985; Lloyd, Hanna, and Wakefield, 1988; Straus et al., 1985; Vojdani and Lapp, 1999). Peripheral blood cells from children affected by postviral fatigue syndrome produced more interferon-alpha than those from controls. In line with this observation, Vojdani and colleagues (1997) found elevated interferon-alpha levels in CFS patients, but Linde and colleagues (1992) and Straus and colleagues (1989) found no difference. Fatigue occurs in more than 70 percent of patients treated with interferon-alpha, and it may be associated with the development of immune-mediated endocrine diseases, in particular hypothyroidism and hypothalamic-pituitary-adrenal axis-related hormonal deficiencies in these patients (Dalakas, Mock, and Hawkins, 1998; Jones, Wadler, and Hupart, 1998).

Interferon-gamma is an immunoregulatory substance, enhancing both cellular antigen presentation to lymphocytes (Zlotnick et al., 1983) and natural killer cell cytotoxicity (Targan and Stebbing, 1982), and causing inhibition of suppressor T-lymphocyte activity (Knop et al., 1982). Two groups have found impaired interferon-gamma production on mitogenic stimulation of peripheral blood mononuclear cells from CFS patients (Klimas et al., 1990; Visser et al., 1998), and one group (Lloyd et al., 1992) found increased production. In contrast with the findings on lymphocyte activation, four groups reported no difference in the levels of circulating interferon-gamma (Linde et al., 1992; Peakman et al., 1997; Straus et al., 1989; Visser et al., 1998). These results are in favor of the Th2 shift described previously, a shift that is not apparent at the level of circulating cytokines.

Interleukin-4. Visser and colleagues (1998) reported that although CD4 T cells from CFS patients produce less interferon-gamma than cells from controls, IL-4 production and cell proliferation are comparable. With CD4 T cells from CFS patients (compared with cells from controls), a ten- to twentyfold lower dexamethasone concentration was needed to achieve 50 percent inhibition of interleukin-4 production and proliferation, an observation that indicates an increased sensitivity to dexamethasone in CFS patients. In contrast to interleukin-4, interferon-gamma production in patients and controls was equally sensitive to dexamethasone. A differential sensitivity of cytokines or CD4 T cell subsets to glucocorticoids might explain an altered immunologic function in CFS patients.

Interleukin-4 acts as a growth factor for various types of lymphoid cells, including B, T, and cytotoxic T cells (Paul and Ohara, 1987), and has been shown to be involved in immunoglobulin isotype selection in vivo (Kuehn, Rajewsky, and Mueller, 1991). Activated T cells are the major source of interleukin-4 production, but mast cells can also produce it, and interleukin-4 has been associated with allergic and autoimmune reactions (Paul and Ohara, 1987). It is also noteworthy that many of the effects of interleukin-4 are antagonized by interferon-gamma, and the decreased production of the latter may underlie a predominance of interleukin-4 over interferon-gamma effects.

Interleukin-6 and soluble interleukin-6 receptor. The levels of spontaneously produced interleukin-6 by both adherent monocytes and nonadherent lymphocytes were significantly increased in CFS patients as compared to controls (Gupta et al., 1997; Gupta, Aggarwal, and Starr, 1999). The abnormality of interleukin-6 expression was also observed at the mRNA level. In terms of circulating interleukin-6, Buchwald and colleagues (1997) found that interleukin-6 was elevated among febrile CFS patients compared to those without this finding and therefore considered it to be an epiphenomenon possibly secondary to infection. Chao and colleagues (1990, 1991) also found elevated levels of interleukin-6 in CFS patients, but five other groups found no difference (Buchwald et al., 1997; Linde et al., 1992; Lloyd et al., 1992; Peakman et al., 1997; See et al., 1997).

Most of the cell types that produce interleukin-6 do so in response to stimuli such as interleukin-1 and tumor necrosis factor (Mizel, 1989). Excessive interleukin-6 production has been associated with polyclonal B-cell activation, resulting in hypergammaglobulinemia and autoantibody production (Van Snick, 1990). As is the case with interleukin-4, interleukin-6 may contribute to activation of CD5-bearing B cells, leading to autoimmune manifestations. Interleukin-6 also synergizes with interleukin-1 in inflammatory reactions and may exacerbate many of the features described previously for interleukin-1.

Cannon and colleagues (1999) found increased interleukin-6 secretion in CFS patients, which is manifested by chronically elevated plasma alpha2-macroglobulin concentrations. Chronic fatigue syndrome patients have higher levels of soluble interleukin-6 receptor (Patarca, Klimas, Sandler, et al., 1995) which enhances the effects of interleukin-6.

Interleukin-10. A study by Gupta and colleagues (1997) revealed that spontaneously produced interleukin-10 by both adherent monocytes and nonadherent lymphocytes, and by phytohemmaglutinin-activated nonadherent monocytes were decreased.

Tumor growth factor-beta. A study by Bennett, Mayes, and colleagues (1997) found that patients with chronic fatigue syndrome had significantly higher levels of bioactive tumor growth factor-beta levels compared to healthy controls and to patients with various diseases known to be associated with immunologic abnormalities and/or pathologic fatigue: major depression, systemic lupus erythematosus, and multiple sclerosis (MS) of both the relapsing/remitting and the chronic progressive types.

Beta-2 microglobulin. Three studies found elevated levels of beta-2 microglobulin in CFS patients (Buchwald et al., 1997; Patarca, Klimas, Sandler, et al., 1995; Patarca, Sandler, et al., 1995) and one study found no difference (Chao et al., 1990). Beta-2 microglobulin is a marker of immune activation.

Soluble CD8. Linde and colleagues (1992) found no elevation of soluble CD8 in CFS patients.

Soluble intercellular adhesion molecule-1. Patarca and colleagues (Patarca, Klimas, Sandler, et al., 1995) found higher levels of soluble intercellular adhesion molecule-1 in CFS patients, an observation that is consistent with the higher expression of intercellular adhesion molecule-1 in monocytes of CFS patients reported by Gupta and Vayuvegula (1991).

The Th1-Type (Cell-Mediated Immunity)/ Th2-Type (Humoral Immunity) Cytokine Imbalance Paradigm in Cancer and Fatigue

T-helper cells are further subclassified into two types (Clerici et al., 1991, 1992; Clerici, Hakim, et al., 1993; Paul and Seder, 1994; Romagnani, 1994). T-helper type 1 (Th1) cells produce a group of cytokines that predominantly stimulate macrophages/monocytes and natural killer cells, the cells best suited to directly attack cancer cells and microbes that hide and replicate in human cells (Whiteside and Herberman, 1989). The type of immune response favored by Th1 cells is therefore called cell-mediated immunity. T-helper type 2 (Th2) cells preferentially stimulate the function of B cells and the production of antibodies. This so-called humoral immunity is best suited to deal with parasites that are too large to be killed by individual macrophages/monocytes or natural killer cells. Parasites need to be coated first with the immunoglobulin bullets to then be attacked by other protein in the blood, such as complement, or by other cells of the immune army. The same strategy can also be used against cancer cells. Undifferentiated T-helper cells that are neither Th1 nor Th2 are designated Th0.

The two types of T-helper cell responses were first documented in mice. The cytokines secreted by Th1-type cells are mainly interleukin-2 and interferon-gamma, while Th2-type cells preferentially secrete interleukin-4, -5, -6, and -10. Some strains of mice differentially succumbed to particular infections based on the type of T-helper response that was predominant in that particular strain (inbreeding of mice strains allowed the selection of strains that would predominantly respond with either a Th1- or a Th2-type response). Although in humans the dichotomy in T-helper cell responses is not as clear-cut as in inbred mice, the Th1/Th2 paradigm is still valid. Human T-helper cell responses have either a Th1- or Th2-type bias, and certain disease states can be associated with a predominance of one or the other T-helper cell type response. For instance, disease progression in AIDS is associated with a shift from a Th1-type predominance to a more undifferentiated Th0-type response (Clerici et al., 1991, 1992; Clerici, Hakim, et al., 1993; Clerici, Lucey, et al., 1993; Graziosi et al., 1994; Maggi, Giudizi, et al., 1994; Maggi, Mazzetti, et al., 1994). The AIDS virus also replicates more readily in Th2- and Th0-type cells.

Based on these observations, several therapeutic interventions for AIDS are aimed at favoring a shift back toward a Th1-type response predominance. Some cytokines, such as interleukin-2 and interleukin-12, have the ability to favor such a shift (Barral-Netto et al., 1995; Cheynier et al., 1992; Gilmore, 1994; Kanagawa et al., 1993; Luzuriaga et al., 1991; Modlin and Nutman, 1993; Morawetz et al., 1994; Paganelli et al., 1995). However, their direct administration to humans or animals, particularly, interleukin-12, is associated with toxicities. As mentioned in Chapter 2, administration of interleukin-2, a strong stimulator of natural killer cells, is used as therapeutic modality in the treatment of patients with certain cancers, such as renal cell carcinoma and melanoma. Interferon-gamma is another Th1-type cytokine with therapeutic potential in cancer.

Other diseases are associated with a predominance of a Th2-type response, many of which, such as AIDS and autoimmune diseases, have been linked with an increased propensity for cancer. As a metaphor for many occasions in human history, the policing and military roles of the bodily army can turn against the body that they are supposed to protect. In these situations, normal components of the body start being recognized as foreign, and diseases, collectively known as autoimmune diseases, ensue. Systemic lupus erythematosus and rheumatoid arthritis are examples of autoimmune diseases, which are characterized by the stimulation of B cells that produce antibodies against the self to produce a sequel of destruction.

Usually a very low level of "autoimmunity" exists in all of us because it is the way that the immune army recognizes our dead cells and gets rid of them, i.e., it is part of the internal cleaning process. In autoimmune diseases, the tight control over this cleaning process is lost. The predominant type of T-helper cell generals that are involved in autoimmune diseases are T-helper type 2 cells. The same is true for allergic reactions and for asthma, which are associated with increased production of one type of immunoglobulin bullets, the E type, in response to environmental factors that are innocuous to most individuals. As detailed in the following subsections, many types of cancer and chronic fatiguing illnesses are associated with a shift to a Th2-type predominance. The latter may therefore be an underlying cause of cancer-related fatigue. Chapter 4 addresses interventions that are being tested in the contexts of cancer, chronic fatiguing illnesses, or both to favor a shift to Th1-type predominance and an improvement in several parameters of clinical symptomatology.

Th2-type predominance in several cancers. As reviewed by Pawelec, Zeuthen, and Kiessling (1997), tumor cells may be able to modulate the immune response away from cell-mediated immunity, as some parasites can. This may not even be a global effect, but restricted to antitumor responses. For instance, although mice transgenic for interleukin-10 (i.e., mice genetically manipulated to express high levels of the Th2-type cytokine interleukin-10) retained their resistance to the parasite *Listeria,* in contrast to their non-genetically manipulated counterparts, they were unable to reject immunogenic tumors (Hagenbaugh et al., 1997). In humans, Smith and colleagues (1994) reported that lung cancer cells constitutively secrete interleukin-10 in vitro, and that anti-interleukin-10 sera increased the production of tumor necrosis factor and interferon by peripheral blood cells cocultured with tumor cells. Kim and colleagues (1995) described secretion of interleukin-10 by basal and squamous cell carcinoma cells and showed that intralesional treatment with interferon-alpha induced tumor regression, associated with down-regulation of interleukin-10 messenger RNA.

Rabinowich and colleagues (1996) noted that in ovarian carcinoma, both tumor cells and tumor-infiltrating lymphocytes expressed elevated levels of interleukin-10 messenger RNA and protein. In breast tumors, messenger RNA for interleukin-10, but not for interleukin-2 and -4, was commonly found (Venetsanakos et al., 1997). Huang and colleagues (1995) reported that both non-small-cell lung cancer cell lines and freshly isolated tumor cells secreted intelerleukin-10, and that exposure of the cells to interleukin-4 or TNF-alpha augmented interleukin-10 secretion. Hishii and colleagues (1995) reported that human glioma cells secreted interleukin-10, which down-regulated HLA-DR expression on monocytes and inhibited interferon-gamma and TNF-alpha effects.

Local T-cell-mediated cytokine expression triggered by contact with basal-cell carcinoma was predominantly of the Th2 type, while that triggered by a benign growth was Th1-type predominant (Yamamura et al., 1993). Yamamoto and colleagues (1995) found that during progression of murine syngeneic tumor, the ability of animal spleen cells to produce interleukin-2, interferon-gamma, and TNF-alpha decreased (Th1-type decrease), whereas the production of tumor growth factor-beta (a suppressive cytokine) increased. Kurt and colleagues (1995) described that tumor-rejecting lymphocytes derived from a secondary tumor were cytotoxic, but those derived from a progressing primary tumor in the same animal were not, although both used the same Vß T-cell receptor. However, the rejection site showed higher expression of interferon-gamma, TNF-alpha, and interleukin-10, while the progressor site showed higher tumor growth factor-beta. The latter observation suggests that although the same T-cell clone able to reject tumors is present in progressing tumors, tumor environment prevents the successful destruction of tumor cells by it. Addition of anti-tumor growth factor-beta-neutralizing antibodies to autologous lymphocyte/tumor cell cocultures increased the frequency of cultures showing positive responses (Vanky et al., 1997). High levels of TGF-beta have been found in serum of cancer patients in direct correlation to the degree of tumor progression; these high levels were reduced upon resection (Tsushima et al., 1996). Colorectal cancers in patients responding to immunotherapy were found not to express tumor growth factor-beta messenger RNA, whereas nonresponders did. The expression of interleukin-1, -6, -8, -10 and TNF-alpha was variable between responders and nonresponders, an observation that underscores the importance of TGF-beta expression (Doran et al., 1997).

Elevated serum interleukin-10 levels have been found in patients with various solid tumors, particularly melanoma (Fortis et al., 1996). Pisa, Halapi, and colleagues (1992) found increased local amounts of interleukin-10 but no interleukin-2 in ovarian tumors. Similarly, Nakagomi and colleagues (1995) found interleukin-10 messenger RNA in freshly isolated renal carcinoma cells, but not in renal carcinoma cell lines, patients' peripheral blood mononuclear cells, or normal kidney tissue; they did not detect interleukin-2, -3, or -4 messenger RNA in any tissue. Yamamura and colleagues (1993) found the Th2-type cytokines interleukin-4, -5, and -10 locally in basal-cell carcinoma lesions, but the Th1-type cytokines interleukin-2, interferon-gamma, and TNF-beta in benign skin lesions. Young and colleagues (1996) noted that freshly excised human head and neck cancers released prostaglandin E2, interleukin-10, and TGF-beta. Taken together, the majority of reports suggest that when tumors and/or tumor-infiltrating lymphocytes express higher levels of the Th2-type cytokines interleukin-10 and TGF-beta, this mostly results in deleterious immunosuppressive effects. Gene therapy models are providing evidence consistent with this conclusion; thus vaccination with an interleukin-10-producing murine tumor transfected with the granulocyte-macrophage colony-stimulating factor gene failed to induce dendritic cell accumulation and tumor rejection unless production of interleukin-10 was prevented using antisense techniques (Qin et al., 1997).

Th2-type cells are thought not to be efficient anticancer effectors. In a mouse lymphoma model, although the presence of tumor-specific cytotoxic T lymphocytes could be demonstrated in both susceptible and resistant hosts, in the susceptible hosts the helper response was dominated by Th2-type phenotype cells and in the resistant hosts the dominant response was of the Th1-type phenotype (Lee, Zeng, et al., 1997). This is a striking finding because although the tumor was immunogenic and even stimulated cytotoxic T lymphocyte responses, the presence of Th2-type responses was overriding and was still associated with fatal outcome. In a comparison of spontaneously regressing with nonregressing melanomas, Lowes and colleagues (1997) found elevated levels of messenger RNA for the Th1-type cytokines interleukin-2, interferon-gamma, and TNF-beta in the former compared to the latter, although they found no differences in Th2-type cytokine messenger RNA levels. In colon cancer patients, a preferential accumulation of Th2-type cells has been reported that might contribute to suppression and blockade of Th1-type effectors (Pellegrini, Berghella, Del Beato, Cicia, et al., 1996). This observation prompted Contasta and colleagues (1996) and Pellegrini and colleagues (Pellegrini, Berghella, Del Beato, Adorno, and Casciani, 1996) to stress the necessity of biotherapeutic treatments that induce Th1-type cell functions in colorectal cancer. Evaluation of Th-type cell patterns may also be of prognostic significance for colorectal cancer (Berghella et al., 1996).

The Th1-type effectors are thought to be of prime importance in most antitumor responses. However, the presumption that Th1-type cytokine patterns indicate host-mediated tumor rejection and that Th2-type cytokine predominance inhibits this process is not universally valid. For example, the Th2-type cytokine interleukin-4 enhanced immunogenicity and induced efficient tumor rejection when expressed in situ (Golumbek et al., 1991). Interleukin-4 is also effective in reversing the decline of cytotoxic T lymphocyte activity observed during in vivo progression of a murine B-cell lymphoma (Santra and Ghosh, 1997). Some evidence even indicates that the Th2-type cytokine interleukin-10 can also enhance tumor rejection (Giovarelli et al., 1995; Richter et al., 1993; Yang et al., 1995). It should be pointed out that, even in those cases, interleukin-10 had many negative effects on other aspects of the host immune system. The observations once again underscore the complexity of the cytokine system, a barrier that has curtailed the rapid development of effective therapeutic interventions. However, although the findings presented previously do not constitute proof, they are highly suggestive of a causal link for a switch from a Th1- to a Th2-type predominant cytokine expression pattern and consequent expression and development of many different tumors.

Th2-type predominance in other fatiguing illnesses. Although chronic fatigue syndrome is an ailment of yet unknown cause, it is characterized in a significant number of patients, mostly among those with an acute onset, i.e., following a flulike illness, by evidence of activation of the immune army. This observation lends support to the hypothesis that chronic fatigue syndrome is caused by an infection that either lingers chronically or leaves an autoimmune sequel. In this respect, it is known that microbes can cause damage either directly or indirectly. As the immune system attacks a microbe, some microbial components may resemble human components, and the body may end up generating antibody bullets that can also recognize bodily components, a process termed *molecular mimicry* that can lead to autoimmune disease manifestations. The process is also favored by genetic predisposition in the form of particular variants of the human leukocyte antigen (HLA) molecules, the proteins that antigen-presenting cells use to present particles to the T cells.

It is curious that although the immune army is activated in a subset of CFS patients, the soldiers of the immune army, particularly the T-cell generals and natural killer cells, function poorly. T cells from CFS patients have a decreased capacity to divide and generate new T cells, and the natural killer cells have significantly decreased "killing" or cytotoxic activity. Besides chronic fatigue syndrome, natural killer cell activity has been shown to be decreased in other fatiguing conditions such as protein calorie malnutrition (Kelley et al., 1994), repeated infections (Holland, 1996), vitamin and trace mineral deficiency (Gogos, Kalfarentzos, and Zoumbos, 1990), autoimmune disorders (Kantor et al., 1992), chemotherapy, and immunotherapy (Villa et al., 1991).

Levy and colleagues (1987) reported that natural killer cell activity is an important predictor of patient baseline prognosis relevant to nodal status in breast cancer patients. Unlike findings in other reports, on reassessment after three months, it was found that natural killer cell activity was not affected by the interim administration of chemotherapy and/or radiotherapy. However, natural killer cell activity levels remained markedly lower in patients with positive nodes than in patients with negative nodes. Although average levels of natural killer cell activity were lower for patients with more tumor burden, there was still a substantial range of natural killer cell activity levels within the node-positive patient group, as well as within the patient group as a whole. In fact, Levy and colleagues (1987) found that they could account for 30 percent of natural killer cell activity level variance at three months follow-up on the basis of baseline natural killer cell activity, fatigue, depression, and lack of social support. Therefore; although neither radiation nor chemotherapy appeared to affect natural killer cell activity, tumor burden was again clearly associated with natural killer cell activity levels, and a significant amount of baseline and three-month natural killer cell activity could be predicted on the basis of central nervous system-mediated effects.

In chronic fatigue syndrome, the repertoire of T-helper cells is also biased, as described earlier for autoimmune diseases and many cancers, toward a Th2-type response. Activated T-helper cell generals from CFS patients produce less Th1-type cytokine interferon-gamma, and more interleukin-5, a Th2-type cytokine. These features combined create a pervasive immunological battlefield-like environment in CFS patients that is Th2-type predominant with compromised cellular immunity and decreased ability of the body to deal with microbes along with the presence of auto-antibodies.

The triggers and maintenance factors of the Th2-type predominance are unknown but could include infections, toxins, prior immunizations, hormonal status changes, or a combination thereof. Potent immunogens can have systemic, long-lasting, nonspecific effects on the nature of the immune response to unrelated antigens. In particular, vaccinations or infections can exert a systemic effect and nonspecifically increase or reduce the Th1/Th2 cytokine ratio balance of the response to other unrelated antigens (Shaheen et al., 1996) and affect (positively or negatively) survival from unrelated diseases (Aaby, 1995; Aaby et al., 1995).

Based on the fact that Persian Gulf War personnel were given multiple Th2-type response-inducing vaccinations, Rook, Stamford, and Zumla, in international published patent number WO-09826790, presented the hypothesis that Gulf War syndrome represents a special case of chronic fatigue syndrome, in which the Th2-inducing stimuli can be identified. Rook and colleagues pointed out four features of the vaccination protocol used for the Persian Gulf War troops that underscore the possibility of induction of a systemic Th2-type switch.

First, pertussis was used as an adjuvant in British troops in the Persian Gulf, and its adjuvanticity is potently Th2-type response inducing (Mu and Sewell, 1993; Ramiya et al., 1996; Smit, Stark, and Myburgh, 1996). This property of pertussis has recently led to discussion of the possibility that its use in children contributes to the contemporary increased prevalence of atopy (Nilsson et al., 1996; Odent, Culpin, and Kimmel, 1994).

Second, Gulf War troops were given Th2-type-inducing immunogens against plague, anthrax, typhoid, tetanus, and cholera. Such a cumulatively large antigen load would tend to drive the response toward a Th2-type response predominance (Aaby, 1995; Bretscher et al., 1992; Hernandez-Pando and Rook, 1994). The measles vaccine, when used at the standard dose, reduced mortality by considerably more than can be accounted for by the incidence of measles in the unvaccinated population. It has been reported that diphtheria, tetanus, and pertussis (DPT) vaccines (Th2-type inducing) do not show this nonspecific protective effect (Aaby et al., 1995). However, when a high-titer measles vaccine was used, the mortality increased, although protection from measles itself was maintained (Aaby, 1995; Aaby et al., 1995). Some evidence shows that this increase in mortality was accompanied by a switch toward a Th2-type response, and dose-related increases in the induction of a Th2-type component are well established for several other immunogens (Bretscher et al., 1992; Hernandez-Pando and Rook, 1994).

Third, the vaccinations were given after deployment of the troops in the war zone, or just before they traveled there, at a time when stress levels would have been high. Immunization in the presence of raised levels of glucocorticoids (i.e., cortisol) drives the cytokine expression response by stimulated lymphocytes toward a Th2-type predominance (Bernton et al., 1995; Brinkmann and Kristofic, 1995; Zwilling, Brown, and Pearl, 1992).

Fourth, Persian Gulf War troops were also exposed to carbamate and organophosphorus insecticides, and these inhibit interleukin-2-driven phenomena essential for normal Th1-type function (Casale et al., 1993). The importance of this component is uncertain. However, it has been rumored that the insecticides were often obtained from local sources in the Persian Gulf, so purity was not known and even more toxic contaminants may have been present.

In terms of untoward effects of vaccines related to fatiguing illnesses, it should be also pointed out that the National Vaccine Injury Compensation Program and the U.S. Court of Federal Claims have accepted a causal relationship between currently used rubella vaccine in the United States and some chronic arthropathy with an onset one week and six weeks after vaccine administration. Fibromyalgia was reported in four out of seventy-two subjects with chronic arthropathy developing between one week and six weeks after the rubella vaccination, and in eleven out of fifty-two individuals in whom chronic arthropathy developed in less than one week or greater than six weeks postvaccination (Weibel and Benor, 1996).

Autoantibodies

Another aspect of the Th2-type immunity predominance is the presence of autoantibodies. The body's defense system, in attacking cancerous tissue or microbial invaders, may develop antibodies and cytotoxic T lymphocytes that cross recognize body components and end up attacking them, the process discussed earlier termed *autoimmunity*. The process happens because of what is termed *molecular mimicry* (Atkinson et al., 1994; Banki et al.,

1992; Blick et al., 1990; Ciampolillo et al., 1989; Dang et al., 1991; Gama Sosa et al., 1997; Garry et al., 1990; Jones and Armstrong, 1995; Lagaye et al., 1992; Perl et al., 1991; Silvestris, Williams, and Dammacco, 1995; Talal, Dauphinée, et al., 1990; Talal, Garry, et al., 1990; Tian, Lehmann, and Kaufman, 1994; Trujillo et al., 1993). Most tumor antigens that have been identified are of embryonic or adult tissue origin, and they behave as cryptic peptides (Barnd et al., 1988, 1989; Boon, Coolie, and Vanden Eynde, 1997; Bouchard et al., 1989; Brausseur et al., 1992; Brichard et al., 1993; Dugan et al., 1997; Gedde-Dahl, 1993; Hines, Jenson, and Barnes, 1995; Ionnides et al., 1993; Jerome et al., 1991; Jung and Schluesener, 1991; Kwon et al., 1987; Lustgarten et al., 1997; Majewski and Jablonska, 1997; Rimoldi, Romero, and Carrel, 1993; Roitt, 1994; Van der Bruggen et al., 1991; Yasumoto, 1995; Yoshino et al., 1994). The activation by immune and/or gene therapy of tumor-specific cytotoxic T lymphocytes that have escaped negative selection in the thymus may also favor autoimmunity (Abdelnoor, 1997; Pawelec, Zeuthen, and Kiessling, 1997). This possibility is underscored by the numerous reports concerning patients who have both cancer and autoimmune disease.

It seems that recognition of self is associated with immune recognition of cancer, and immunotherapeutic measures taken to treat cancer enhance the occurrence of autoimmune diseases. For instance, in a clinical trial where interleukin-2 was used to treat patients with melanoma, vitiligo was more common in patients who responded to treatment than in those who did not respond (Rosenberg and White, 1996). In another study, mice immunized with modified gp75 (a tumor antigen belonging to the tyrosinase family) rejected a metastatic melanoma and developed patchy pigmentation in their coats (Naftzger et al., 1996). Paraneoplastic neurological syndromes are rare conditions associated with certain cancers, such as small-cell lung cancer. Antineuronal antibodies have been detected in patients and are believed to be produced against tumor antigens that cross-react with neuronal antigens (Lang and Vincent, 1995; Zenone, 1992).

It remains to be determined whether autoimmunity plays a role in cancer-related fatigue, or at least in some cases of it. Some indirect evidence suggests that this may be the case for other fatiguing illnesses. One research team (Konstantinov et al., 1996) found that approximately 52 percent of sera from CFS patients react with nuclear envelope antigens. Some sera immunoprecipitated the nuclear envelope protein lamin B1, an observation that favors an autoimmune component in chronic fatigue syndrome (Poteliakhoff, 1998). Another report (Von Mikecz et al., 1997) documented a high frequency (83 percent) of autoantibodies to insoluble cellular antigens (vimentin and lamin B1) in chronic fatigue syndrome, a unique feature that might help to distinguish chronic fatigue syndrome from other rheumatic autoimmune diseases.

Several studies have documented the presence of the following in CFS patients: rheumatoid factor (Jones, 1991; Jones and Straus, 1987; Jones et al., 1985; Kaslow, Rucker, and Onishi, 1989; Prieto et al., 1989; Salit, 1985; Straus et al., 1985; Tobi et al., 1982), antinuclear antibodies (Bates et al., 1995; Gold et al., 1990; Jones, 1991; Jones and Straus, 1987; Jones et al., 1985; Prieto et al., 1989; Salit, 1985; Straus et al., 1985; Tobi et al., 1982; Von Mikecz et al., 1997), antithyroid antibodies (Behan, Behan, and Bell, 1985; Tobi et al., 1982; Weinstein, 1987), anti-smooth-muscle antibodies (Behan, Behan, and Bell, 1985), antigliadin, cold agglutinins, cryoglobulins, and false serological positivity for syphilis (Behan, Behan, and Bell, 1985; Straus et al., 1985). However, no circulating antimuscle and anti-central nervous system antibodies were found in ten CFS patients (Plioplys, 1997a), and one group (Rasmussen et al., 1994) found no significant differences in the number of positive tests for autoantibodies in CFS patients.

One team (Itoh et al., 1997) found that among children who chronically complain of nonspecific symptoms such as headache, fatigue, abdominal pain, and low-grade fever, those who were antinuclear antibody (ANA) positive (approximately 50 percent of cases) tended to have general fatigue and low-grade fever, while gastrointestinal problems, such as abdominal pain, diarrhea, and orthostatic dysregulation symptoms, were commonly seen in ANA-negative patients. Children who were unable to go to school more than one day a week were seen significantly more among ANA-positive patients than among negative patients. Based on these observations, the authors concluded that autoimmunity may play a role in childhood chronic nonspecific symptoms and proposed a new disease entity: the autoimmune fatigue syndrome (AIFS) in children.

The features shared between chronic fatigue syndrome and autoimmune diseases may complicate diagnosis. For instance, three cases of dermatomyositis had been erroneously diagnosed as chronic fatigue syndrome because of the presence of elevated titers of serum Epstein-Barr virus antibodies (Fiore, Giacovazzo, and Giacovazzo, 1997). In one study, one-third of CFS patients with sicca symptoms fulfilled the diagnostic criteria for Sjögren's syndrome, but they were "seronegative," differing from the ordinary primary Sjögren's syndrome (Nishikai et al., 1996).

Twenty-eight of eighty patients with sudden deafness and progressive hearing losses (approximately half of whom had phospholipid antibodies that can cause venous or arterial vasculopathies, or serotonin and ganglioside antibodies) displayed symptoms typical for fibromyalgia and chronic fatigue disorders, including fatigue, myalgia, arthralgia, depressions, sicca symptoms, and diarrhea (Lindal et al., 1997). The authors recommend questioning patients suffering from inner ear disorders for symptoms typical for fibromyalgia or chronic fatigue syndrome, since these diseases are often closely related to inner ear disorders. If symptoms are present, antibodies should be tested against phospholipids, serotonin, and gangliosides.

Fatigue is commonly associated with connective tissue and rheumatologic autoimmune disorders, and some patients with autoimmune disorders have been erroneously diagnosed with chronic fatiguing illnesses such as chronic fatigue syndrome (Fiore, Giacovazzo, and Giacovazzo, 1997; Nishikai et al., 1996). Patients with primary Sjögren's syndrome report more fatigue than healthy controls on all the dimensions of the Multidimensional Fatigue Inventory and, when controlling for depression, significant differences remain on the dimensions of general fatigue, physical fatigue, and reduced activity (Asim and Turney, 1997; Barendregt et al., 1998). Although fatigue in patients with systemic lupus erythematosus does not correlate with disease activity, it is correlated with fibromyalgia, depression, and lower overall health status (Wang, Gladman, and Urowitz, 1998). Fatigue is a major symptom in patients with ankylosing spondylitis and, unlike systemic lupus erythematosus, it is more likely to occur with active disease but may occur as a lone symptom (Jones et al., 1996). Fatigue is also common in osteoarthritis and rheumatoid arthritis, associated with measures of distress, and is a predictor of work dysfunction and overall health status (Wolfe, Hawley, and Wilson, 1996). Several studies (Huyser et al., 1998; Riemsma et al., 1998; Stone et al., 1997) have reported that rheumatoid arthritis-related fatigue is strongly associated with psychosocial variables, apart from disease activity per se.

Studies of lymph node cells from CFS patients (Fletcher et al., 2000) also reveal changes in phenotypic distributions that are similar to those found in several autoimmune diseases. In this respect, although Tedla and colleagues (1999) reported that the majority of the CD4+ and CD8+ T lymphocytes obtained from both lymph nodes and peripheral blood of control subjects were immunologically naive (CD45RA+), Fletcher and colleagues (2000) found that in both lymph nodes and peripheral blood of CFS patients a greater proportion of lymphocytes had the "memory" phenotype (CD45RO+). Klimas and colleagues (1990) had previously reported a decreased proportion of CD4+CD45RA+ cells in the peripheral blood compartment of CFS patients. CD4+CD45RA+ lymphocytes are associated with suppressor/cytotoxic cell induction (Morimoto et al., 1985), and CD45RA+ lymphocytes preferentially home into lymph nodes (Mackay, Martson, and Dudler, 1990; Mackay, 1992; Westemann and Pabst, 1996). Although one group (Natelson, LaManca, et al., 1998) found no significant change in the proportions of CD4+CD45RA+ and CD4+CD45RO+ cells in

CFS patients, another group also described a decrease in the number of CD4+CD45RA+ lymphocytes in two patients with severe, chronic Epstein-Barr virus infection (Franco et al., 1987). One of the two patients showed a persistent diminished number of cells despite clinical improvement with interleukin-2 treatment. Several publications have also associated decreased proportions in the CD45RA+ subset of lymphocytes with autoimmune diseases such as systemic lupus erythematosus, procainamide-induced lupus, rheumatoid arthritis, Sjögren's syndrome, and multiple sclerosis (Alpert et al., 1987; Emery et al., 1987; Klimas et al., 1992; Morimoto et al., 1985; Sato et al., 1987; Sobel et al., 1988).

Among patients with chronic fatigue syndrome, elevated levels of circulating immune complexes have been reported in four studies (Bates et al., 1995; Behan, Behan, and Bell, 1985; Borysiewicz et al., 1986; Straus et al., 1985). However, the studies by Natelson, LaManca, and colleagues (1998) and Mawle and colleagues (1997) revealed no abnormality in the level of circulating immune complexes (i.e., Raji cell and C1q binding). Depressed levels of complement, another feature of active autoimmune diseases, have also been reported in up to 25 percent of CFS patients (Behan, Behan, and Bell, 1985; Borysiewicz et al., 1986; Mawle et al., 1997; Natelson, LaManca, et al., 1998; Straus et al., 1985). Buchwald and colleagues (1997) found elevated levels of the inflammation marker C-reactive protein among CFS patients.

Multiple sclerosis, another autoimmune disease, encompasses a variety of symptom complexes including paroxysmal symptoms such as trigeminal neuralgia, paroxysmal dysarthria and ataxia, paresthesia and pain, paroxysmal itching, and akinesia (Taylor, 1998), as well as symptoms such as seizures, adventitious movements, and complications related to pregnancy and fatigue (Taylor, 1998). Fatigue is one of the most common findings in multiple sclerosis (Bergamaschi et al., 1997; Dulli and Schutta, 1996; Ford, Trigwell, and Johnson, 1998; Krupp and Pollina, 1996; Poser, 1996; Tola et al., 1998). Multiple sclerosis patients with progressive illness, of greater age, and those with higher Expanded Disability Status Scale scores have more fatigue (Stuifbergen and Rogers, 1997). This aspect is not affected by age of onset, duration of illness, gender, or index of progression. In patients with multiple sclerosis and in patients with chronic fatigue syndrome, subjective fatigue severity is related to impairment in daily life, low sense of control over symptoms, and strong focusing on bodily sensations (Vercoulen, Hommes, et al., 1996).

In chronic fatigue syndrome, but not in multiple sclerosis, there is a relationship between low levels of physical activity and attributing symptoms to a physical cause and between subjective fatigue severity and physical activity. One study (Tantucci et al., 1996) concluded that excessive "physiological" fatigue contributes to the symptom of fatigue in multiple sclerosis and is central in origin. However, since the degree of exercise-induced fatigue did not correlate with the baseline complaint of fatigue, other factors must also have been operating to produce the full range of clinical symptoms. An increase of metabolic cost of exercise did not occur in multiple sclerosis patients with mild disability, an observation that suggests a lack or a low degree of spasticity and/or ataxia elicited by the effort. Thus exertional capacity in multiple sclerosis appears to be limited mainly by poor training (Tantucci et al., 1996).

Fatigue in multiple sclerosis is secondary to central, neurogenic factors and does not seem to involve any myogenic factors such as might be related to muscle changes secondary to the long-standing disorder (Latash et al., 1996). The subjective feeling of tiredness ("fatigue") may be related to a dissociation between central motor commands ("effort") and their mechanical consequences. One study (Fukuzawa et al., 1996) showed that acylcarnitine deficiency and fatty acid metabolic dysfunction in mitochondria were not relevant to the excessive fatigue in patients with multiple sclerosis. Central fatigue in multiple sclerosis may also be secondary to impaired drive to the primary motor cortex, and several lines of evidence strongly suggest that this is not secondary to a lack of motivation (Latash et al., 1996). In this respect, one study (Sheean et al., 1997) showed that pyramidal dysfunction leads to increased fatigability. Other neuroendocrine factors may contribute to fatigue. For instance, correlations with C-reactive protein and gadolinium-enhanced brain MRI scans suggest that activation of the HPA axis in MS patients is secondary to an active inflammatory stimulus (Wei and Lightman, 1997). Psychological factors such as focusing on bodily sensations and low sense of control play a role in the experience of fatigue in multiple sclerosis and chronic fatigue syndrome (Deatrick, Brennan, and Cameron, 1998; Djaldetti et al., 1996; Iriarte, Carreno, and De Castro, 1996; Taylor and Taylor, 1998).

The treatment of multiple sclerosis includes two main areas: immunotherapies and management of the effects or symptoms resulting from multiple sclerosis (Rosenblum and Saffir, 1998). It should be noted that immunotherapy with interferon-beta-1b is associated with fatigue, and a study showed that only fatigue and depression were significantly associated with discontinuation of therapy (Neilley et al., 1996). Several new therapies, including tizanidine, intrathecal baclofen, botulinum toxin injections gabapentin, ondansetron, thalamic stimulation, and lamotrigine, increase our treatment options (Metz, 1998). Smoked cannabis has been reported to improve (in descending rank order) spasticity, chronic pain of extremities, acute paroxysmal phenomenon, tremor, emotional dysfunction, anorexia/weight loss, fatigue states, double vision, sexual dysfunction, bowel and bladder dysfunctions, vision dimness, dysfunctions of walking and balance, and memory loss (Consroe et al., 1997). A study (Sheean et al., 1998) suggests that 3,4-diamino-pyridine (25 to 60 mg/day for three weeks) may play a role in the symptomatic treatment of fatigue in multiple sclerosis. However, the mechanism behind such a benefit in fatigue remains unclear and the discrepancy between subjective and more objective responses underlines the probable multifactorial nature of the pathogenesis of this symptom in multiple sclerosis. An extended outpatient rehabilitation program for persons with definite progressive multiple sclerosis appears to effectively reduce fatigue and the severity of symptoms associated with multiple sclerosis (Di Fabio et al., 1998; LaBan et al., 1998).

Major Histocompatibility Complex Genes

The major histocompatibility complex (MHC) proteins are involved in antigen processing/presenting, a phenomenon that eventually leads to the generation of the immune response. Certain MHC gene alleles are found with increased frequency among patients with autoimmune diseases. The possible autoimmune etiology of chronic fatigue syndrome is further underscored by the significant association between chronic fatigue syndrome and the presence of histocompatibility locus antigen DQ3 (HLA-DQ3) (Keller et al., 1994), albeit the study that reached this conclusion needs to be expanded to a much larger population.

In terms of the possible link between cancer, cancer-related fatigue, and MHC alleles, the occurrence of a number of tumor types has also been associated with the presence of certain major histocompatibility alleles (Abdelnoor, 1997). Wank and Thomsen (1991) observed that the DQW03 allele was more frequent in patients with invasive cervical cancer than in the general population. Lee and colleagues (1996) reported a strong association between HLA-DQB1*0301 and advanced-stage melanoma, and gastric adenocarcinoma. HLA-DRB1*04, -DR*11, and in particular -DQB1*03 alleles were strongly associated with susceptibility to cervical intraepithelial neoplasia (Odunsi et al., 1996). Apple and colleagues (1994) reported an association between the DRB1*1501-DQB1*0602 haplotype and human papilloma virus (HPV)-positive invasive cervical carcinoma in Hispanic women. They also reported a negative association with DRB1*13 alleles. On the other hand, Sastre-Garau and colleagues (1996) reported that no correlation exists between HLA-DR-DQ alleles and susceptibility to HPV-positive carcinoma of the cervix in French women. However, they suggested that DR13 may offer a protective effect against HPV-associated lesions of the cervix. The discrepancy in the results obtained between their study on French women and that obtained by Apple and colleagues (1994) on Hispanic women was suggested to be secondary to differences in allele frequencies in the normal populations. Whereas the frequency of DRQ1B1*0301 in Hispanics was 7 percent, the frequency in French women was 19 percent.

In this context, it is worth noting that in establishing an association between a MHC phenotype and a disease, the frequencies of a MHC allele in the normal population and in the diseased population are used to calculate the relative risk. A relative risk greater than 1 is suggestive of an association. Frequencies of a number of MHC alleles vary among different ethnic groups. Therefore, an established MHC allele-disease association in one ethnic group does not necessarily apply to other ethnic groups. For instance, there is a strong association between HLA-B27 and ankylosing spondylitis among people of European descent. However, this strong association does not exist among African Americans and Lebanese (Abdelnoor and Abdelnoor, 1993; Abdelnoor and Heneine, 1985; Malak and Abdelnoor, 1997).

Macrophage Activation (Neopterin)

Another association between immune system activation and cancer-related fatigue or chronic fatigue syndrome has been put forth around monocytes/macrophages and the interaction between the immune and nervous systems. Human monocyte/macrophages, in response to cytokines such as interferon-gamma, produce and release a compound known as neopterin (Werner et al., 1990; Furukawa et al., 1995). Humans and primates uniquely share substantial amounts of neopterin in body fluids, and neopterin has been used as a marker for monocyte/macrophage activation in these species (Barak, Mezerbach, and Gruener, 1989; Fuchs et al., 1988). Neopterin derivatives belong to the cytotoxic arsenal of the activated human macrophage, and in high doses increase oxidative stress through enhancement of radical-mediated effector functions and programmed cell death by TNF-alpha, although it has an opposite effect at low doses (Baier-Bitterlich et al., 1995; Fuchs et al., 1994; Fuchs, Baier-Bitterlich, and Wachter, 1995). Serum and urinary neopterin levels are significantly elevated in cancer patients (Melichar et al., 1995; Iwagaki et al., 1995; Kuzmits, Ludwig, et al., 1986; Rokos et al., 1980; Hausen and Wachter, 1982; Mura et al., 1986; Stea, Halpern, and Smith, 1981; Andondonskaja-Renz and Zeitler, 1984). Moreover, Park and colleagues (1995) documented that measurement of preoperative serum neopterin levels helped to discriminate between benign and malignant tumors and was related to ovarian cancer survival. Urinary neopterin levels in cancer patients correlate significantly with urinary *N*-acetyl-beta-D-glucosaminidase and urinary zinc, both indicators of renal tubular dysfunction (Melichar et al., 1995).

A negative correlation between serum levels of neopterin and those of the neurotransmitter precursor amino acid tryptophan was also found among cancer and AIDS patients, an observation which indicates activity of indoleamine 2,3-dioxygenase, a tryptophan-degrading enzyme (Iwagaki et al., 1995). The enzyme converts L-tryptophan to L-kynurenine, kynurenic acid, and quinolinic acid. Quinolinic acid is a neurotoxic metabolite that accumulates within the central nervous system following immune activation and is also a sensitive marker for the presence of immune activation within the central nervous system (Heyes et al., 1995; Shaskan et al., 1992; Saito, 1995). Direct conversion of L-tryptophan into quinolinic acid by brain tissue occurs in conditions of central nervous system inflammation, but not by normal brain tissue, a process that may be related to fatigue in post-polio syndrome and cancer-related fatigue (Heyes et al., 1995; Andondonskaja-Retz and Zeitler, 1984). Elevated serum levels of neopterin correlate with the presence of brain lesion and with neurological and psychiatric symptoms in patients with AIDS dementia complex (Lutgendorf, Antoni, et al., 1995; Lutgendorf, Klimas, et al., 1995; Sonnerborg et al., 1990). It is worth noting in this context that Buchwald, Umali, and colleagues (1996) found subcortical lesions consistent with edema and demyelination by magnetic resonance scans in 78 percent of CFS patients as compared to 20 percent of controls.

Buchwald and colleagues (1997) and Chao and colleagues (1990, 1991) found elevated levels of neopterin in CFS patients, and Linde and colleagues (1992) and Patarca, Lutgendorf, and colleagues (1994) found no difference. A report of nine CFS cases showed significantly elevated serum neopterin levels in association with high cognitive difficulty scale scores (Lutgendorf, Antoni, et al., 1995; Lutgendorf, Klimas, et al., 1995), and neopterin levels have been shown to correlate with levels of many other medications that have been found to be dysregulated in chronic fatigue syndrome, including members of the tumor necrosis factor family (Buchwald et al., 1997; Patarca, Lutgendorf, et al., 1994; Patarca, Klimas, Sandler, et al., 1995).

Viral Reactivation and Microbial Attack

Viruses

Several families of viruses have been studied in association with fatiguing illnesses, and it has been proposed that reactivation of certain viruses may play a role in their pathophysiology but may not be their primary cause (Ablashi, Handy, et al., 1998; Ablashi, Josephs, et al., 1998; Ablashi et al., 2000; Archard et al., 1988; Bode, Fersyt, and Czech, 1993; Braun, Dominguez, and Pellett, 1997; Cuende et al., 1997; DeFreitas et al., 1991; Fohlman, Friman, and Tuvemo, 1997; Galbraith, Nairn, and Clements, 1997; Gunn et al., 1997; Hellinger et al., 1988; Hill, 1996; Holmes et al., 1997; Jacobson et al., 1997; Jones, 1985; Jones et al., 1985; Kitani et al., 1996; Levine, 1999; Levy et al., 1990; Martin, 1996a,b, 1997; Mendoza Montero, 1990; Miller et al., 1991; Nakaya et al., 1996, 1997; Salvatore et al., 1998; Sauder et al., 1996; Schmaling and Jones, 1996; Stitz et al., 1993; White et al., 1998).

Endogenous retroviruses. Viral reactivation has also been proposed to play a role in cancer and fatigue. For instance, conserved and analogous transmembrane segments of retroviral and hepatitis virus envelope proteins (Cianciolo, Kipnis, and Snyderman, 1984; Elfassi, Patarca, and Haseltine, 1986; Patarca and Haseltine, 1984) can down-regulate TNF-alpha gene expression through induction of de novo synthesis of transcription suppressors (Haraguchi et al., 1993) and dampen immune responses in general, thus increasing susceptibility to neoplasia development and progression (Foulds et al., 1993; Harrell et al., 1986; Oostendorp et al., 1992; Snyderman and Cianciolo, 1984; Stöger et al., 1993). Induction of endogenous retroviral-like particles by several agents could also favor neoplastic growth and fatigue (Anders et al., 1994; Fiegl et al., 1995).

The relevance of endogenous retroviral components is underscored by experiments with components of exogenous retroviruses. For instance, intracerebroventricular administration of the outer segment, gp120, of the HIV envelope protein induces dose-dependent enhanced non-rapid eye movement and rapid eye movement (REM) sleep without affecting body temperature. Heat inactivation of gp120 results in the loss of its sleep- and fatigue-promoting effects (Opp et al., 1996). Gp120 also stimulates production of sleep- and fatigue-promoting cytokines such as interleukin-1beta and TNF-alpha from human and rat glial cells in vitro and in freely moving rats (Opp et al., 1996).

Although some studies looked into a possible link between retroviruses and chronic fatigue syndrome, no conclusive evidence has been garnered (DeFreitas et al., 1991; Gunn et al., 1997).

Lentiviruses. Although structures consistent in size, shape, and character with various stages of a lentivirus replicative cycle were observed by electron microscopy in twelve-day peripheral blood lymphocyte cultures from ten of seventeen CFS patients and not in controls, attempts to identify a lymphoid phenotype containing these structures failed and the results of reverse transcriptase assay from culture supernatant fluids were equivocal (Holmes et al., 1997).

Chronic fatigue is a common and troubling symptom in patients with HIV infection and AIDS, and it results in significant disability with an adverse impact on activities of daily living and overall quality of life (Breitbart et al., 1998; Rose et al., 1998; Soucy, 1997; Walker, McGown, et al., 1997). The etiology of HIV infection-associated fatigue remains complex and is most likely multifactorial. Recognizable causes and correlates for which interventions can be beneficial include anemia, pain, infection/fever, hormonal or nutritional deficiencies, depression/anxiety, sleep disturbances, and excessive inactivity or rest (Breitbart et al., 1998; Rose et al., 1998; Soucy, 1997; Walker, McGown, et al., 1997). It should also be noted that against a background of HIV-infection-related fatigue, some forms of therapy such as that with interleukin-2 dramatically increase the experience of fatigue (Grady, Anderson, and Chase, 1998). Poor sleep, daytime fatigue, and loss of cognitive ability exist during all stages of HIV infection, symptoms that worsen with disease progression. Data from several research groups support a role of somnogenic inflammation-related peptides whose levels are elevated in HIV infection, such as TNF-alpha. Although the literature is in conflict regarding an effect of HIV infection on growth hormone secretion, growth hormone axis dysregulation and treatment with growth hormone may be important in some complications of HIV infection, such as the wasting syndrome (Darko, Mitler, and Miller, 1998). Fatigue declines significantly among responders to testosterone therapy in HIV seropositive men with clinical hypogonadism (Wagner and Rabkin, 1998; Wagner, Rabkin, and Rabkin, 1998).

Herpesviruses. Viruses from the herpesvirus family have also been associated with both cancer and fatigue (Braun, Dominguez, and Pellett, 1997; Fox et al., 1992; Pisa, Cannon, et al., 1992; Iyengar et al., 1991; Mendoza Montero, 1990; Mitterer et al., 1995; Rea et al., 2001; Tedeschi et al., 1995; Whelton, Salit, and Moldofsky, 1992). For instance, acute illness secondary to infection with Epstein-Barr virus, a herpesvirus that is associated with Burkitt's lymphoma and nasopharyngeal carcinoma in certain geographic locations, is characterized by nonspecific somatic and psychological symptoms, particularly fatigue and malaise (Bennett et al., 1998; Katz et al., 2001; Stephan et al., 2001; Tosato et al., 1985; Vujosevic and Gvozdenovic, 1994). Although improvement in several symptoms occurs rapidly, fatigue commonly remains a prominent complaint at four weeks, and resolution of fatigue is associated with improvement in cell-mediated immunity. A shift to humoral immunity predominance in EBV-infected patients would favor reactivation of the virus and the possible concurrent recurrence of fatigue.

Serologically proven acute infectious illness secondary to Epstein-Barr virus is associated with a range of nonspecific somatic and psychological symptoms, particularly fatigue and malaise rather than anxiety and depression (Bennett et al., 1998). Although improvement in several symptoms occurs rapidly, fatigue commonly remains a prominent complaint at four weeks, and resolution of fatigue is associated with improvement in cell-mediated immunity. A prospective cohort study of 250 primary care patients also revealed a higher incidence and longer duration of an acute fatigue syndrome and a higher prevalence of chronic fatigue syndrome after glandular fever as compared to after an ordinary upper respiratory tract infection (White et al., 1998). In another study, anti-EBV titers were higher among CFS patients and were associated with being more symptomatic (Schmaling and Jones, 1996). However, testing of 548 chronically fatigued individuals, including patients with chronic fatigue syndrome, for antibodies to thirteen viruses (herpes simplex virus 1 and 2, rubella, adenovirus, human herpesvirus 6, Epstein-Barr virus, cytomegalovirus, and Coxsackie B virus types 1 through 6) in patients found no consistent differences in any of the seroprevalences compared with controls (Buchwald, Ashley, et al., 1996).

In terms of other herpesviruses, the prevalence of antibodies directed against human herpesvirus 6 is higher in sera from patients with certain malignancies such as B-cell lymphomas, or with Sjögren's syndrome, sarcoidosis, AIDS, or chronic fatigue syndrome (Ablashi, Josephs, et al., 1998). Some studies suggest an association between human herpesvirus 6 (HHV-6) (*Roseolovirus* genus of the betaherpesvirus subfamily) and chronic fatigue syndrome (Braun, Dominguez, and Pellett, 1997; Cuende et al., 1997; Levy et al., 1990; Marsh et al., 1996). One study found that a high proportion of CFS patients (50 percent by antibody testing and up to 80 percent by nested-PCR detection of viral DNA but not RNA) were infected with HHV-6 but with low viral load. The results do not support HHV-6 reactivation in CFS patients (Cuende et al., 1997). Other studies have addressed a possible association between HHV-7 and chronic fatigue syndrome. Use of the supernatant fluid from HHV-7 infected cells as antigen in immunoassays yielded high and low HHV-7 antibody titers in sera from chronic fatigue patients and healthy donors as controls, respectively (Ablashi, Handy, et al., 1998).

The role of herpesviruses and their reactivation in chronic fatiguing illnesses remains to be elucidated.

Stealth viruses. Cloned DNA obtained from the culture of an African green monkey, simian cytomegalovirus-derived stealth virus contains multiple discrete regions of significant sequence homology to portions of known human cellular genes (Martin, 1998). The stealth virus has also been cultured from several CFS patients, and a cytopathic stealth virus was also cultured from the cerebrospinal fluid of a nurse with chronic fatigue syndrome. The findings lend support to the possibility of replicative RNA forms of certain stealth viruses (Martin, 1997). Review of the clinical histories and brain biopsy findings of three patients with severe stealth virus encephalopathy showed that the patients initially developed symptoms consistent with chronic fatigue syndrome (Martin, 1996b). One patient has remained in a vegetative state for several years, while the other two patients have shown significant, although incomplete, recovery. Histological and electron microscopic studies have revealed vacuolated cells with distorted nuclei and various cytoplasmic inclusions suggestive of incomplete viral expression. No significant inflammatory response was noted. Viral cultures provided further evidence of stealth viral infections occurring in these patients (Martin, 1996b). Partial sequencing of stealth virus segments isolated from a CFS patient revealed a fragmented genome and sequence microheterogeneity, observations which suggest that both the processivity and the fidelity of replication of the viral genome are defective (Martin, 1996a). An unstable viral genome may provide a potential mechanism of recovery from stealth viral illness.

Enteroviruses. Enteroviruses (Coxsackie virus A and B, echovirus, poliovirus) belong to a group of small RNA viruses, picornaviruses, which are widespread in nature. Enteroviruses cause a number of well-known diseases and symptoms in humans, from subclinical infections and the common cold to poliomyelitis with paralysis. Serologic and molecular biology techniques have demonstrated that enteroviral genomes, in certain situations, persist after the primary infection, which is often silent. Persistent enteroviral infection or recurrent infections and/or virus-stimulated autoimmunity might contribute to the development of diseases with hitherto unexplained pathogenesis, such as post-polio syndrome, dilated cardiomyopathy, juvenile (type 1) diabetes, and possibly some cases diagnosed as chronic fatigue syndrome (Archard et al., 1988; Fohlman, Friman, and Tuvemo, 1997; Galbraith, Nairn, and Clements, 1997; Hill, 1996; Miller et al., 1991). However, several studies have failed to document persistent enteroviral infection in chronic fatigue syndrome (Buchwald, Ashley, et al., 1996).

Parvovirus B19. The spectrum of disease caused by parvovirus B19 has been expanding in recent years because of improved and more sensitive methods of detection. Some evidence suggests that chronic infection occurs in patients who are apparently not immunosuppressed. A young woman with recurrent fever and a syndrome indistinguishable from chronic fatigue syndrome was found to have persistent parvovirus B19 viremia, which was detectable by PCR despite the presence of IgM and IgG antibodies to parvovirus B19 (Jacobson et al., 1997). Testing of samples from this patient suggested that in some low viremic states, parvovirus B19 DNA is detectable by nested PCR in plasma but not in serum. The patient's fever resolved with the administration of intravenous immunoglobulin.

Ross River virus. A prospective investigation revealed that serologically proven acute infectious illness secondary to Ross River virus is associated with a range of nonspecific somatic and psychological symptoms, particularly fatigue and malaise rather than anxiety and depression (Bennett et al., 1998). Although improvement in several symptoms occurs rapidly, fatigue commonly remains a prominent complaint at four weeks. Resolution of fatigue is associated with improvement in cell-mediated immunity as measured by delayed-type hypersensitivity skin responses.

Borna disease virus. Borna disease virus (BDV) is a neurotropic, nonsegmented, negative-sense, single-stranded RNA virus. Natural infection with this virus has been reported to occur in horses and sheep. Recent epidemiological data suggest that BDV may be closely associated with neuropsychiatric disease (depression and schizophrenia) in humans (Bode, Fersyt, and Czech, 1993; Kitani et al., 1996; Levine, 1999; Nakaya et al., 1996, 1997; Salvatore et al., 1998; Sauder et al., 1996; Stitz et al., 1993). In Japanese patients with chronic fatigue syndrome, the prevalence of BDV infection is up to 34 percent. Furthermore, anti-BDV antibodies and BDV RNA were detected in a family cluster with chronic fatigue syndrome. These results suggest that BDV or a related agent may contribute to or initiate chronic fatigue syndrome, although the single etiologic role of BDV is unlikely (Bode, Fersyt, and Czech, 1993; Kitani et al., 1996; Levine, 1999; Nakaya et al., 1996, 1997; Salvatore et al., 1998; Sauder et al., 1996; Stitz et al., 1993).

Bacteria

It should be pointed out that besides viruses, bacteria or fragments thereof could play a role in fatigue etiology. For instance, lysozyme is an enzyme involved in resistance to infections that is able to digest bacterial proteins into fragments. Fragments of bacterial cell wall peptidoglycan known as muramyl peptides exert many effects on the immune system and the central nervous system, and appear to contribute to nonspecific resistance to infection, fever, fatigue, and the pathogenesis of bacterial infection (Burman et al., 1991).

Borrelia. Despite antibiotic treatment, a sequel of Lyme disease may be a post-Lyme disease syndrome (PLS), which is characterized by persistent arthralgia, fatigue, and neurocognitive impairment (Bujak, Weinstein, and

Dornbush, 1996; Diamantis, 1996; Ellenbogen, 1997; Ravdin et al., 1996). Although patients with chronic fatigue syndrome and post-Lyme disease syndrome share many features, including symptoms of severe fatigue and cognitive impairment, patients with PLS show greater cognitive deficits than patients with chronic fatigue syndrome compared with healthy controls. This is particularly apparent among patients with post-Lyme disease syndrome without premorbid psychiatric illness (Gaudino, Coyle, and Krupp, 1997). Schutzer and Natelson (1999) pointed out that CFS patients lacking antecedent signs of Lyme disease—erythema migrans, Bell's palsy, or large-joint arthritis—are not likely to have laboratory evidence of *Borrelia* infection. Treib and colleagues (2000) conducted a prospective double-blind study of 156 healthy young males testing for *Borrelia* antibodies. Seropositive subjects who had never suffered from clinically manifest Lyme borreliosis or neuroborreliosis showed chronic fatigue and malaise significantly more often than seronegative recruits. Treib and colleagues (2000) therefore proposed examining whether an antibiotic therapy should be considered in patients with chronic fatigue syndrome or chronic fatiguing illnesses and positive *Borrelia* serology.

Chlamydia. Some authors have proposed a link between *Chlamydia* bacteria and chronic fatigue syndrome (Bottero, 2000; Chia and Chia, 1999).

Mycoplasma. Multiplex PCR analysis to detect the presence of *Mycoplasma* genus DNA sequences in 100 CFS patients revealed that 52 percent were infected with *Mycoplasma* genus as compared to 15 percent of healthy individuals. *Mycoplasma fermentans, M. hominis,* and *M. penetrans* were detected in 32, 9, and 6 percent of the CFS patients, but only in 8, 3, and 2 percent of the healthy control subjects, respectively (Choppa et al., 1998). An analysis based on the use of forensic polymerase chain reaction or polymerase chain reaction found that 52 to 63 percent of chronic fatigue syndrome/fibromyalgia patients (from a total of 1,000) had mycoplasmal infections, whereas 9 to 15 percent of 450 controls tested positive (Choppa et al., 1998; Nicolson, Nasralla, and Haier, 1998; Nicolson et al., 2000; Vojdani et al., 1998; Vojdani and Franco, 1999). Nasralla, Haier, and Nicolson (1999) found multiple mycoplasmal infections by PCR in forty-eight of ninety-one chronic fatigue syndrome/fibromyalgia patients with a positive serological test for mycoplasmal infection, with double infections being detected in 30.8 percent and triple infections in 22 percent, but only when one of the species was *Mycoplasma pneumoniae* or *M. fermentans.* Patients infected with more than one mycoplasmal species generally had a longer history of illness, suggesting that they may have contracted additional mycoplasmal infection with time (Nasralla, Haier, and Nicolson, 1999).

Rickettsiae. Several links have been proposed since 1991 between chronic fatigue syndrome and chronic Rickettsial infection (Jadin JG, 1962; Jadin CL, 1999, 2000), including the following:

1. Chronic fatigue syndrome and Rickettsial infection present with a similar symptomatology.
2. Chronic fatigue syndrome was reported in Incline, Nevada, in 1984 (Mauff and Gon, 1991) and developed into epidemic proportions. Rocky Mountain spotted fever originated from the same place in 1916 (Jadin, 1953). Drury described the spirochete *Borrelia duttoni,* in 1702 as causing recurrent Malgach fever. In 1975, *Borrelia burgdorferi* was found in Connecticut, giving birth to a new name, Lyme disease.
3. A link has been established between chronic fatigue syndrome and Florence Nightingale (Hennessy, 1994), who worked surrounded by lice, fleas, and ticks during the Crimean War. Soldiers were presenting with epidemic typhus, the common disease of wars, regularly reported since the time of Hannibal.
4. Lymphocyte studies conducted on sheep with tickborne diseases (Woldehiwe, 1991), chronic fatigue syndrome patients, and patients with Q-fever endocarditis (Drancourt and Levy, 1990) have shown similar results.
5. Chronic fatigue syndrome was proposed to overlap with post-Q-fever syndrome (Marmion et al., 1996).

Q-fever is a zoonotic condition caused by *Coxiella burnetti* and associated with high levels of interleukin-6. Although improvement in several symptoms occurs rapidly, resolution of fatigue takes longer and is associated with improvement in cell-mediated immunity as measured by delayed-type hypersensitivity skin responses (Penttila et al., 1998). Several authors claim that the recovery rate associated with treatment of chronic fatigue syndrome patients with tetracyclines is 84 to 96 percent (Bottero, 2000; Jadin, 1998; Tarbleton, 1995).

Yersinia. A study based on the detection of antibodies to various *Yersinia* outer membrane proteins (YOPs) in serum samples from eighty-eight chronic fatigue syndrome patients and seventy-seven healthy age- and gender-matched controls concluded that *Yersinia enterocolitica* is unlikely to play a major role in the etiology of chronic fatigue syndrome (Swanink et al., 1998).

Fungi

Sorenson (1999) places chronic fatigue syndrome among the diseases associated with inhalation of fungal spores.

Reaction to Foreign Substances: The Case of Silicone
Breast Implants

A comparative examination of complaints of patients with breast cancer with and without silicone implants revealed that many of the symptoms examined, such as arthralgias, myalgias, and fatigue, are present in middle-aged women regardless of silicone implants and underlying disease (Berner et al., 2002). Moreover, although some authors in older studies have suggested a link with fibromyalgia or soft tissue rheumatism (Bridges et al., 1996; Cuellar et al., 1995; Fuchs, Johnson, and Sergent, 1995; Levenson, Greenberger, and Murphy, 1996; Solomon, 1994; Vasey, 1997; Vasey and Aziz, 1995; Young et al., 1995), immunologic and other sequels of silicone breast implantation such as collagen vascular diseases or fibromyalgia have not been confirmed in large studies and reviews (Blackburn, Grotting, and Everson, 1997; Brown, Lagone, and Brinton, 1998; Friis et al., 1997; Lai et al., 2000; Levine et al., 2000; Martin, 1999; Nyren et al., 1998; Peters et al., 1997; Thomas et al., 1997; Wolfe, 1999; Wolfe and Anderson, 1999).

Although some authors have also suggested a link with chronic fatigue syndrome, immunological sequels of silicone breast implantation have not been confirmed in large studies either. Nonetheless, there is a report of a fifty-five-year-old woman who developed severe fatigue, peripheral blood eosinophilia, and hyperimmunoglobulinemia A after rupture of a silicone breast implant during closed manual manipulation to lyse fibrotic tissue. The effects of silicone breast implant rupture lasted over nineteen years (Levenson, Greenberger, and Murphy, 1996).

Several reports have discussed the possible breast implant-associated induction of autoimmunity, in particular antipolymer antibodies whose presence has also been reported in fibromyalgia (Angell, 1997; Edlavitch, 1997; Ellis, Hardt, and Atkinson, 1997; Everson and Blackburn, 1997; Korn, 1997; Lamm, 1997; Romano, 1996; Silverman et al., 1996). However, many studies have failed to find evidence for autoimmunity or other immunological abnormalities. For instance, Blackburn, Grotting, and Everson (1997) found that the levels of interleukin-6, interleukin-8, TNF-alpha, soluble intercellular adhesion molecule-1, and soluble interleukin-2 receptor were not different in silicone breast implant disease patients from those seen in normal subjects and were significantly less than those seen when examining chronic inflammatory disorders such as rheumatoid arthritis or systemic lupus erythematosus.

Although Young and colleagues (1995) have found a higher frequency of HLA-DR53 among symptomatic breast implant patients and Bridges and colleagues (1996) reported 5 percent positivity for antinuclear antibodies among silicone breast implant patients, these findings have not panned out in larger analyses. Nonetheless, some studies have found that breast implants appear to be more common in patients with fibromyalgia than in those without it. This observation has led some authors to postulate that a common predisposing set of psychosocial characteristics may be shared between those who have fibromyalgia and those who undergo silicone breast implantation (Wolfe and Anderson, 1999).

Berner and colleagues (2002) performed a matched-pair analysis of ninety-six women with breast cancer (thirty-two with silicone implants and sixty-four without implants) and found no correlation between silicone implants and the symptoms of chronic fatigue syndrome or any other described silicone-induced disease. The authors concluded that the symptoms reported are present with the same frequencies in middle-aged women regardless of silicone implants and underlying disease. Moreover, although uncontrolled case series have reported neurological problems believed to be associated with silicone breast implants, one review report (Rosenberg, 1996) failed to find any evidence that silicone breast implants are causally related to the development of any neurological diseases. This study found that although neurological symptoms were frequently endorsed, including fatigue (82 percent), memory loss and other cognitive impairment (76 percent), and generalized myalgias (66 percent), most patients (66 percent) had normal neurological examinations. Findings reported as abnormal were mild and usually subjective, including sensory abnormalities in 23 percent, mental status abnormalities in 13 percent, and reflex changes in 8 percent. No pattern of laboratory abnormalities was seen, either in combination or in attempts to correlate them with the clinical situation. Laboratory studies appeared to be randomly chosen without an attempt to confirm or correlate with a particular diagnosis.

Rosenberg (1996) also reported that diagnoses by physicians endorsing the concept that silicone breast implants cause illness included "human adjuvant disease" in all cases, memory loss and other cognitive impairment ("silicone encephalopathy") and/or "atypical neurological disease syndrome" in 73 percent, "atypical neurological multiple sclerosis-like syndrome" in 8 percent, chronic inflammatory demyelinating polyneuropathy in 23 percent, and some other type of peripheral neuropathy in 18 percent. There was no coherence in making these diagnoses; the presence of any symptoms in these women was sufficient to make these diagnoses. After review of the data, no neurological diagnosis could be made in 82 percent. Neurological symptoms could be explained in some cases by depression (sixteen cases), fibromyalgia (nine cases), radiculopathy (seven cases), anxiety disorders (four cases), multiple sclerosis (four cases), multifocal motor neuropathy (one case), carpal tunnel syndrome (one case), dermatomyositis (one case), and other psychiatric disorders (one case).

Environmental Toxins

Environmental toxins have been studied as potential causes of chronic fatigue syndrome.

Chlorinated Hydrocarbons

A study of the potential relationships between chlorinated hydrocarbon contamination in human serum and red/white blood cell profiles and an assessment of cellular response patterns to high and low serum organochlorine levels revealed that patients with unexplained and persistent fatigue had significantly higher levels of DDE (1,1-dichloro-2,2-bis (p-chlorophenyl) ethene) and different specific blood cell responses to organochlorines compared with controls. The red cell distribution width was elevated in the high DDE group and it was the most important discriminant parameter for differentiating between the high and low DDE groups (Dunstan, Donohoe, et al., 1996; Dunstan, Roberts, et al., 1996). Nonetheless, there is no clear association between chronic fatigue syndrome and chlorinated hydrocarbons.

Dental Amalgam Fillings

In a study of ninety-nine self-referred patients complaining of multiple somatic and mental symptoms attributed to dental amalgam fillings, one-third of the patients reported symptoms of chronic fatigue syndrome compared with none of eighty in a dental control sample (patients with dental amalgam fillings seen in an ordinary dental practice) and only 2 and 6 percent, respectively, in the two clinical comparison samples (ninety-three and ninety-nine patients with known chronic medical disorders seen in alternative and ordinary medical family practices, respectively). The authors attributed the higher frequency of chronic fatigue syndrome symptomatology to the observation of higher mean neuroticism and lower lie scores in the dental amalgam group as compared to the comparison groups (Malt et al., 1997). In contrast to the latter conclusion, another report described a patient who suffered from several complaints, which were attributed to her amalgam fillings, and analysis of mercury in plasma and urine showed unexpectedly high concentrations, 63 and 223 nmol/L, respectively. Following removal of the amalgam fillings, the urinary excretion of mercury became gradually normalized and her symptoms declined (Langworth and Stromberg, 1996).

Lead Poisoning

Lead poisoning can also masquerade as chronic fatigue syndrome (Mesch, Lowenthal, and Coleman, 1996).

ENDOCRINE FACTORS

Fatigue states share many of the somatic symptom characteristics seen in recognized endocrine disorders (Anisman et al., 1996; Baschetti, 1997c; Demitrack, 1997, 1998; Jones, Wadler, and Hupart, 1998; Poteliakhoff, 1998; Sterzl and Zamrazil, 1996). Moreover, defects in the hypothalamic-pituitary axis have been observed in chronic fatiguing illnesses and in autoimmune, rheumatic, and chronic inflammatory diseases, all of which are commonly associated with fatigue. For instance, prolactin levels are often elevated in patients with systemic lupus erythematosus and other autoimmune diseases, post-polio fatigue syndrome, and chronic fatigue syndrome (Anisman et al., 1996; Demitrack, 1997, 1998). Patients with chronic fatigue syndrome with chronic facial pain show a high comorbidity with other stress-associated syndromes such as interstitial cystitis. The clinical overlap between these conditions may reflect a shared underlying pathophysiologic basis involving dysregulation of the hypothalamic-pituitary-adrenal stress hormone axis in predisposed individuals (Korszun et al., 1998).

Although hypothyroidism with a modest elevation of thyroid-stimulating hormone has been reported in approximately 7 percent of CFS cases (Borysiewicz et al., 1986; Buchwald and Komaroff, 1991; Kaslow, Rucker, and Onishi, 1989; Kroenke et al., 1988; Lane, Manu, and Matthews, 1988; Prieto et al., 1989) and several studies have documented the presence of antithyroid antibodies (Behan, Behan, and Bell, 1985; Dinarello, 1988; Tobi et al., 1982), CFS patients usually remained fatigued after correction of their hypothyroidism (Buchwald and Komaroff, 1991). Interleukin-1 inhibits tyrotropin release (Weinstein, 1987), and several cytokines, including interleukin-1 (Weinstein, 1987), interleukin-6, and interferon-alpha (Jones, Wadler, and Hupart, 1998), have been shown to be cytotoxic to thyroid cells, properties that could mediate the hypothyroidism seen in some CFS cases. In this respect, fatigue occurs in more than 70 percent of patients treated with interferon-alpha and may be associated with the development of immune-mediated endocrine diseases, in particular hypothyroidism and hypothalamic-pituitary-adrenal axis-related hormonal deficiencies (Jones, Wadler, and Hupart, 1998).

A case-control study (Harlow et al., 1998) analyzed data collected in self-administered questionnaires on menstrual, reproductive, and medical histories of 149 women being seen for nongynecological conditions with and without chronic fatigue syndrome. Women with chronic fatigue syndrome reported increased gynecologic complications and a lower incidence of premenstrual symptomatology, both of which could be explained by the higher number of self-reported cases of irregular cycles, periods of amenorrhea, and sporadic bleeding between menstrual periods, and the higher frequency of histories of polycystic ovarian syndrome, hirsutism, and ovarian cysts among women with chronic fatigue syndrome as compared to controls.

Besides fatigue, many of the adverse effects commonly associated with chemotherapy, such as nausea and vomiting, are also characteristic of adrenal insufficiency. It is conceivable that chemotherapy drugs may directly or indirectly impact the activity of the hypothalamic-pituitary-adrenal axis. In this respect, in a study of twenty-three chemotherapy-naive women with histologically confirmed ovarian cancer, Morrow, Hickok, and colleagues (2002) reported a reduction in serum levels of the adrenal hormone cortisol after platinum-based chemotherapy for cancer. Because the reduction in cortisol was seen only in the presence of the cytotoxic drug, it is likely that the effect of the drug is direct and does not involve overt psychological or circadian mechanisms. The possible role of these factors in some forms of cancer-related fatigue is discussed in the following sections.

Hypothalamic-Pituitary-Adrenal Stress System

The diagnosis and treatment of cancer and living with cancer itself can be associated with significant stress. The word *stress* is derived from the Latin *stringere,* which means to strangle or tightly bind (Jencks, 1977). Although stress increasingly has become a part of the vocabulary of the physician, the mental health professional, and the layperson, there is a lack of consensus about its precise definition (Elliot and Eisdorfer, 1982). McLean (1979) stated that stress is the reaction to any physical, psychological, emotional, cognitive, or behavioral sources of stimulation that result in an emergency fight-or-flight response. Sklar and Anisman (1981) defined stress as the psychophysiological outcome of exposure to a demanding or harmful condition, and they found that tumor growth is intensified after long exposure to uncontrollable stress. Basso and colleagues (1992) also found that chronic variable stress facilitates tumor growth.

Irie and colleagues (Irie, Asami, Nagata, Miyata, and Kasai, 2001) investigated the relationship between work-related factors, including psychological stress, and the formation of 8-hydroxydeoxyguanosine (8-OH-dG), a molecule that reflects oxidative DNA damage and therefore is potentially a risk factor for occupational carcinogenesis. Fifty-four nonsmoking and nondrinking workers were chosen to exclude the influence of cigarette smoking and alcohol drinking, which have associations with the formation of 8-OH-dG. Levels of 8-OH-dG in female, but not in male, subjects were significantly related to perceived workload, perceived psychological stress, and the impossibility of alleviating stress. The authors concluded that, at least in female workers, psychological stress and perceived overwork appear to be related to the pathogenesis of cancer via the formation of 8-OH-dG. The results were confirmed in another study by the same group in 362 healthy workers (Irie, Asami, Nagata, Ikeda, et al., 2001) which also revealed that the levels of 8-OH-dG increased reliably in the female subjects who had poor stress-coping behaviors, particularly wishful thinking strategy. There were also positive relationships of the 8-OH-dG levels to average working hours, a self-blame coping strategy, and recent loss of a close family member in male subjects. These findings among healthy adults not only evince a stress-cancer linkage, but also suggest possible sex differences in the mechanisms of stress-related cancer initiation (Irie, Asami, Nagata, Ikeda, et al., 2001; Irie, Asami, Nagata, Miyata, and Kasai, 2001).

Besides cancer, stress is also known to be a major contributor to coronary heart disease, lung ailments, accidental injuries, suicide, and infectious diseases (Charlesworth and Nathan, 1984; Kasl, Evans, and Niederman, 1979; Meyer and Haggarty, 1962). Therefore, interest is growing in the field of psychoneuroimmunology, a discipline that is contributing novel interventions for prevention and treatment of cancer and its associated manifestations.

As reviewed by Sadigh (2001), scientific research in the field on mind-body medicine suggests that there is a significant positive correlation between stress levels and a variety of complicating physical and psychological symptoms (Girdano, Everly, and Dusek, 1997). Some of the complications include fatigue, depression, panic attacks, gastrointestinal symptoms, and alcoholism (Selye, 1976). Sackheim and Weber (1982) noticed that a variety of conditions such as chronic pain, musculoskeletal pain syndrome, and rheumatic pain appeared to be significantly affected by chronic stress (Basso et al., 1992). Individuals with heightened catecholamine and cardiovascular reactions to stress are also more likely to show suppression in their immune functions in response to a twenty-minute laboratory stressor (Manuck et al., 1991). Meyer and Haggarty (1962) found that infectious diseases caused by common bacteria such as *Streptococcus* have been related to stress.

As an example of the interrelatedness of immune and central nervous systems, stress is known to decrease natural killer cell activity. Partly replicating previous data in healthy volunteers, Lekander, Fredrikson, and Wik (2000) found that natural killer cell activity in fibromyalgia patients correlated negatively with right hemisphere activity in the secondary somatosensory and motor cortices as well as the thalamus. Moreover, natural killer cell activity was negatively and bilaterally related to activity in the posterior cingulate cortex. These findings illustrate the premise that immune parameters are related to activity in brain areas involved in pain perception, emotion, and attention (Lekander, Fredrikson, and Wik, 2000). Natural killer cells, which are mostly large granular lymphocytes that are constitutively cytocidal against tumor-transformed and virus-infected cells (Patarca, Fletcher, and Podack, 1995), also have impaired activity in CFS patients (Barker et al., 1994; DuBois, 1986; Gupta and Vayuvegula, 1991; Kibler et al., 1985; Klimas et al., 1990; Morrison, Behan, and Behan, 1991; Ojo-Amaise, Conley, and Peters, 1994; See et al., 1997; Straus et al., 1985; Whiteside and Friberg, 1998).

Based on the interrelations of the immune, endocrine, and central nervous systems, some authors have entertained the possibility that stress could modulate these bodily systems to induce fatigue (Beh, 1997; Cleare and Wessely, 1996; Glaser and Kiecolt-Glaser, 1998; Korszun et al., 1998). Stress, whether psychological or physical, activates the hypothalamic-pituitary-adrenal axis and thereby leads to a variety of changes, including increased production of cortisol (Selye, 1982). The HPA axis begins with the hypothalamus, a major regulatory center in the brain that closely interacts with the master hormonal regulator, the pituitary gland, located at the base of the brain. The hypothalamus interacts with the pituitary gland via the production of the corticotropin-releasing factor. Once a stressful stimulus is perceived and corticotropin-releasing factor is released, the pituitary gland stimulates the outer layer of the adrenal gland (the adrenal cortex) through the secretion of adrenocorticotropic hormone. As a result of the stimulation of the adrenal cortex, specialized hormones known as glucocorticoids (such as cortisol and corticosterone) are poured into the bloodstream.

Acute stress in the form of excessive exercise and deprivation of food and sleep result in a falling ratio of dehydroepiandrosterone (DHEA) to cortisol. DHEA tends to promote cell-mediated immunity and restores immune functions in aged mice and humans through correction of dysregulated cytokine release (Daynes and Araneo, 1989; Daynes, Meikle, and Araneo, 1991; Daynes et al, 1990, 1993, 1995; Garg and Bondade, 1993; Morales et al., 1994; Suzuki, Suzuki, et al., 1991), while the glucocorticoid cortisol enhances humoral immunity (Fisher and Konig, 1991; Guida, O'Hehir, and Hawrylowicz, 1994; Padgett, Sheridan, and Loria, 1995; Wu et al., 1991). A falling ratio of DHEA to cortisol correlates directly with a fall in delayed-type hypersensitivity responsiveness (a cell-mediated immunity marker), and there is a simultaneous rise in serum immunoglobulin E levels, a humoral immunity marker (Bernton et al., 1995).

An example of the effect of acute stress on cell-mediated to humoral immunity predominance switching is the increase in the levels of antibody directed against Epstein-Barr virus among students reacting in a stressed manner to their exams. Epstein-Barr virus is usually controlled by cell-mediated immunity, and loss of control results in virus replication and increased antibody production by the body (Zwilling, Brown, and Pearl, 1992). As explained previously, viral reactivation can contribute to fatigue. Similarly, peripheral blood leukocytes from medical students during examination periods showed lower production of cytokines involved in cell-mediated immunity (Glaser et al., 1993). Cohen, Tyrrell, and Smith (1991) also described an association between psychosocial stressors, immunomodulation, and the incidence and progression of rhinovirus infections in healthy controls. Here, the rates of respiratory infections and clinical colds increased in a dose-response fashion with increases in psychological stress across all five of the cold viruses studied. Acute stress imposed by natural disasters has also been associated with exacerbation of chronic fatiguing illnesses (Lutgendorf, Antoni, et al., 1995; Lutgendorf, Klimas, et al., 1995).

Under conditions of chronic stress, the continued overstimulation of cortisol production may result in a depletion of cortisol which in turn may result in adrenal insufficiency. Symptoms include fatigue, weakness, diabetic-like symptoms, and immune dysfunction. Indeed, one of the most common debilitating symptoms of cortisol insufficiency is debilitating fatigue, followed by joint pain, muscle pain, swollen lymph nodes, allergic responses, and finally disturbances in mood and sleep (Baxter and Tyrell, 1981). In fact, patients with chronic fatigue syndrome or with fibromyalgia tend to have low circulating cortisol levels (Griep, Boersma, and De Kloet, 1993; Scott and Dinan, 1998; Strickland et al., 1998). In these cases hydrocortisone has been used as a therapeutic intervention with some improvement of symptoms; however, the degree of adrenal suppression precludes its practical use (McKenzie et al., 1998).

Patients with fibromyalgia or chronic fatigue syndrome with chronic facial pain show a high comorbidity with other stress-associated syndromes (irritable bowel syndrome, premenstrual syndrome, and interstitial cystitis). The clinical overlap between these conditions may reflect a shared underlying pathophysiologic basis involving dysregulation of the hypothalamic-pituitary-adrenal stress hormone axis in predisposed individuals (Anisman et al., 1996; Baschetti, 1996b, 1997c, 1999a,c-d; Demitrack, 1997, 1998; Heim, Ehlert, and Hellhammer, 2000; Jeffcoate, 1999; Jones, Wadler, and Hupart, 1998; Korszun et al., 1998; Poteliakhoff, 1998; Pruessner, Hellhammer, and Kirschbaum, 1999; Scott and Dinan, 1999; Scott, Medbak, and Dinan, 1999; Scott, Salahuddin, et al., 1999; Scott, The, et al., 1999; Sterzl and Zamzaril, 1996).

Several reports have provided replicated evidence of disruptions in the integrity of the hypothalamic-pituitary-adrenal axis in CFS patients. It is notable that the pattern of the alteration in the stress response apparatus is not reminiscent of the well-understood hypercortisolism of melancholic depression but, rather, suggests a sustained inactivation of central nervous system components of this system. In this respect, one report (Scott and Dinan, 1998) documented a significantly lower urinary free cortisol (UFC) excretion in CFS patients and a significantly higher UFC in patients with depression as compared to controls. A subgroup of CFS patients with comorbid depressive illness retained the pattern of UFC excretion of those with chronic fatigue syndrome alone, an observation that points to a different pathophysiological basis for depressive symptoms in chronic fatigue syndrome. A study (Strickland et al., 1998) further confirmed cortisol hyposecretion in saliva as well as plasma of CFS patients compared to patients with depression and controls.

Study of the detailed, pulsatile characteristics of the hypothalamic-pituitary-adrenal axis in CFS patients reveals a reduction of hypothalamic-pituitary-adrenal axis activity secondary, in part, to impaired central nervous system drive (Demitrack and Crofford, 1998). A diminished output of neurotrophic adrenocorticotropin hormone, in response to administration of 100 micrograms of ovine corticotropin-releasing hormone causing a reduced adrenocortical secretory reserve that is inadequately compensated for by adrenoreceptor up-regulation is suggested to explain the reduced cortisol production in CFS patients (Scott, Medbak, and Dinan, 1998b). Using the 1 microgram ACTH test, another study provided further evidence for a subtle pituitary-adrenal insufficiency (lower delta cortisol value) in CFS patients compared to controls (Scott, Medbak, and Dinan, 1998b). Measurement of adrenocorticotropin hormone and cortisol responses following the administration of the opiate antagonist naloxone revealed that naloxone-mediated activation of the hypothalamic-pituitary-adrenal axis is attenuated in chronic fatigue syndrome, an observation that renders excessive opioid inhibition of the hypothalamic-pituitary-adrenal axis an unlikely explanation for its dysregulation in this disorder (Scott et al., 1998).

Several studies disagree with these findings. One study (MacHale et al., 1998) found a significantly decreased diurnal change in cortisol levels, nonsignificant lower levels of morning cortisol, and higher levels of adrenocorticotropin hormone and evening cortisol among CFS patients as compared to controls. Although a relationship between adrenocorticotropical function and disability in chronic fatigue syndrome (general health and physical functioning, functional improvement over the past year, and current social functioning) was found, no causal connection was apparent. Another study (Young et al., 1998) failed to document a reduction in the basal activity of the hypothalamic-pituitary-adrenal axis in measurements of salivary and urinary cortisol over a twenty-four-hour period. One study (Wood et al., 1998) found slightly but significantly higher mean levels of salivary cortisol (hourly sampling over a sixteen-hour period) in CFS patients as compared to controls.

Other work also implicates alterations in central serotonergic tone in the overall pathophysiology of hypothalamic-pituitary-adrenal axis dysregulation (Sharpe, Hawton, Clements, and Cowen, 1997). One study (Dinan et al., 1997) found that release of adrenocorticotropin hormone (but not cortisol) in response to ipsapirone (20 mg orally) challenge was significantly blunted in patients with chronic fatigue syndrome and concluded that serotonergic activation of the hypothalamic-pituitary-adrenal axis is defective in chronic fatigue syndrome.

In terms of the growth hormone/insulin-like growth factor (IGF)-1 (somatomedin C) axis, one study found that, in contrast to patients with fibromyalgia, in whom levels of somatomedin C have been found to be reduced, levels in patients with chronic fatigue syndrome were found to be elevated. Thus, despite the clinical similarities between these two conditions, they may be associated with different abnormalities of sleep and/or of the somatotropic neuroendocrine axis (Bennett, Mayes, et al., 1997; Berwaerts, Moorkens, and Abs, 1998; Buchwald, Umali, and Stene, 1996). Another study (Allain et al., 1997) found attenuated basal levels of IGF-I and IGF-II in CFS patients and a reduced growth hormone response to hypoglycemia. Insulin levels were higher and IGF-binding protein-1 (IGFBP-1) levels were lower in CFS patients compared with controls. Unlike the latter reports, no significant differences were observed among any of the patient groups (chronic fatigue syndrome, fibromyalgia, and patients with both) and controls in the mean concentration of either IGF-I and IGFBP-1 in another study (Vara-Thorbeck et al., 1996).

The implications of observations of neuroendocrine dysfunction are areas of intense research and interesting correlations, and therapeutic interventions are being formulated. For instance, one group (Cannon et al., 1998) found that the previously described relationships between basal circulating neutrophil numbers and plasma progesterone concentrations, and between exercise-induced neutrophilia and urinary cortisol and plasma creatine kinase concentrations, in healthy women were not observed in CFS women. These observations suggest that normal endocrine influences on the circulating neutrophil pool may be disrupted in CFS patients. Moreover, the differential sensitivity of cytokine expression by CD4 T-cell subsets to glucocorticoids in CFS patients might explain an altered immunologic function in these patients (Visser et al., 1998).

Since both changes in endocrine and immune status variables are observed in chronic fatigue syndrome, it is noteworthy that during acute febrile illness immune-derived cytokines initiate an acute phase response, which is characterized by fever, inactivity, fatigue, anorexia, and catabolism. Profound neuroendocrine and metabolic changes also take place: acute phase proteins are produced in the liver, bone marrow function and the metabolic activity of leukocytes are greatly increased, and specific immune reactivity is suppressed. Defects in regulatory processes that are fundamental to immune disorders and inflammatory diseases may lie in the immune system, the neuroendocrine system, or both. Defects in the hypothalamic-pituitary-adrenal axis have been observed in autoimmune and rheumatic diseases and chronic inflammatory disease. Prolactin levels are often elevated in patients with systemic lupus erythematosus and other autoimmune diseases, whereas the bioactivity of prolactin is decreased in patients with rheumatoid arthritis. Levels of sex hormones and thyroid hormone are decreased during severe inflammatory disease. Defective neural regulation of inflammation likely plays a pathogenic role in allergy and asthma, in the symmetrical form of rheumatoid arthritis, and in gastrointestinal inflammatory disease.

A better understanding of neuroimmunoregulation holds the promise of new approaches to the treatment of immune and inflammatory diseases with the use of hormones, neurotransmitters, neuropeptides, and drugs that modulate these regulators (Anisman et al., 1996). For instance, an article (Bruno, Creange, and Frick, 1998) proposes a possible common pathophysiology and treatment with replacement of depleted brain dopamine for post-polio fatigue and chronic fatigue syndrome based on the clinically significant deficits on neuropsychologic tests of attention, histopathologic and neuroradiologic evidence of brain lesions, impaired activation of the hypothalamic-pituitary-adrenal axis, increased prolactin secretion, and EEG slow-wave activity seen in both conditions. Some therapeutic attempts have not yielded clear-cut results but have provided further insight into the neuroendocrinology of chronic fatigue syndrome. For instance, acute administration of the serotonin receptor agonist buspirone (0.5 mg/Kg orally) in eleven male patients with chronic fatigue syndrome and a group of matched healthy controls showed that CFS patients had significantly higher plasma prolactin concentrations and experienced more nausea in response to buspirone than did controls (Sharpe et al., 1996). However, the growth hormone response to buspirone did not distinguish CFS patients from controls. These data question whether the enhancement of buspirone-induced prolactin response in chronic fatigue syndrome is a consequence of increased sensitivity of post-synaptic serotonin receptors, but open the possibility that it could reflect changes in dopamine function (Sharpe et al., 1996). Although hydrocortisone treatment (13 mg/m^2 of body surface every morning and 3 mg/m^2 every afternoon for twelve weeks) in a randomized, placebo-controlled, double-blind therapeutic trial was associated with some improvement in symptoms of chronic fatigue syndrome (as assessed by the Wellness Scale), the degree of adrenal suppression (twelve out of thirty patients) precludes its practical use for chronic fatigue syndrome (McKenzie et al., 1998).

Changes in neuroendocrine transmitters such as serotonin, substance P, growth hormone, and cortisol suggest that dysregulation of the autonomic and neuroendocrine systems are associated with fibromyalgia (Bellometti and Galzigna, 1999; Bradley, McKendree-Smith, and Alarcon, 2000; Clauw and Chrousos, 1997; Crofford, Engleberg and Demitrack, 1996; Dessein et al., 2000; Griep et al., 1998; Heim, Ehlert, and Hellhammer, 2000; Millea and Holloway, 2000; Pillemer et al., 1997; Russell, 1998; Scott and Dinan, 1999). Almost all of the hormonal feedback mechanisms controlled by the hypothalamus are altered in fibromyalgia. This dysregulation is evinced by elevated basal values of adrenocorticotropic hormone, follicle-stimulating hormone (FSH), and cortisol, as well as lowered basal values of insulin-like growth factor-1 (IGF-1, somatomedin C), free triiodothyronine (FT3), and estrogen (Bennett, Mayes, et al., 1997; Clauw and Chrousos, 1997; Griep et al., 1998; Neeck, 2000; Riedel, Layka, and Neeck, 1998).

In fibromyalgia patients, the systemic administration of corticotropin-releasing hormone (CRH), growth hormone-releasing hormone (GHRH), thyrotropin-releasing hormone (TRH), and luteinizing hormone-releasing hormone (LHRH) leads to increased secretion of ACTH and prolactin, whereas the degree to which thyroid-stimulating hormone (TSH) can be stimulated is reduced (Neeck and Riedel, 1999; Netter and Hennig, 1998; Riedel, Layka, and Neeck, 1998). The stimulation of the hypophysis with LHRH in female fibromyalgia patients during their follicular phase results in a significantly reduced luteinizing hormone response (Neeck and Riedel, 1999; Riedel, Layka, and Neeck, 1998).

Based on these observations, it has been proposed that the alterations in set points of hormonal regulation that are typical for fibromyalgia patients can be explained as a primary stress activation of hypothalamic CRH neurons caused by chronic pain or other factors (Crofford and Demitrack, 1996; Lentjes et al., 1997; Neeck, 2000; Netter and Hennig, 1998; Oye, Morland, and Gustafsson, 1996; Stanton, 1999; Torpy and Chrousos, 1996;

Winfield, 1999). In addition to the stimulation of pituitary ACTH secretion, CRH activates somatostatin at the hypothalamic level, which in turn inhibits the release of GH and TSH at the hypophyseal level. The lowered estrogen levels could be accounted for both via an inhibitory effect of the CRH on the hypothalamic release of LHRH or via a direct CRH-mediated inhibition of the FSH-stimulated estrogen production in the ovary. Serotonin (5-HT), precursors such as tryptophan (5-HTP), drugs that release 5-HT or act directly on 5-HT receptors stimulate the hypothalamic-pituitary-adrenal axis, indicating a stimulatory serotonergic influence on HPA axis function. Therefore, activation of the HPA axis may reflect an elevated serotonergic tonus in the central nervous system of fibromyalgia patients.

Administration of interleukin-6 (3 µg/Kg of body weight subcutaneously), a cytokine capable of stimulating CRH, to thirteen female fibromyalgia patients yielded exaggerated norepinephrine responses and heart rate increases, as well as delayed ACTH release (Torpy et al., 2000). These observations are consistent with a defect in hypothalamic CRH neuronal function and abnormal regulation of the sympathetic nervous system. The excessive heart rate response after interleukin-6 injection in fibromyalgia patients may be unrelated to the increase in norepinephrine, or it may reflect an alteration in the sensitivity of cardiac beta-adrenoreceptors to norepinephrine. These responses to a physiologic stressor support the notion that fibromyalgia may represent a primary disorder of the stress system (Torpy et al., 2000).

Not all studies agree with the assessment of endocrine function described previously. For instance, in a study of fifteen premenopausal women with fibromyalgia, Samborski and colleagues (1996) failed to find significant differences in the levels of ACTH, substance P, and TSH in patients as compared to controls. Adler and colleagues (1999) reported that although twenty-four-hour urinary free cortisol levels and diurnal patterns of ACTH and cortisol were normal, as also found by Maes and colleagues (1998), there was a significant (approximately 30 percent) reduction in the ACTH and epinephrine responses to hypoglycemia in women with fibromyalgia compared with controls. Prolactin, norepinephrine, cortisol, and dehydroepiandrosterone responses to hypoglycemia were similar in the two study groups. In subjects with fibromyalgia, the epinephrine response to hypoglycemia correlated inversely with overall health status as measured by the fibromyalgia impact questionnaire. Adler and colleagues (1999) concluded that fibromyalgia patients have an impaired ability to activate the hypothalamic-pituitary portion of the hypothalamic-pituitary-adrenal axis as well as the sympathoadrenal system, leading to reduced ACTH and epinephrine responses to hypoglycemia.

The role of the hypothalamic-pituitary-adrenal axis and other related neuroendocrinological axes in cancer-related fatigue needs to be addressed in well-planned studies. However, as mentioned earlier, it is not a simple task, as evidenced by the contradictory results obtained by several studies within the context of different chronic fatiguing illnesses (Akkus, Delibas, and Tamer, 2000; Allain et al., 1997; Anderberg, 2000a; Anisman et al., 1996; Bennett, Mayes, et al., 1997; Bennett, Cook, et al., 1997; Berwaerts, Moorkens, and Alos, 1998; Buchwald, Umali, and Stene, 1996; Cleare et al., 2000; Crofford-Engleberg, and Demitrack, 1996; Crofford and Demitrack, 1996; De Becker et al., 1999; Demitrack, 1997; Demitrack and Crofford, 1998; Dinan et al., 1997; Hapidou and Rollman, 1998; Korszun et al., 2000; MacHale et al., 1998; Ostensen, Rugelsjoen, and Wigers, 1997; Patarca, 2000; Scott and Dinan, 1999; Raphael and Marbach, 2000; Scott, Medbak, and Dinan, 1999; Scott, Salahuddin, et al., 1999; Scott, The, et al., 1999; Sharpe et al., 1996; Sharpe, Hawton, Clements, and Cowen, 1997; Strickland et al., 1998; Torpy and Chrousos, 1996; Vara-Thorbeck et al., 1996; Wood et al., 1998; Young et al., 1998).

The complexity of establishing associations between endrocrinological changes and cancer-related fatigue stems from the fact that the latter changes vary according to the type of treatment and cancer present. Some changes show no association with fatigue. For instance, following chemotherapy or radiation therapy, a significant proportion of men have biochemical evidence of Leydig cell dysfunction, defined by a raised luteinizing hormone level in the presence of a low/normal testosterone level. Howell and colleagues (2000) postulated that mild testosterone deficiency may account for some of the long-term side effects of treatment, and they therefore assessed fatigue, mood, and sexual function by questionnaire in thirty-six patients with Leydig cell dysfunction (group 1), and also in a group of thirty patients (group 2) with normal hormone levels who underwent the same treatment for cancer. There was no significant difference in anxiety and depression scores between the two groups. Fatigue scores were significantly higher in both groups compared with normal men, but there were no significant differences in any of the fatigue subscales between the two groups. The authors concluded that mild Leydig cell insufficiency following treatment with cytotoxic chemotherapy with or without radiation therapy is not associated with higher levels of fatigue and anxiety but may result in reduced sexual function.

Other components of the nervous system such as the sympathetic nervous system may also be involved in neuroendocrinological imbalances associated with fatigue in cancer and other contexts. For instance, a study was conducted on the prevalence of fatigue assessed in a nonspecific preexamination questionnaire by 431 patients, each subsequently diagnosed as having one of eight neurological or endocrine disorders. The study revealed that although fatigue commonly results from delayed orthostatic hypotension and all forms of hypocortisolism, it is less common in patients with acute orthostatic hypotension, both idiopathic and secondary to multiple system atrophy, which is more commonly present with lightheadedness or syncope (Baschetti, 1996a; Beard, 1996). Autonomic dysfunction is covered in the next subsection.

NEUROLOGICAL FACTORS

Autonomic Dysfunction

The autonomic nervous system is a major mediator of the visceral response to central influences such as psychological stress. Autonomic dysfunction may therefore represent the physiological pathway that accounts for many of the extraintestinal symptoms seen in irritable bowel syndrome patients and some of the frequent gastrointestinal complaints reported by patients with fatiguing illnesses, such as chronic fatigue syndrome and fibromyalgia (Tougas, 1999). However, sympathetic dysautonomia may present differentially among the latter syndromes since denervation hypersensitivity of the pupil is not apparent in CFS patients (Sendrowski, Buker, and Gee, 1997).

Several studies have reported a close association between chronic fatigue syndrome and disturbances in the autonomic regulation of blood pressure and pulse, which are evident as neurally mediated hypotension or the postural tachycardia syndrome (Chester, 1997b; De Lorenzo and Kakkar, 1996; De Lorenzo, Hargreaves, and Kakkar, 1996b, 1997; Freeman and Komaroff, 1997; Klonoff, 1996; Rowe and Calkins, 1998; Streeten and Anderson, 1998; Wilke et al., 1998). The latter two conditions can be induced by using tilt-table testing, which involves laying the patient horizontally on a table and then tilting the table upright to seventy degrees for forty-five minutes while monitoring blood pressure and heart rate. Persons with neurally mediated hypotension or the postural tachycardia syndrome will develop lowered blood pressure and higher heart rate (palpitations) under these conditions, as well as other characteristic symptoms such as lightheadedness, weakness, visual dimming, or a slow response to verbal stimuli. Resumption of a supine posture relieves the latter symptoms.

Many CFS patients show signs of abnormal vasovagal or vasodepressor responses to upright posture as evinced by their experience of lightheadedness or worsened fatigue when they stand for prolonged periods or when in warm places, such as in a hot shower. Autonomic impairment in CFS pediatric patients is suggested by depression of heart rate variability indices, even when compared to children with syncope or controls. Sympathovagal balance does not shift toward enhanced sympathetic modulation of heart rate with head-up tilt and there is blunting in the overall heart rate variability response with syncope during head-up tilt (Stewart, Weldon, et al., 1998).

Power analyses of heart rate variability have revealed that the basal autonomic state of fibromyalgia patients is characterized by increased sympathetic and decreased parasympathetic tones (Cohen et al., 2000) and a deranged sympathetic response to orthostatic stress (Kelemen et al., 1998; Martinez-Lavin et al., 1997; Martinez-Lavin and Hermosillo, 2000). As is the case with chronic fatigue syndrome (Wilke et al., 1998), Bou-Holaigah and colleagues (1997) identified a strong association between fibromyalgia and neurally mediated hypotension. During stage one of upright tilt test, twelve of twenty fibromyalgia patients (60 percent), but no controls, had an abnormal drop in blood pressure. Among those with fibromyalgia, all eighteen who tolerated upright tilt for more than ten minutes reported worsening or provocation of their typical widespread fibromyalgia pain during stage one, while controls were asymptomatic (Bou-Holaigah et al., 1997). Spectral analysis of heart rate variability may therefore be useful to identify fibromyalgia patients who have dysautonomia.

In terms of the reasons for the presence of orthostatic intolerance and other symptoms of autonomic dysfunction, chronic fatigue syndrome is also associated with changes in neuroendocrine function, such as hypocortisolism, and several reports have explored the links between neuroendocrine function disturbances, fatigue, and autonomic dysfunction. A study on the prevalence of fatigue assessed in a nonspecific preexamination questionnaire by 431 patients, each subsequently diagnosed as having one of eight neurological or endocrine disorders, revealed that although fatigue commonly results from delayed orthostatic hypotension and all forms of hypocortisolism, it is less common in patients with acute orthostatic hypotension, both idiopathic and secondary to multiple system atrophy, which is more commonly present with light-headedness or syncope (Baschetti, 1996a; Beard, 1996). The Addison-type overtraining syndrome provides another example of a link between hypocortisolism, fatigue, and autonomic dysfunction (Lehmann et al., 1998). During heavy endurance training or overreaching periods, a reduced adrenal responsiveness to ACTH is no longer compensated by an increased pituitary ACTH release, and the pituitary ACTH release also decreases with a concomitantly decreased intrinsic sympathetic activity and sensitivity of target organs to catecholamines. This is indicated by decreased catecholamine excretion during night rest, decreased beta-adrenoreceptor density, decreased beta-adrenoreceptor-mediated responses, and increased resting plasma norepinephrine levels and responses to exercise. These observations can explain persistent performance incompetence in affected athletes (Lehmann et al., 1998). A study of vagal power during walking in CFS patients reported that in each of four periods of walking in one of three periods of rest, CFS patients had significantly less vagal power than the control subjects despite there being no significant groupwise differences in mean heart rate, tidal volume, minute volume, respiratory rate, oxygen consumption, or total spectrum power. Furthermore, patients had a significant decline in resting vagal power after periods of walking. These results suggest a subtle abnormality in vagal activity to the heart in patients with the chronic fatigue syndrome and may explain, in part, their postexertional symptom exacerbation (Cordero et al., 1996).

One study suggests that orthostatic intolerance and other symptoms of autonomic dysfunction in chronic fatigue syndrome may be explained by cardiovascular deconditioning, a postviral idiopathic autonomic neuropathy, or both (Freeman and Komaroff, 1997). Besides impaired vasomotor tone, deconditioning, and autonomic neuropathy, hypovolemia may be a factor that could be influenced by hormonal or cytokine imbalances. Psychosomatic factors may also influence the occurrence of orthostatic dysregulation in young men as suggested by a study where the percentage classed in categories suggestive of emotional or psychological disturbance, according to the personality test, was 42.1 percent in those with orthostatic dysregulation and 8.9 percent in the controls (Nozawa et al., 1997).

In contrast to these data, some groups argue that the findings of increased heart rate and higher low-frequency power after tilting, which point to sympathetic overactivity and no parasympathetic abnormalities, provide no real explanation for the fatigue and intolerance to physical exertion in CFS patients (De Becker et al., 1998). Furthermore, several studies have failed to document an association between autonomic function impairment and chronic fatigue syndrome. One study of nineteen CFS patients and eleven controls showed that autonomic function, as assessed by an analysis of heart rate variability during a two-stage tilt-table test while wearing a Holter monitor, does not differ in the baseline supine state, nor in response to upright tilt among CFS patients and healthy controls (Yataco et al., 1997). Another report argued that many CFS patients examined by the tilt test had orthostatic symptoms prior to the examination, it is not certain that cardiovascular dysregulation is present in CFS patients without orthostatic symptoms, and it is also not clear whether such a dysregulation would be the effect of physical inactivity or a manifestation of a subtle form of autonomic neuropathy (Smit et al., 1998). One study reported that although higher heart rate and lower spectral indices of blood pressure variability while supine were found in CFS patients, analysis of RR-interval variability could not detect major alterations in autonomic function in chronic fatigue syndrome (Duprez et al., 1998). Another study documented the absence in chronic fatigue syndrome of denervation hypersensitivity of the sympathetic system, as assessed by a standardized supersensitivity test of pupil size (1.0 percent topical phenylephrine) (Sendrowski, Buker, and Gee, 1997).

Despite the negative associations described, some interventions in cases of proven abnormal tilt test results have been beneficial. For instance, in a case comparison study with follow-up of eight weeks of a group of seventy-eight CFS patients and thirty-eight healthy controls (De Lorenzo, Hargreaves, and Kakkar, 1997), patients with orthostatic hypotension by tilt test assessment at entry were offered therapy with sodium chloride (1,200 mg) in a sustained-release formulation for three weeks, prior to resubmission to the tilt-table testing, and clinical and laboratory evaluation. An abnormal response to upright tilt was observed in twenty-two of seventy-eight patients with chronic fatigue syndrome. After sodium chloride therapy for eight weeks, tilt-table testing was repeated on the twenty-two patients with an abnormal response at baseline. Of these twenty-two patients, ten redeveloped orthostatic hypotension, while eleven did not show an abnormal response to the test and reported an improvement of CFS symptoms. However, these CFS patients who again developed an abnormal response to tilt test had a significantly reduced plasma renin activity (0.79 pmol/mL per hour) compared with both healthy controls (1.29 pmol/mL per hour) and those eleven CFS patients (1.0 pmol/mL per hour) who improved after sodium chloride therapy (De Lorenzo, Hargreaves, and Kakkar, 1997). Another intervention involves the selective alpha-adrenergic agonist midrodrine, administration of a single dose of which before hemodialysis has been proven to be an effective therapy for intradialytic hypotension where autonomic dysfunction is thought to play a significant role (Cruz, Mahnensmith, and Perazella, 1997). There is one report of successful head-up tilt-guided therapy (Handa, Sra, and Akhtar, 1997). Controlled therapeutic trials for chronic fatigue syndrome are underway.

The role of autonomic dysfunction in some forms of cancer-related fatigue and other chronic fatiguing illnesses remains to be determined.

The Vagal Afferent Hypothesis

In addition to supplying a number of visceral organs (heart, stomach) with efferent parasympathetic fibers, the vagus nerve also has a high percentage (90 percent in the abdominal vagus) of afferent fibers conveying information from the viscera to the brainstem. As reviewed by Morrow, Andrews, and colleagues (2002), evidence from animal studies suggests that some vagal afferents could be involved in the genesis of fatigue sensations by modulation of somatic muscle tone.

The modulation of somatic muscle tone by vagal afferent activation was first reported in 1937 by Schweitzer and Wright (1937), who showed that electrical stimulation of the central terminus of the vagus caused a reduction in the magnitude of the knee-jerk reflex. Further studies showed that activation of a population of vagal afferents supplying the lungs J (juxtapulmonary capillary)-receptors (Paintal, Damodaran, and Guz, 1973) and pulmonary C-fibers (Coleridge and Coleridge, 1984) caused reflex inhibition of somatic motor activity in decerebrate and anesthetized cats. In a mesencephalic cat, activation of pulmonary receptors attenuated or abolished walking (Kalia, 1973; Pickar, Hill, and Kaufman, 1993). More recently, activation of vagal afferents by a 5-hydroxytryptamine 3 (5-HT3) receptor agonist reduced steady state exercise-induced EMG activity in conscious rats (DiCarlo, Collins, and Chen, 1994). Intravenous injection of a thromboxane A2 receptor agonist can inhibit the knee-jerk reflex in anesthesized cats (Pickar, 1998). Other studies in the rat have shown that activation of abdominal vagal afferents reduced reflex activation of skeletal muscles (Kawasaki, Kodama, and Matsushita, 1983). In dog studies, shielding the abdomen prevented performance decrement caused by gamma radiation (Malakhovski, Small, and Bokk, 1990).

Although the hypothesis has not been universally accepted, it has been proposed that the physiological function of the reflex pulmonary afferent suppression of somatic muscle activation is to limit exercise by detecting the pulmonary congestion resulting from exercise (Davies et al., 1987; Paintal, 1973, 1995). The function of the abdominal vagal afferent suppression of somatic muscle activity has not been identified. It should be noted that the evidence for these vagosomatic inhibitory reflexes in humans is scant; a recent study was unable to demonstrate suppression of somatic muscle activity by pulmonary C-fiber activation, although the explanation may reside in technical rather than physiological considerations (Gandevia et al., 1998; Widdicombe, 1998). Further studies of this reflex are required in humans. Although there are numerous differences in the physiological response to exercise in humans and animals, on teleological grounds it appears likely that a reflex from the lungs to the somatic muscles will be identified in humans when appropriate experimental conditions are identified.

If a vagosomatic inhibitory reflex is identified in humans then it could have a role in the genesis of lethargy, weakness, and fatigue associated with cancer and its treatment. Studies in animals have shown that vagal afferent C-fibers can be stimulated by 5-HT, substance P, cytokines (e.g., interleukin-1beta), and prostaglandins (Forsyth et al., 1999; Gandevia et al., 1998). If they were secreted in appropriate locations (e.g., lungs, gut mucosa, liver) where vagal afferents terminate, they could evoke a reflex decrease in skeletal muscle tone. This decrease in tone would be perceived as either an inability to complete a motor task or as a feeling that more effort (i.e., central drive) was needed to complete the task that was usually required or anticipated. Activation of such a pathway would be anticipated to give rise to feelings of weakness rather than fatigue.

Studies performed predominantly in rats have suggested an additional role for abdominal vagal afferents, which may also be relevant to the genesis of "sickness syndrome"; that of signaling information about peripheral pathogenic information to the brain. Following intraperitoneal injection of either bacterial polysaccharide or interleukin-1beta a "sickness syndrome" is induced. The initial phase takes the form of hyperalgesia/allodynia, increased activity, and fever, and the later phase, of hypoalgesia, decreased activity, increased sleep, and either fever or hypothermia. Abdominal vagotomy attenuates or abolishes the hyperalgesia, increased sleep, reduced activity, and fever (Hansen and Krueger, 1998; Kapas et al., 1998; Opp and Toth, 1998).

As summarized by Morrow, Andrews, and colleagues (2002), a considerable body of data from animal studies shows that vagal afferents have the ability to generate many features of the sickness syndrome. This nonspecific host response to the invasion of a pathogenic organism and the release of proinflammatory mediators has many features in common with the symptoms observed in patients with cancer, including those under treatment. It is not unreasonable to suggest that vagal afferent activation contributes to the genesis of symptoms, including fatigue, in humans. The influence of the vagal afferents may be extensive: intraperitoneal injection of interleukin-1beta in rats increased induction of interleukin-1beta mRNA in the brainstem, hippocampus, and hypothalamus. This induction was either reduced or abolished by abdominal vagotomy (Hansen, Taishi, et al., 1998). The authors proposed that the induction of brain cytokines is a critical step in the pathway by which vagal-mediated signals result in centrally controlled symptoms of the acute-phase response. The importance of this fatigue is twofold. First, it is hypothesized that central cytokines and 5-HT are involved in the pathogenesis of fatigue, and second, one of the areas in which brain cytokines are induced by vagal activation is the hypothalamus, which together with the pituitary gland has often been implicated in the genesis of fatigue (Demitrack, 1998).

Sleep and Circadian Rhythms

Sleep difficulty is a prominent concern of cancer patients (Lee KA, 2001). Davidson and colleagues (2002) assessed the prevalence of reported sleep problems in patients attending six clinics at a regional cancer center, sleep problem prevalence in relation to cancer treatment, and the nature of reported insomnia (type, duration, and associated factors). They conducted a cross-sectional survey in which a brief sleep questionnaire was offered over a period of three months to all patients attending clinics for breast, gastrointestinal, genitourinary, gynecologic, lung, and nonmelanoma skin cancers. Response rate was 87 percent; the final sample size was 982 patients. The most prevalent problems were excessive fatigue (44 percent of patients), leg restlessness (41 percent), insomnia (31 percent), and excessive sleepiness (28 percent). The lung clinic had the highest prevalence of sleep problems. The breast clinic had a high prevalence of insomnia and fatigue. Recent cancer treatment was associated with excessive fatigue and hypersomnolence. Insomnia commonly involved multiple awakenings (76 percent of cases) and duration of cancer greater than or equal to six months (75 percent of cases). In 48 percent of cases, insomnia onset was reported to occur around the time of cancer diagnosis (falling within the period six months prediagnosis to eighteen months postdiagnosis). The most frequently identified contributors to insomnia were thoughts, concerns, and pain/discomfort. Variables associated with increased odds of insomnia were fatigue, age (inverse relationship), leg restlessness, sedative/hypnotic use, low or variable mood, dreams, concerns, and recent cancer surgery (Davidson et al., 2002).

In cancer patients, as in other medically ill patients, sleep that is inadequate or unrefreshing may be important not only to the expression of fatigue, but also to the patient's quality of life and tolerance to treatment, and may influence the development of mood disorders and clinical depression. In fact, the most reliable effect of sleep deprivation on performance and self-reports in healthy subjects is a worsening of mood, often characterized by fatigue, loss of vigor, irritability, and depression (Pilcher and Huffcutt, 1996). Studies of sleep restriction in healthy young adults showed evidence of progressive increases in fatigue, stress, and exhaustion, and diurnal variation in mood, with worsening mood in the evening hours (Dinges et al., 1997; Wood and Magnello, 1992).

Objectively recorded sleep and biological rhythms have not been well investigated in cancer patients, but it appears that most cancer patients may in fact not be getting a good night's sleep. Moore and Dimsdale (2002) proposed that part of the fatigue typically experienced by cancer patients can be attributed to disruption of sleep by opioid medications they are taking. Research is needed to assess the sleep and next-day consequences that can be expected from typical doses of different types of pain medications. Larsen and colleagues (1999) reported that long-term opioid therapy produces a slight (nonsignificant) impairment of psychomotor performance in patients with cancer pain or nonmalignant chronic pain. These effects become significantly more pronounced with increasing age and in patients with cancer pain, indicating a higher susceptibility of the elderly toward opioids. These results indicate that, particularly in older patients receiving long-term opioid treatment for cancer or noncancer pain, careful evaluation of the effects on psychomotor function is necessary to estimate the patient's ability to perform his or her daily activities.

Broeckel and colleagues (1998), Bower and colleagues (2000), and Okuyama and colleagues (Okuyama, Akechi, Kugaya, Okamura, Imoto, et al., 2000; Okuyama, Akechi, Kugaya, Okamura, Shima, et al., 2000) reported that more severe fatigue among cancer patients was associated with poorer quality of sleep. Ancoli-Israel, Moore, and Jones (2001) posit that some degree of cancer-related fatigue experienced during the day may relate to sleep/wake cycles or to the quality and quantity of sleep obtained at night. Different components or dimensions of fatigue (physical, attentional/cognitive, emotional/affective, etc.) are probably associated in some way with disrupted sleep and desynchronized sleep/wake rhythms. These associations may change in measurable ways prior to treatment, during treatment, and after treatment completion.

In a study of fourteen women with stage I or II breast cancer receiving four cycles of chemotherapy, Berger and Higginbotham (2000) found fluctuating patterns of disturbed sleep, mild-to-moderate symptom distress, lowered activity, and moderate fatigue. Sleep, symptom distress, activity, and health status cluster in patterns associated with either lower or higher fatigue. Patients experienced the highest levels of fatigue and symptom distress during the first four days after treatment 3. Patterns of sleep (total rest, sleep latency, wake after sleep onset, and sleep efficiency) differed from established norms. Mean activity levels ranged from 65 to 80 percent of norms during and following treatments. Correlates of fatigue were greater symptom distress, lower activity, and poorer physical and social health status; variables representing disturbed sleep trended toward associations with fatigue (Berger and Higginbotham, 2000).

Faithfull and Brada (1998) assessed nineteen patients who received high-dose cranial irradiation as treatment for primary brain tumors. Following treatment, sixteen patients developed somnolence syndrome, a collection of symptoms consisting of drowsiness, lethargy, and fatigue. Time series analysis identified a cyclical pattern to the symptoms, with a period of drowsiness and fatigue occurring from day eleven to day twenty-one and from day thirty-one to day thirty-five after radiotherapy (Faithfull, 1997). The principal symptoms were those of excessive drowsiness, feeling clumsy, an inability to concentrate, lethargy, being mentally slow, and fatigue. Patients treated with accelerated (eleven individuals) compared with more conventional (eight individuals) fractionation experienced more severe drowsiness and fatigue, although there was no difference in the pattern or the incidence of symptoms. Interview data suggested that patients frequently attributed their symptoms of somnolence to "flu or other ailments." The unexplained and overwhelming nature of the symptoms was a cause of anxiety (Faithfull and Brada, 1998).

Outpatients receiving radiation therapy for bone metastasis reported moderate amounts of pain and fatigue (Miaskowski and Lee, 1999). Average pain scores did not vary significantly over a forty-eight-hour period. However, patients reported significantly lower fatigue scores in the morning compared to the evening. In addition, patients experienced significant sleep disturbances, with a mean sleep efficiency index of 70.7 percent (estimated using wrist actigraphy). Patients with lower Karnofsky Performance Status scores reported more sleep disturbances. Moreover, patients who had received a higher percentage of their radiation treatment reported more sleep disturbances (Miaskowski and Lee, 1999).

Evidence is accumulating that not only sleep but also circadian rhythms are often disturbed in cancer patients, probably owing to a variety of causes. For instance, data suggest that hot flashes in postmenopausal breast cancer survivors do not follow the same circadian pattern as seen in healthy, naturally postmenopausal women (Carpenter et al., 2001). Roscoe and colleagues (2002) assessed seventy-eight female breast cancer patients for fatigue, depression, overall mood, and circadian rhythm at their second and fourth on-study chemotherapy cycles and reported that circadian rhythm disruption is involved in the experience of fatigue and depression in cancer patients.

The rest/activity rhythm reflects endogenous circadian clock function. Mormont and Waterhouse (2002) investigated the relationship between the individual rhythm in activity and quality of life in 200 patients with metastatic colorectal cancer. The authors reported that the rest/activity circadian rhythm appeared to be an objective indicator of physical welfare and quality of life, and that circadian function may be one of the biological determinants of quality of life in cancer patients. The distribution of the rest/activity cycle parameters and that of quality-of-life scores was independent of sex, age, primary tumor, number of metastatic sites, and prior treatment.

The rest/activity circadian cycle has been used as a reference for chemotherapy administration at specific times to improve tolerability and efficacy (Mormont et al., 2000). A study in 200 metastatic colorectal cancer patients showed that survival at two years was fivefold higher in patients with marked activity rhythm than in those with rhythm alteration. Moreover, circadian rhythms in activity and in white blood cell counts as well as performance status were jointly prognostic of response. Patients with marked rest/activity rhythms also had better quality of life and reported significantly less fatigue. Therefore, individual rest/activity cycle provides an independent prognostic factor for cancer patients' survival and tumor response as well as a quantitative indicator for quality of life (Mormont and Waterhouse, 2002; Mormont et al., 2000).

To identify indicators involving circadian activity/rest cycles associated with higher levels of cancer-related fatigue, Berger and Farr (1999) performed a prospective, descriptive, repeated measures study of seventy-two women free of unstable chronic illnesses and during the first three chemotherapy cycles after surgery for stage I/II breast cancer. The authors reported that women who were less active and had increased night awakenings reported higher cancer-related fatigue levels at all three cycle midpoints, with the strongest association being number of night awakenings. During the third chemotherapy cycle, women who were less active during the day, took more naps, and spent more time resting during a twenty-four-hour period experienced higher cancer-related fatigue. The study therefore concluded that women whose sleep is disrupted at cycle midpoints are at risk for cancer-related fatigue. The cumulative effects of less daytime activity, more daytime sleep, and night awakenings are associated with higher cancer-related fatigue levels. Therefore, assessment of cancer-related fatigue and night awakenings at the midpoints of each chemotherapy cycle and development of appropriate interventions to promote daytime activity and nighttime rest are key to managing fatigue and preventing loss of biologic rhythmicity (Berger and Farr, 1999).

An alternative explanation for disrupted sleep cycles in cancer patients is provided by autonomic dysfunction as per studies in other chronic fatiguing illnesses detailed in the previous subsection. In this respect, individuals with fibromyalgia have diminished twenty-four-hour heart rate variability secondary to an increased nocturnal predominance of the low-frequency band oscillation consistent with an exaggerated sympathetic modulation of the sinus node (Martinez-Lavin et al., 1998). This abnormal chronobiology could explain the sleep disturbances and fatigue that occur in this syndrome and may also be relevant to cancer-related fatigue.

Another line of study relates to melatonin. Blood levels of melatonin (N-acetyl-5-methoxy tryptamine), a mainly pineal hormone that is involved in synchronizing circadian rhythms, are not affected by sleep or wakefulness and may therefore serve as a reliable marker of circadian phase when unmasking and free-running studies are difficult to conduct. Because of an apparent absence of a secretory or storage mechanism, melatonin levels in blood are regulated by the rate of melatonin production (Weaver, 1999).

For both early-stage breast and ovarian cancer patients receiving chemotherapy for the first time, Payne (2002) reported a significant change in nighttime levels of melatonin. The study included a total of only seventeen patients and, although not significant, daytime melatonin levels changed over time from baseline to six months. A similar melatonin-based desynchronization of circadian systems has been postulated in the etiology of fibromyalgia, and the use of exogenous melatonin has become widespread among patients with fibromyalgia and chronic fatigue syndrome (Webb, 1998). However, Korszun and colleagues (1999) found that although nighttime plasma melatonin levels were significantly higher in fibromyalgia patients compared to controls, there were no differences in the timing of cortisol and melatonin secretory patterns and no internal desynchronization of the two rhythms in fibromyalgia patients compared to controls.

Raised plasma melatonin concentrations have been documented in several other conditions that are associated with dysregulation of neuroendocrine axes, and increased melatonin levels may represent a marker of increased susceptibility to stress-induced hypothalamic disruptions (see subsection on endocrine factors). Although the data indicate that there is no rationale for melatonin replacement therapy in fibromyalgia patients, in a preliminary four-week pilot study of treatment with melatonin (3 mg at bedtime) in nineteen fibromyalgia patients, Citera and colleagues (2000) reported significant improvements after thirty days in median values for the tender point count and severity of pain at selected points, patient and physician global assessments, and sleep. Also, unlike Korszun and colleagues (1999), Wikner and colleagues (1998) found a 31 percent lower nighttime melatonin secretion in eight fibromyalgia patients as compared to healthy subjects and proposed that this deficiency may contribute to impaired sleep at night, fatigue during the day, and changed pain perception. However, Press and colleagues (1998) found that nocturnal urine 6-sulphatoxymelatonin levels were similar in thirty-nine fibromyalgia patients and controls.

Although a number of studies have reported reduced melatonin concentrations in depressed patients (Arendt, 1989; Claustrat et al., 1984; Beck-Friis et al., 1985), most of the studies have included small numbers of subjects, poorly matched controls, and infrequent melatonin sampling. The best-controlled studies of melatonin in depressed patients found neither reduced levels nor phase alterations in patients with endogenous depression (Rubin et al., 1992; Thompson, Rubin, and Fefer, 1987).

Melatonin is another hormone whose role as a mediator of fatigue, through its effects on sleep, in cancer and other contexts remains controversial. There is even controversy on the role of melatonin in the regulation of sleep because of differences in the way experiments were carried out and the questions about sleep that were addressed. Different studies have administered melatonin at different times of the day, have used different routes of administration, have used different doses of melatonin from the physiological to the pharmacological, have examined sleep in normal controls and in subjects with a wide variety and often unclearly defined sleep problems, and have used a wide variety of outcome measures of treatment ranging from subjective alertness to subjective appraisal of sleep to EEG measurements (Mendelson, 1997; Turek and Czeisler, 1999).

Gonzalez and colleagues (1991) investigated the therapeutic potential of orally administered melatonin in patients with advanced melanoma. Forty-two patients received melatonin in doses ranging from 5 mg/m^2/day to 700 mg/m^2/day in four divided doses. Two were excluded from analysis. After a median follow-up of five weeks, six patients had partial responses and six other patients had stable disease. Sites of response included the central nervous system, subcutaneous tissue, and lung. The median response duration was thirty-three weeks for the partial responders. There was a suggestion of a dose-response relationship. Although the toxicity encountered was minimal, it is noteworthy that it consisted primarily of fatigue in seventeen of forty patients (Gonzalez et al., 1991). In fact, Kendler (1997) points out that since tolerance, fatigue, and other side effects have been reported, melatonin use on consecutive nights should be avoided and only the lowest effective hypnotic dose should be taken.

As mentioned previously, nonrestorative sleep is a prominent feature of fibromyalgia. Unrefreshing sleep occurs in 76 to 90 percent of fibromyalgia patients compared with 10 to 30 percent of controls (Campbell et al., 1983; Green, 1999; Hemmeter et al., 1995; Hench, 1996; Kempenaers et al., 1994; Lugaresi et al., 1981; Moldofsky, 1989b; Moldofsky et al., 1975; Reilly and Littlejohn, 1993; Roizenblatt et al., 2001; Schaefer, 1995; Smythe, 1995; Smythe and Moldofsky, 1977; Wolfe and Cathey, 1983; Wolfe et al., 1990; Yunus et al., 1981). Fibromyalgia patients report early-morning awakenings, awakening feeling tired or unrefreshed, insomnia, as well as mood and cognitive disturbances; they may also experience primary sleep disorders, including sleep apnea (Harding, 1998).

Sleep disturbances contribute to overnight pain and stiffness exacerbation and increased pain sensitivity in fibromyalgia and other chronic musculoskeletal pain conditions (Affleck et al., 1996; Agargun et al., 1999; Croft, Schollum, and Silman, 1994; Greenberg et al., 1995; Hemmeter et al., 1995; Hirsch et al., 1994; Kryeger, 1995; Kryger and Shapiro, 1992; Leigh et al., 1998; Mahowald et al., 1989; Moldofsky and Scarisbrick, 1976; Older et al., 1998; Roizenblatt et al., 1997; Scharf et al., 1998; Walsh, Hartman, and Schweitzer, 1994; Wittig et al., 1982). Poor sleep is also associated with psychological distress and cognitive dysfunction (Affleck et al., 1996; Côte and Moldofsky, 1997; Hansotia, 1996; Hyyppa and Kronholm, 1995; Paiva et al., 1995; Phillips and Cousins, 1986; Pilowski, Crettenden, and Townly, 1985; Shaver et al., 1997).

Among the disruptions in sleep architecture in fibromyalgia patients, there is evidence for prolonged sleep latencies (Branco, Atalaia, and Paiva, 1994; Horne and Shackeel, 1991), low sleep efficiency (Touchon et al., 1988; Wittig et al., 1982), an increased amount of stage 1 non-rapid eye movement (non-REM) sleep (Anch et al., 1991; Branco, Atalaia, and Paiva, 1994; Harding, 1998; Moldofsky et al., 1975; Sergi et al., 1999; Shaver et al., 1997), the presence of alpha EEG activity during non-REM sleep (Branco, Atalaia, and Paiva, 1994; Drewes, Gade, et al., 1995; Drewes, Nielsen, et al., 1995; Flanigan, Morehouse, and Shapiro, 1995; Harding, 1998; MacFarlane et al., 1996; Moldofsky et al., 1975; Perlis et al., 1997; Roizenblatt et al., 1997, 2001; Ware, Russell, and Campos, 1986), a reduction in slow-wave sleep (Branco, Atalaia, and Paiva, 1994; Drewes, Gade, et al., 1995; Drewes, Nielsen, et al., 1995; Drewes et al., 1996; Horne and Schackeel, 1991; Touchon et al., 1988) and in REM percentages (Branco, Atalaia, and Paiva, 1994), an increased number of arousals (Branco, Atalaia, and Paiva, 1994; Clauw et al., 1994; Harding, 1998; Horne and Schackeel, 1991; Molony et al., 1986; Shaver et al., 1997; Staedt et al., 1993; Touchon et al., 1988), periodic breathing (Sergi et al., 1999) and arterial oxygen desaturations (Alvarez-Lario et al., 1996), and restless leg movements (Atkinson et al., 1988; Wittig et al., 1982; Yunus and Aldag, 1996).

Lentz and colleagues (1999) reported that disruption of slow-wave sleep in healthy volunteers, without reducing total sleep or sleep efficiency, for several consecutive nights is associated with decreased pain threshold, increased discomfort, fatigue, and the inflammatory flare response in skin. Also, deep pain induced during sleep in normal controls causes the alpha frequency rhythm, termed alpha-delta sleep anomaly, that is seen in fibromyalgia and in normal controls during stage 4 sleep deprivation (Fischler, LeBon, et al., 1997; Harding, 1998). These results suggest that disrupted sleep is probably an important factor in the pathophysiology of symptoms in fibromyalgia.

The association between sleep disturbances and pain and other fibromyalgia symptoms has been challenged by several studies. Older and colleagues (1998) found that three nights of delta-wave sleep interruption caused no significant lowering of pain thresholds or serum insulin-like growth factor 1 in healthy volunteers. The authors therefore concluded that the low levels of IGF-1 seen in fibromyalgia patients may result from chronic rather than acute delta-wave sleep interruption, or may be dependent on factors other than disturbances of delta-wave sleep. Tischler and colleagues (1997) also reported that sleep abnormalities and fibromyalgia in primary Sjögren's syndrome patients are frequent and that their etiology might involve other mechanisms besides joint pain or sicca symptomatology. Donald and colleagues (1996) reported that although fibromyalgia was uncommon (2.7 percent) in patients with a primary complaint of disturbed sleep and, in particular, patients with sleep apnea, reduced physical activity was strongly associated with reported pain symptoms.

Fatigue is present in a broad range of sleep disorders, and several investigators have addressed the question of whether chronic fatigue syndrome may be related to sleep disorders. In this respect, home polysomnography showed significantly higher levels of sleep disruption by both brief and longer awakenings in eighteen CFS teenagers, aged eleven to seventeen, as compared to controls (Stores, Fry, and Crawford, 1998). In another study (Morriss, Wearden, and Battersby, 1997), CFS patients reported significantly more naps and waking by pain, a similar prevalence of difficulties in maintaining sleep, and significantly less difficulty getting off to sleep compared to depressed patients. Although sleep continuity complaints preceded fatigue in only 20 percent of CFS patients, there was a strong association between relapse and sleep disturbance. Certain types of sleep disorders were associated with increased disability or fatigue in CFS patients, and disrupted sleep appeared to complicate the course of chronic fatigue syndrome. For the most part, sleep complaints in this study were either attributable to the lifestyle of CFS patients or seemed inherent to the underlying condition of chronic fatigue syndrome. They were generally unrelated to depression or anxiety in chronic fatigue syndrome.

This conclusion stands in contrast to the finding by another group that short rapid eye movement latency is associated with depression in the CFS population (Morehouse et al., 1998). Yet another study (Fischler, LeBon, et al., 1997) found that although the percentage of stage 4 sleep was significantly lower in 49 CFS patients, no association was found between sleep disorders and the degree of functional status impairment. Moreover, the mean REM latency and the percentage of subjects with a shortened REM latency were similar in chronic fatigue syndrome and controls.

The differences in findings by these several groups may be reconciled by the possibility that sleep changes are differentially distributed among subsets of CFS patients. For instance, one study (Ambrogetti et al., 1998) found that only a subgroup of CFS patients had significant daytime sleepiness and REM sleep abnormalities. Nonetheless, it should be noted that daytime sleepiness and perceived fatigue are independent phenomena (Lichstein et al., 1997), and fatigue should be considered an independent symptom of sleep disturbance. Moreover, although sleep abnormalities may play a role in the etiology of chronic fatigue syndrome, they seem unlikely to be an important cause of daytime fatigue in the majority of patients (Sharpley et al., 1997).

As discussed for cancer-related fatigue, besides sleep abnormalities, alterations in circadian rhythms could contribute to chronic fatigue syndrome symptomatology. In one study (Van de Luit et al., 1998), CFS patients had circadian rhythms that were synchronous but of increased amplitudes, and systolic blood pressures consistently below 100 mm Hg during the nighttime (one hypertensive CFS patient was excluded). Although positive inotropic compounds may be beneficial in such patients as shown by a reduction in nighttime hypotension by Inopamil (200 mg daily), melatonin (4 mg daily) increased nighttime hypotension. In a second study (Williams, Pirmohamed, et al., 1996), although there were no differences between the two groups in the amplitude, mean value or timing of the peak (acrophase) of the circadian rhythm of body core temperature, or in the timing of the onset of melatonin secretion, CFS patients did not show the significant correlation between the timing of the temperature acrophase and the melatonin onset seen in controls.

The dissociation of circadian rhythms can explain the finding of a study that used continuous twenty-four-hour recordings of core body temperature, with an ingestible radio frequency transmitter pill and a belt-worn receiver-logger. The study showed that CFS patients have normal core body temperatures despite frequent self-reports of subnormal body temperature and low-grade fever (Hamilos et al., 1998). Dissociation of circadian rhythms could be secondary to the sleep deprivation and social disruption, and/or the reduction in physical activity that typically accompany chronic fatigue syndrome. By analogy with jet lag and shift working, circadian dysrhythmia could be an important factor in initiating and perpetuating the cardinal symptoms of chronic fatigue syndrome, notably fatigue, and impaired concentration and intellectual abilities.

Cognition

Many cancer patients experience impairments of neurocognitive function, including memory loss, distractibility, difficulty in performing multiple tasks (multitasking), and a myriad of other symptoms. The etiologies of these problems are diverse and include the direct effects of cancer within the central nervous system, indirect effects of certain cancers (e.g., paraneoplastic brain disorders), and both diffuse and highly specific effects of cancer treatments on the brain. In addition to these cancer-related causes, patients may have coexisting neurological or psychiatric disorders that affect their cognition and mood. Careful assessment of patients complaining of neurocognitive or behavioral problems is essential to providing appropriate interventions and maximizing their ability to carry out usual activities (Meyers, 2000).

Although fatigue, cognitive dysfunction, and mood disturbance, including depression, are very common in cancer patients, a cause-effect relationship among the three entities is recognized but poorly understood (Valentine and Meyers, 2001). Factors that contribute to this poor understanding are the subjective nature of the symptoms, multiple potential causes, and a lack of reliable assessment tools. Moreover, the nature and magnitude of cognitive changes may vary with time, as illustrated as follows by the effects of cancer treatment.

Assessment of cognitive and motor performance of bone marrow transplant patients prior to, during, and following intensive toxic chemoradiotherapy showed slight but significant changes in neuropsychological capacity when compared to baseline levels and controls, particularly near the beginning of treatment (Parth et al., 1989). A number of patients who have undergone adjuvant chemotherapy for operative primary breast carcinoma have reported impaired cognitive function, namely concentration and memory, sometimes even years after completion of therapy (Schagen et al., 1999). Schagen and colleagues (2001) suggest that there is neurophysiological support for cognitive dysfunction as a late complication of high-dose systemic chemotherapy in breast cancer. However, this cognitive impairment is unaffected by anxiety, depression, fatigue, and time since treatment, and not related to the self-reported complaints of cognitive dysfunction.

Other studies underscore the independent manifestation of objective cognitive dysfunction and fatigue. Severe fatigue was a problem for almost 40 percent of the sample of breast cancer survivors studied by Servaes, Verhagen, and Bleijenberg (2002b,c). Although severe fatigue was related to physical, psychological, social, cognitive, and behavioral factors, Servaes, Verhagen, and Bleijenberg (2002b,c) found no differences between severely fatigued disease-free breast carcinoma survivors, nonseverely fatigued disease-free breast carcinoma survivors, and women in a control group with regard to daily self-reported and objective physical activity. However, the severely fatigued disease-free patients reported more impairment in neuropsychological functioning on daily questionnaires compared with nonseverely fatigued disease-free patients and women in the control group. In contrast to the latter finding, no differences were found between these three groups on a standardized concentration task. Moreover, on a standardized reaction time task, no significant differences were found between the two groups of disease-free breast carcinoma survivors. However, women in the severely fatigued group had a significantly longer reaction time compared with women in the control group. From this study, Servaes,

Verhagen, and Bleijenberg (2002b,c) concluded that fatigue is correlated strongly with daily self-reported neuropsychological functioning, but not with objective neuropsychological functioning, in a laboratory setting.

Ahles and colleagues (2002) compared the neuropsychologic functioning of long-term survivors (five years postdiagnosis, not presently receiving cancer treatment, and disease free) of breast cancer and lymphoma who had been treated with standard-dose systemic chemotherapy (thirty-five breast cancer and twenty-six lymphoma cases) or local therapy only (thirty-five breast cancer and twenty-two lymphoma cases). Multivariate analysis of variance, controlling for age and education, revealed that survivors who had been treated with systemic chemotherapy scored significantly lower on the battery of neuropsychological tests compared with those treated with local therapy only, particularly in the domains of verbal memory and psycho-motor functioning. Survivors treated with systemic chemotherapy were also more likely to score in the lower quartile on the Neuropsychological Performance Index and to self-report greater problems with working memory on the Squire Memory Self-Rating Questionnaire. Therefore, data from this study support the hypothesis that systemic chemotherapy can have a negative impact on cognitive functioning as measured by standardized neuropsychological tests and self-report of memory changes. However, analysis of the Neuropsychological Performance Index suggests that only a subgroup of survivors may experience long-term cognitive deficits associated with systemic chemotherapy (Ahles et al., 2002).

Armstrong and colleagues (1993) used a comprehensive neuropsychological battery to evaluate five patients with low-grade brain tumors prior to radiation therapy and then at three-month intervals up to nine months post-completion of radiation therapy. Although all patients showed deterioration in long-term memory at a mean of 1.5 months postcompletion of radiation therapy regardless of tumor site, functional measures of fatigue and mood did not correlate significantly with the long-term memory scores. Based on the results of the latter study and those of a similar one conducted on twenty patients with low-grade primary brain tumors who were treated with radio-therapy (Armstrong et al., 2000), the authors suggest that the deficit in long-term memory, which rebounded a few months after completion of therapy, may be secondary to white matter changes associated with the early-delayed effects of radiation therapy (Fiegler et al., 1986; Garwicz et al., 1975). This conclusion is substantiated by a more recent study in which Armstrong and colleagues (2002) examined the effects of radiation therapy on the cognitive and radiographic outcomes of twenty-six patients with low-grade, supratentorial, brain tumors. Assessments were performed six weeks after surgery and immediately before radiation therapy, and there-after yearly up to six years. There was no evidence of a general cognitive decline or progression of white matter changes after three years. Results argue for limited damage from radiation therapy at the frequently used doses and volumes in the absence of other clinical risk factors.

Multiple factors related to cancer, its treatment, and the demands of a life-threatening illness increase the risk for loss of concentration and attentional fatigue (Cimprich, 1995). Attentional fatigue usually follows intense use of mental effort and is manifested as a decreased capacity to concentrate, that is, to direct attention (Cimprich, 1992). Women treated for breast cancer have shown attentional fatigue manifested as a decreased capacity to concentrate or direct attention in daily life activities (Cimprich, 1998). Older age and more extensive surgery increase the likelihood of loss of attention secondary, in part, to greater risk of attentional fatigue. In a study of forty-five women, Lehto and Cimprich (1999) reported that preoperative anxiety is a clinically significant issue in women newly diagnosed with breast cancer regardless of age and extent of anticipated surgery. Higher anxiety requires use of attentional resources and initially may act to reduce perceptions of effectiveness in attentional functioning. Older women who have high anxiety combined with both subjective and objective decline in attentional functioning may be at particularly high risk for attentional fatigue.

Cognitive function items are increasingly included in quality-of-life measures, and cancer patients often report complaints of concentration and memory difficulties. However, Cull and colleagues (1996) assessed a sample of adult lymphoma patients, disease free and six or more months after treatment, and found no significant difference between complainers and noncomplainers in sociodemographic or clinical characteristics or in their performance on standard neuropsychometric tests of concentration and memory. Those reporting concentration and memory difficulties had significantly higher scores on measures of anxiety, depression, and fatigue. Cull and colleagues (1996) concluded that the observation calls into question the validity of including cognitive function items in self-report quality-of-life measures, and that patients who report concentration and memory difficulties should be screened for a clinically significant and potentially remediable mood disorder.

In a study of twenty-nine patients with cancer pain admitted to a palliative care unit, Klepstad and colleagues (2002) reported that although patients who complained from difficulties with concentration or memory did not score differently from noncomplainers on objective assessments of cognitive function, they had a significantly higher level of fatigue. In a previous study, Klepstad, Borchgrevink, and Kaasa (2000) concluded that in cancer patients with reduced health-related quality of life, the start of morphine therapy had no major influence on aspects of health-related quality of life other than pain.

Besides cognitive difficulties, delirium is also a common complication in patients with advanced cancer. Seventy-one of 104 patients studied by Lawlor and colleagues (2000) met DSM-IV criteria for a first episode of delirium. Loge and Kaasa (2000) point out that neuropsychiatric conditions such as delirium, dementia, and amnestic disorder are prevalent (more than 20 percent), especially in the terminal phase of cancer illness. Anxiety and depressive symptoms are also common and may be caused by the patient's medical condition. Probably less than 10 percent have anxiety or depressive disorders.

An understanding of fatigue in cancer patients may benefit from studies of chronic fatigue syndrome and other nonmalignant diseases indicating that cognitive impairment varies with physical and mental fatigue, and that symptoms of depression experienced by patients with physical illnesses and primary mood disorders are qualitatively different. Although chronic fatigue syndrome and major depression and dysthymia have distinct clinical features, these disorders have slowed motor and cognitive processing speed (reaction time tasks and working memory tests) in common (Marshall et al., 1997). Nonetheless, the ability of patients with chronic fatigue syndrome to attend to verbal versus figural stimuli and the mood ratings were different from those reported in studies of patients with depression (Marshall et al., 1996).

A relationship exists between cognitive impairment and functional disability in chronic fatigue syndrome that cannot be explained entirely on the basis of psychiatric factors (Christodoulou, DeLuca, et al., 1998; DeLuca et al., 1997a; Wearden and Appleby, 1996, 1997). The most consistently documented neuropsychological impairments in chronic fatigue syndrome are in the areas of complex information processing speeds and efficiency (Fry and Martin, 1996a). Although general intellectual abilities and higher-order cognitive skills are intact, one study (Michiels, Cluydts, and Fischler, 1998) reported that patients with chronic fatigue syndrome performed poorer on recall of verbal information across learning trials. This phenomenon may be secondary to poor initial learning and not only to a retrieval failure. Emotional factors influence subjective report of cognitive difficulty, whereas their effect on objective performance remains uncertain.

Fry and Martin (1996a) hypothesized that idiosyncratic cognitive processes are associated with chronic fatigue syndrome and may play a role in the maintenance of the disorder; one study concluded that slowed speed of information processing and motor speed were related to low levels of physical activity (Vercoulen et al., 1998); and another study associated cognitive dysfunction with psychological distress in chronic fatigue syndrome (Kane,

Gantz, and DiPino, 1997). Although the neuropathological processes underlying cognitive dysfunction in chronic fatigue syndrome are not yet known, preliminary evidence suggests the involvement of cerebral white matter and independence from mood disturbances (Fairhurst, Waterman, and Lynch, 1997; Tiersky et al., 1997). An organic brain dysfunction within a defined neural substrate in patients with chronic fatigue syndrome is suggested by the observation of an impaired acquisition of the eyeblink response and normal sensitivity and responsivity to acoustic or airpuff stimuli (Servatius et al., 1998).

One study found that deficits in cognitive functioning in patients with chronic fatigue syndrome are more likely to be found on naturalistic than on laboratory tasks (Lakein et al., 1997), and another found that a metamemory deficit is not the cause of the memory problems reported by patients with chronic fatigue syndrome (Vollmer-Conna et al., 1997). At least a subset of patients with chronic fatigue syndrome had a slower learning rate of verbal and visual material and impaired delayed recall of verbal and visual information (DiPino and Kane, 1996; Michiels et al., 1996). In one study, patients with chronic fatigue syndrome were differentially impaired on the auditory relative to the visual processing task, while patients with multiple sclerosis were equally impaired on both versions of the task (Johnson et al., 1996).

After physically demanding exercise, subjects with chronic fatigue syndrome demonstrate impaired cognitive processing (as assessed by the Symbol Digit Modalities Test, Stroop Word Test, and Stroop Color Test) compared with healthy individuals (LaManca et al., 1998). Patients with chronic fatigue syndrome also show specific sensitivity to the effects of exertion at the level of effortful cognitive functioning (focused and sustained attention), a feature that may indicate reduced working memory capacity, a greater demand to monitor cognitive processes, or both (Blackwood et al., 1998; Joyce, Blumenthal, and Wessely, 1996). In patients with chronic fatigue syndrome, everyday cognitive tasks may require excessive processing resources leaving patients with diminished spare attentional capacity or flexibility (Marcel et al., 1996). Self-efficacy is shown to be a significant predictor of CFS symptoms beyond the variance determined by demographic variables and distress (Findley et al., 1998).

Many observations suggest that chronic fatigue syndrome could derive from residual damage to the reticular activating system (RAS) of the upper brainstem and/or to its cortical projections (Gonzalez, Cousins, and Doraiswamy, 1996; Lange et al., 1998). It should be pointed out that, although larger right greater than left asymmetry in regional cerebral blood flow is found at the parietotemporal level in chronic fatigue syndrome patients as compared to healthy controls (Fischler et al., 1996, 1998), no significant correlations are found between frontal tracer uptake and right-left parieto-temporal asymmetry on the one hand, and clinically relevant chronic fatigue syndrome dimensions on the other (Fischler et al., 1998). Damage to RAS could be produced by a previous viral infection, leaving functional defects unaccompanied by any gross histological changes. In animal experiments, activation of the RAS can change sleep state and activate or stimulate cortical functions. RAS lesions can produce somnolence and apathy. Studies by modern imaging techniques have not been entirely consistent (Greco et al., 1997), but generally many magnetic resonance imaging (MRI) studies suggest that small, discrete patchy brainstem and subcortical lesions can often be seen in chronic fatigue syndrome. Regional blood flow studies by single photon-emission computed tomography (SPECT) have been more consistent (Richardson and Campos Costa, 1998). They have revealed blood flow reductions in many regions, especially in the hind brain. Similar lesions have been reported after poliomyelitis and in multiple sclerosis—in both of which conditions chronic fatigue is characteristically present (Roelcke et al., 1997). In the well-known post-polio fatigue syndrome, lesions predominate in the RAS of the brainstem. If similar underlying lesions in the RAS can eventually be identified in chronic fatigue syndrome, the therapeutic target for chronic fatigue syndrome would be better defined than it is at present. In this respect, [18F]fluorine-deoxyglucose (18FDG) positron emission tomography (PET) showed specific metabolism abnormalities in CFS patients (hypometabolism in right mediofrontal cortex and brainstem) as compared with both healthy controls and depressed patients (Tirelli et al., 1998). The most relevant abnormality is brainstem hypometabolism, which has been also reported in SPECT studies, and seems to be a marker for the in vivo diagnosis of chronic fatigue syndrome (Nixon, 1996a,b).

A central nervous system dysfunction in chronic fatigue syndrome has been proposed based on the observation of a significant prolongation of central motor conduction time as assessed from recordings of motor-evoked potentials from the musculus abductor pollicis brevis and digiti minimi (Hilgers, Frank, and Bolte, 1998). The direct involvement of the central nervous system in the onset of chronic fatigue syndrome is underscored by the observation of gait abnormalities in CFS patients (Saggini et al., 1998). The "Prolonged Decay Test," a modified impedenzometric technique that explores any alterations of stapedial contraction, yielded significantly different clinico-audiological results in CFS patients as compared to controls and was proposed by the authors of the study as a new diagnostic test for chronic fatigue syndrome (Neri et al., 1996). On the other hand, denervation hypersensitivity of the pupil, as a test for sympathetic oversensitivity, does not occur in CFS patients, and the use of 1.0 percent topical phenylephrine had no diagnostic value in detecting CFS patients versus normals (Sendrowski, Buker, and Gee, 1997).

Brain Injury

In one study, patients with brain injury were found to experience significant levels of fatigue, and the Fatigue Impact Scale provided the most comprehensive examination of fatigue (LaChapelle and Finlayson, 1998). One proposal under investigation is that type I Chiari malformation or spinal cord compression by protrusion of cerebellar tonsils may underlie some cases of chronic fatigue syndrome.

Ion Channelopathy

A study (Watson et al., 1998) measured resting energy expenditure by indirect calorimetry and measurement of total body potassium in eleven women with chronic fatigue syndrome and in eleven healthy women found that five out of eleven CFS subjects had resting energy expenditure above the upper limit of normal as defined by the control group data. These findings were suggested to be consistent with an up-regulation of the sodium-potassium pump in chronic fatigue syndrome. Possible abnormalities in ion channel metabolism in chronic fatigue syndrome are being investigated by the same group of researchers.

Regulation of Respiration

Because hyperventilation can produce substantial fatigue, it might be hypothesized that hyperventilation plays a causal or perpetuating role in chronic fatigue syndrome. However, in one study (Bazelmans, Bleijenberg, et al., 1997), CFS patients and non-CFS patients known to experience hyperventilation offered substantial complaints of fatigue and hyperventilation, both to a similar degree. Hyperventilation in chronic fatigue syndrome should probably be regarded as epiphenomenon, a conclusion that is underscored by studies that found no abnormality in the regulation of respiration in subjects with chronic fatigue syndrome (Baschetti, 1997b; De Lorenzo, Hargreaves, and Kakkar, 1996a; Lavietes, Bergen, and Natelson, 1998).

PSYCHOLOGICAL AND PSYCHIATRIC FACTORS

Suffering has a physical foundation that can be caused by the illness itself or by treatment of the illness. Kuuppelomaki and Lauri (1998) reported that the primary sources of physical suffering among cancer patients were fatigue, pain, and the side effects of chemotherapy. The causes of psychological suffering lie in the physiological changes associated with the disease and with the imminence of death. Psychological suffering was most typically manifested in depression, which most of the patients suffered during the initial stages of the disease, when the disease metastasized, and when they were in particularly poor condition. General deterioration and fear of infections very much restrict the social life of cancer patients, causing them to withdraw into their home or the hospital.

As reviewed by Holland (2002), the formal beginnings of psychooncology date to the mid-1970s, when the stigma making the word *cancer* unspeakable was diminished to the point that the diagnosis could be revealed and the feelings of patients about their illness could be explored for the first time. However, a second stigma has contributed to the late development of interest in the psychological dimensions of cancer: negative attitudes attached to mental illness and psychological problems, even in the context of medical illness. It is important to understand these historical underpinnings because they continue to color contemporary attitudes and beliefs about cancer and its psychiatric comorbidity and psychosocial problems. Over the last quarter of the twentieth century, psychooncology became a subspecialty of oncology with its own body of knowledge contributing to cancer care.

In the new millennium, a significant base of literature, training programs, and a broad research agenda have evolved with applications at all points on the cancer continuum: behavioral research in changing lifestyle and habits to reduce cancer risk; study of behaviors and attitudes to ensure early detection; study of psychological issues related to genetic risk and testing; symptom control (anxiety, depression, delirium, pain, and fatigue) during active treatment; management of psychological sequels in cancer survivors; and management of the psychological aspects of palliative and end-of-life care.

As pointed out in the endocrine factors section, links between psychological and physiological domains of relevance to cancer risk and survival are being actively explored through psychoneuroimmunology. Research in these areas will occupy the research agenda for the first quarter of the twenty-first century. At the start of the third millennium, psychooncology has come of age as one of the youngest subspecialties of oncology, as one of the most clearly defined subspecialties of consultation-liaison psychiatry, and as an example of the value of a broad multidisciplinary application of the behavioral and social sciences.

Behavior

Broeckel and colleagues (1998) found that more severe fatigue among breast cancer patients was associated with greater use of catastrophizing as a coping strategy. The feelings, such as frustration, anger, irritability, anxiety, demoralization, and profound change in mood, associated with cancer-related fatigue and other fatiguing illness can also impair recovery from fatigue (Surawy et al., 1995). Besides their role in the intensity and duration of cancer-related fatigue, one study stressed the role of behavioral factors in the presence of cancer-related fatigue. Upon investigation of why some individuals with lung or colorectal cancer develop fatigue whereas others do not, Olson and colleagues (2002) found that an adaptive behavioral mode labeled gliding characterized those who reported little or no fatigue, even when hemoglobin levels were low, while three other nonadaptive behavioral modes (inertia, disorganization, and overexertion) characterized those who reported fatigue.

The findings underscore the importance of behavioral coping and adaptation strategies in the prognosis of patients with cancer and cancer-related fatigue, and point to the relevance of cognitive-behavioral interventions (covered in Chapter 4) alone or in combination with other approaches for cancer and cancer-related fatigue, as well as chronic fatiguing illnesses (Ray, Jefferies, and Weir, 1997). The universality of these conclusions is undermined by a longitudinal study of fifty individuals with stages III and IV adenocarcinoma of the lung over four consecutive combination chemotherapy courses. The study revealed that although perceived stress was moderately high only at the time of pretreatment and four coping strategies were used (seeking social support, planful problem solving, self-control, and positive reappraisal), no relationships existed between coping strategies and side effects from chemotherapy, coping and perceived stress, mood and side effects, and perceived stress and side effects (Chernecky, 1999).

Other studies have looked into the coping strategies used by cancer patients and how they relate to their level of fatigue. In a study of twenty-one patients with malignant glioma who were interviewed in the course of radiation therapy, Petz and colleagues (2001) found that the coping strategies of patients were comparable with those of other cancer patients. They were mainly characterized by "self-encouragement," "compliance," and "trust in the treating physician." Anxiety was low and showed no significant changes. Although depressivity was higher than in the normal population, it showed no significant changes in the course of therapy. Quality-of-life scores remained constant, despite an increase of fatigue (Petz et al., 2001).

Hosaka and colleagues (1995) reported that coping methods such as active-cognitive, active-behavioral, and avoidance were more frequently used after Japanese women were diagnosed with cancer than before. There were also positive correlations between active-reliance behavior and tension/anxiety and depression, between cognitive-passive behavior and depression and lack of vigor, between passive/resignation behavior and anger/hostility and confusion, and between avoidance/solitary behavior and anger/hostility, fatigue, depression, lack of vigor, and confusion. Hosaka and colleagues (1995) concluded that a diagnosis of cancer causes a patient to more frequently use avoidance behavior as well as active coping styles, and these passive/avoidance coping styles are often correlated with negative emotions. These results imply that patients with breast cancer need support considering the relationship between passive/avoidance coping styles and negative emotions.

Lutgendorf and colleagues (2000) reported that although extensively treated patients with gynecological cancers reported more fatigue and less vigor, their depression and anxiety levels did not differ from early-stage patients. Patients using avoidant coping reported poorer physical and emotional well-being, along with greater anxiety, depression, fatigue, and total mood disturbance. Those using active coping reported better social well-being, better relationships with their doctors, and less overall distress.

Stanton and Snider (1993) followed 117 women age forty or over regarding personality, cognitive appraisal, coping, and mood variables before breast biopsy, after diagnosis, and, for those who had cancer, after surgery. Upon biopsy, thirty-six received a cancer diagnosis, and eighty-one received a benign diagnosis. The two groups did not differ on appraisals, coping, or affect before diagnosis. With prebiopsy affect controlled, cancer patients reported more negative affect postbiopsy than did benign patients. Postsurgery, cancer patients expressed less vigor and more fatigue than benign patients, but the groups did not differ on other negative emotions. Prebiopsy, psychosocial predictors accounted for 54 and 29 percent of the variance in negative and positive emotion, respectively. Prebiopsy variables also predicted postbiopsy and postsurgery mood; cognitive-avoidance coping was a particularly important predictor of high distress and low vigor (Stanton and Snider, 1993).

A descriptive, retrospective, mailed survey of eighty-two women previously treated for gynecologic cancer revealed that women described a range of psychosocial difficulties including depression, anxiety, and fear of dying (Steginga and Dunn, 1997). Physical side effects included fatigue, pain, bladder dysfunction, and vaginal problems. Women most often described emotional support from family members as assisting them to cope with difficulties. The most commonly described personal coping strategy was the use of positive thinking; the others are listed as follows:

- active-behavioral
- active-cognitive
- avoidance
- catastrophizing
- compliance
- planful problem solving
- positive thinking
- positive reappraisal
- seeking social support
- self-control
- self-encouragement
- trust in the treating physician

Descriptions of how health care professionals were helpful reflected their roles within the health care system (Steginga and Dunn, 1997).

Although several researchers have found that coping styles and stress, as detailed in the endocrine factors section of this chapter, are related to illness and immune function (Cohen and Williamson, 1991), it should be kept in mind that no definitive evidence links psychological states to specific diseases of the immune system (Bower, 1991). Despite this caveat, several studies in chronic fatiguing illnesses underscore the relevance of the associations described between psychological factors and cancer-related fatigue and suggest that further studies are warranted. For instance, a study by Clements and colleagues (1997) reported that most patients with chronic fatigue syndrome believed that they could control their symptoms to some degree but could not alter the course of the underlying disease process. The coping methods they described were resting, avoiding activity, and reducing activity. Personal experience of feeling worse after activity was a major factor in the adoption of rest and avoidance (Clements et al., 1997; Ray, Jefferies, and Weir, 1995). A study by Fischler, Dendale, and colleagues (1997) also emphasizes a major contribution of avoidance behavior to functional status impairment in chronic fatigue syndrome.

Pelcovitz and colleagues (1995) studied behavior problems and family functioning in a sample of ten adolescent girls with chronic fatigue syndrome, ten matched healthy adolescent girls, and ten adolescents with childhood cancer in remission. Based on the adolescent girls' reports, the CFS group had significantly higher scores than the cancer and healthy comparison adolescent girls on somatic complaints and also significantly higher scores than the cancer controls on internalizing symptoms and depression. Parent reports resulted in significantly higher scores in the CFS group than the adolescent girls from the healthy comparison groups on internalizing scores and somatic complaints. There were no significant differences on any family variables (Pelcovitz et al., 1995).

Several authors emphasize that somatization plays an important role in chronic fatigue syndrome, both etiologically and in the perpetuation of symptoms (Bennett, 1997; Chagpar, 1996; Cheung and Lim, 1997; Holland, 1997; Robbins, Kirmayer, and Hemami, 1997; Simpson, 1997; Wessely, 1997; Wessely et al., 1996). Katon and Walker (1993) found that the prevalence of somatization disorder in patients with chronic fatigue syndrome averages 10 to 15 percent, at least three times higher than in other medical populations. Somatization, defined as one or more medically unexplained symptoms, is presumably related to underlying emotional or social difficulties. Somatizing patients avoid the blame that would be associated with a psychological attribution by focusing on bodily symptoms (Goldberg and Bridges, 1988). For instance, Wessely and Powell (1989) found that 86 percent of patients with postviral fatigue attributed their illness to physical factors, whereas only 14 percent of depressive patients attributed their illness to such factors.

In contrast to the studies mentioned, other investigations have not supported a somatization model for CFS symptomatology. A study by Wood and colleagues (1994) that exposed chronic fatigue patients to a stressful task found no evidence for the hypothesis that participants with chronic fatigue syndrome respond to stress with physical rather than psychological symptoms. In addition, Ray and colleagues (1992) found no significant relationship between indices of perceived chronic fatigue syndrome illness severity (e.g., frequency of symptoms, course of illness, disability, severity of illness) and emotional distress. The absence of a relationship between these two variables may be one reason why people with chronic fatigue syndrome attribute their illness to physical rather than psychological causes.

Finally, if people with chronic fatigue syndrome present physical complaints to mask their psychological problems, then an inverse relationship should exist between the number of depression and anxiety symptoms and the number of reported somatic symptoms (Katon and Walker, 1993). However, this relationship has not been found; rather, people who become distressed report more somatic, depression, and anxiety symptoms concurrently (Katon and Russo, 1992; Katon and Walker, 1993; Lutgendorf, Antoni, et al., 1995).

Personality

In a prospective observational study of 101 French patients with upper aerodigestive tract cancer, Allison, Guichard, and Gilain (2000) documented that dispositional optimism is associated with better health-related quality of life, including less fatigue. Before treatment, optimists reported better role, cognitive, and emotional function; less pain and fatigue; and a better global rating of health-related quality of life than did pessimists. Following treatment, optimists reported better role and cognitive functioning, less pain, and better global health-related quality of life than did pessimists. Pessimists reported a greater deterioration in the role domain following treatment than did optimists. At no point did pessimists rate health-related quality of life better than optimists.

Some investigators have studied the relationships between personality factors and fatigue states (Abbey, 1993). Montgomery (1983) found that individuals with complaints of chronic fatigue in the absence of infection had higher levels of introversion and neuroticism. Negative perfectionism and neuroticism have been implicated as vulnerability factors in the development of chronic unexplained fatigue (Magnusson, Nias, and White, 1996). Albus (1997) even proposes that specific somatic factors (e.g., cancer or viruses) seem to be less important for onset of fatigue than certain personality traits such as depresiveness and workaholism. Albus (1997) posits that the latter traits lead to an increased vulnerability to unspecific psychological or biological stressors that may cause chronic fatigue by complex psychosomatic interferences. In a correlational study of fatigue and psychosocial variables, a less definite diagnosis by a general practitioner and the tendency of the patient to attribute symptoms to physical disorders rather than to psychological factors were significant predictors of chronic fatigue (Cope et al., 1994). Personality traits that negatively influence fatigue include:

- pessimism,
- introversion,
- depresiveness,
- neuroticism,
- workaholism, and
- negative perfectionism.

In one study (Johnson, DeLuca, and Natelson, 1996), subjects with chronic fatigue syndrome, mild multiple sclerosis, and depression as well as sedentary healthy controls were administered a structured psychiatric interview to determine axis I psychiatric disorders and two self-report instruments to assess axis II personality disorders and the personality trait of neuroticism. The study revealed that the depressed group had significantly more personality disorders and elevated neuroticism scores compared with the other three groups. The CFS and multiple sclerosis subjects had intermediary personality scores that were significantly higher than healthy controls. The CFS group with concurrent depressive disorder (34 percent of the CFS group) was found to account for most of the personality pathology in the CFS sample (Johnson, DeLuca, and Natelson, 1996b). Another study (Saltzstein et al., 1998) reported the finding of a mixture of neurotic and healthy defenses, and a low proportion of defenses associated with personality disorders in chronic fatigue syndrome. Psychological adaptation to chronic fatigue syndrome is similar to adaptive coping in other chronic illnesses: subjective perceptions of health status can predict functional status. Personality traits may therefore influence the perpetuation of symptomatology in chronic fatigue syndrome and other chronic fatiguing illnesses, including cancer-related fatigue.

Psychosocial Adaptation

In a survey of 101 cured cancer patients, Ehrmann-Feldman and colleagues (1987) reported the following problems faced by cancer patients returning to work: fatigue (30 percent), absenteeism (14 percent), psychological problems (12 percent), social stigma (12 percent), and discrimination by an employer (10 percent). In a descriptive, retrospective, mailed survey of eighty-two women previously treated for gynecologic cancer, Steginga and Dunn (1997) concluded that women's existing social supports may be most important in determining how they cope with gynecologic cancer.

While psychosocial factors may play a role in fatigue symptomatology amplification, they are unlikely to be the main cause for fatigue. However, psychosocial adjustment is also affected by fatigue. In a study on the relationships between fatigue and hope to psychosocial adjustment in 122 Korean women with breast cancer who received postsurgical chemotherapy or radiation therapy, E. H. Lee (2001) reported that after controlling for hope, fatigue uniquely accounted for 38 percent of the variance in psychosocial adjustment. After controlling for fatigue, hope uniquely accounted for 7 percent of the variance in psychosocial adjustment. However, there was no significant interaction between fatigue and hope in accounting for the variance in psychosocial adjustment. The findings inform clinicians of the importance of fatigue and hope so that they may consider these factors when planning care for women with breast cancer, especially in women receiving chemotherapy or radiation therapy (Lee EH, 2001).

Content analysis of interviews of eighty-four patients from the first year after bone marrow transplantation identified three areas of psychosocial morbidity: (1) physical problems, which included fatigue, appearance, troubles in eating, and physical restrictions; (2) psychological problems, which included fears about the future, sense of loss of control, anxiety, and depression; and (3) community reintegration problems, which included difficulty in returning to former social roles, separation from home, family, and friends, difficulty in resuming social relations, dealing with stigmatization, problems with family and children, and financial and employment difficulties (Baker et al., 1999).

The cultural context obviously colors psychosocial adaptation in cancer patients. Im, Lee, and Park (2002) explored cultural meanings of breast cancer among South Korean women through a descriptive longitudinal study. The themes that emerged through the analysis process included (1) "I did wrong," (2) "I cannot ask male physicians," (3) "I don't want to show the operation site to my husband," and (4) "I do household tasks by myself." The overriding theme was marginalization of the women within the context of their patriarchal culture. The findings suggest that culture is an important context circumscribing women's health/illness experience (Im, Lee, and Park, 2002).

Evaluation of late psychosocial sequels in 100 long-term survivors of Hodgkin's disease in the population of Calvados, France, revealed these patients to be more often childless, fewer divorces or separations, fewer changes in relationships with friends, similar proportions at work but less ambitious professional plans, and greater difficulties in borrowing from banks (Joly et al., 1996). There was also a slight increase in the number of visits to a general practitioner and greater consumption of medical resources (mainly thyroid extracts). Therefore, the study demonstrated that French long-term Hodgkin's disease survivors have good global health status and good psychological, familial, and professional status, but difficulties in borrowing from banks remain a major limitation in daily life. Although physical, role, and cognitive functioning impairments persist that might limit their activities, Hodgkin's disease survivors seem to have learned to cope with problems related to their disease and its treatment (Joly et al., 1996). Psychosocial problems that may aggravate fatigue include the following:

- work absenteeism,
- altered physical appearance or disabilities,
- social stigmatization,
- social marginalization,
- discrimination, and
- financial constraints.

The role of psychosocial factors and psychosocial amplification on fatigue is exemplified in a study (Goodwin, 1997) of 131 couples with wives with chronic fatigue syndrome, where marital adjustment scores, wives' conflict scores, and husbands' self-empathy scores were associated with wives' chronic fatigue syndrome scores. Wives with higher education, lengthier marriages, dyads with higher marital adjustment, and wives with less conflict and more support were predictive of lower problematic chronic fatigue syndrome symptoms. Another study (Cope et al., 1996) investigated psychosocial morbidity, coping styles, and health locus of control in 64 cases with and without chronic fatigue identified from a cohort of primary care patients recruited six months previously with a presumed, clinically diagnosed viral illness. A significant association between chronic fatigue and psychosocial morbidity, somatic symptoms, and escape-avoidance coping styles was shown. Chronic illness can also be associated with a social process of marginalization that affects, for instance, employment of those affected (Ware, 1998). A study of 117 adult cancer patients revealed that females and patients who reported more communication problems with friends or relatives reported more anxiety in medical situations (Friedman et al., 1994). Female patients and patients who reported more communication problems with friends or relatives also reported more chemotherapy-related problems.

In fibromyalgia, psychosocial factors are relevant at different levels as predisposing, triggering and stabilizing "chronifying" factors (Affleck et al., 1998; Anderberg, 1999; Eich et al., 2000; Rosenfeld and Walco, 1997; Walker, Keegan, et al., 1997). Hallberg and Carlsson (1998) found that individuals with insecure attachment styles are overrepresented among patients with chronic pain. Wolfe and Hawley (1998) pointed out that psychosocial distress and psychological abnormality occur frequently in fibromyalgia patients (Jamison, 1999a,b). Patterns of decreased levels of education and increased rates of divorce, obesity, and smoking have been noted in clinical and epidemiological studies (Neumann and Buskila, 1998). Ostensen and Schei (1997) reported that smoking was significantly more frequent for Norwegian women reporting fibromyalgia. Anxiety and depression in fibromyalgia were also associated with higher consumption of cigarettes (Kurtze, Gundersen, and Svebak, 1998, 1999). Tobacco use may therefore adversely affect fibromyalgia (Aaron and Buchwald, 2000; Jay, 2000).

Links of physical and sexual abuse to fibromyalgia have been noted as well. Anderberg and colleagues (2000) and Anderberg (2000b) documented that stressful life events in childhood/adolescence and in adulthood seem to be very common in those who have fibromyalgia. Furthermore, these life events were experienced as more negative than the life events experienced by healthy controls. Goldberg, Pachas, and Keith (1999) found that 64.7 percent of fibromyalgia patients studied had childhood traumatic events that are significantly related to chronic pain. Winfield (2000) also pointed out that adverse experiences during childhood are among the antecedents of fibromyalgia. Walker, Keegan, and colleagues (1997) documented that patients with fibromyalgia as compared to those with rheumatoid arthritis had significantly higher lifetime prevalence rates of all forms of victimization as well as combinations of adult and childhood trauma. Finestone and colleagues (2000) reported more chronic pain symptoms among women with a history of childhood sexual abuse, and Alexander and colleagues (1998) found that greater pain and fatigue characterized abused patients.

Turk and colleagues (1998) suggest that customizing fibromyalgia treatment based on patients' psychosocial needs will lead to enhanced treatment efficacy. The same appears logically valid for the treatment of cancer-related fatigue.

Mood

Mood is typically defined as the pervasive and sustained emotional climate that colors one's perception of the world (American Psychiatric Association, 1994) and is usually defined in terms of the subject's own perception. Fatigue is one of the most common presenting symptoms of depression (Hayes, 1991; Thase, 1991). However, there is not necessarily a cause-and-effect relationship between the two. In a study of 250 cancer patients who were interviewed before treatment, two weeks after treatment, and nine months later, Visser and Smets (1998) found that fatigue and depression do not follow the same course over time. Just after radiotherapy, fatigue had either increased or remained stable, depending on the dimension under consideration. Depression, in contrast, decreased. Nine months later fatigue had decreased, whereas levels of depression remained stable. Concurrent relations between fatigue and depression were mostly moderate. There was no strong evidence for a cause-and-effect relationship between depression and fatigue. Depression showed highest concurrent relationships with quality of life, especially before treatment (Visser and Smets, 1998).

As reviewed by Morrow, Andrews, and colleagues (2002), the close link between fatigue and depression in cancer patients suggests that a common mechanism could underlie the development of both. In this respect, tumor necrosis factor could alter central serotonin (5-HT) levels directly, both by increasing neuronal release of serotonin and by up-regulating 5-HT transporter expression, the main mechanism for removal of 5-HT from the synaptic space. Peripherally, TNF also increases circulating levels of tryptophan, a necessary precursor for serotonin synthesis. Serotonin may have a complex regulatory feedback loop with tumor necrosis factor. One hypothesis theorizes that this feedback loop becomes dysfunctional in the face of the greatly increased cytokine cascade produced by cancer and aggressive treatment. In particular, Morrow, Andrews, and colleagues (2002) believe that chronic TNF stimulation results in augmented and self-maintained levels of 5-HT transporter. In the face of disease, the brain may not synthesize adequate levels of 5-HT to overcome the increased transporter expression.

Aass and colleagues (1997, 1998) reported that fatigue predicted depression and correlated with anxiety and depression in a study of 716 unselected hospitalized and ambulatory cancer patients at a Norwegian hospital. In the ambulatory population, the prevalence of anxiety and depression was 13 and 9 percent. A history of previous psychiatric problems and impaired social life were correlated with both anxiety and depression. Female gender, impaired physical activity, and impaired social role function were additional predictive parameters for anxiety (Aass et al., 1997, 1998). The results of a study in 200 cancer patients suggest that there is a relationship between pain and mood in oncology outpatients and that health care professionals need to assess for mood disturbances in this population and develop appropriate treatment strategies (Glover et al., 1995). In a sample of 263 cancer patients who were undergoing chemotherapy, insomnia, fatigue, depression, and anxiety were positively correlated with one another and negatively correlated with quality of life (Redeker, Lev, and Ruggiero, 2000). Although overall depression levels were low in this sample, these findings suggest that insomnia and fatigue are related to depression and that depression is more closely associated with quality of life than are insomnia and fatigue.

Depression and anxiety occur more frequently in cancer of the pancreas than they do in other forms of intraabdominal malignancies and other cancers in general (Passik and Roth, 1999). Yet the etiology of psychiatric symptoms in patients with cancer of the pancreas may not be traced solely to poor prognosis, pain, or existential issues related to death and dying. In as many as half of patients that go on to be diagnosed with the disease, symptoms of depression and anxiety precede knowledge of the diagnosis. This observation has raised speculation that mood and anxiety syndromes are related to disruption in one of the physiologic functions of the pancreas. In fact, Passik and Roth (1999) presented a patient who had no prior psychiatric history and developed panic attacks just prior to diagnosis of her cancer; her symptoms resolved following resection of the tumor.

A cross-sectional, questionnaire-based survey of sixty patients with primary brain tumors showed a high burden of depressive symptoms, with 38 percent of the sample scoring in the clinically depressed range (Pelletier et al., 2002). Fifty percent of the sample could be classified as struggling with existential issues. Although scores reflecting depression, fatigue, emotional distress, and existential problems were interrelated, the presence of depressive symptoms was the single most important independent predictor of quality of life in this cohort of brain tumor patients (Pelletier et al., 2002). Suzuki and colleagues (1998) reported that patients with brain tumors feel disability to cope with social life. On discharge, they showed a better mood state compared to that on admission, but the mood state turned for the worse again during the follow-up period.

To evaluate the correlation between fatigue and physical impairment, Dimeo, Stieglitz, and colleagues (1997) assessed maximal physical performance with a treadmill test, and mental state with two questionnaires, the Profile of Mood States (POMS) and the Symptom Check List (SCL-90-R), in a successive series of seventy-eight cancer patients with solid tumors or hematological malignancies. Although a weak association between fatigue and maximal physical performance was found, intensity of fatigue showed a strong correlation with several indicators of psychological distress such as depression, somatization, and anxiety. Furthermore, patients with lower levels of physical performance had significantly higher scores for depression, somatization, and anxiety, and significantly lower scores for vigor than their counterparts whose physical performance was higher. Dimeo, Stieglitz, and colleagues (1997) concluded that fatigue in cancer patients may be related to mood disturbance but appears to be independent of physical performance. Moreover, low physical performance can be viewed as an independent predictor of mental distress in cancer patients.

A survey of 149 testicular cancer patients, with no evidence of disease for three or more years, revealed that patients felt significantly less exhausted after a working day, were more satisfied with life, and felt stronger and more fit than the controls. On the other hand, the patients reported a significantly higher incidence of anxiety and depression than the normal population. The results indicate that patients treated for a malignant disease may have greater fluctuations in mood and affect than the general population (Kaasa et al., 1991).

In a study of 580 adult survivors of childhood acute lymphoblastic leukemia, Zeltzer and colleagues (1997) found that survivors had higher total mood scores (which indicates greater negative mood) than sibling controls and reported more tension, depression, anger, and confusion, but not more fatigue or less vigor. Female, minority, and unemployed survivors reported the highest total mood disturbance.

In an outpatient medical oncology department, approximately 25 percent of 201 participants had borderline or clinical levels of anxiety and depression (Newell et al., 1999). Although relatively low levels of perceived needs were reported, physical and psychological needs were the most common. Major depressive disorders or generalized anxiety disorders were estimated in 16 percent of the 190 cancer patients attending the European Institute of Oncology in Milan (Bredart et al., 1999). Independent predictors of psychological distress were female gender, experience of disturbance in family and social life due to illness, nausea and vomiting, and perception of being in a poor state of health, while physical functioning, fatigue, and pain were not predictors (Bredart et al., 1999). A similar disparity of results in terms of associations between fatigue and mood disorders among different studies is seen in other fatiguing illnesses.

Although there is overlap between chronic fatigue syndrome and depression, and depression is commonly observed in chronic fatigue syndrome (De Portugal et al., 1996; Johnson, DeLuca, and Natelson, 1996; Moss-Morris et al., 1996), CFS patients and those with acute infection report less severe mood disturbance than patients with depression and, in turn, patients with depression present less somatic complaints. Moreover, as detailed in the endocrine factors section, chronic fatigue syndrome is characterized by hypocortisolism, while hypercortisolism is associated with depression. These observations suggest that the pathophysiological processes in patients with chronic fatigue syndrome and acute infection are not simply secondary to depressed mood (Johnson et al., 1996; Vollmer-Conna et al., 1997).

While in one study (Terman et al., 1998) a subgroup of patients with chronic fatigue syndrome showed seasonal variation in symptoms resembling those of seasonal affective disorder, with winter exacerbation, and light therapy was suggested as a treatment alternative, another study (Garcia-Borreguero et al., 1998) found that CFS patients exhibit an abnormally reduced seasonal variation in mood and behavior, and would not be expected to benefit from light therapy.

Offenbächer, Glatzeder, and Ackenheil (1998) found clinically relevant depression in 27 percent of 304 fibromyalgia patients studied. Meyer-Lindenberg and Gallhofer (1998) proposed that the subgroup of fibromyalgia patients with depressive symptoms may be pragmatically classified as suffering from somatized depression, and Keel (1998) pointed out that fibromyalgia patients most often present with persistent somatoform pain disorder (ICD-10) and dysthymia than with major psychiatric disorders. In a multicenter study of seventy-three individuals, Epstein and colleagues (1999) found that fibromyalgia patients exhibited high levels of some lifetime or current psychiatric disorders (mainly depression, 22 percent, and panic disorders, 7 percent) and significant current psychological distress. A study by Aaron and colleagues (1996) yielded similar results. Current anxiety level appears to be an important correlate of functional impairment in fibromyalgia patients (Epstein et al., 1999). Repeated traumatic experiences during childhood and as adults can be discovered in many cases, a finding that helps in understanding some of the difficulties met in psychotherapy with fibromyalgia patients (Keel, 1998).

Although antidepressant treatment is generally beneficial in fibromyalgia, improvement in symptomatology does not necessarily correlate with treatment of comorbid psychiatric conditions (Dunne and Dunne, 1995; Gruber, Hudson, and Pope, 1996; Hudson and Pope, 1996), an observation that curtails those who favor a psychiatric etiology of diffuse pain syndromes. In this respect, a study by Katz and Kravitz (1996) suggests that the tendency toward depression in fibromyalgia patients may be a manifestation of a familial depressive spectrum disorder (alcoholism and/or depression in family members), not simply a "reactive" depression secondary to the pain, fatigue, and other symptoms.

Drawing from the experiences described and others, research on mood disorders in association with cancer and its associated symptoms, or other fatiguing illnesses, will benefit from several recommendations made by a panel on neuropsychiatric syndromes and psychological symptoms of the National Cancer Institute of Canada Workshop on Symptom Control and Supportive Care in Patients with Advanced Cancer (Breitbart et al., 1995). The recommendations include the following:

1. adoption of uniform terminology (taxonomy of disorders) and diagnostic classification systems
2. utilization of existing validated tools and measures in prevalence and intervention research
3. development of new tools and measures that are more applicable and relevant to the palliative care setting
4. encouragement for studies of the prevalence of neuropsychiatric symptoms and syndromes
5. promotion of intervention studies utilizing pharmacologic and nonpharmacologic treatments for depressive disorders and cognitive disorders in advanced cancer patients
6. expansion of the focus of such research to other neuropsychiatric disorders (for example, anxiety disorders, post-traumatic stress disorders, and sleep disorders), symptoms (fatigue and tension), and related issues (suicidal ideation and desire for hastened death) (Breitbart et al., 1995)

HEMATOLOGICAL FACTORS

Anemia

Fatigue is considered the cardinal symptom of anemia (Cella, 1997, 1998, 2002; Glaus and Muller, 2000; Koeller, 1998; La Verde and Arienti, 2002; Sobrero et al., 2001; Yount, Lai, and Cella, 2002). Anemia is a common disorder in cancer patients, occurring in 10 to 40 percent of cases, depending upon the tumor type and chemotherapy or radiotherapy used (Coiffier, 2000; Groopman and Itri, 1999; Monti et al., 1996; Shasha and Harrison, 2001; Thomas, 1998a). Anemia is present in nearly all patients with leukemia at some time in the disease and in 50 percent of patients with lymphoma after chemotherapy. Cancer-related anemia appears to result from a range of factors, including chronic inflammation, blood loss, nutritional deficiencies, hemolysis, bone marrow infiltration by malignant cells, low serum levels of erythropoietin (the hormone that stimulates red blood cell production), and a decrease of bone marrow responsiveness to erythropoietin (Coiffier, 2000).

The most common cause of cancer-related anemia is suppression of erythropoietin production and erythropoiesis; in many cases (approximately 50 percent of them) these abnormalities are reversible with recombinant erythropoietin therapy (Oster, Herman, and Gamm, 1990; Yount, Lai, and Cella, 2002; see also Chapter 4). However, causes for anemia in malignant disorders are multiple and diverse, ranging from simple hemodilution to hematophagic histiocytosis (Spivak, 2000).

Inadequate erythropoietin levels consequent to renal impairment and the effect of inflammatory cytokines cause anemia associated with multiple myeloma. The degree of anemia can have prognostic importance, as is the case with multiple myeloma, or be a significant indicator of disease stage, as noted with chronic lymphocytic leukemia. Anemia results in fatigue, exhaustion, dizziness, headache, shortness of breath, and decreased motivation, thereby seriously affecting a patient's quality of life (Littlewood, 2002; Littlewood and Mandelli, 2002; Littlewood et al., 2002).

By decreasing the oxygen-carrying capacity of the blood, anemia may result in tumor hypoxia and may have a negative influence on the outcome of radiotherapy for various malignancies, even for small tumors not normally assumed to be hypoxic (Harrison, Shasha, and Homel, 2002). The antitumor activity of radiation is mediated via its interaction with oxygen to form labile free radicals; therefore, the intratumoral oxygen level has an important influence on the ability of radiation therapy to kill malignant cells. Because a high proportion (about 50 percent) of cancer patients undergoing radiotherapy are anemic prior to or during treatment, strategies to correct anemia and/or the resultant tumor hypoxia are increasingly being considered to be an important component of treatment (Harrison, Shasah, and Homel, 2002).

Fatigue and anemia contribute not only to a suboptimal response to treatment modalities such as radiation, but also to decreased performance status and poor patient compliance with treatment (Ramalingam and Belani, 2002). Anemia is a common complication in patients with hematological malignancies, with incidence rates ranging up to 63 percent (Cella, 2002). In myelodysplastic syndromes, anemia is an essential feature of the disease. The decrease in hemoglobin may lead to several symptoms such as fatigue, exhaustion, and impaired quality of life, and it may worsen prognosis (Ludwig, 2002). Fatigue and anemia also cause significant morbidity and impaired quality of life among patients with lung cancer. Effects of anemia in cancer patients include the following:

- fatigue,
- exhaustion,
- impaired quality of life,
- decreased performance status,
- worse prognosis,
- suboptimal response to radiation therapy, and
- poor patient compliance with treatment.

At the clinical level, the relationship between anemia and fatigue is universally accepted (Cella, 1997, 1998, 2002; Glaus and Muller, 2000). However, the pathogenesis of anemia-related fatigue remains unclear. Some authors suggest that abnormalities in energy metabolism play a role in inducing fatigue. In cancer patients, this effect may be exacerbated by the increased metabolic needs associated with tumor growth. Although anemia is clearly a factor that contributes to the severity of disease-related fatigue among cancer patients (Glaspy, 2001), hemoglobin levels explain only part of the difference compared with fatigue among the general U.S. population.

Implementation of survey instruments that assess the effects of fatigue and other (nonfatigue) symptoms of anemia on the patient's well-being and quality of life has shown a direct effect of hemoglobin levels on fatigue and other quality-of-life parameters (Cella, 2002; Cella and Bron, 1999; Lind et al., 2002; Monti et al., 1996). In this line, Payne (2002) reported that the physiologic trajectory of fatigue from baseline to three months indicated a significant change over time in hemoglobin levels in early-stage breast cancer patients receiving chemotherapy for the first time. Thus amelioration of anemia and fatigue should be considered a primary end point of antineo-plastic and supportive-care treatment of cancer patients. Accordingly, the search for new simplified methods of assessment of fatigue and other anemia-related symptoms and their treatment outcomes should be strongly encour-aged (Sobrero et al., 2001).

Other studies found less strong associations between hemoglobin levels and fatigue. For instance, Holzner and colleagues (2002) investigated the relationship between hemoglobin levels and the subjective experience of fa-tigue and quality of life in sixty-eight cancer patients (twenty-five colo-rectal, twenty-six lung, and seventeen ovarian cancer) with mild or no ane-mia undergoing chemotherapy. Compared with healthy subjects, cancer patients experienced significantly higher levels of subjective fatigue. Corre-lations between hemoglobin values and quality-of-life subscales were mod-erate, with a tendency to increase during chemotherapy. Hemoglobin values alone, however, did not fully account for the observed fatigue. Other symp-toms, especially pain, shortness of breath, and sleep disturbances, also showed an association with perceived fatigue. This study therefore con-cluded that hemoglobin values only partially explain subjectively experi-enced fatigue and quality of life in cancer patients (Holzner et al., 2002).

Through a discriminant analysis approach, Cella and colleagues (2002) differentiated anemic cancer patients from the general population with high sensitivity and reasonable specificity. The latter differentiation was achieved thanks to the distinct distributions of fatigue scores of 2,369 anemic cancer patients compared with those for the 1,010 individuals drawn from the gen-eral U.S. population and the substantial sample sizes of these two groups. Cella and colleagues (2002) concluded that although fatigue is a symptom most anyone can relate to, the fatigue of cancer patients, particularly those who are anemic, is decidedly worse, thereby stressing the need for interven-tions targeting this common and life-disrupting symptom.

In a study of 375 anemic cancer patients with a median age of sixty-one years, age as a covariate in multiple linear regression analysis failed to reach significance for most measures of function and quality of life, includ-ing measures of energy, activities, mental health, general cancer-related quality of life, and overall quality of life. Additional analysis suggests that other factors, including cancer progression, hemoglobin change, and base-line hemoglobin levels, are much more important in determining change in functional and quality-of-life scores (Aapro, Cella, and Zagari, 2002). However, it should be stressed that attention to anemia in the elderly is im-portant because it can lead to weakness, fatigue, limitations in activity, and may increase cardiovascular risk.

Anemia is a correctable pathologic finding in elderly people (Aapro, Cella, and Zagari, 2002). Recent studies of the effect of erythropoietin in an aging population support the hypothesis that anemia is associated with pathologic factors and not with normal aging. While older individuals admitted to hospitals are more likely to be anemic, these same individuals have a bone marrow mass and numbers of cultured progenitor cells that are similar to those of the younger population. Therefore, the predicted response to erythropoietin, and thus the function of the bone marrow and cellular progenitors, is maintained.

A high prevalence and frequent severity of low red blood cell mass was found among patients with chronic fatigue syndrome, an observation which suggests that a reduction in oxygen-carrying power of the blood reaching the brain may contribute to chronic fatigue syndrome symptomatology (Streeten and Bel, 1998). Studies underway are aimed at detecting possible abnormalities in erythropoietin production in chronic fatigue syndrome and at assessing the influence of cytokines such as tumor necrosis factor, which are known to inhibit erythropoietin production (Jelkman, Wolff, and Fandrey, 1995) and whose serum levels are increased in a subset of CFS patients (Patarca, Klimas, Lutgendorf, et al., 1994).

MUSCULOSKELETAL FACTORS

Skeletal Muscle Wasting

St. Pierre, Kasper, and Lindsey (1992) proposed that one physiologic mechanism of cancer-related fatigue may involve changes in skeletal muscle protein stores or metabolite concentration. Skeletal muscle wasting, which occurs as part of cancer cachexia, is one of the mechanisms that contribute to fatigue (Al-Majid and McCarthy, 2001). A reduction in skeletal muscle protein stores may result from endogenous tumor necrosis factor or from tumor necrosis factor administered as antineoplastic therapy. This muscle wasting would require patients to exert an unusually high amount of effort to generate adequate contractile force during exercise performance or during extended periods of sitting or standing. This additional effort could result in the onset of fatigue. However, Kasper and Sarna (2000) documented that although quadricep muscle size and strength increased in some women undergoing adjuvant chemotherapy for breast cancer, the subjective experiences of fatigue did not necessarily decrease.

A study by Bruera and colleagues (1988) found that although patients with advanced breast cancer have abnormal muscle electrophysiology that is not secondary to abnormal nutritional status or decreased muscle mass, muscle electrophysiology did not correlate with tumor mass or performance status, including fatigue level. Koczocik-Przedpelska, Bombicki, and Bik (1994) tested the effect of tumor on neuromuscular function in rats and compared it to the neoplastic neuromyopathy in cancer patients. Neurogenic atrophy with destruction of motor units was apparent in rats transplanted with epithelioma Guerin as well as with benzopyrene induced fibrosarcoma, while a decrease of sensory nerve excitability was apparent in cancer patients.

Cancer-related fatigue may develop or become exacerbated during exercise as a consequence of changes in the concentration of skeletal muscle metabolites. These biochemical alterations may interfere with force that is produced by the muscle contractile proteins (St. Pierre, Kasper, and Lindsey, 1992). Alterations in the muscular energetic systems caused by cancer and its treatment may also underlie cancer-related fatigue (Dimeo, 2001).

Low Cysteine-Glutathione Syndrome

Cancer patients may also exhibit the combination of skeletal muscle wasting or muscle fatigue, abnormally low plasma cysteine and glutamine levels, low natural killer cell activity, and increased rates of urea production, a complex of abnormalities that has been tentatively called "low cysteine-glutathione syndrome" (Droge and Holm, 1997). The latter symptoms are also found in patients with human immunodeficiency virus infection, major injuries, sepsis, Crohn's disease, ulcerative colitis, chronic fatigue syndrome, and to some extent in overtrained athletes. The coincidence of these symptoms in diseases of different etiologies suggests a causal relationship. The low natural killer cell activity in most cases is not life threatening but may have untoward consequences on disease progression in, for instance, cancer and HIV infection because natural killer cells are an important line of defense against cancer cells and microbial-infected cells.

Cysteine is an essential amino acid that is utilized in the biosynthesis of the peptide glutathione. In vitro studies in persistently HIV-infected cells have demonstrated that cysteine and *N*-acetylcysteine raise intracellular glutathione levels and inhibit HIV replication. This may be secondary to blocking the effects of tumor necrosis factor on HIV-infected cells (Droge et al., 1991; Kalebic et al., 1991; Mihm et al., 1991). Among the clues about the role of cysteine and glutathione in the development of skeletal muscle wasting one may mention that cysteine level is regulated primarily by the normal postabsorptive skeletal muscle protein catabolism; cysteine level itself is a physiological regulator of nitrogen balance and body cell mass; and cysteine-mediated regulatory circuitry is compromised in various catabolic conditions, including old age (Droge and Holm, 1997).

Muscle Physiology in Chronic Fatigue Syndrome

In twenty-one CFS patients, the deep (muscle) versus superficial (skin, subcutis) sensitivity to pain was explored by measuring pain thresholds to electrical stimulation unilaterally in the deltoid, trapezius, and quadriceps, and overlying skin and subcutis in comparison with normal subjects (Vecchiet et al., 1996). Thresholds in patients were normal in skin and subcutis, but significantly lower than normal (hyperalgesia) in muscles in all sites. The selective muscle hypersensitivity also corresponded to fiber abnormalities at muscle biopsy (quadriceps) performed in nine patients that were absent in normal subjects (four cases): morphostructural alterations of the sarcomere, fatty degeneration and fibrous regeneration, inversion of the cytochrome oxidase/succinate dehydrogenase ratio, pleio/polymorphism and monstruosity of mitochondria, reduction of some mitochondrial enzymatic activities, and increments of common deletion of 4,977 bp of mitochondrial DNA 150 to 3,000 times the normal values. By showing both sensory (diffuse hyperalgesia) and anatomical (degenerative picture) changes at the muscle level, the results suggested a role played by peripheral mechanisms in the genesis of CFS symptoms (Lodi, Taylor, and Radda, 1997; Vecchiet et al., 1996).

The findings described are underscored by a study (Lane, Barrett, Taylor, et al., 1998) using phosphorus magnetic resonance spectroscopy on forearm muscles of ten subanaerobic threshold exercise test (SATET)-positive patients (abnormal increase in plasma lactate following a short period of moderate exercise), nine SATET-negative patients, and thirteen sedentary volunteers. This study showed no differences in resting spectra between these groups, but, at the end of exercise, intracellular pH in the SATET-positive patients was significantly lower than in both the SATET-negative cases and controls. The SATET-positive patients also showed a significantly lower ATP synthesis during recovery. These observations indicate impaired mitochondrial oxidative phosphorylation in SATET-positive test individuals and, since some CFS patients have a SATET-positive test, they may have a peripheral component to their fatigue. In this respect, although muscle histometry (proportions of types 1 and 2 muscle fibers and muscle fiber atrophy) in CFS patients did not show the changes that would be seen as a result of inactivity (shift to predominance of type 2 muscle fibers and fiber atrophy), those patients with abnormal lactate responses to exercise (subanaerobic threshold exercise test) had a significantly lower proportion of mitochondria-rich type 1 muscle fibers (Lane, Barrett, Woodrow, et al., 1998). Another study (McCully et al., 1996) confirmed that oxidative muscle metabolism, as measured by the maximal rate of postexercise phosphocreatine (PCr) resynthesis using the adenosine diphosphate (ADP) model, is reduced in chronic fatigue syndrome patients compared to sedentary controls and a single bout of strenuous exercise does not cause a further reduction in oxidative metabolism.

NUTRITIONAL FACTORS

In a prospective, observational study of forty-five adults with primary cancer of the lung receiving outpatient primary or adjuvant radiation therapy, Beach and colleagues (2001) reported that although fatigue and nutrition are major problems for patients with lung cancer, nutritional changes do not correlate with fatigue. However, in a review of records of 455 pediatric cancer patients to investigate the relationship of nutritional status at time of first referral to various measurements of disease and survival, Donaldson and colleagues (1981) found that initial symptoms of weight loss, anorexia, fatigue, and early satiety were all directly correlated. In addition, improved survival was related to good nutritional status for children with localized disease, whereas those with advanced disease had a poorer survival regardless of their nutritional status. Nutritional status therefore appears to have prognostic implications among children with cancer (Donaldson et al., 1981). Besides the role of cysteine deficiency in certain cases discussed above, some studies suggest that other nutritional deficiencies may also be pertinent to cancer-related fatigue.

Another possibility, namely impaired detoxification of nutrients or environmental agents, has been postulated to be associated with both cancer and fatigue (Racciatti et al., 2001; Thorn and Kerekes, 2001). The human body is exposed to a wide array of xenobiotics in an individual's lifetime, from food components to environmental toxins to pharmaceuticals, and relies on complex enzymatic mechanisms to detoxify these substances. These mechanisms exhibit significant individual variability and are affected by environment, lifestyle, and genetic influences. The scientific literature suggests an association between impaired detoxification and certain diseases, including cancer, Parkinson's disease, fibromyalgia, and chronic fatigue syndrome (Sorenson, 1999). Data regarding these hepatic detoxification enzyme systems and the body's mechanisms of regulating them suggests the ability to efficiently detoxify and remove xenobiotics can affect these and other chronic disease processes (Liska, 1998).

Carnitine Deficiency

At doses greater than 50 g/cm^2 or in combination with cisplatin, the alkylating agent ifosfamide can cause temporary and permanent damage to the proximal renal tubule (Smeitink et al., 1988). Ifosfamide and cisplatin therefore can cause urinary loss of carnitine, which is a fundamental molecule for energy production in mammalian cells. Carnitine is essential for energy production by mitochondria, cellular organelles that are energy factories. Carnitine deficiency may be a factor in ifosfamide chemotherapy-related fatigue, and carnitine supplementation has been associated with improvement of fatigue in postchemotherapy patients (Graziano et al., 2002).

It is worth noting that Kuratsune and colleagues (1998) reported a serum acylcarnitine deficiency in Japanese and Swedish patients with chronic fatigue syndrome or with chronic hepatitis C but not in those with hematological malignancies, chronic pancreatitis, hypertension, diabetes mellitus, or psychiatric diseases.

Phosphate Deficiency

Nephrotoxicity associated with use of ifosfamide, alone or in combination with cisplatin, results in a reduced threshold for phosphate reabsorption. The consequences are metabolic acidosis, renal phosphate loss, hypercalciuria, and, in severe cases, hypophosphatemic osteomalacia (Smeitink et al., 1988). Phosphate diabetes, i.e., phosphate depletion secondary to abnormal renal absorption of phosphate by the proximal tubule, has been associated with chronic fatigue (De Lorenzo, Hargreaves, and Kakkar, 1998; Laroche and Tack, 1999). In this respect, based on measurements of phosphate reabsorption by the proximal renal tubule, phosphate clearance, and renal threshold phosphate concentration, nine out of 87 chronic fatigue syndrome patients in one study (De Lorenzo, Hargreaves, and Kakkar, 1998) also fulfilled the diagnostic criteria for phosphate diabetes (phosphate depletion secondary to abnormal renal reabsorption of phosphate by the proximal tubule). Studies are needed to investigate if the possible beneficial effects of vitamin D and oral phosphate supplements should be considered in the management of fatigue in this and other contexts of cancer-related fatigue.

Magnesium Deficiency

As mentioned in Chapter 2, magnesium deficiency can be apparent as a chronic fatiguing illness that may even predispose to cancer (Aleksandrowicz and Skotnicki, 1982; Bois, 1968; Bois and Beaulnes, 1966; Hass et al., 1981). Cancer therapy may also affect mineral levels, and it is therefore important to monitor and manage for possible mineral deficiencies.

Although chronic sleep deprivation causes a deficiency of intracellular magnesium and decreased exercise tolerance, which can be improved by oral magnesium administration (Tanabe et al., 1998), one study found no association between magnesium deficiency, chronic fatigue syndrome, or fibromyalgia (Moorkens et al., 1997). Magnesium deficiency may be present in a subset of patients with spasmophilia, and some groups are investigating whether magnesium supplementation may benefit CFS patients (Laylander, 1999a,b; Seelig, 1998).

Low Serum Albumin Levels

Low serum albumin was found to be a laboratory value predictor for severe fatigue in patients with hematological malignancies: leukemia and non-Hodgkin's lymphoma (Wang et al., 2002). As discussed in Chapter 4, hypolbuminemia can be addressed with appropriate nutritional interventions.

High Cerebrospinal Fluid Homocysteine Levels

One study found that increased homocysteine levels in the central nervous system characterize patients fulfilling the criteria for both chronic fatigue syndrome and fibromyalgia. A significant positive correlation occurred between both high cerebrospinal fluid-homocysteine and low vitamin B_{12} levels and fatigability. Vitamin B_{12} deficiency causes a deficient remethylation of homocysteine and probably contributed to the increased homocysteine levels found (Regland et al., 1997).

Vitamins C and B_{12}, and Folate

In terms of the potential usefulness of vitamins in chronic fatigue syndrome treatment, a group (Kodama, Kodama, and Murakami, 1996a,b) in Japan indicated that a megadose vitamin C drip infusion treatment enhanced the activity of endogenous glucocorticoids in such a way as to improve the clinical course of allergy and autoimmune disease. This group studied patients with chronic pneumonia who fit the diagnostic criteria for chronic fatigue syndrome and tested two kinds of vitamin C infusion sets, with and without concomitant oral intake of erythromycin and chloramphenicol, for treatment of the pneumonia. The dehydroepiandrosterone-annexed vitamin C infusion set (expected to enhance the endogenous activities of both glucocorticoids and gonadal steroids) was effective in patients with chronic pneumonia and CFS-like symptoms when used in combination with antibiotics while the annex-free vitamin C set was effective only in patients with the common cold (Kodama, Kodama, and Murakami, 1996a,b).

Whether certain forms of vitamin supplementation are useful in chronic fatigue syndrome remains to be determined. One group reported ineffectiveness of high-dose vitamin B_{12} injections in one CFS patient (Wiebe, 1996). Although a subset of chronic fatigue syndrome patients was reported to be deficient (Jacobson et al., 1993), a common genetic variant affecting folate metabolism was not overrepresented in chronic fatigue syndrome (Harmon et al., 1997) and a trial of liver extract-folic acid-cyanocobalamin did not yield significant effects (Kaslow, Rucker, and Onishi, 1989).

Amino Acids

Studies in animals and human subjects have revealed a role for the serotonergic system in fatigue after exercise, and these results may be useful to understanding postexertional fatigue in chronic fatigue syndrome. Tryptophan is converted to the neurotransmitter 5-hydroxytryptamine in the brain and an increase in the concentration of serotonin can result in physical and mental fatigue during prolonged exercise and can also affect sleep (Bianchi, Grossi, and Bargossi, 1997; Cunliffe, Obeid, and Powell-Tuck, 1997, 1998; Gastmann and Lehmann, 1998; Newsholme and Blomstrand, 1996; Struder et al., 1998; Tanaka et al., 1997; Yamamoto et al., 1997). A study showed that fatigue during endurance exercise in normal individuals was increased by pharmacological augmentation of the brain serotonergic activity by serotonin reuptake inhibitors (Struder et al., 1998). The entry of tryptophan in the brain is influenced by the plasma level of free tryptophan (that not bound to albumin) and, from competition for entry into brain, by the plasma level of branched chain amino acids. Animal studies have shown that tryptophan ingestion and the resulting raised plasma free tryptophan to competitor amino acid ratios leads to an increased subjective and central fatigue. Oral administration of branched amino acids could prevent the increase in serotonin level during exercise and therefore delay physical and mental fatigue, but results from different reports on athletes are contradictory and the ergogenic value of amino acids needs further investigation (Gastmann and Lehmann, 1998; Newsholme and Blomstrand, 1996; Struder et al., 1998). Although L-glutamine was proposed to have an ergogenic effect during exercise considering its base generating potential, a study provided evidence that although low plasma and muscle glutamine concentrations may occur coincident with chronic fatigue syndrome, they may not be directly causative of fatigue or other symptoms since normalization of glutamine levels with supplementation was not associated with clinical improvement (Rowbottom, Keast, Pervan, et al., 1998). The results are consistent with the finding that acute ingestion of L-glutamine does not enhance either buffering potential or high-intensity exercise performance in trained males (Haub et al., 1998).

High doses of creatine supplementation improve performance during repeated sprint runs in well-trained handball players (Aaserud et al., 1998; Greenhaff, 1996). Further studies are needed to clarify whether low doses of creatine supplementation, after a period with supplementation of high doses, are able to maintain improved performance. Studies in chronic fatigue syndrome patients are also needed.

Low muscle glycogen levels secondary to consecutive days of extensive exercise have been shown to cause fatigue and thus decrements in performance. Low muscle glycogen levels could also lead to oxidation of the branched amino acids and central fatigue. Research on swimmers has shown that those who were nonresponsive to an increase in their training load had low levels of muscle glycogen and consumed insufficient energy and carbohydrates. However, cyclists who increased their training load for two weeks, but also increased carbohydrate intake to maintain muscle glycogen levels, still met the criteria of overreaching (short-term overtraining) and might have met the criteria for overtraining had the subjects been followed for a longer period of time. Thus some other mechanism than reduced muscle glycogen levels must be responsible for the development and occurrence of overtraining (Snyder, 1998). Despite these results, particular forms of carbohydrate supplementation may be beneficial in chronic fatigue syndrome since addition of a glyconutrient compound (dietary supplement that supplies the crucial eight monosaccharides required for synthesis of glycoproteins) to peripheral blood cells of CFS patients in vitro significantly increased the expression of the glycoproteins CD5, CD8, and CD11a, enhanced natural killer cell activity, and decreased the percentage of apoptotic cells (all three parameters were deficient at baseline) (See et al., 1998).

A study of urine specimens from twenty CFS patients revealed increases in aminohydroxy-*N*-methylpyrrolidine (referred to as chronic fatigue symptom urinary marker 1, or CFSUM1), tyrosine, beta-alanine, aconitic acid, and succinic acid and reductions in an unidentified urinary metabolite, CFSUM2, alanine, and glutamic acid. CFSUM1, beta-alanine, and CFSUM2 were found by discriminant function analysis to be the first, second, and third most important metabolites, respectively, for discriminating between CFS and non-CFS subjects. The abundances of CFSUM1 and beta-alanine were positively correlated with symptom incidence, symptom severity, core chronic fatigue syndrome symptoms, and symptom core list (SCL)-90-R somatization, an observation that suggests a molecular basis for chronic fatigue syndrome (McGregor et al., 1996a). In a second report by the same group, severe fatigue was the only symptom with 100 percent sensitivity and specificity and CFSUM1 excretion was the primary metabolite for expression of this symptom. All symptom indices analyzed (symptom indices of total symptom incidence, chronic fatigue syndrome core symptoms, cognitive, neurological, musculoskeletal, gastrointestinal, infection-related, and genitourinary symptom indices, as well as a visual analog pain scale of average pain intensity) had elevated responses in the CFS patients and significant correlations with changes in the urinary excretion of metabolites. CFSUM1 and beta-alanine were the first and second metabolites correlated with the chronic fatigue syndrome core symptom index, and CFSUM1 was primarily associated with infection-related and musculoskeletal indexes whereas beta-alanine was primarily associated with gastrointestinal and genitourinary indexes (McGregor et al., 1996b).

The ATP Hypothesis

As reviewed by Morrow, Andrews, and colleagues (2002), the fact that many cancer patients describe feelings of weakness in association with the fatigue that they experience during and after treatment supports the hypothesis that abnormalities of generation or use of adenosine triphosphate (ATP) could be an underlying mechanism of fatigue. Research has demonstrated a relationship between fatigue and physical performance ability in cancer patients (Akechi et al., 1999; Dimeo, Stieglitz, et al., 1997), who often describe their fatigue as a feeling of lack of energy (Forsyth et al., 1999; Nail and Winningham, 1995).

ATP is the source of energy for most cellular functions, including membrane transport (of sodium, potassium, and other ions), synthesis of chemical compounds (such as proteins), and mechanical work (e.g., muscle contraction, ciliary movement, and ameboid motion). Most cellular ATP is formed in mitochrondria when hydrogen atoms, released in the citric acid cycle, subsequently undergo oxidation to form water, in a process called oxidative phosphorylation. Splitting of one or both of ATP's high-energy phosphate bonds to form adenosine diphosphate (ADP) or adenosine monophosphate (AMP) quickly provides needed energy for cellular functioning.

ATP can be quickly replenished from ADP and AMP, provided adequate food energy, particularly in the form of glucose, is available. Patients with cancer, especially those under treatment, often report alterations in appetite ranging from a mild decrease in desire for food, sometimes manifest as a distaste for particular food items, to full-blown anorexia, resulting in decreased energy intake. Treatment with chemotherapy, accompanied by nausea in more than 50 percent of patients and vomiting in up to 25 percent, can lead to decreased food intake in the days immediately after infusion of the chemotherapy agents. Fatigue associated with receipt of chemotherapy often follows a similar time pattern, gradually increasing in severity in the days following treatment, reaching a peak seven to ten days after treatment, and then slowly improving until the next cycle of chemotherapy begins.

In one study of patients with chronic fatigue syndrome, increased 2'-5' A synthetase and RNase L activity led to depleted cellular ATP, which was thought to be a pivotal lesion responsible for severe fatigue, cognitive difficulties or other disturbances (Forsyth et al., 1999). Other investigators have also found impaired synthesis of ATP and defective muscle energy metabolism along with impaired voluntary activation of skeletal muscle during sustained intense exercise in a proportion of patients with chronic fatigue syndrome (Lane, Barrett, Taylor, et al., 1998), suggesting the presence of a central component of fatigue, possibly associated with decreased effort, reduced motivation, or impaired concentration (Kent-Braun et al., 1993). Reduced ATP concentration owing to impaired oxidative phosphorylation may also be involved in feelings of fatigue and weakness in patients with chronic renal failure (Pastoris et al., 1997).

Altered muscle metabolism, as a result of decreased synthesis of various proteins or accumulation of certain metabolites, for example, may also contribute to cancer-related fatigue (Cella et al., 1998). ATP concentrations may be relatively low in certain areas of tumors themselves (Feller et al., 1994; Karczmar et al., 1989, 1991; Tamulevicius and Streffer, 1995). Compromised blood supply to tumors results in oxygen-depleted areas of the tumors, associated with deprivation of nutrients and energy and a hostile metabolic microenvironment (i.e., severe tissue acidosis), including decreased ATP in tumor cells (Karczmar et al., 1991) and lymphocytes (Robins et al., 1991). Incubation of malignant cell lines with cytostatic drugs has resulted in marked decreases in intracellular ATP levels, the degree of decrease varying with the strength of the cytostatic drugs (Kuzmits, Rumpold, et al., 1986). In an in vivo study, lymphocyte ATP decreased following surgery in nine of thirteen patients, and the decrease was associated with cancer spread and presence of immunosuppressive tumors (Mukherjee and Sahasrabuddhe, 1982).

Nicotinamide adenine dinucleotide (NAD) is a key coenzyme in the process of oxidative phosphorylation and is therefore important in the formation of ATP (Pastoris et al., 1997). In a randomized, double-blind, crossover study, Forsyth and colleagues (1999) compared the ability of NADH, the reduced form of the coenzyme nicotinamide adenine dinucleotide, and placebo, to ameliorate symptoms of chronic fatigue syndrome, including fatigue, cognitive dysfunction, and sleep disturbance. Eight of twenty-six patients (31 percent) showed at least 10 percent improvement in their source on a questionnaire measuring fatigue, memory, ability to concentrate, sleep disturbance, and mood and reported decreased fatigue, decreased symptoms overall, and improved quality of life while taking the study drug, compared with two of the twenty-six (8 percent) taking placebo (Forsyth et al., 1999).

Similarities in the quality and degree of fatigue in patients with chronic fatigue syndrome, other diseases associated with this symptom, and cancer, especially in patients undergoing chemotherapy, and the correspondence between appetite changes and the course of postchemotherapy fatigue, suggest a reasonable hypothesis that at least a portion (Haskell, 1994; Haskell and Lee, 1994; Haskell et al., 1996; Mansur-Garza and Ishikawa, 1994) of the fatigue associated with chemotherapy of cancer could be related to alterations in energy metabolism. Repletion of intracellular stores of ATP, for example by giving NADH, might be expected to ameliorate feelings of lack of energy and promote enhanced physical performance. Such research tools as assessment of physical activity using Actigraphy and appraisal of cellular metabolic activity (e.g., ATP, creatine phosphate, and lactate levels) in vivo using NMR or in muscle biopsy samples could be used for further evaluation of this hypothesis.

Chapter 4

Treatment of Chronic Fatiguing Illnesses

The National Comprehensive Cancer Network (NCCN) Fatigue Practice Guidelines Panel has reviewed the available evidence and the consensus of practitioners regarding the management of cancer-related fatigue and has developed clinical practice guidelines (Mock, 2001b; Mock et al., 2000). The guidelines propose a treatment algorithm in which patients are evaluated regularly for fatigue, using a brief screening instrument, and are treated as indicated by their fatigue level. The goal is to identify and treat all patients with fatigue that causes distress or interferes with daily activities or functioning. Management of fatigue begins with primary oncology team members who perform the initial screening and either provide basic education and counseling or expand the initial screening to a more focused evaluation for moderate or higher levels of fatigue.

At the initial screening point the patient is assessed for the five primary factors known to be associated with fatigue: pain, emotional distress, sleep disturbance, anemia, and hypothyroidism. If any of these conditions are present, it should be treated according to practice guidelines, and the patient's fatigue should be reevaluated regularly. If none of the primary factors is present or the fatigue is unresolved, a more comprehensive assessment is indicated, with referral to other care providers as appropriate. The comprehensive assessment should include a thorough review of systems, review of medications, assessment of comorbidities, nutritional/metabolic evaluation, and assessment of activity level. Management of fatigue is cause specific when conditions known to cause fatigue can be identified and treated. When specific causes, such as infection, fluid and electrolyte imbalances, or cardiac dysfunction, cannot be identified and corrected, nonpharmacologic and pharmacologic treatment of the fatigue should be considered.

Nonpharmacologic interventions may include a moderate exercise program to improve functional capacity and activity tolerance, restorative therapies to decrease cognitive alterations and improve mood state, and nutritional and sleep interventions for patients with disturbances in eating or sleeping. Pharmacologic therapy may include drugs such as antidepressants for depression or erythropoietin for anemia. A few clinical reports of the use of corticosteroids and psychostimulants suggest the need for further research on these agents as potential treatment modalities in managing fatigue. Basic to these interventions, the effective management of cancer-related fatigue involves an informed and supportive oncology care team that assesses patients' fatigue levels regularly and systematically and incorporates education and counseling regarding strategies for coping with fatigue, as well as using institutional fatigue management experts for referral of patients with unresolved fatigue (Mock, 2001b; Mock et al., 2000).

The Mersey Palliative Care Audit Group also developed guidelines for the assessment and management of fatigue (Coackley et al., 2002). These guidelines were produced following a regional survey, which looked at both the educational needs of nurses and the impact of fatigue on patients with advanced cancer. However, Servaes, Verhagen, and Bleijenberg (2002) point out that although most intervention studies to reduce fatigue appear to be successful, follow-up analyses are lacking and it is hard to draw conclusions with regard to the relationships between fatigue and disease- and treatment-related characteristics, because these relationships are seldom properly investigated. Although gaps exist in our knowledge and further research is needed to support proposed practice guidelines for fatigue, there is a developing body of knowledge and consensus of clinicians and other health care workers regarding the management of fatigue in cancer patients (Cognis, 1999). Current practice guidelines are therefore based on a combination of research and expert clinical judgment (Nail, 2002; Wharton, 2002). Treatment of other chronic fatiguing illnesses follows a similar approach and the strategies overlap. The following sections, as outlined here, will cover in further detail the interventions mentioned previously as well as other possible treatments for fatigue and chronic fatiguing illnesses, some based on treatment of related diseases.

    I. Graded exercise
   II. Graded activity (energy management) therapy
  III. Sleep therapy
  IV. Cognitive-behavioral therapy
   V. Nutritional therapy
     A. Carnitine supplementation
     B. Cysteine supplementation alone or with vitamin C
     C. Electrolyte supplementation
     D. Alcohol consumption
  VI. Pharmacological therapy
     A. Erythropoietin
     B. Treatment of underlying disease such as cancer and paraneoplastic syndromes

C. Methylphenidate
D. Selective serotonin reuptake inhibitors (SSRIs)
E. Monoamine oxidase inhibitors (MAOIs)
F. Amantadine
G. Corticosteroids
VII. Complementary and alternative therapy
    A. Herbal therapy
        1. *Aloë vera (Aloë vulgaris, Aloë barbadensis)*
        2. *Echinacea (E. angustifolia, E. pallida, E. purpurea,* purple coneflower)
        3. Erkang
        4. Hochu-ekki-to (TJ-41:bu-zhong-yi-qi-tang)
        5. *Syngnathus acus*
        6. Hedgehog hydnum
        7. Juzen-taiho-to
        8. Lentinan
        9. *Panax ginseng*
        10. *Tinospora cordifolia*
        11. *Rhodiola rosea*
        12. Kavosporal forte
        13. *Astragalus membranaceus*
          a. Limitations and precautions with herbal medicine
        14. Homeopathy
        15. Massage therapy
        16. Acupuncture
        17. Melatonin
        18. Neurofeedback
VIII. Immunotherapy
    A. Cytokine antagonists
    B. Therapies that shift cytokine expression patterns
        1. Lymph node cell-based therapy
        2. *Mycobacterium vaccae*
        3. Staphylococcal vaccine
        4. Sizofiran
IX. Antimicrobial therapies
    A. Historical background
    B. Acyclovir and related antiherpetic drugs
    C. Ampligen
    D. 2CVV
    E. Epstein-Barr virus vaccine
    F. Immunovir (inosine pranobex)

G. Influenza virus vaccine alone or in combination with other vaccines
H. Thimerosal
 I. Staphylococcal vaccine
 J. Stealth virus vaccine
K. SPV-30
 L. Transfer factors against herpesviruses

GRADED EXERCISE

In cancer patients, exercise is a feasible and potentially beneficial intervention to combat distressing cancer-related fatigue by helping to prevent its appearance and reduce its intensity (Al-Majid and McCarthy, 2001; Dimeo, 2001, 2002; Evans, 2002; Friendenreich and Courneya, 1996; Mock et al., 1998; Nail, 2002; Pinto and Maruyama, 1999). In fact, graded aerobic exercise has been shown in randomized controlled trials to be an effective intervention in specific patient groups (Irwin et al., 2002; Stone, 2002). Therefore, an aerobic exercise program of precisely defined intensity, duration, and frequency can be prescribed as therapy for primary fatigue in cancer patients (Dimeo, Rumberger, and Keul, 1998). Koch (2002) pointed out that an active aerobic training program can improve physical performance and fitness in a short time as part of rehabilitation after surgery for gastrointestinal malignant tumors.

Courneya and Friedenreich (1999) reviewed twenty-four empirical studies published between 1980 and 1997 on physical exercise following cancer diagnosis. Although eighteen of the studies were interventions (i.e., quasi-experimental or experimental), most of these were preliminary efficacy studies that suffered from the common limitations of such designs. Overall, however, the studies consistently demonstrated that physical exercise has a positive effect on quality of life following cancer diagnosis, including physical and functional well-being (e.g., functional capacity, muscular strength, body composition, nausea, fatigue) and psychological and emotional well-being (e.g., personality functioning, mood states, self-esteem, and quality of life).

In a pilot study undertaken to test the effects of a twenty-eight-day exercise intervention on levels of fatigue in advanced cancer patients, all participants were able to increase their activity levels with no increase in reported fatigue (Porock et al., 2000). Furthermore, a trend was noted in all patients toward increased quality-of-life scores and decreased anxiety scores. All participants described a sense of satisfaction in attaining increased activity levels. The preliminary pilot results also suggest that patients who initially report the highest levels of fatigue may achieve the largest decrease in fatigue scores (Porock et al., 2000).

Dimeo and colleagues (1996) reported that fatigue and loss of physical performance in patients undergoing bone marrow transplantation can be corrected with adequate rehabilitative measures. In their study, twenty patients entered the six-week rehabilitation program, consisting of walking on a treadmill. Patients started the training program thirty (+/– 12) days (range eighteen to forty-two) post-bone marrow transplantation. By the end of the program, the authors observed a significant improvement in maximal physical performance and maximum walking distance, and a significant lowering of the heart rate with equivalent workloads. All participants of the program reached a peak performance (calculated in metabolic equivalents [METs]) more than sufficient for carrying out all basic activities of daily living. These results contrast with literature reports discussed in previous chapters which indicate that spontaneous recovery of physical functioning after bone marrow transplantation can take many months and that about 30 percent of patients experience long-lasting impairment of physical performance.

In another study, Dimeo and colleagues (1999) reported on a group of cancer patients receiving high-dose chemotherapy followed by autologous peripheral blood stem cell transplantation (training group of twenty-seven individuals) who followed an exercise program during hospitalization. The program was comprised of biking on an ergometer in the supine position following an interval-training pattern for thirty minutes daily. Patients in the control group (thirty-two individuals) did not train. By the time of hospital discharge, fatigue and somatic complaints had increased significantly in the control group but not in the training group. Furthermore, by the time of hospital discharge, the training group had a significant improvement in several scores of psychological distress (obsessive-compulsive traits, fear, interpersonal sensitivity, and phobic anxiety); this outcome was not observed in the control group. The study concluded that aerobic exercise reduces fatigue and improves symptoms of psychological distress in cancer patients undergoing chemotherapy (Dimeo et al., 1999).

Dimeo, Tilmann, and colleagues (1997) also evaluated the feasibility and effects of aerobic training in the rehabilitation of cancer patients after completing high-dose chemotherapy. Sixteen patients participated in a specially designed rehabilitation program for six weeks. The patients entered the program, which consisted of walking on a treadmill, shortly after completing treatment. Sixteen patients who did not train served as controls. At the time of discharge from the hospital, maximum physical performance and hemoglobin concentration were similar for both groups. After seven weeks, improvement in maximum physical performance and hemoglobin concentration were significantly higher for the training group. By the second examination, no patient in the training group but four controls (25 percent) reported fatigue and limitations in daily activities secondary to low physical performance. Aerobic exercise therefore improves the physical performance of cancer patients recovering from high-dose chemotherapy. Dimeo, Tilmann, and colleagues (1997) recommend that to reduce fatigue, this group of patients should be counseled to increase physical activity rather than rest after treatment.

A multi-institutional pilot study explored the effects of a home-based moderate walking exercise intervention on fatigue, physical functioning, emotional distress, and quality of life in fifty-two women during breast cancer treatment (Mock et al., 2001). Women who exercised at least ninety minutes per week on three or more days reported significantly less fatigue and emotional distress, as well as higher functional ability and quality of life, than women who were less active during treatment. Therefore, this pilot study suggests that a home-based walking exercise program is a potentially effective, low-cost, and safe intervention to manage fatigue and to improve quality of life during adjuvant chemotherapy or radiation therapy for breast cancer (Mock et al., 2001).

Based on an experimental, two-group pretest, posttest study of forty-six women beginning a six-week program of radiation therapy for early-stage breast cancer, Mock and colleagues (1997) found that the exercise group scored significantly higher than the usual-care group on physical functioning and symptom intensity, particularly fatigue, anxiety, and difficulty sleeping. The authors concluded that a self-paced, home-based walking exercise program can help manage symptoms and improve physical functioning during radiation therapy. Moreover, in a study of fourteen women receiving adjuvant chemotherapy for breast cancer (86 percent stage II) following surgical treatment, measures of physical performance, psychosocial adjustment, and symptom intensity revealed improved adaptation in subjects who completed the walking/support group program as compared to standard care (Mock et al., 1994).

Schwartz, Mori, and colleagues (2001) examined the relationship between a home-based moderate-intensity exercise intervention and fatigue over the first three cycles of chemotherapy in seventy-two women receiving either cyclophosphamide, methotrexate, and fluorouracil or doxorubicin and cyclophosphamide for breast cancer. Exercise significantly reduced daily fatigue, and as the duration of exercise increased, the intensity of fatigue declined. There was a significant carryover effect of exercise on fatigue, but the effect lasted only one day. This study underscores the effectiveness of a low- to moderate-intensity regular exercise program in maintaining functional ability and reducing fatigue in women with breast cancer receiving chemotherapy (Schwartz, Mori, et al., 2001).

In seventy-eight women who had recently received a diagnosis of breast cancer and who were beginning adjuvant chemotherapy, Schwartz (2000b) studied the effects of a home-based exercise study during the first four cycles of chemotherapy. Women who adhered to the exercise program maintained their body weight, while nonexercisers steadily gained weight. There were no differences in incidence or intensity of nausea or anorexia between the exercisers and nonexercisers. Women who exercised over the four cycles of chemotherapy improved their functional ability (mean 23 percent) compared to the nonexercisers, who showed significant declines in functional ability (mean –15 percent). Therefore, exercise may be an effective intervention to minimize weight gain in women with breast cancer who are receiving adjuvant chemotherapy. Preventing weight gain in these patients may be important in preventing recurrent disease and other comorbidities associated with excess weight (Schwartz, 2000a,b).

The study confirmed findings of a previous smaller study of thirty-one breast cancer patients, in which Schwartz (1999) also concluded that women who adopted the exercise program (60 percent) showed significant increases in functional ability and less weight gain. It should be pointed out that the maximum effect of exercise on quality-of-life outcomes may be mediated by fatigue. In this respect, Schwartz (2000a) also reported that exercise appears to reduce the levels of average and worst fatigue and may help women recognize their pattern of fatigue. In this respect, the most common pattern of fatigue after chemotherapy demonstrated a sharp rise in fatigue. However, several women demonstrated a chaotic pattern with erratic and wide swings in their fatigue. Women who adopted exercise experienced fewer days of high fatigue levels and more days of low levels of fatigue for both average and worst levels of fatigue. In contrast, women who did not exercise experienced more bad days (high fatigue) and fewer good days (low fatigue). Exercise may therefore also reduce the intensity of fatigue by reorganizing women's interpretation of fatigue (Schwartz, 2000a).

Schwartz (1998a) performed a cross-sectional, descriptive survey of 219 cancer survivors, the majority of whom were physically active before diagnosis and continued to exercise during their treatments with modifications in their activity level. Respondents exercised an average of nine hours per week. Sixty-nine percent of the respondents experienced problems with cancer-related fatigue during treatment, with 52 percent describing their cancer-related fatigue as affecting their whole body. Although 26 percent of the respondents felt most fatigued before exercise, exercise and rest were the most commonly used strategies for managing their symptoms. Patients with non-Hodgkin's lymphoma experienced significantly different cancer-related fatigue than patients with breast or prostate cancer and reported fewer benefits from exercise (Schwartz, 1998a).

Graydon and colleagues (1995) reported that sleep and exercise were among the most effective fatigue-reducing strategies (as assessed by the Pearson Byars Fatigue Feeling Checklist and the Fatigue Relief Scale) used by women patients receiving treatment for cancer, either chemotherapy (forty-five patients studied) or radiation therapy (fifty-four patients studied). Progressive resistance exercise training has been demonstrated to greatly increase strength, improve protein balance, and increase muscle mass even in very frail and old men and women (Evans, 2002). Exercise has also been shown to decrease the levels of many inflammatory and blood clotting markers that are associated with congestive heart failure, diabetes, and the geriatric syndrome of frailty, which is characterized by fatigue, muscle weakness, weight loss, declines in activity, and slow or unsteady gait (Walston et al., 2002).

Evidence suggests that endurance exercise also ameliorates cancer-related fatigue. However, no compelling evidence supports the assertion that exercise-induced reduction in fatigue is related to preservation of muscle mass. Although resistance exercise attenuates muscle wasting associated with a variety of catabolic conditions, its effects on cancer-induced muscle wasting have not been adequately studied (Al-Majid and McCarthy, 2001). Moreover, Kasper and Sarna (2000) documented that although quadricep muscle size and strength increased in some women undergoing adjuvant chemotherapy for breast cancer, the subjective experiences of fatigue did not necessarily decrease. A similar dissociation between fatigue and muscle strength appears to also be present in chronic fatigue syndrome. Although many CFS patients experience "relapses" of severe symptoms following even moderate levels of exertion, most studies report CFS patients to have normal muscle strength and either normal or slightly reduced endurance (McCully, Sisto, and Natelson, 1996). Histological and metabolic studies report that CFS patients have either no impairment or mild impairment of mitochondria and oxidative metabolism compared with sedentary controls (McCully, Sisto, and Natelson, 1996). Normal muscle metabolism during exercise and no muscle damage after physical activity have been reported in fibromyalgia patients (Mengshoel, Vollestad, and Forre, 1995; Mengshoel, 1996). Moreover, Miller, Allen, and Gandevia (1996) reported that muscle contractile failure, poor motivation, and reflex pain inhibition are not important in the pathogenesis of fatigue in fibromyalgia patients.

Benefits of exercise in patients with chronic fatiguing illnesses include:

1. Reduction of:
   - Fatigue
   - Anxiety and psychological distress
   - Difficulty sleeping
   - Weight gain
   - Levels of inflammatory and blood clotting factors
2. Improvement of:
   - Activity levels
   - Protein balance
   - Recovery time of physical functioning
   - Muscle mass

Several groups also suggest that exercise training programs are beneficial (if "relapses" can be avoided) in fatiguing illnesses, such as chronic fatigue syndrome, although few controlled studies have been performed (Baschetti, 1998; Elliot, Goldberg, and Loveless, 1997; Franklin, 1997; Fulcher and White, 1997; Goudsmit, 1997, 1998; Lapp, 1997; Michael, 1998; Sadler, 1997; Shepherd and MacIntyre, 1997). A randomized controlled trial (Fulcher and White, 1997) to test the efficacy of a graded aerobic exercise program in sixty-six CFS patients with control treatment crossover after the first follow-up examination supports the use of appropriately prescribed graded aerobic exercise in the management of CFS patients. Studies have also documented that extended outpatient rehabilitation programs with exercise for persons with definite progressive multiple sclerosis (MS) appear to effectively reduce fatigue and the severity of other symptoms (DiFabio et al., 1998; LaBan et al., 1998).

As reviewed by Manu (2000), the beneficial effects of exercise in patients with chronic fatigue syndrome are evinced in several studies. One such trial was performed at the National Sports Medicine Institute and St. Bartholomew's Hospital, London, in which CFS patients without psychiatric disorders or sleep disturbances were randomly assigned to receive a twelve-week program of either graded aerobic exercise or a combination of relaxation therapy and flexibility training (Fulcher and White, 1997). Analysis by intention to treat showed that severity of fatigue, functional capacity, and fitness improved in 52 percent of patients enrolled in the aerobic exercise program compared with 27 percent of the control group. Graded exercise was also effective when tested in a twenty-eight-week trial conducted at the Whittington Hospital by faculty members of the University of Manchester, United Kingdom (Wearden et al., 1998). Using a four-cell design that compared exercise with treatment with the antidepressant fluoxetine (Prozac) and placebo, the study showed that exercise was effective in reducing the severity of fatigue, improving functional work capacity, and favorably influencing the health perception of this group of CFS patients. In all of these studies, and in additional research measuring immunological parameters (Lloyd et al., 1994; LaManca et al., 1999), graded aerobic exercise to exhaustion was well tolerated.

Measurement of physical activity after strenuous exercise in women with chronic fatigue syndrome compared to sedentary healthy volunteers who exercised no more than once per week revealed that although marked exertion produces changes in activity, these changes are apparent later than self-reports would suggest and that they are not so severe that CFS patients cannot compensate (Sisto et al., 1998). One study (Sisto et al., 1996) found that, compared with normal controls, women with chronic fatigue syndrome have an aerobic power indicating a low normal fitness level with no indication of cardiopulmonary abnormality. The CFS group would withstand a maximal treadmill exercise test without a major exacerbation in either fatigue or other symptoms of their illness. Similarly, Nielens, Boisset, and Masquelier (2000) found that cardiorespiratory fitness, as expressed by a submaximal work capacity index, seems normal, despite increased perceived exertion scores, in thirty female fibromyalgia patients compared with sixty-seven age- and sex-matched healthy individuals. Moreover, the observation that the performance decrements associated with the development of chronic fatigue syndrome in an elite ultra-endurance athlete were the result of detraining rather than an impairment of aerobic metabolism may be indicative of central, possibly neurological, factors influencing fatigue perception in CFS sufferers (Rowbottom, Keast, Green, et al., 1998). In this respect, a study (Samii et al., 1996) of the effects of exercise on motor-evoked potentials elicited by transcranial magnetic stimulation (TMS) found that postexercise cortical excitability is significantly reduced in patients with chronic fatigue syndrome and in depressed patients compared with that of normal subjects. Whether a similar phenomenon may play a role in cancer-related fatigue remains to be determined.

Exercise programs alone or in combination with other interventions have also proven useful in the treatment of fibromyalgia (Buckelew et al., 1998; Deuster, 1996; Dominick et al., 1999; Wigers, Stiles, and Vogel, 1996). The type, duration, and intensity of the exercise program deserve special consideration. Training has shown little benefit with regard to pain but has improved the physical fitness of the patients. Since pain may be exacerbated by physical activity, many patients become physically inactive, with possible development of reduced physical fitness. In the long run, fibromyalgia patients who exercise report fewer symptoms than sedentary patients do.

Thus, exercise should be aimed at preventing physical inactivity and improving patients' physical fitness (Mengshoel, 1996). Similar to cancer, physical therapy for fibromyalgia is aimed at reducing pain, fatigue, deconditioning, muscle weakness, sleep disturbances, and other disease consequences (Mengshoel, 1997). A review by Offenbächer and Stucki (2000) concluded that, based on evidence from randomized controlled trials, cardiovascular fitness training significantly improves cardiovascular fitness, both subjective and objective measures of pain, as well as subjective energy and work capacity, and physical and social activities. Moreover, based on anecdotal evidence of small observational studies, physiotherapy may reduce overloading of the muscle system, improve postural fatigue and positioning, and condition weak muscles.

A study of fifty-eight fibromyalgia patients by Mannerkorpi and colleagues (2000) concluded that six months of exercise in a temperate pool combined with a six-session education program improve physical function, grip strength, pain severity, social functioning, psychological distress, and quality of life. Gowans and colleagues (1999) found similar efficacy for a six-week exercise and educational program tested on forty-one subjects. Meiworm and colleagues (2000) reported a positive effect for twelve weeks of aerobic endurance exercise (jogging, walking, cycling, or swimming) on pain parameters, cardiovascular status, fitness, and well-being of twenty-seven fibromyalgia patients compared to sedentary patient controls. A study of thirty-eight fibromyalgia patients by Martin and colleagues (1996) showed that an exercise program that included aerobic, flexibility, and strengthening elements had no adverse effects and was effective in the short term. Ramsay and colleagues (2000) found that although there was no improvement in pain in a study of seventy-four fibromyalgia patients following either a supervised twelve-week aerobic exercise class or unsupervised home aerobic exercises, there was some significant benefit in psychological well-being in the exercise class group and perhaps a slowing of functional deterioration. Based on a limited study, Meyer and Lemley (2000) suggest that individuals with fibomyalgia can adhere to low-intensity walking programs two to three times per week, possibly reducing fibromyalgia impact on daily activities. Self-help programs that include stretching exercises are also beneficial (Han, 1998).

In a randomized controlled 2 × 2 factorial trial conducted from April 1999 to September 2001 among 1,092 Persian Gulf War veterans who reported at least two of three symptom types (fatigue, pain, and cognitive) for more than six months and at the time of screening, Donta and colleagues (2003) reported that cognitive-behavioral therapy and/or exercise can provide modest relief for some of the symptoms of Gulf War syndrome and other chronic multisystem illnesses. Exercise alone or in combination with cognitive-behavioral therapy significantly improved fatigue, distress, cognitive symptoms, and mental health functioning, while cognitive-behavioral therapy alone significantly improved cognitive symptoms and mental health functioning. Neither treatment had a significant impact on pain. The percentage of veterans with improvement in physical function at one year was 11.5 percent for usual care, 11.7 percent for exercise alone, 18.4 percent for cognitive-behavioral therapy plus exercise, and 18.5 percent for cognitive-behavioral therapy alone (Donta et al., 2003).

Exercise is beneficial not only for the treatment of fatigue in a variety of contexts including cancer but also, as has been covered in many biomedical reviews over the years, for the prevention and treatment of cancer itself (Albanes, Blair, and Taylor, 1987; Ames, Gold, and Willett, 1995; Bartram and Wynder, 1989; Calabrese, 1990; Colditz and Frazier, 1995; Francis, 1996a,b; Friendenreich and Rohan, 1995; Gammon and John, 1993; Hackney, 1996; Hickson, Ball, and Falduto, 1989; Hoffman-Goetz, 1994; Hoffman-Goetz and Husted, 1994; Holmes and Willett, 1995; Irwin et al., 2002; Jákó, 1995; Kelsey and Gammon, 1991; Kohl, LaPorte, and Blair, 1988; Kramer and Wells, 1996; Kuller, 1995; Lee, 1994, 1995; Love and Vogel, 1997; MacFarlane and Lowenfels, 1994; Marti, 1992; Marti and Minder, 1989; Mettlin, 1988; Noble, 1984; Paffenbarger, Lee, and Wing, 1992; Potter, 1995; Potter et al., 1993; Sandler, 1996; Shephard, 1986, 1990, 1992, 1993, 1995, 1996; Shephard and Futcher, 1997; Shephard and Bouchard, 1996; Shephard and Shek, 1996a,b; Simopoulos, 1990; Sternfeld, 1992; Weisburger and Wynder, 1987; Zaridze and Boyle, 1987).

As concluded from a series of meta-analyses of published work by Shephard and Futcher (1997), regular physical activity protects animals against cancer from a variety of sources: subcutaneous, intraperitoneal or intragastric carcinogens, intravenous infusion of tumor cells, or tumor implantation. A study in mice that received intravenous injections of syngeneic B16 melanoma cells thirty minutes postexercise suggests that prolonged exercise has a protective effect against lung tumor metastases and enhances alveolar macrophage antitumor cytotoxicity in vitro (Davis, Kohut, et al., 1998). In humans, regular exercise reduces susceptibility to all-cause cancer, colonic adenomas, colon but not rectal cancers, breast cancers, uterine tumors, prostate and testicular tumors, and possibly lung cancers. At most tumor sites, the average response of women is similar to that of men, but because of a limited number of studies, the effect in women is commonly nonsignificant. The relative effects of occupational and leisure activity are generally similar, an observation which suggests that the optimum response of cancer defense mechanisms is obtained from moderate levels of energy expenditure (Shephard and Futcher, 1997). A few reviews have also considered the beneficial interactions between exercise, immune function, and cancer (Hoffman-Goetz, 1994; Lee, 1995; Liesen and Uhlenbruck, 1992; Shephard and Shek, 1995, 1996a,b).

Winningham (1991, 2000) points out that unnecessary bed rest and prolonged sedentarism can contribute significantly to the development of fatigue and may result in rapid and potentially irreversible losses in energy and functioning among cancer patients. Walking is an important self-care activity that can counter some of the debilitating effects of disease, treatment, and inactivity. By teaching self-care techniques, such as keeping a walking diary and pulse monitoring to regulate activity, nurses can help patients develop safe activity practices (Winningham, 1991, 2000).

Durstine and colleagues (2000) point out that exercise prescription for persons with chronic disease and/or disability should place emphasis on the patient's clinical status, and, as a result, the exercise mode, intensity, frequency, and duration are usually modified according to his or her condition. The types of exercise and activities prescribed for patients with cancer and cancer-related fatigue should be adapted to their current capability and to goals that are realistic, achievable, and increased in a stepwise manner (Fulcher and White, 1998; Cox, 1999). It is recommended that, at least initially, sessions should be carried out by a qualified exercise therapist and supported by written instructions. Exercise intensity and duration should be adapted for the individual and progress determined by response (Fulcher and White, 1998; McCully, Sisto, and Natelson, 1996). The initial aim is to establish a regular pattern of exercise, usually walking, for a small amount per day (such as five minutes), with the exercise routine scheduled into the daily routine of activity and rest (Fulcher and White, 1998; Sharpe, Hawton, Simkin, et al., 1997). Exercise target heart rates are calculated for each patient and monitored throughout treatment to assess cardiovascular response (Fulcher and White, 1998; McCully, Sisto, and Natelson, 1996). The type of exercise is increased in duration and/or intensity as improvement is noted (Fulcher and White, 1998). Several types of exercise, such as swimming, cycling, jogging, walking, or rowing, all of which primarily involve large muscle groups, have been found to be beneficial in fatiguing illnesses (Klug, McAuley, and Clark, 1989). Exercise should preferably not be done within three to six hours of sleep time.

Pickett and colleagues (2002) randomly assigned fifty-two patients with newly diagnosed breast cancer to one of two treatment arms: usual care or usual care plus exercise. Those assigned to the exercise group received a standardized, self-administered, home-based brisk walking intervention in addition to usual care. Each day subjects completed self-report diary forms that elicited information about activity levels and the occurrence of symptoms and side effects during cancer treatment. Analyses of self-reported daily activity levels revealed a diffusion of treatment effect. Fifty percent of the usual-care group reported maintaining or increasing their physical activity to a moderate intensity level, while 33 percent of the exercise group did not exercise at the prescribed levels. Analyses of self-reported disease symptoms and treatment side effects did not reveal clinically meaningful differences between the two groups. Therefore, the results of this study suggest that women who exercised regularly before receiving a breast cancer diagnosis attempted to maintain their exercise programs. Women who lead sedentary lifestyles may benefit from a structured exercise program that includes information and support related to exercise adherence strategies (Pickett et al., 2002).

Courneya, Blanchard, and Liang (2001) applied the theory of planned behavior to understand factors that influence the motivation to exercise after a cancer diagnosis. The authors used a prospective design and assessed exercise adherence among twenty-four breast cancer survivors attending a twice-weekly, twelve-week training program in preparation for a dragon boat race competition. Analyses indicated that the key underlying beliefs were support from physician, spouse, and friends, and confidence in being able to attend the training class when having limited time, no one to exercise with, fatigue, and other health problems. Based on this preliminary study, it was concluded that the theory of planned behavior may provide a good framework on which to base interventions designed to promote exercise in breast cancer survivors (Courneya, Blanchard, and Liang, 2001).

At this point it is worth remembering that too much of a good thing can also be harmful and that exercise, as a therapeutic tool, should be done in moderation. The most important aspects of an exercise program are consistency and grading (Cox, 1999; Royal Colleges of Physicians, General Practitioners, and Psychiatrists, 1996; Sharpe, Hawton, Simkin, et al., 1997). Patients need to be encouraged not to overexert themselves in an attempt to speed up the recovery process, as this could lead to exacerbation of symptoms and consequent avoidance of future exercise or activity (Joyce and Wessely, 1996; Royal Colleges, 1996). Exercise taken to the extreme can be deleterious, as illustrated by the overtraining syndrome, a condition which affects mainly endurance athletes and is characterized by chronic fatigue, underperformance, and an increased vulnerability to infection leading to recurrent infections (Budgett, 1998; Hawley and Reilly, 1997). Although symptoms normally resolve in six to twelve weeks with a very careful exercise regimen and regeneration strategies, they may continue much longer or recur if athletes return to hard training too soon. Psychological, endocrinological, physiological, and immunological factors may all play a role in the failure to recover from exercise in the overtraining syndrome. One study (Lehmann et al., 1998) found that the parasympathetic, Addison-type overtraining syndrome represents the dominant modern type of this syndrome and that functional alterations of the pituitary-adrenal axis and sympathetic system can explain persistent performance incompetence in affected athletes. Another study (Gabriel et al., 1998) found that overtraining does not lead to clinically relevant alterations of immunophenotypes in peripheral blood and an immunosuppressive effect could not be detected. Data from one study (Derman et al., 1997) indicated that skeletal muscle disorders may play a role in the development of symptoms experienced by the athlete with chronic fatigue, which one group termed the "fatigue athlete myopathic syndrome" and another the "Olympic fatigue syndrome."

GRADED ACTIVITY (ENERGY MANAGEMENT) THERAPY

Although the terms exercise and activity are often used interchangeably, they are not the same (Sharpe, Hawton, Simkin, et al., 1997). *Activity* is defined as anything that stimulates or overstimulates the brain in terms of physical, cognitive, or emotional effort (Cox, 2000). Thus, talking, watching television, reading, and even eating are regarded as activities, and each of them requires a different amount of energy. Although regular physical activity is associated with important physical and mental health benefits, an estimated 53 million U.S. adults are inactive during their leisure time—the period most amenable to efforts to increase physical activity. The presence of chronic conditions, especially those associated with disabilities such as cancer, may reduce levels of leisure time physical activity.

In the past, patients suffering from cancer and other chronic diseases were told to avoid physical activity in order to rest and reduce discomfort. Thune and Smeland (2000) reviewed the literature and found a total of thirty-eight studies that focused on the importance of physical activity in the treatment and rehabilitation of cancer patients. Studies that assessed the effects of physical activity on quality of life following cancer diagnosis consistently suggested that physical activity may improve quality of life for cancer patients and influence fatigue. No information was provided on whether physical activity increases survival. The authors pointed out that limitations of the clinical studies they reviewed included small sample size, lack of adjustment for possible confounders, and short intervention spans (Thune and Smeland, 2000).

Many clinicians and therapists advocate a gradual increase not only in leisure time but in all daily and weekly activities to manage fatigue, and some suggest that it should be accompanied by attention to psychological factors to increase effectiveness (Sharpe, Hawton, Simkin, et al., 1997; Wilson, Hickie, Lloyd, and Wakefield, 1994). To examine the relationship between low-energy reporting with demographic and lifestyle factors, Caan and colleagues (2000) examined data from 1,137 women diagnosed with stage I, stage II, or stage IIIA primary, operable breast cancer, and enrolled in the Women's Healthy Eating and Living Study. The authors found that women who had a body mass index (BMI) greater than thirty were almost twice as likely to be low-energy reporters. Women with a history of weight gain or weight fluctuations were one-and-a-half times as likely to be low-energy reporters as those who were weight stable or weight losers. Age, ethnicity, alcohol intake, supplement use, and exercise level were also related to low-energy reporting (Caan et al., 2000).

In sixty-nine women who had lived with primary or recurrent lung cancer for more than twelve months, had non-small-cell limited disease, and most not currently receiving treatment, the most prevalent disruptions in physical function were reduced energy (59 percent), difficulty with household chores (33 percent), and interference with work (28 percent) (Sarna, 1993a-c, 1994). One-third of the sample had serious limitations in three or more activities. Approximately 26 percent of the sample had severe limitations in moderate activities, 20 percent in walking short distances, and 16 percent in walking one flight of stairs. Only one-quarter were satisfied with their level of activity. Physical function varied by income category, with those with the lowest income having the poorest function (Sarna, 1994). In terms of other factors, Sarna (1993a-c) measured disruptions in physical activities (functional status) over a one-month period in twenty-four patients with non-small-cell lung cancer. Prior weight loss was significantly associated with baseline functional status. Age was not significantly associated with degree of functional disruption, although 42 percent of the sample was aged sixty-five years or older. Serious fatigue was experienced by 79 percent of the subjects, and 44 percent had difficulty with household chores. Pain improved in the treated subjects over time. Despite no significant differences at baseline, untreated subjects had more limitations in physical activities than treated subjects over time. Careful monitoring of physical difficulties may therefore help health care professionals focus interventions and decrease the physical distress associated with illness and treatment (Sarna, 1993a-c, 1994).

In a study of seven adult subjects with cancer who received a six-week course of external beam radiation therapy to the trunk (including breast, chest, or abdomen), Sarna and Conde (2001) showed that, contrary to expectations, activity increased during treatment while fatigue decreased. The authors concluded that the observation supports the benefits of increasing physical activity during cancer treatment. Harpham (1999) recommends that cancer patients should be reassured that the fatigue they feel is real, and by learning personal energy conservation, they should be able to improve their abilities to function, to socialize, to interact with others, and ultimately to adjust to a "new normal" baseline.

In prospective, descriptive, repeated measures of seventy-two women who were receiving chemotherapy after surgery for stage I or II breast cancer, Berger (1998) found that activity levels were significantly different over time in a mirror-image pattern of fatigue. Based on these observations, the author suggests that examination of the inverse relationship between fatigue and activity will assist health care professionals in the development and testing of interventions to modify fatigue. Women should be instructed to monitor the intensity of fatigue and encouraged to maintain activity levels balanced with efficient rest periods (Berger, 1998). In a pilot study, Barsevick and colleagues (2002) showed that an energy conservation and activity management intervention moderates the expected rise in fatigue secondary to cancer therapy. The intervention is supported by patient adherence and by their self-reports of its usefulness and plans to continue using energy conservation and activity management skills. A full-scale clinical trial is needed to evaluate the efficacy of this approach.

Davies and colleagues (2002) performed a typology study of fatigue in twenty children with cancer and in eighteen parents and found that energy, as an overriding phenomenon, was a core concept in the descriptions of fatigue. Children with cancer may experience three subjectively distinct types of fatigue which represent different levels of energy: typical tiredness, treatment fatigue, and shutdown fatigue. Children managed their dwindling energy and minimized further energy loss through strategies of replenishing, conserving, and preserving. Children's use of these strategies was influenced by temperament, lifestyle, environmental factors, and treatment modalities (Davies et al., 2002). Holley and Borger (2001) evaluated the acceptability and efficacy of a rehabilitation group intervention in twenty people with six different types of cancers (fifteen receiving some form of therapy) experiencing cancer-related fatigue. From this preliminary study, the authors concluded that the intervention, which consisted of eight weekly, ninety-minute sessions with educational and sharing components focused on energy management, is appropriate and beneficial for patients with cancer experiencing fatigue, even for those patients who are very debilitated.

The purpose of energy grading patients' activities is to enable sustained and consistent activity on a daily and weekly basis. The idea is that patients do not have all of their high-energy activity together (peak) but that these activities are spread throughout the day and week, interspersed with medium and low-level activities, a scheme that enables a more paced used of their energy and therefore reduction in fatigue (Cox, 1999). It is important that the patient's baseline is established before further activity is introduced, to ensure that he or she has reduced the peaks and troughs pattern, and therefore is starting to build up activity again from a firm foundation (Cox, 1999). Rest also needs to be scheduled into each day, regardless of the severity of symptoms (Cox and Findley, 1998; Sharpe, Hawton, Simkin, et al., 1997). However, it should be pointed out that energy management-oriented therapies are different from the "rest cure." As reviewed by Cox (2000), the rest cure as a treatment for fatiguing illnesses has a long history (Wessely, 1991), and although it may relieve symptoms in the short term, in the long run it creates problems by reducing exercise tolerance and producing increased weakness, muscle wasting, and cardiac and respiratory difficulties, together with increased sensitivity to activity (Greenleaf and Kozlowski, 1982; Sharpe and Wessely, 1998).

Further studies are needed to generalize and substantiate the preliminary findings described for the use of graded activity interventions in cancer patients. Also, patients with other fatiguing illnesses have benefited from occupational therapy interventions. In this respect, it is important to distinguish between the terms *occupation* and *activity,* which are often used interchangeably (Cox, 2000; Creek, 1997; Golledge, 1998). Creek (1997) defines *activity* as the performance by an individual for a specific purpose on a particular occasion and *occupation* as a sphere of action over a period of time that is perceived by the individual as part of their social identity; occupation has meaning for the individual and forms part of their personal framework.

In a study of the sociomedical situation of 459 adult disease-free long-term survivors of Hodgkin's disease three to twenty-three years after first-line curative treatment, Abrahamsen and colleagues (1998) documented that most long-term Hodgkin's disease survivors had adapted well to their sociomedical situation except for a high number of permanently disabled patients. These authors found that fatigue and long-term disablement after first-line treatment were predictors for permanent disablement, and therefore suggested that by focusing more on factors predisposing for permanent disablement and early treatment for these, more patients may be helped to return to their jobs.

Cancer patients are now more often long-term survivors, and their needs for returning to social and productive activities have become a primary focus of intervention. Capodaglio and colleagues (1997) assessed an evaluation test for predicting endurance capacity in breast cancer patients after surgery, aimed at optimizing return to work or previous daily activities, and at monitoring changes during rehabilitation. In addition to the measures of the circumferences in the arm-forearm and the manual muscle strength test, a 0 to 100 constant scale for shoulder function, and an instrumental evaluation of daily/occupational upper limb activities (Lido WorkSET) were included. The authors monitored the mechanical parameters, the perception of effort, pain, or discomfort, and the range of movement while performing a three-minute steady daily/occupational task chosen by the subject. Patients were asked to perform the three-minute test at three different intensities ("moderate," "somewhat hard," "hard") until the perception of fatigue, pain, or discomfort was rated greater than 3 on the 10-point Borg's scale. The "power-duration" product (Watt × min) defined by the three tests represented the individual tolerable workload, since subjective indicators of pain/discomfort remained within tolerable limits during the exertion. On this basis, patients were encouraged to return to levels of daily physical activities compatible with the individual tolerable workload. Although no statistical analysis was performed, the second evaluation confirmed that the "guided" daily activity in a two-month period increased patients' capacities and "trust" in their physical capacity (Capodaglio et al., 1997).

Occupational interventions also help address the many nuances inherent to the return of patients to intellectual activities. Despite normal levels of physical activity, fatigue was the area of highest distress identified among adolescent cancer survivors pursuing postsecondary education (Griffith and Hart, 2000). Although help, from family, friends, and teachers, was seen as supportive, lack of knowledge about their disease was cited most frequently by this same group as interfering with their coping. The adolescent cancer survivors demonstrated more discipline, stamina, and commitment than was expected. However, stigmatization of patients by professional health workers was evident and needs to be addressed (Griffith and Hart, 2000). In this respect, school intervention programs for children and adolescents with cancer have been developed in France to improve the psychosocial adaptation of these children to normal life through school integration (Bouffet et al., 1996; Bouffet, Zucchinelli, et al., 1996). Based on the observation that sixty percent of the thirty French children with incurable cancer studied demonstrated a genuine desire to attend school until the advanced stages of their disease, Bouffet and colleagues (1996; Bouffet, Zucchinelli, et al., 1997) point out that school attendance should even be part of palliative care for the terminally ill child with cancer.

Some cancers impinge more directly on intellectual abilities. Brain tumor patients experience changes in function and quality of life during their disease course, and rehabilitation services may offer a unique opportunity to influence functional outcome and more closely assess quality of life in these individuals (Huang et al., 2001). Rehabilitation professionals are essential for the comprehensive care of cancer patients throughout the phases of their disease: treatment planning, treatment, remission, recurrence, and end of life (Gerber, 2001; Gillis, Cheville, and Worsowicz, 2001). Rehabilitation professionals must be trained to manage problems associated with cancer and its treatments. Research about what are effective and efficient rehabilitation treatments must be done to determine how best to treat cancer patients throughout the various phases of their illness. Physicians and patients must be alerted to the importance of rehabilitation interventions to the overall function of these patients (Gerber, 2001; Gillis, Cheville, and Worsowicz, 2001; Schmidt, 2001).

These arguments also extend to terminally ill cancer patients. Disability in advanced cancer patients often results from bed rest, deconditioning, and neurological and musculoskeletal complications of cancer or cancer treatment (Santiago-Palma and Payne, 2001). Fatigue is the common symptom of terminally ill patients. Rehabilitation and palliative care have emerged as two important parts of comprehensive medical care for patients with advanced disease (Van Harten et al., 1998). Both disciplines have a multidisciplinary model of care that aims to improve patients' levels of function and comfort. There is scarce evidence that rehabilitation interventions can impact function and symptom management in terminally ill patients. However, clinical experience suggests that the application of the fundamental principles of rehabilitation medicine is likely to improve their care. Physical function and independence should be maintained as long as possible to improve patients' quality of life and reduce the burden of care for the caregivers (Santiago-Palma and Payne, 2001).

SLEEP THERAPY

Graydon and colleagues (1995) reported that sleep and exercise were among the most effective fatigue-reducing strategies (as assessed by the Pearson Byars Fatigue Feeling Checklist and the Fatigue Relief Scale) used by women patients receiving treatment for cancer, either chemotherapy (forty-five studied) or radiation therapy (fifty-four studied). Curt and colleagues (2000) reported that among the 379 cancer patients they interviewed, bed rest and relaxation were the most common treatment recommendations by physicians (37 percent of cases). In a study of seventy-six women with breast cancer receiving external radiation therapy, the most frequently reported self-relief strategies for fatigue were "sit" and "sleep" (Irvine et al., 1998).

As covered in Chapter 3, sleep disturbances among cancer patients can occur for many reasons. Moore and Dimsdale (2002) proposed that part of the fatigue typically experienced by cancer patients can be attributed to disruption of sleep by opioid medications they are taking, and that research is needed to assess the sleep and next-day consequences that can be expected from typical doses of different types of pain medications. In cancer patients, as in other medically ill patients, sleep that is inadequate or unrefreshing may be important not only to the expression of fatigue, but also to the patients' quality of life and their tolerance to treatment, and it may influence the development of mood disorders and clinical depression (Ancoli-Israel, Moore, and Jones, 2001).

The results of a study by Berger and colleagues (2002) underscore that adopting behaviors to promote sleep may assist in maintaining sleep and managing fatigue during chemotherapy. Berger and colleagues (2002) conducted a prospective, repeated measures, quasi-experimental feasibility study of an intervention designed to promote sleep and modify fatigue in twenty-five women with stage I-II breast cancer receiving four cycles of doxorubicin-based adjuvant breast cancer chemotherapy. Each woman developed, reinforced, and revised an individualized sleep promotion plan (ISPP) with four components: sleep hygiene, relaxation therapy, stimulus control, and sleep restriction techniques. A daily diary, the Pittsburgh Sleep Quality Index, a wrist actigraph, and the Piper Fatigue Scale were used to collect data two days before and seven days after each treatment. Adherence rates with the components of the ISPP varied during treatments one through four: sleep hygiene (68 to 78 percent), relaxation therapy (57 to 67 percent), stimulus control (46 to 67 percent), and sleep restriction (76 to 80 percent). Mean sleep and wake outcomes at baseline, peak, and rebound times were that

1. sleep latency remained brief (less than thirty minutes per night),
2. time awake after sleep onset exceeded the desired less than thirty minutes per night,
3. sleep efficiency scores remained stable at 85 to 90 percent,
4. total rest time remained stable at eight to ten hours per night,
5. subjective ratings of feelings on arising were stable, and
6. nighttime awakenings were eight to ten per night.

Fatigue outcomes were that fatigue was stable two days after each treatment and mean daily fatigue intensity was lower at treatment three than at treatment one but rebounded at treatment four. The study showed that the intervention was feasible, adherence rates improved over time, and most sleep and wake patterns were consistent with normal values. Berger and colleagues (2002) stress that revisions of the protocol will focus on decreasing nighttime awakenings.

Davidson and colleagues (2001) described and examined, in twelve cancer patients with insomnia, the initial efficacy of a six-session sleep therapy program that included stimulus-control therapy, relaxation training, and other strategies aimed at consolidating sleep and reducing cognitive-emotional arousal. Significant improvement over baseline was observed at weeks four and eight in the number of awakenings, time awake after sleep onset, sleep efficiency, sleep quality ratings, and scores on European Organization for Research and Treatment of Cancer (EORTC) QLQ-C30 for role functioning and insomnia. Total sleep time and fatigue were significantly improved at week eight. The preliminary evidence therefore suggests that this sleep therapy program is associated with improved sleep, reduced fatigue, and enhanced ability to perform activities in relatively well individuals attending a cancer center (Davidson et al., 2001). Further studies in larger and other cancer patient populations are needed.

More studies are needed to support the role of sleep therapy in the management of cancer-related fatigue. Harding (1998) recommends that before prescribing pharmacological compounds aimed at modifying sleep, adequate pain control and sleep habits should be achieved; tricyclic antidepressants, trazodone, zopiclone, and SSRIs may be required (Touchon, 1995).

COGNITIVE-BEHAVIORAL THERAPY

Less direct evidence than that available for exercise supports the use of psychological interventions in the management of cancer-related fatigue (Stone, 2002). Based on a review of studies published before 1992, Trijsburg and colleagues (1992) concluded that tailored counseling had been shown to be effective with respect to distress, self-concept, (health) locus of control, fatigue, and sexual problems. Structured counseling showed positive effects with respect to depression and distress. Behavioral interventions and hypnosis were effective with respect to specific symptoms such as anxiety, pain, nausea, and vomiting.

Evidence indicates that psychotherapeutic intervention can augment natural killer (NK) cell activity and lymphokine-activated killer (LAK) cell activity in patients with malignant melanoma and with locally advanced, nonmetastatic breast cancer, respectively (Greer, 1999, 2000). How are these effects accomplished? Cognitive-behavioral therapy is based on the notion that certain cognitions and behavior may perpetuate symptoms and disability. Thoughts, feelings, and actions interlink with one another; what we do influences thoughts and feelings and, equally, the way we think can affect actions and feelings (Surawy et al., 1995). As summarized by Sadigh (2001), people are not aware that there is an intimate interaction between our thoughts, feelings, and behaviors. A negative thought can almost instantly have emotional manifestations, which may in turn influence the way one behaves. This is especially important to keep in mind when one is experiencing fatigue. At times some fatigue may result in anxiety, fear, frustration, and even helplessness. This may result in behavior that may actually worsen the fatigue. The behavior will cause more negative thoughts and feelings, which makes one feel trapped in a vicious cycle with no end in sight.

The major task of cognitive-behavioral therapy is to assist people to become aware of their faulty thoughts (cognitions) and to teach them ways of modifying or replacing these thoughts with more constructive ones, which will bring about a change in feelings and behaviors. Cognitive-behavioral therapy is therefore based on the theory that inaccurate unhelpful beliefs, ineffective coping behavior, negative mood states, social problems, and pathophysiological process all interact to perpetuate illness (Cox, 2000). As detailed in Chapter 3, psychoneuroimmunology teaches us about the interconnections among the different bodily systems, so how we feel and behave will end up affecting our immune, endocrine, nervous, and other bodily systems, and vice versa.

When studying why some individuals with lung or colorectal cancer develop fatigue whereas others do not, Olson and colleagues (2002) found that an adaptive behavioral mode labeled *gliding* characterized those who reported little or no fatigue, even when hemoglobin levels were low, while three other nonadaptive behavioral modes (inertia, disorganization, and overexertion) characterized those who reported fatigue. A randomized trial of a cognitive-behavioral therapy program developed specifically for patients with cancer evinced that patients who feel helpless/hopeless or who are otherwise emotionally distressed could be induced, by gentle encouragement, to adopt a fighting spirit (Greer, 1999, 2000). This trial showed that fighting spirit was associated with substantial improvement in the patients' quality of life. Another five-year prospective study of women with breast cancer and men and women with lymphoma also showed that fighting spirit was significantly associated with a favorable disease outcome (Greer, 1999, 2000). In a study of 294 breast cancer survivors, Dow and colleagues (1996) reported good outcomes in hopefulness, having a life purpose, and having a positive change after cancer treatment.

In an assessment of 176 childhood cancer survivors, Zebrack and Chesler (2002) found that patients rate themselves high on happiness, feeling useful, life satisfaction, and their ability to cope as a result of having had cancer, but their hopefulness is tempered by uncertainty. Whereas the salience of spiritual and religious activities appears to be low, having a sense of purpose in life and perceiving positive changes as a result of cancer are associated with positive quality of life. A lower valence of physical concerns reflects the vitality and positive life outlook of a young population (Zebrack and Chesler, 2002).

Counseling of patients and their families has a very positive effect. Elmberger, Bolund, and Lutzen (2000) interviewed nine women with children aged four to twenty-three living at home at the time of diagnosis. By the process of constant comparative analysis, the main theme that seemed to capture how the lives of these women had changed was transforming the exhausting-to-energizing process in being a good parent in the face of cancer. This theme is related to Meleis's concept of health-illness transition. The findings here indicate the need for family counseling, with special attention paid to the single parent with cancer (Elmberger, Bolund, and Lutzen, 2000).

Singer and Schwarz (2002) state that there is a high need for psychosocial counseling in daily clinical practice. Good precare is just as important as good aftercare to reduce anxiety and pain and to increase well-being. Addressing information and support in a timely fashion is important in providing success to psychosocial aftercare. In randomized clinical trials, Oyama and colleagues (2000) showed that the bedside wellness system, a virtual reality system, is effective for decreasing stress and improving mental well-being and should help relieve the side effects and mental disorders of patients during cancer chemotherapy.

Informing patients about their conditions is of paramount importance to help address fears and expectations. Kim, Roscoe, and Morrow (2002) conducted a randomized clinical trial with 152 patients to examine the effects of an informational intervention on the severity of side effects resulting from radiation therapy for prostate cancer. They also examined negative affect both as a predictor and as an outcome variable. The informational intervention, given to patients at the first and fifth treatments, was based upon self-regulation theory and provided patients with specific, objective information about what to expect during their radiation treatments. Patients in the comparison group received general information at the same point in time. The results showed that patients in the informational intervention group reported significantly fewer problems with sleep and fatigue (marginally significant) as compared to those in the comparison group. Negative affect was not influenced by group assignment. Baseline negative affect was not related to symptom development, although the development of side effects was associated with an increase in negative mood. The results suggest that patients could benefit from increased knowledge about what to expect during their radiation treatments (Kim, Roscoe, and Morrow, 2002).

Developing interventions to maintain or restore attentional capacity during demanding phases of illness helps promote effective functioning in people with cancer. Cimprich (1993) tested the effects of an experimental intervention aimed at maintaining or restoring attentional capacity in thirty-two women during the three months after surgery for localized (stage I or II) breast cancer. The intervention was designed to minimize or prevent attentional fatigue through regular participation in activities that engage fascination and have other restorative properties. Analysis of data showed a significant interaction of experimental intervention and time on attentional capacity. Specifically, subjects in the intervention group showed significant improvement in attentional capacity over the four assessment time points, while the nonintervention group showed a pattern of inconsistent performance over time (Cimprich, 1993).

Badger, Braden, and Mishel (2001) reported that self-help interventions were particularly helpful, relative to their fatigue experience, among 169 women receiving treatment for breast cancer and reporting a high level of depression burden. On the other hand, depression burden did not significantly influence the side effect burdens of nausea or pain, the burden of difficulty concentrating or experiencing anxiety, the number of side effects, or perceived severity of side effects. The interventions significantly reduced the fatigue, pain, and nausea burden in women with breast cancer. Badger, Braden, and Mishel (2001) therefore concluded that every woman who is undergoing cancer treatment should be assessed for depression and depression burden, and that self-help interventions are effective and convenient treatments that reduce side effects and promote quality of life in women with breast cancer. It should be noted, however, that other authors have concluded that self-care behaviors are not sufficient for fatigue management (Richardson and Ream, 1997).

Given and colleagues (2002) conducted a randomized clinical trial of an eighteen-week, ten-contact nursing intervention utilizing problem-solving approaches to symptom management and improving physical functioning and emotional health. Fifty-three patients, who reported pain and fatigue at baseline while undergoing an initial course of chemotherapy, were included in the experimental arm and sixty in the control arm. Interviews conducted at ten and twenty weeks revealed that patients who received the intervention reported a significant reduction in the number of symptoms experienced and improved physical and social functioning as compared to those who did not. Fewer patients in the experimental arm reported both pain and fatigue at twenty weeks. Based on the findings, the authors concluded that behavioral interventions targeted to patients with pain and fatigue can reduce symptom burden, improve the quality of the daily life of patients, and demonstrate the "value-added" role of nursing care for patients undergoing chemotherapy.

Fawzy and colleagues (1990) evaluated the immediate and long-term effects on psychological distress and coping methods of a six-week, structured, psychiatric group intervention for postsurgical patients with malignant melanoma. The intervention consisted of health education, enhancement of problem-solving skills, stress management (e.g., relaxation techniques), and psychological support. Despite good prognosis, most patients had high levels of psychological distress at baseline, comparable with other patients with cancer. However, at the end of brief psychiatric intervention, the thirty-eight experimental subjects, while not without some distress, exhibited higher vigor and greater use of active-behavioral coping than the twenty-eight controls. At six months' follow-up, the group differences were even more pronounced. The intervention-group patients then showed significantly lower depression, fatigue, confusion, and total mood disturbance as well as higher vigor. They were also using significantly more active-behavioral and active-cognitive coping than the controls. These results indicate that a short-term psychiatric group intervention for patients with malignant melanoma effectively reduces psychological distress and enhances longer-term effective coping (Fawzy et al., 1990).

Fawzy (1995) determined if a psychoeducational nursing intervention including (1) health education, (2) stress management, and (3) the teaching of coping skills could enhance the coping behavior and affective state of newly diagnosed stage I/II malignant melanoma patients. The secondary purpose was to determine if this intervention could be implemented by a nurse and integrated into the overall patient care program. Sixty-one patients were randomized to a control condition or an experimental condition that received an educational manual plus three hours of individual nurse teaching. Despite randomization, experimental patients had significantly higher baseline distress. By three months, there was a complete reversal of the baseline trend in Profile of Mood States (POMS) total mood disturbance (TMD), suggesting that the experimental subjects were experiencing less distress over time. Between-group analysis of change scores found significant decreases in experimental subjects for POMS TMD, fatigue, and Brief Symptom Index (BSI) somatization. Within-group analysis found significant experimental decreases for BSI somatization, anxiety, General Severity Index, and Positive Symptom Distress Index as well as for POMS anxiety, fatigue, confusion, vigor, and TMD. No significant changes were found for controls. Experimental patients were using significantly fewer ineffective passive resignation coping strategies than controls at three months.

In a randomized controlled clinical trial of patients with breast cancer who underwent autologous bone marrow/peripheral blood stem cell transplantation, Gaston-Johansson and colleagues (2000) assessed a coping strategy program composed of preparatory information, cognitive restructuring, and relaxation with guided imagery. Randomization placed fifty-two patients in the coping strategy program treatment group and fifty-eight patients in the control group. The coping strategy program was found to be effective in significantly reducing nausea as well as nausea combined with fatigue seven days after the autologous bone marrow transplantation, when the side effects of treatment were most severe. The cognitive strategy program-treated group experienced mild anxiety as compared with the control group who reported moderate anxiety (Gaston-Johansson et al., 2000).

Ream, Richardson, and Alexander-Dann (2002) conducted a pilot study on eight patients to test an intervention named the "Beating Fatigue" program that is aimed at facilitating patients' coping with fatigue during chemotherapy. The intervention has four elements: assessment/monitoring, education, coaching in the management of fatigue, and provision of emotional support. Overall, patients were very positive about the program and perceived the opportunity to talk to someone about fatigue as the most beneficial strategy within the program, although individual patients varied in which aspect they most preferred. Data from the pilot work supported the view that a multifaceted approach to the management of cancer-related fatigue is appropriate because it enables an intervention package to be tailored to an individual's requirements. The approach appeared both feasible and practical. Although numeric data were limited, some evidence did indicate that the approach had the capacity to lessen fatigue and enhance emotional well-being (Ream, Richardson, and Alexander-Dann, 2002).

In a study of fifty-four women with metastatic carcinoma of the breast who were offered weekly group therapy during one year (with or without self-hypnosis training directed toward enhancing their competence at mastering pain and stress related to cancer), both treatment groups demonstrated significantly less self-rated pain sensation and suffering than the control sample (Spiegel and Bloom, 1983). Those who were offered the self-hypnosis training as well as group therapy fared best in controlling the pain sensation. Pain frequency and duration were not affected. Changes in pain measures were significantly correlated with changes in self-rated total mood disturbance and with its anxiety, depression, and fatigue subscales (Spiegel and Bloom, 1983).

In a study of twenty-four patients, Forester and colleagues (1993) reported that group therapy may enhance quality of life for cancer patients undergoing radiotherapy by reducing their emotional and physical distress. The degree to which patients acknowledge the diagnosis of malignancy may be a factor in their initial distress level and their response to radiotherapy and group therapy. Moreover, patient gender and knowledge of diagnosis affected the pattern and magnitude of the response to psychotherapy (Forester, Kornfeld, and Fleiss, 1985; Forester et al., 1993). According to self-regulation theory, inadequate management of the symptom of fatigue may lead to increased fatigue distress among patients with cancer. Reuille (2002) described a theory-based educational intervention developed to help patients manage their fatigue more effectively, with the goal of decreasing the distress that fatigue causes for patients receiving outpatient cancer treatment. The intervention is designed to be delivered before the patient's first cancer treatment.

Among psychosocial interventions for reducing treatment-related side effects, relaxation and imagery have been most investigated in controlled trials. Luebbert, Dahme, and Hasenbring (2001) used meta-analytic methods to synthesize published, randomized intervention-control studies aiming to improve patients' treatment-related symptoms and emotional adjustment by relaxation training. Mean weighted effect sizes were calculated for twelve categories: treatment-related symptoms (nausea, pain, blood pressure, pulse rate) and emotional adjustment (anxiety, depression, hostility, tension, fatigue, confusion, vigor, overall mood). Significant positive effects were found for the treatment-related symptoms. Relaxation training also proved to have a significant effect on the emotional adjustment variables depression, anxiety, and hostility. In addition, two studies point to a significant effect of relaxation on the reduction of tension and amelioration of the overall mood. Intervention features of the relaxation training, the time the professional spent with the patient overall (intervention intensity), and the schedule of the intervention (offered in conjunction with or independent of medical treatment to the cancer patient) were relevant to the effect of relaxation on anxiety. The interventions offered independently of medical treatment proved to be significantly more effective for the outcome variable anxiety. Relaxation seems to be equally effective for patients undergoing different medical procedures (chemotherapy, radiotherapy, bone marrow transplantation, hyperthermia). According to these results, Luebbert, Dahme, and Hasenbring (2001) conclude that relaxation training should be implemented into the clinical routine for cancer patients in acute medical treatment.

Beneficial outcomes reported for cognitive-behavioral therapy in patients include the following:

- Adopting a fighting spirit
- Maintaining or restoring attentional capacity
- Adequately addressing fears and expectations
- Appropriately confronting family and social situations
- Improving quality of life
- Reducing psychological distress
- Enhancing long-term effective coping

Servaes and colleagues (2002) reported some similarities but also many differences between severely fatigued breast cancer survivors and females with chronic fatigue syndrome, an observation which suggests that cognitive-behavioral therapy to reduce fatigue after treatment for cancer should also differ in certain aspects from cognitive-behavioral therapy as it has been developed for patients with chronic fatigue syndrome. As reviewed by Manu (2000), cognitive-behavioral therapy has been thoroughly studied in patients with chronic fatigue syndrome but has yielded contradictory results. In the first trial, Australian investigators were unable to demonstrate improvement in global well-being, physical capacity, and functional status; when favorable changes occurred they were considered to be nonspecific and secondary to the propensity to remission that characterizes the natural history of this illness (Lloyd et al., 1993).

Similar results were reported by investigators from the State University of New York at Stony Brook, who observed that cognitive-behavioral therapy did not change the severity of fatigue experienced by a group of patients with chronic fatigue syndrome, despite reduced depression-symptom scores. In contrast, in a control group of patients with primary depression, this therapy improved the severity of fatigue and fatigue-related thinking as it corrected the impact of depression and stress (Friedberg and Krupp, 1994). Positive results have been reported by a group of British clinicians from the King's College Hospital, London, who obtained improvement in at least three times as many patients treated according to a program of cognitive restructuring and graded activity than in a control group that had received relaxation therapy (Deale et al., 1997). A confirmation of these results was offered by a trial of cognitive-behavioral therapy conducted in Oxford, England, during which patients with chronic fatigue syndrome were helped to achieve gradual and consistent increases in activity by learning to try strategies other than avoidance (Sharpe, Hawton, Simkin, et al., 1997).

Although it is clear that a decrease in activity avoidance behavior had greater impact on the outcome than changing the patients' beliefs about the cause of their illness (Deale, Chalder, and Wessely, 1998), analysis of the data produced by the four trials suggests that the therapeutic agent may have been the increase in physical activity per se rather than the supportive, interpersonal, or psychodynamic dimensions of the cognitive-behavioral intervention. This conclusion is consistent with the benefits of graded exercise and graded activity described in other sections previously, and many advocate the inclusion of psychotherapeutic interventions in combination with other treatment modalities in the management of cancer-related fatigue and other complications of cancer and cancer treatment.

Although poor outcomes for patients with chronic fatigue syndrome in a longitudinal outcome study (Wilson, Hickie, Lloyd, Hadzi-Pavlovic, et al., 1994) and in cognitive-behavioral therapy treatment programs (Butler et al., 1991; Sharpe, Hawton, Simkin, et al., 1997) were associated with patient attribution of physical causes for chronic fatigue syndrome, most of this research used the definition by Holmes and colleagues (1988) of chronic fatigue syndrome, which requires eight or more minor symptoms. Therefore, individuals might have been selected who had a higher likelihood of having somatization and other psychiatric disorders (Katon and Russo, 1992).

It should be noted that, besides cancer-related fatigue and chronic fatigue syndrome, cognitive-behavioral therapy alone or in combination with other approaches appears to also offer a viable alternative for the management of fibromyalgia and arthritis pain (Bradley and Alberts, 1999; Callahan and Balock, 1997; Keefe and Caldwell, 1997). In a pilot study of twenty fibromyalgia patients, Singh and colleagues (1998) showed that a mind-body approach (cognitive-behavioral therapy—eight weekly sessions, two and a half hours each, with three components: an educational component focusing on the mind-body connection, a portion focusing on relaxation response mechanisms, primarily mindfulness meditation techniques, and a qigong movement therapy session) resulted in a significant reduction in pain, fatigue, and sleeplessness, as well as improved function, mood state, and general health. Similar positive results were obtained by Decker, Cline-Elsen, and Gallagher (1992) who studied the impact of stress reduction by relaxation training and imagery in eighty-two outpatients who were undergoing curative (seventy-three patients) or palliative (nine patients) radiotherapy. Significant reductions were noted in the treatment group in tension, depression, anger, and fatigue.

A study by Nicassio and colleagues (1997) also underscored the value of a ten-week psychoeducational intervention in decreasing the psychological and behavioral effect of fibromyalgia by reducing dysfunctional coping and helplessness. However, in randomized clinical trial comparisons in 131 fibromyalgia patients, Goosens and colleagues (1996) and Vlaeyen and colleagues (1996) found that the addition of a cognitive component to the educational intervention led to significantly higher health care costs (Goosens et al., 2000; Maetzel, Ferraz, and Bombardier, 1998; Ruof, Hulsemann, and Stucki, 1999) and no additional improvement in quality of life compared to the educational intervention alone.

NUTRITIONAL THERAPY

Although progress has been made in improving the nutritional status of cancer patients (Cushman, 1986; Grant and Kravits, 2000; Persson et al., 2002; Tchekmedyian, 1995), more studies are needed to support the role of nutritional interventions in the management of fatigue and other cancer-related symptoms (Giuliani and Cestaro, 1997; Kadar et al., 1998). For instance, although evidence may not yet support the benefits of a particular diet intervention, based on results from a pilot clinical trial, Bye, Ose, and Kaasa (1995) suggest that diet intervention during radiotherapy might influence patients' ability to cope with diarrhea by giving them more control over their own situation.

Kalman and Villani (1997) point out that knowledge of fatigue models can help dietitians identify potential causes of fatigue, such as activity-rest patterns, and identification can lead dietitians to early intervention. Understanding cancer treatment factors, such as nausea and decreased participation in activities of daily living, that are believed to play a part in fatigue form another level on which dietitians can provide intervention. Through intervention, dietitians, working with patients and other members of the multidisciplinary team, may increase the understanding and appreciation of fatigue as well as provide relief from it. Efforts to maintain nutritional status can decrease or prevent some of the fatigue associated with cancer and its treatment. Therefore, the goal of clinical dietitians who work with a fatigued patient with cancer is to use nutrition management to minimize therapeutic side effects and maximize the patient's nutritional parameters (Kalman and Villani, 1997). In some particular instances, described as follows, particular dietary interventions may be pertinent to management of cancer-related fatigue and that of other chronic fatiguing illnesses.

Carnitine Supplementation

Graziano and colleagues (2002) documented a potential role for levocarnitine (or L-carnitine) supplementation for the treatment of chemotherapy-induced fatigue in nonanemic cancer patients. Ifosfamide and cisplatin cause urinary loss of carnitine, which is a fundamental molecule for energy production by the cellular organelles termed mitochondria in mammalian cells. Restoration of the carnitine pool with oral levocarnitine, 4 grams daily, for seven days in fifty patients (cisplatin-based chemotherapy in forty-four patients and ifosfamide-based in six patients) led to amelioration of fatigue in forty-five patients, an improvement that was sustained until the next cycle of chemotherapy (Graziano et al., 2002). Further confirmation in a placebo-controlled trial is warranted.

Some studies suggest that orally administered L-carnitine is also an effective medicine in treating the fatigue seen in a number of chronic neurological diseases (Bowman et al., 1997; Plioplys and Plioplys, 1997). Treatment of thirty CFS patients with L-carnitine yielded a statistically significant clinical improvement in twelve of eighteen studied parameters after eight weeks of treatment. None of the clinical parameters showed any deterioration. The greatest improvement took place between four and eight weeks of L-carnitine treatment. One patient was unable to complete eight weeks of treatment because of diarrhea. L-carnitine is therefore a safe and well-tolerated medicine that improves the clinical status of CFS patients (Plioplys and Plioplys, 1997).

Cysteine Supplementation Alone or with Vitamin C

Droge and Holm (1997) suggested that cysteine supplementation combined with disease-specific treatments may be a useful therapy in those patients with demonstrated low cysteine-glutathione syndrome, which is characterized, as covered in Chapter 3, by muscle wasting. However, Dimeo (2001) points out that cancer-induced skeletal muscle wasting may occur despite normal food intake and may not be prevented by nutritional supplementation.

Many patients, particularly those with HIV infection, use *N*-acetyl-cysteine (NAC), the *N*-acetyl derivative of cysteine as a nutritional supplement. *N*-acetylcysteine is utilized in its aerosolized form as a mucolytic treatment for bronchitis in Europe, while in the United States it is administered intravenously or by mouth (Mucomyst) for the management of acetaminophen (Tylenol) overdose. *N*-acetylcysteine use lacks significant toxicity (occasional dyspepsia, diarrhea) and is widely available in foreign markets and in buyer's clubs nationwide.

Cysteine is a sulfur-containing amino acid. Parcell (2002) points out that sulfur is the sixth most abundant macromineral in breast milk and the third most abundant mineral based on percentage of total body weight. The sulfur-containing amino acids (SAAs) are methionine, cysteine, cystine, homocysteine, homocystine, and taurine. Dietary SAA analysis and protein supplementation may be indicated for vegan athletes, children, or patients with HIV, because of an increased risk for SAA deficiency in these groups. Methylsulfonylmethane (MSM), a volatile component in the sulfur cycle, is another source of sulfur found in the human diet. Increases in serum sulfate may explain some of the therapeutic effects of MSM, dimethylsulfoxide (DMSO), and glucosamine sulfate. Organic sulfur, as SAAs, can be used to increase synthesis of *S*-adenosylmethionine (SAMe), glutathione (GSH), taurine, and *N*-acetylcysteine. MSM may be effective for the treatment of allergy, pain syndromes, athletic injuries, and bladder disorders. Other sulfur compounds such as SAMe, DMSO, taurine, glucosamine or chondroitin sulfate, and reduced glutathione may also have clinical applications in the treatment of a number of conditions such as depression, fibromyalgia, arthritis, interstitial cystitis, athletic injuries, congestive heart failure, diabetes, cancer, and AIDS. The author suggests that the low toxicological pro-files of these sulfur compounds, combined with promising therapeutic effects, warrant continued human clinical trials (Parcell, 2002).

Similar to cysteine or its *N*-acetyl derivative, vitamin C (ascorbic acid) is also able to raise intracellular glutathione levels, an activity that may allow for synergistic activity when ascorbate is combined with cysteine supple-mentation (Jariwalla and Harakek, 1992).

Electrolyte Supplementation

Magnesium supplementation may also aid in improvement of fatigue in those patients with marginal or more significant deficiency of this mineral (Seelig, 1998). Phosphate deficiency secondary to chemotherapy should also be monitored and addressed with appropriate supplementation. A word of caution about magnesium and fatiguing illnesses in general: Experience with magnesium supplementation and chronic fatiguing illnesses stems from the proposal by some authors that, for instance, chronic fatigue syn-drome may be secondary to magnesium deficiency (Cox, Campbell, and Dowson, 1991; Seelig, 1998). However, four different laboratories have shown that the concentration of magnesium is normal in patients with chronic fatigue syndrome (Clague, Edwards, and Jackson, 1992; Deulofue et al., 1991; Gantz, 1991; Hinds et al., 1994). In addition, studies using in-travenous loading with magnesium have been unable to demonstrate that chronic fatigue syndrome is a magnesium-deficient state (Clague, Edwards, and Jackson, 1992; Hinds et al., 1994). Therefore, magnesium supple-mentation should be used only when justified by pertinent laboratory test results.

Alcohol Consumption

A study of 191 patients with head and neck cancers concluded that alco-hol drinking was associated with significantly better physical and role func-tioning, and better global health-related quality of life, plus less fatigue, pain, problems swallowing, dry mouth, and feelings of illness (Allison, 2002). The author of the study recommends that, despite alcohol's role as an etiological factor, it may be reasonable to drink a little as one recovers from head and neck cancer. It has also been suggested that moderate alcohol con-sumption helps decrease levels of inflammatory markers that contribute to disability and mortality (Stewart, 2002). However, the study findings are limited by the study's design and sample bias. Alcohol consumption may also exacerbate certain symptoms. For instance, alcohol consumption may exacerbate symptomatology in fibromyalgia (Eisinger, 1998). Moreover, alcohol intolerance was reported by 60 percent of CFS patients and by 21 percent of depressed patients in a comparative study (Komaroff, Fagioli, Geiger, et al., 1996).

PHARMACOLOGICAL THERAPY

Erythropoietin

Very little evidence supports the use of pharmacological treatment of cancer-related or cancer-treatment-related fatigue (Burks, 2001), with the possible exception of erythropoietin therapy for anemic patients undergoing chemotherapy (Demetri, Gabrilove, et al., 2002; Gabrilove et al., 2001; Griggs and Blumberg, 1998; Johansson et al., 2001; Libretto et al., 2001; Littlewood, 2001, 2002; Littlewood et al., 2001, 2002; Meadowcroft et al., 1998; Nail, 2002; Osterbor, 2000; Sabbatini, 2000; Stone, 2002; Scagliotti and Novello, 2001; Turner et al., 2001). As pointed out in Chapter 3, anemia occurs in a significant number of patients with cancer and is associated with symptoms of fatigue, dizziness, headache, and decreased health-related quality of life (Ludwig, 2002; Yount, Lai, and Cella, 2002).

As reviewed by Crawford (2002), in the 1990s, randomized, placebo-controlled trials in anemic cancer patients demonstrated that recombinant human erythropoietin resulted in an improvement in hemoglobin and hematocrit, a reduction in transfusion requirements, and improvement in quality-of-life end points. Based on these trials, recombinant erythropoietin was approved for the treatment of anemia in patients with nonmyeloid malignancies in whom the anemia was caused by the effect of chemotherapy. The clinical indication was to decrease the need for transfusion in patients for whom anemia was not secondary to other reversible causes. Despite this broad indication, the incorporation of recombinant human erythropoietin in clinical practice was limited because of a variety of factors, including physician perception that mild-to-moderate anemia in the cancer patient was generally asymptomatic and did not warrant intervention.

Subsequent to this trial, three large open-label, prospective trials of recombinant erythropoietin were performed in the community setting in anemic cancer chemotherapy patients. All three trials replicated the results of the original randomized study, but with a much larger database of more than 7,000 patients. Most important, these trials were able to define the major impact of hemoglobin level on quality of life. Patients on these trials who improved their hemoglobin greater than 2 g/dL or achieved a hemoglobin level greater than or equal to 12 g/dL had the greatest improvement in symptoms of energy, activities of daily living, and overall quality of life. Furthermore, a once-per-week dosing schedule was found to be comparable to three-times-weekly administration of erythropoietin. A European randomized, placebo-controlled trial confirmed these quality-of-life results, and a meta-analysis of other randomized clinical trials firmly supports the role of erythropoietin therapy in improving hemoglobin levels and reducing transfusion requirements. Based on this aggregate of data, the use of erythropoietin in the treatment of mild-to-moderate anemia has become a standard of care (Crawford, 2002).

Clinical trials have also demonstrated the ability of epoetin alfa to increase hemoglobin concentration, decrease transfusion requirements, and significantly increase quality of life in a variety of clinical settings (Baron et al., 2002; Buchsel, Murphy, and Newton, 2002; Cella and Bron, 1999; Coiffier, 2000; Demetri, Gabrilove, et al., 2002; Dempke and Schmoll, 2001; Fallowfield et al., 2002; Gabrilove et al., 2001; Griggs and Blumberg, 1998; Henry, 1997, 1998a,b; Itri, 2002; Johansson et al., 2001; Lavey, 1998; Littlewood et al., 2001, 2002; Ludwig, 1999; Leitgeb et al., 1994; Osterbor, 2000; Scagliotti and Novello, 2001; Stovall, 2001; Straus, 2002; Turner et al., 2001; Yount, Lai, and Cella, 2002).

Lappin, Maxwell, and Johnston (2002) point out that recent research indicates that erythropoeitin has pleiotropic effects on the body well beyond the maintenance of red cell mass, and its effects on relieving fatigue and improving quality of life may involve other effects. In this respect, erythropoietin receptors have been detected in many different cells and tissues, a feature that provides evidence for autocrine, paracrine, and endocrine functions of erythropoietin. For instance, apart from its endocrine function, erythropoietin may have a generalized role as an antiapoptotic agent that is associated with enhancement of muscle tone, mucosal status, and gonadal and cognitive function (Lappin, Maxwell, and Johnston, 2002).

Demetri (2001) points out that despite objectively defined benefits, less than 50 percent of anemic patients undergoing cytotoxic chemotherapy receive erythropoietin, in contrast to patients with chronic renal failure on dialysis, where anemia is universally and aggressively treated to more optimal hemoglobin values. Several barriers may limit more widespread use of erythropoietin, including inconvenience associated with frequent dosing; failure of a large proportion (40 to 50 percent) of patients to respond; relatively slow time to response; absence of reliable early indicators of response; and current lack of rigorous pharmacoeconomic data demonstrating cost-effectiveness.

In the face of the issues raised with erythropoietin administration, it is worth remembering that before the introduction of recombinant human erythropoietin (epoetin alfa), red blood cell transfusions were the traditional treatment for improvement of hemoglobin levels. Transfusions, however, are associated with several adverse events and risks, have only transient effects, and have a limited capacity to ameliorate the symptoms of anemia. On the other hand, epoetin alfa represents a physiologic treatment option, especially in the long-term treatment of cancer- and cancer treatment-associated anemia, and is well tolerated, with response rates as high as 80 percent. Because persistent fatigue is the most common complaint of patients following hysterectomy, Bachmann (2001) suggested that the use of epoetin alfa also should be considered to preoperatively correct anemia in patients with benign or malignant gynecological disorders.

Darbepoetin alfa (Aranesp) is an erythropoiesis-stimulating glycoprotein that has been shown, in dose-finding studies, to be safe and clinically active when administered to patients with cancer every one, two, or three weeks (Kallich et al., 2002; Smith, Jaiyesimi, et al., 2001; Valley, 2002). Vansteenkiste and colleagues (2002) conduced a phase III multicenter, double-blind, placebo-controlled study on 320 anemic patients with lung cancer receiving chemotherapy who were randomly assigned to receive darbepoetin alfa or placebo injections weekly for twelve weeks. They found that patients with chemotherapy-associated anemia can safely and effectively be treated with weekly darbepoetin alfa therapy. Darbepoetin alfa decreased blood transfusion requirements, increased hemoglobin concentration, and decreased fatigue as assessed by Functional Assessment of Cancer Therapy (FACT)-Fatigue scores.

However, as pointed out earlier, not every patient responds to epoetin alfa (Ludwig, 2002). For example, epoetin alfa is less effective in the treatment of the anemia of myelodysplastic syndrome, but it appears to be synergistic with granulocyte-colony stimulating factor. As a corollary, failure of the anemia of cancer to respond to recombinant erythropoietin is in itself a poor prognostic sign (Ludwig et al., 1994). Although recombinant erythropoietin therapy is effective even with concomitant chemotherapy or if the marrow is affected by tumor, identification of the tumors for which chemotherapy alone will alleviate the associated anemia is important (Spivak, 2000). Regrettably, it should also be noted that erythropoietin has become an illegal performing-enhancing drug among endurance athletes, which can be fatal as a result of hemoconcentration and dangerously high hematocrit levels (Lippi and Guidi, 2000).

Treatment of Underlying Disease Such As Cancer and Paraneoplastic Syndromes

Osoba and colleagues (1985) reported that the majority of forty-eight patients with recurrent and advanced stage (III and IV) non-small-cell lung cancer treated with a combination of bleomycin, etoposide, and *cis*-diamminedichloroplatinum experienced relief of fatigue, cough, hemoptysis, and pain associated with their disease. There was a good correlation between objective responses and palliation of symptoms. Fatigue also improved in 45 percent of eighty patients with advanced non-small-cell lung cancer treated with gemcitabine plus cisplatin in a phase II trial (Jassem et al., 2002). In another study, fatigue improved significantly among 400 women with human epithelial growth factor receptor (HER)-2/neu-over-expressing, metastatic breast cancer after completion of combined trastuzumab (Herceptin; Genentech) and chemotherapy (Osoba et al., 2002). Higher proportions of patients receiving the combined therapy achieved improvement in global quality of life than did patients treated with chemotherapy alone. Higher proportions of the combined therapy group also achieved improvement in physical and role functioning and in fatigue as compared with the chemotherapy group, but the differences were not statistically significant. There were no differences in the proportions of patients in the two groups that reported worsening (Osoba et al., 2002).

A randomized phase III trial on the impact of azacytidine on the quality of life of 191 patients with myelodysplastic syndrome revealed that patients on azacytidine experienced significantly greater improvement in fatigue, dyspnea, physical functioning, positive affect, and psychological distress over the course of the study period than those in the supportive care arm (Kornblith et al., 2002). Particularly striking were improvements in fatigue and psychological state in patients treated with azacytidine compared with those receiving supportive care for patients who remained in the study through at least day 106, corresponding to four cycles of azacytidine. Significant differences between the two groups in quality of life were maintained even after controlling for the number of red blood cell transfusions. Therefore, improved quality of life for patients treated with azacytidine coupled with significantly greater treatment response and delayed time to transformation to acute myeloid leukemia or death compared with patients on supportive care establishes azacytidine as an important treatment option for myelodysplastic syndrome (Kornblith et al., 2002).

Treatment of paraneoplastic syndromes may also aid in improvement and resolution of fatigue (Schweiger and Hsiang, 2002). For instance, the paraneoplastic syndrome of serum-inappropriate antidiuretic hormone has significant overlap with chronic fatigue disorders, and its treatment, namely salt loading and/or direct inhibition of arginine vasopressin, has been proposed as a therapeutic approach in individuals with chronic fatigue disorders, even in the absence of cancer (Peroutka, 1998). In fact, one study showed that, among CFS patients with evidence of autonomic dysfunction, a beneficial response to salt loading (1,200 mg of sodium chloride in a sustained-release formulation for three weeks) could be seen (De Lorenzo, Hargreaves, and Kakkar, 1997).

Health care professionals need to recognize that fatigue can be the result of complications associated with therapeutic modalities and that direct interventions may preclude debilitating fatigue. For instance, patients on the antiemetic arm of a clinical trial in which vomiting was better controlled showed significantly less increase in fatigue after receiving chemotherapy (Pater et al., 1997). However, antiemetics such as ondansetron, tropisetron, and metoclopramide can also cause fatigue (Fraschini et al., 1991; Nukariya et al., 1996). The choice of antiemetic may therefore be important in terms of fatigue induction. A randomized, double-blind, controlled clinical trial comparing octreotide administration in the management of nausea, vomiting, and abdominal pain versus conservative treatment for inoperable bowel obstruction in sixty-eight patients with far advanced cancer revealed statistically significant differences in favor of octreotide use in fatigue and anorexia between the two groups at different evaluation time points (Mystakidou et al., 2002). Octreotide is also useful in the treatment, but not the prevention, of chemotherapy-induced diarrhea. Besides antiemetics, antiulcer medications can also cause fatigue (Piper, 1995).

Wang and colleagues (2001) reported that preoperative chemoradiation therapy for patients with rectal cancer was associated with progressive fatigue during therapy, with uncontrolled diarrhea being the only predictor for increased fatigue. Eighteen percent of patients experienced severe fatigue before chemoradiation in association with uncontrolled pain. Based on the identified predictors for fatigue, Wang and colleagues (2001) suggested more active pain management before chemoradiation and bowel management during chemoradiation as possible means to reduce cancer-related fatigue in these patients. However, pain control medications such as opioids may also be associated with fatigue as a side effect (Petzke et al., 2001).

A randomized, double-blind, crossover study showed that treatment with megestrol acetate, a medication aimed at cachexia, results in rapid and significant improvement of symptoms, including fatigue, in terminally ill patients; the effects are not secondary to nutritional changes (Bruera et al., 1998). Other approaches to address the untoward effects of cancer treatment may also prove beneficial to the management of cancer-related fatigue. For instance, a phase III randomized, placebo-controlled, double-blind study of administration of a spleen peptide preparation (Polyerga) during chemotherapy (cisplatin/carboplatin, 5-fluorouracil) of patients with head and neck cancer revealed, among other beneficial effects, a reduction of the generally observed increase of fatigue/inertia during chemotherapy cycles (Borghardt et al., 2000). Further studies are warranted.

Methylphenidate

Psychostimulants such as methylphenidate have been proposed for treatment of fatigue in cancer patients. Sarhill and colleagues (2001) reported a prospective, open-label, pilot study of the successful use of methylphenidate to treat fatigue in nine of eleven consecutive patients with advanced cancer. Seven had received radiation or chemotherapy, a median of three weeks (range from one to thirty weeks) prior to methylphenidate. A rapid onset of benefit was noted, even in the presence of mild anemia. Sedation and pain also improved in some. Only one patient had side effects severe enough to stop the medication (Sarhill et al., 2001). Similar results were obtained in a pilot study of the use of methylphenidate for the treatment of depression in HIV-infected patients; improvement was noted both in depression and fatigue scores in a statistically significant proportion of patients (Breitbart et al., 2001). A phase II, open-label, prospective study of methylphenidate for depression in forty-one patients with advanced cancer showed efficacy; in addition, anorexia, fatigue, concentration, and sedation improved in some patients (Homsi et al., 2001). The study confirms previous observations by the same researchers in a smaller group of patients (Homsi et al., 2000).

Schwartz, Thompson, and Masood (2002) performed a pilot study of the effectiveness of aerobic exercise (four days a week for fifteen to thirty minutes) and methylphenidate (20 mg sustained-release tablet every morning) in the management of interferon-induced fatigue in twelve patients with melanoma compared to historic controls (patients with melanoma receiving only interferon-alpha). Sixty-six percent of patients adhered to exercise and methylphenidate; all adhered to exercise. Fatigue was lower for the exercise and methylphenidate group as compared to the historic controls. Functional ability increased six percent for all patients and nine percent for the exercise and methylphenidate group. Cognitive function was stable for the exercise and methylphenidate group, while the exercise-only group showed marked cognitive slowing. Although this study suggests that the combination of aerobic exercise and methylphenidate may have a positive effect on fatigue, cognitive function, and functional ability, a larger sample size in a randomized trial is needed to more rigorously evaluate the results of exercise and methylphenidate alone or in combination.

Chaturvedi and Maguire (1998) evaluated eighty-one adequately treated cancer patients, disease-free or with residual disease, using a controlled, prospective, follow-up design. Patients were included in the index group (sixty individuals) if they had persistent somatic complaints or unexplained nature or severity of somatic complaints, or in the control group (twenty-one individuals) if they did not report somatic complaints. Common somatic complaints in the index group were pain (19 percent), fatigue (17 percent), sensory symptoms (30 percent), and mixed symptoms (27 percent). Subjects in the index group significantly more often had depressive or anxiety disorder (19 percent) and atypical somatoform disorder (15 percent). Evaluation at four to six months revealed that treatment of patients with psychotropic medications and counseling led to a significant reduction in the number of somatic symptoms, including fatigue, and in anxiety and depression scores.

Despite the pilot studies described, consensus is lacking on the effectiveness of methylphenidate or other psychostimulants, and these drugs have not proven to be widely effective in the management of fatigue in cancer patients (McNeil, 2001; Nail, 2002; Sugawara et al., 2002).

Selective Serotonin Reuptake Inhibitors

A pilot trial of the selective serotonin reuptake inhibitor paroxetine (Paxil) for the treatment of hot flashes and associated symptoms in thirteen women with breast cancer revealed significant improvements not only in hot flashes but also in general, emotional, and mental fatigue (Weitzner et al., 2002). Rates of clinically significant depressive symptomatology also decreased, and sleep quality improved significantly as well. The incidence of clinical depression improved from 39 percent at baseline to 8 percent after treatment. These preliminary data suggest that the antidepressant paroxetine can be helpful in the treatment of hot flashes and associated fatigue, sleep disturbance, and depression in women with breast cancer treated with chemotherapy (Weitzner et al., 2002). Passik and colleagues (2002) also point out that fluoxetine in combination with appropriate follow-up is useful in the treatment of depression in cancer patients. Further controlled studies are needed to more fully evaluate this preliminary observation.

In this respect, it is worth noting that in a study of forty patients with malignant melanoma eligible for interferon-alpha treatment who were randomly assigned to receive either paroxetine or placebo in a double-blind design, Capuron and colleagues (2002) documented that symptoms of depression, anxiety, cognitive dysfunction, and pain were more responsive, whereas symptoms of fatigue and anorexia were less responsive, to paroxetine treatment. These results are in line with the reduced risk of major depression in patients with malignant melanoma undergoing interferon-alpha therapy and pretreated with the antidepressant paroxetine (Capuron et al., 2002).

Although antidepressants are commonly prescribed for other fatiguing illnesses, such as fluoxetine (Prozac) for patients with chronic fatigue syndrome, valid studies published so far have shown a lack of demonstrable improvement among patients (Vercoulen, Swanink, Zitman, et al., 1996; Wearden et al., 1998). Moreover, several studies have failed to demonstrate a serotonergic deficiency among patients with chronic fatigue syndrome (Cleare et al., 1995; Yatham et al., 1995). Use of monoamine oxidase inhibitors, such as phenelzine and selegiline, in patients with chronic fatigue syndrome has also met with disappointing results (Natelson et al., 1996; Natelson, Cheu, et al., 1998).

The experience with antidepressants appears to be more promising with fibromyalgia. O'Malley and colleagues (2000) performed a meta-analysis of published English-language, randomized, placebo-controlled trials (sixteen identified, thirteen of which were deemed appropriate for data extraction). The authors concluded that antidepressants, regardless of class (three assessed: tricyclics, SSRIs, and *S*-adenosylmethionine), are efficacious in treating many symptoms of fibromyalgia (fatigue, sleep, pain, and well-being, but not trigger points). Patients were more than four times as likely to report overall improvement; they also reported moderate reductions in individual symptoms, particularly pain. In the five studies in which the assessment was adequate for an effect independent of depression, only one study found a correlation between symptom improvement and depression scores. Whether this effect is independent of depression needs further study. A previous meta-analysis by O'Malley and colleagues (1999) had arrived at similar conclusions.

Arnold, Keck, and Welge (2000) also reviewed twenty-one randomized, controlled clinical trials, identified sixteen involving tricyclic agents, and performed meta-analysis with the nine of the sixteen studies that were considered suitable. Compared with placebo, tricyclic agents were associated with effect sizes that were substantially larger than zero for all measurements of physician and patient overall assessment, pain, stiffness, tenderness, fatigue, and sleep quality. The largest improvement was associated with measures of sleep quality; the most modest improvement was found in measures of stiffness and tenderness. Other review articles suggest that antidepressants play an important role in the drug treatment of chronic pain and fibromyalgia (Baraczka et al., 1997; Fishbain, 2000; Godfrey, 1996; Johnson, 1997; Lautenschlager, 2000; Maes et al., 1999; Touchon, 1995). However, moclobemide, a reversible inhibitor of monoamine oxidase, seems to be ineffective and inferior to amitriptyline for pain (Hannonen et al., 1998).

Bellometti and Galzigna (1999) reported that mud packs together with antidepressant treatment (trazodone) are able to influence the hypothalamic-pituitary-adrenal axis, stimulating increased serum levels of adrenocorticotropic hormone, cortisol, and beta-endorphin. The discharge of corticoids in the blood and the increase in beta-endorphin serum levels are followed by a reduction in pain symptoms, which is closely related to an improvement in functional ability, depression, and quality of life. It seems that the synergistic association between a pharmacological treatment (trazodone) and mud packs acts by helping the physiological responses to achieve homeostasis and to rebalance the stress response system.

Monoamine Oxidase Inhibitors

Based on the striking similarity of the clinical manifestations produced by use of the drug reserpine and the symptoms seen in patients with chronic fatigue syndrome, it was theorized that chronic fatigue syndrome was a disorder of reduced central sympathetic drive. Because of the pharmacology of control of this central sympathetic system, it was postulated that CFS symptoms would respond quickly to low-dose treatment with a monoamine oxidase inhibitor. A randomized, double-blind placebo-controlled study (Natelson et al., 1996) using phenelzine (Nardil), a nonspecific MAOI (15 mg every other day for two weeks and then daily), in a chronic fatigue syndrome population without a diagnosis of lifetime or current psychiatric disorder or of depressed mood in the range of clinically depressed patients showed a small but significant pattern of improvement compared to worsening in twenty self-report vehicles of CFS symptoms, illness severity, mood, or functional status. Although the data support the hypothesis of reduced sympathetic drive, an alternative hypothesis of pain alleviation is also possible. Inspired by the previous trial, a six-week trial (Natelson, Cheu, et al., 1998) of selegiline (5 mg daily), a specific MAOI B receptor inhibitor, was carried out in twenty-five CFS patients. Results of the trial showed a small but significant therapeutic effect in chronic fatigue syndrome (as reflected by tension/anxiety, vigor, and sexual relations variables) which appears independent of an antidepressant effect.

Amantadine

Amantadine is one of the most effective medicines for treating the fatigue seen in multiple sclerosis patients, and isolated reports suggest that it may also be effective in treating patients with chronic fatigue syndrome (Bowman et al., 1997; Plioplys and Plioplys, 1997). However, in one study, treatment of thirty CFS patients with amantadine for two months revealed that amantadine was poorly tolerated by CFS patients. Chronic fatigue syndrome patients, as compared to controls or patients with other diseases, are known to have different sensitivities to many medications. Only fifteen of the thirty patients were able to complete eight weeks of treatment; the others had to stop the medication because of side effects. Moreover, in those patients who completed eight weeks of treatment, there was no statistically significant difference in any of the studied clinical parameters (Plioplys and Plioplys, 1997). There are no reports on the use of amantadine in cancer-related fatigue.

Corticosteroids

Corticosteroids are valuable pharmacological adjuncts utilized in the management of the diverse symptoms observed in terminally ill patients, including asthenia and fatigue, bone, neuropathic, and hepatic pain, and anorexia, and serve as an adjunct for the treatment of nausea and vomiting (Rousseau, 2001). If relief of suffering is the goal and mandate of palliative care, high-dose corticosteroids should be utilized in terminally ill patients for quickly reducing pain and improving quality of life for both patients and family members. In patients with a limited life expectancy of days to several weeks, long-term side effects will not occur and therefore should not preclude the continuous use of corticosteroids until the patient's death. Strang (1997) points out that if anorexia, nausea, and a negative body image are major concerns and if the patient has a life expectancy of more than three months, megestrol acetate is a reasonable treatment option (Tait and Aisner, 1989). However, if the central problem is fatigue and a low Karnofsky index (a measure of functional status), especially in a patient with a short expected survival, megestrol acetate, which is not inexpensive, is not likely to be of significant help.

COMPLEMENTARY AND ALTERNATIVE THERAPY

Herbal Therapy

Herbal therapy is gaining recognition within the health care community, and although it is grouped with alternative medicine treatments, it fits the definition of conventional allopathic, as opposed to homeopathic, medicine (Onopa, 1999). In fact, herbs were being used as medical treatments long before the advent of modern medicine, and some derivatives, such as aspirin, reserpine, and digitalis, have become mainstays of human pharmacotherapy. The current categorization of herbal medicine under alternative medical practices may stem from the fact that, as a modern discipline, phytotherapy is in its infancy regarding educational standards, credentialing, standardization, regulation of products, and clinical applications within the conventional health care system (Belew, 1999; Dashina and Krikorova, 1999; De Smet, 1997; Donaldson, 1998; Ernst and Weihmayr, 1998a-c; Gahlinger, 1999; Jobst, 1999; Kori-Lindner, 1999; Kottke, 1998; Lee, 1999; Li, 1997; McIntyre, 1999a,b; Mishkin, 1999; Moyad, 1999a,b; Nowak and Zlatic, 1999; Petri, 1999; Smith, Boyd, and Kirking, 1999; Thacker and Booher, 1999; Weintraub, 1999; Winkelaar, 1999; Winslow and Kroll, 1998). Nonetheless, herbal medicine lends itself well to standard clinical and basic science evaluation methods. In line with the current trend toward an evidence-based approach to integrative medicine, this section summarizes the knowledge and experience garnered from published case reports, randomized controlled clinical trials, and meta-analyses on the use of herbal medicine, with emphasis on those herbs most commonly used for the treatment of fatigue and chronic fatiguing illnesses. Potential applications and pharmacological interactions of herbal products that have not been subjected to clinical trials for the treatment of fatigue or chronic fatiguing illnesses are also addressed.

The use of herbal medicine is widespread and growing (Beal, 1998; Belew, 1999; Chandola et al., 1999; Dalzell, 1999; Guirguis, 1998; Prophet, 1999), with as many as three in ten Americans in a given year using botanical remedies for preventive or therapeutic purposes (Barrett, Kiefer, and Rabago, 1999; Cirigliano and Sun, 1998; Eisenberg et al., 1998; Higuchi et al., 1999; Norton, 1998; Plotnikoff and George, 1999; Rawsthorne et al., 1999; Stevenson, 1999; Winston and Dattner, 1999). Profits from the herbal remedy market now exceed $10 billion annually in the United States and are expected to increase (Cirigliano and Sun, 1998; Eisenberg et al., 1998; Glaser, 1999; Satake, 1998). Conventional medical literature also documents the widespread use of herbal remedies in many other countries, including Germany, Italy, Japan, Canada, Ecuador, Mexico, Paraguay, Belize, the West Indies, Nepal, Nigeria, Tanzania, West Africa, and Thailand (Bull and Melian, 1998; Catania, 1998; Chanecka, 1998; Disayavanish and Disayavanish, 1998; Firenzuoli and Gori, 1999; Greenwood, 1998; Halberstein, 1997; Harrison, 1998; Heinrich et al., 1998; Kikwilu and Hiza, 1997; Kraft, 1999; Manandhar, 1998; Miles, 1998; Nwosu, 1998; Sanyaolu, Fagberro, and Beyioku, 1997; Taddei-Bringas et al., 1999; Wong et al., 1998). The high cost, therapeutic limitations, and side effects of conventional medications have been a key factor in fueling the revival of herbal remedies, which have been used for centuries for a variety of ailments (Biswas et al., 1996; Duke, 1985; Durrigl and Fatovic-Ferencic, 1999; Theophrastus, 1916).

More than 3,000 species of herbs used in treating cancer since 2838 B.C. are known to biomedicine (Kaegi, 1998; LeMoine, 1997; Onopa, 1999). In fact, many of the pharmacological principles of the currently used anti-cancer agents were initially isolated from plants. Of new major anticancer drugs, four of the most promising are either obtained directly from plants or are modified from plant lead compounds: *Taxus brevifolia* (Taxol and Taxotere); *Camptotheca acuminata* (the water soluble campothecin analog topotecan hydrochloride) Hycamtin; *Podophyllum peltatum* (the podo-phyllotoxin analog Vumon); and *Catharanthus roseus* (Oncovin and the vincristine analog vinorelbine or Navolbine) (Pelley and Strickland, 2000).

Many plant products are under investigation. Muthu marunthu is an herbal formulation comprising eight various plant ingredients, and has been claimed to possess an antitumor effect based on tumor weight reduction in methylcholanthrene-induced fibrosarcoma rats after muthu marunthu treatment (Palani et al., 1999). Rasayanas are immunostimulating preparations used extensively in indigenous medical practice, and studies in mice demonstrated that they enhance the proliferation of spleen and marrow cells, humoral immunity, antibody-dependent complement-mediated tumor cell lysis, and natural killer cell activity in normal as well as in tumor-bearing animals. Brahma rasayana was found to have the maximum activity (Kumar, Kuttan, and Kuttan, 1999a,b). The herbal preparation termed PC-SPES, which is a refined powder of eight different medicinal plants, causes a dramatic decrease in prostate-specific antigen level in some prostate cancer patients with advanced disease and has significant antitumor effects on MAT-LyLu-induced tumorigenesis and metastasis in Copenhagen rats, in general refractory to most conventional therapy (Tiwari et al., 1999).

One study demonstrated that *Scutellaria barbata, Hedyotis diffusa* Willd., xi huang wan, green tea, and tea polyphenol all had antimutagenic effects, to some extent (Han, Hu, and Xu, 1997). Green tea can induce apoptosis of rat glioma cells (Serenelli et al., 1997). Chinese herbal medicine was shown to be effective in treating different complications (fever, lung infection, jaundice) post-bone marrow transplantation in patients with leukemia and could accelerate the recovery of patients (Li, Qian, and Feng, 1997). Xuefu zhuyu tang decoction showed coordinative effect with radiotherapy on primary hepatocellular carcinoma; it could enhance the radiosensitivity of liver cancer cells, increase the radiation tolerance of normal hepatocytes, and reduce the side effects of radiotherapy (Han, Chen, and Zhai, 1997). One study indicated that combined treatment of Chinese herbal medicine and cord blood infusion is an effective method in treating aplastic anemia (Li, Gan, and Ji, 1996). Sho-saiko-to displayed antitumor and antimetastatic effects on melanoma with regulation of the balance of matrix metalloproteinase and tissue inhibitor of the matrix metalloproteinase levels (Kato et al., 1998). Many components from dietary or medicinal plants have been identified that possess substantial chemopreventive properties. An example is curcumin (*Curcuma longa* Linn., Zingiberaceae), which has been shown to inhibit tumor promotion in experimental carcinogenesis. *Alpinia oxyphylla* Miquel, another plant of the ginger family used in Oriental herbal medicine, contains diarylheptanoids whose structures are analogous to that of curcumin and possess potential chemopreventive and antitumorigenic activities (Lee, Park, et al., 1998). Juzen-taiho-to has antimetastatic effects that are partly associated with its shimotsu-to-derived constituents (Onishi et al., 1998).

Examples of herbal remedies reported to have antitumor activity include the following:

- *Taxus brevifolia* (Taxol, Taxotere)
- *Camptotheca acuminata* (Topotecan)
- *Podophyllum peltatum* (Vumon)
- *Catharanthus roseus* (Oncovin, Vinorelbine)
- Muthu marunthu
- Rasayanas (brahma rasayana)
- PC-SPES
- *Scutellaria barbata*
- *Hedyotis diffusa* Willd.
- *Curcuma longa* (curcumin)
- Xi huang wan
- Green tea
- Xuefu zhuyu
- Sho-saiko-to
- Juzen-taiho-to

The following subsections summarize the published experience with herbal remedies for the treatment of fatigue and chronic fatiguing illnesses, experiences that open the door for testing in the context of cancer-related fatigue. Other herbal medicines that could be included under the general category of adaptogens (i.e., agents that increase resistance to physical, chemical, and biological stress and build up general vitality, including the physical and mental capacity for work) are not discussed because of lack of clinical trials or other evidence of effect on fatigue. Among these one may mention eleuthero, sarsaparilla, sassafras, ashwagandha, and cordyceps.

Aloë vera (Aloë vulgaris and Aloë barbadensis)

The aloe plants are native to eastern and southern Africa. Gel from the inner central zone of the leaves and latex from pericyclic cells are used for medicinal purposes (Hadley and Petry, 1999). Primary active components include anthraquinones, saccharides, prostaglandins, and fatty acids. One study showed that freeze-dried *Aloë vera* gel extract or a combination of freeze-dried *Aloë vera* gel extract and additional plant-derived saccharides resulted in a remarkable reduction in initial symptom severity in patients with chronic fatigue syndrome and fibromyalgia, with continued improvement in the period between initial assessment and follow-up (Dykman et al., 1998). Further research is needed to verify these results, specifically crossover designs in well-defined populations. As detailed in the following paragraphs, aloe plants and their individual chemical components perform a variety of activities that could underlie their use for cancer-related fatigue and other cancer-associated pathologies.

Acemannan, the major carbohydrate fraction of *Aloë vera* gels, acts as an immune stimulant by activating macrophages and stimulating cytokine production and nitric oxide release, surface molecule expression, and cell morphologic changes (Yagi et al., 1999; Zhang and Tizard, 1996). In one study, the production of the cytokines interleukin-6 and tumor necrosis factor-alpha was dependent on the dose of acemannan provided. Nitric oxide (NO) production, cell morphologic changes, and surface antigen expression were increased in response to stimulation by a mixture of acemannan and interferon-gamma (Chauhan et al., 1998). Analysis of the products of aloemannan metabolism suggests that the immunomodulation of aloemannan may come from not only neutral polysaccharides but also contaminated hexosamine in aloemannan (Vazquez et al. 1996).

Muktashukti bhasma, an Ayurvedic compound that consists of *Aloë vera,* pearl, and vinegar, inhibited acute and subacute inflammation in albino rats, being one-third to one-half as potent as aspirin. The anti-inflammatory activity of the compound is attributed to its ability to cause inhibition of prostaglandins, histamine, and serotonin, and also by stabilization of the lysosomal membranes (Chauhan et al., 1998). *Aloë vera* gel alone has shown anti-inflammatory activity in rats through decreased carrageenan-induced edema and neutrophil migration and inhibition of cyclooxygenase-dependent prostaglandin E2 production from arachidonic acid (Vazquez et al., 1996). Moreover, a new anti-inflammatory agent identified as 8-[C-beta-D-[2-O-(E)-cinnamoyl] glucopyranosyl]-2-(R)-2-hydroxy-propyl]-7-methoxy-5-methylchromone has been isolated from *Aloë barbadensis* Miller and shown to have a potency similar to hydrocortisone (Hutter et al., 1996).

Cutaneous exposure to ultraviolet B radiation suppresses the induction of T-cell-mediated responses such as contact and delayed type hypersensitivity by altering the function of immune cells in the skin and causing the release of immunoregulatory cytokines. Extracts of crude *Aloë barbadensis* gel, tamarind xyloglucans, and aloe poly/oligosaccharides prevent this photosuppression (Byeon et al., 1998; Lee, Han, et al., 1997; Strikland et al., 1999). The ability of aloe gel to prevent suppression of contact hypersensitivity responses to hapten decayed rapidly after manufacture (Byeon et al., 1998). Moreover, two phase III randomized trials failed to find any effect of *Aloë vera* gel against radiation therapy-induced dermatitis (Williams, Burk, et al., 1996).

Aloë vera has several important therapeutic properties, including anti-cancer effects, as demonstrated by the effects of *Aloë vera* administration in a rat pleural tumor model (Corsi et al., 1998). *Aloë vera* gel extract and vitamin C supplementation reduce the severity of hepatocarcinogenesis induced in male Sprague-Dawley rats by diethylnitrosamine and 2-acetylamino-fluorene (Shamaan et al., 1998). *Aloë barbadensis* Miller (polysaccharide fraction) has an inhibitory effect on benzo[a]pyrene (B[a]P)-DNA adduct formation, which might also have a chemopreventive effect by inhibition of B[a]P absorption (Kim and Lee, 1997). Freeze-dried whole leaves of kidachi aloe chemoprevent hepatocarcinogenesis by *trans*-beta-carotene by inhibiting formation of 2-amino-3-methylimidazol[4,5-f]quinoline (IQ)-DNA adducts (Uehara et al., 1996). *Aloë vera* gel has angiogenic activity, and it increases proliferation of calf pulmonary artery endothelial (CPAE) cells, induces CPAE cells to invade type 1 collagen gel and form capillary-like tubes, increases invasion of CPAE cells into matrigel, and enhances mRNA expression in CPAE cells of proteolytiic enzymes that are key participants in the regulation of extracellular matrix degradation such as urokinase-type plasminogen activator, matrix metalloproteinase-2 (MMP-2), and membrane-type MMP (Lee, Lee, et al., 1998). Preliminary clinical studies have shown that melatonin may induce some benefits in untreatable metastatic solid tumor patients, and a preliminary study suggests that natural cancer therapy with melatonin plus *Aloë vera* extracts may produce some therapeutic benefits, at least in terms of stabilization of disease and survival, in patients with advanced solid tumors for whom no other standard effective therapy is available (Lissoni et al., 1998).

Aloë vera influences the wound-healing process by enhancing collagen turnover in the wound tissue as demonstrated by increased biosynthesis of collagen and its degradation, increase in the urinary excretion of hydroxyproline, and elevated levels of lysyl oxidase as indication of increased crosslinking of newly synthesized collagen (Chithra, Sajithlal, and Chandrakasan, 1998b). Both topical application and oral administration of *Aloë vera* increase the collagen content, particularly that of type III collagen, of the granulation tissue as well as its degree of crosslinking (Chithra, Sajithlal, and Chandrakasan, 1998a). Aloe appears to expedite wound contraction in Sprague-Dawley rats and neutralize the wound-retardant effect seen with the topical antimicrobial mafenide acetate alone. This effect appears to be secondary to an increased collagen activity, which is enhanced by a lectin, and consequently improves the collagen matrix and enhances the breaking strength, activities that probably counteract the toxicity on keratinocytes and fibroblasts associated with some antibacterial agents (Heggers et al., 1996).

Both topical and oral treatments with *Aloë vera* have a positive influence on the synthesis of glycosaminoglycans and thereby beneficially modulate wound healing (Chithra, Sajithlal, and Chandrakasan, 1998c). *Aloë vera* treatment of wounds in diabetic rats may enhance the process of wound healing by influencing phases such as inflammation, fibroplasia, collagen synthesis and maturation, and wound contraction. These effects may also be secondary to the reported hypoglycemic effects of the aloe gel (Chithra, Sajithlal, and Chandrakasan, 1998d). A glycoprotein fraction of leaf gel from *Aloë barbadensis* Miller promotes proliferation of human normal dermal and baby hamster kidney cells (Yagi et al., 1997). Aloe appears to have a wound-healing advancement factor. It appears that aloe's effect of preventing dermal ischemia by reversing the effects of thromboxane synthetase (TxA2) may act synergistically with nitric oxide or, alternatively, aloe could be an oxygen radical scavenger. NO is a potent vasodilator that is thought to be an endothelium-dependent relaxing factor and a regulator of blood pressure and regional blood flow. It affects vascular smooth muscle proliferation and inhibits platelet aggregation and leukocyte adhesion. NO's activities may underlie the use of many systemic and topical therapeutic agents, such as growth hormone, platelet-derived growth factor, fibroblast growth factor, epidermal growth factor, and insulin-like growth factor, as vulnerary (wound-healing) agents (Heggers et al., 1997). It is noteworthy that extracts from the parenchymatous leaf gel and the rind of the *Aloë barbadensis* Miller were shown to contain seven electrophoretically identifiable superoxide dismutases (SODs). The specific activities of SODs in the *Aloë vera* rind and gel are comparable to those of spinach leaves and of rabbit liver (Sabeh, Wright, and Norton, 1996).

A gel containing *Aloë vera,* silicon dioxide, and allantoin had an inconsistent effect on healing of recurrent aphthous ulcers (Garnick, Singh, and Winkley, 1998). Although some studies appear to show that topical and orally administered *Aloë vera* preparations in patients with chronic venous leg ulcers may aid healing, larger research studies are needed (Atherton, 1998). A double-blind, placebo-controlled study showed clinical efficacy and tolerability of topical *Aloë vera* extract 0.5 percent in a hydrophilic cream to cure patients with psoriasis vulgaris (Syed et al., 1996).

Lyophylized *Aloë barbadensis* at concentrations of 7.5 percent and 10 percent proved to be spermicidal secondary to multiple microelements (boron, barium, calcium, chromium, copper, iron, potassium, magnesium, manganese, phosphorus, and zinc), which were toxic to the tail and caused instant immobilization. The compound did not irritate or cause ulceration of rabbit vaginal epithelium. These results suggest the possibility of using lyophilized *Aloë barbadensis* as an effective and safe vaginal contraceptive. Lyophilized *Aloë barbadensis* had no antiviral effect (Fahim and Wang, 1996).

Aloe is contraindicated in children younger than twelve years old and in older persons with suspected intestinal obstruction, inflammatory bowel disease, or pregnancy. Caution is indicated when used in conjunction with cardiac glycosides (Hadley and Petry, 1999). Reflex engorgement of pelvic blood vessels can increase menstrual bleeding and may increase the risk of spontaneous abortion. Crampy abdominal pain or diarrhea may occur, but rarely allergies (Ishii et al., 1998; Izzo et al., 1999). With long-term use, diarrhea may cause electrolyte imbalance, especially potassium deficiency, which may be increased by the simultaneous use of thiazide diuretics, corticosteroids, or licorice root. Basal calcium-dependent nitric oxide synthase activity in the rat colon was dose-dependently inhibited by aloe and aloin, the active ingredient of aloe (Izzo et al., 1999). *Aloë vera* gel contains toxic low molecular weight (LMW) compounds, and every effort must be made to limit the amount of these toxins in commercially prepared *Aloë vera* gel products (Avila et al., 1997; Brusick and Mengs, 1997; Chung et al., 1996; Dykman et al., 1998; Muller et al., 1996).

Echinacea (E. angustifolia, E. pallida, E. purpurea, Purple Coneflower)

In one study (See et al., 1997), an extract of *Echinacea purpurea* was evaluated for its capacity to stimulate cellular immune function by peripheral blood mononuclear cells (PBMCs) from normal individuals and patients with chronic fatigue syndrome. PBMCs isolated on a Ficoll-Hypaque density gradient were tested in the presence or absence of varying concentrations of the extract for natural killer cell cytotoxic activity directed against K562 cell targets and antibody-dependent cellular cytotoxicity (ADCC) directed against human herpesvirus 6-infected H9 cells. Echinacea, at concentrations greater than or equal to 0.1 micrograms/Kg, significantly enhanced NK cell function in both groups. Similarly, the addition of the herb significantly increased ADCC of PBMCs from subject groups. Thus, an extract of *Echinacea purpurea* enhances cellular immune function of PBMCs from normal individuals as well as from patients with depressed cellular immunity and chronic fatigue syndrome (See et al., 1997). As detailed in Chapter 3, depressed cellular immunity may be a factor in cancer-related fatigue and cancer etiology or progression.

Echinacea is native to central parts of the United States, and its root and aerial parts are used medicinally (Hadley and Petry, 1999). The active components are believed to be polysaccharides, flavonoids, caffeic acids, essential oils, polyacetylenes, and alkyl amides. Several studies support the immunomodulatory role of echinacea (Melchart et al., 1995). Meta-analyses of sixteen published studies concluded that echinacea may be effective for treating and preventing the common cold; however, more rigorous studies are needed (Gunning and Steele, 1999; Linde, 1999; Pepping, 1999). In fact, other studies found radically different results (Grimm and Muller, 1999; Melchart et al., 1998).

The German Commission E monographs list autoimmune diseases as contraindications for use of echinacea. Although echinacea can stimulate the production of cytokines by human cell lines in vitro, it remains to be determined whether the cytokines expressed would help perpetuate an autoimmune state or would switch the prevalent cytokine expression program to a more desirable one. If used beyond eight weeks, echinacea could cause hepatotoxicity and, therefore, should not be used with other known hepatotoxic drugs, such as anabolic steroids, amiodarone, methotrexate, and ketoconazole. Because of its immunostimulatory activity, echinacea should not be given with immunosuppressants (e.g., corticosteroids and cyclosporine) (Miller LG, 1998). A woman with atopy experienced anaphylaxis after taking, among other dietary supplements, a commercial extract of echinacea.

Patients with atopy should be cautioned about the risk of developing life-threatening reactions to echinacea (Mullins, 1998).

Erkang

Shi-quan-da-bu-tang is a traditional Chinese herbal medicine formula used to increase vital energy and strengthen health and immunity. It also has the ability to attack tumor tissue. The erkang capsule is a modified formula of shi-quan-da-bu-tang, with the addition of four other herbs to increase the adaptogen effects and ergogenic properties. Results from a study in mice indicated that the erkang-treated group had significant differences in fatigue, mortality, body weight change, cold temperature endurance, and immune function-related organ weight change, as compared to control animals (Wu et al., 1998).

Hochu-ekki-to (TJ-41:Bu-zhong-yi-qi-tang)

In one study, hochu-ekki-to was administered in 2.5 g doses three times a day to 162 patients who complained of anorexia or lassitude because of genitourinary cancer (Kuroda et al., 1985). The efficacy rate was 63 percent. The rate of effectiveness on anorexia was 48.4 percent and on lassitude was 36.6 percent. Side effects were observed in twelve patients (7.4 percent), but most of them were mild gastrointestinal disorders. No severe adverse effects were noted.

Restraint stress impairs antitumor immune responses through its suppressive effect on the Th1 (cellular-mediated immunity)-type cytokine production from CD4+ T cells. Oral administration of hochu-ekki-to (TJ-41:bu-zhong-yi-qi-tang), a traditional Chinese herbal medicine, restored the antitumor T-cell responses in stress-burdened, tumor-bearing mice by normalizing the serum levels of corticosterone and interleukin-12, as well as the expression of costimulatory molecules such as CD80 and CD86 (Li et al., 1999). In another study, hochu-ekki-to was also shown to induce innate immunity against murine cytomegalovirus, which at the early phase of infection is mediated by natural killer cells and macrophages (Hossain et al., 1999).

Syngnathus acus

Li and colleagues (2001) listed anticancer, fatigue resisting, immunity improvement, and systolic function enhancement effects for *Syngnathus acus* L., a traditional Chinese medicine from the sea. Investigations on this remedy are needed.

Hedgehog Hydnum

Hedgehog hydnum (*Hydnum repandum* L.) powder or extract given for sixty days had a significant effect on raising physical stamina and delaying fatigue in mice (Lu et al., 1996).

Juzen-taiho-to

Juzen-taiho-to is a *kampo* (Japanese and Chinese traditional) medicine and is a nourishing agent, a so-called hozai (in Japanese), that is used for improving disturbances and imbalances in the homeostatic condition of the body (Saiki, 2000). This drug is administered to patients in various weakened conditions, including postsurgery patients and patients with chronic illnesses, where it can alleviate general symptoms such as extreme fatigue, pale complexion, loss of appetite, dry or scaly skin, night sweating, and dryness of the mouth. Currently, juzen-taiho-to is often administered to cancer patients and has been shown to possess various biological activities, such as enhancement of phagocytosis, cytokine induction, antibody production, induction of the mitogenic activity of spleen cells, antitumor effects when combined with surgical excision, antitumor effects with or without other drugs, and protection against the deleterious effects of anticancer drugs as well as radiation-induced immunosuppression and bone marrow toxicity (Saiki, 2000).

Juzen-taiho-to (TJ-48) is prepared by extracting a mixture of ten kinds of medicinal plants (Yamada, 1989) (*Rehmannia glutinosa, Paeonia lactiflora, Ligusticum wallichii, Angelica sinesis, Glycyrrhiza uralensis, Poria cocos, Atractylodes macrocephala, Panax ginseng, Astragalus membranaceus,* and *Cinnamomum cassia*) that tone the blood and vital energy and strengthen health and immunity. This prescription has long been used traditionally against anemia, anorexia, extreme exhaustion, and fatigue. In fact, juzen-taiho-to and shi-quan-da-bu-tang (Ten Significant Tonic Decoction) were formulated by Taiping Hui-Min Ju (Public Welfare Pharmacy Bureau) during the Chinese Song Dynasty in A.D. 1200 (Zee-Cheng, 1992). In a screening and evaluation of 116 Chinese herbal formularies (kampo), juzen-taiho-to was selected as the most effective as a potent biological response modifier (Zee-Cheng, 1992). TJ-48 may now provide new advantages with little toxicity in combination with chemotherapy (mitomycin, cisplatin, cyclophosphamide, and fluorouracil) or radiation therapy, and promising results have been obtained in terms of preventing leukemia in cancer patients who have taken antitumor agents.

As illustration of the activities described earlier, it is worth mentioning that the combination of TJ-48 and mitomycin C (MMC) produces significantly longer survival in p-388 tumor-bearing mice than MMC alone, and TJ-48 decreases the diverse effects of MMC such as leukopenia, thrombopenia, and weight loss. However, mechanisms of the pharmacological action are still unclear. One of the possible mechanisms of the action of TJ-48 may be some effects on immune responses. TJ-48 augments antibody production, activates macrophages, and reduces MMC-induced immunosuppression in mice. TJ-48 shows mitogenic activity in splenocytes, but not in thymocytes, and an anticomplementary activity (Yamada, 1989).

Anticomplementary activity and mitogenic activity were both observed in the high-molecular polysaccharide fraction but not in the low-molecular weight fraction. Of several polysaccharide fractions in TJ-48, only the pectic polysaccharide fraction (F-5-2) showed potent mitogenic activity. F-5-2 was also shown to have the highest anticomplementary activity. However, the polygalacturonan region is essential for the expression of the mitogenic activity, but the contribution of the polygalacturonan region to the anticomplementary activity is less. F-5-2 activates complement via alternative complement pathways and induces the proliferation of B cells but does not differentiate those cells from antibody-producing cells (Yamada, 1989).

Hozai have also been used to improve the physical condition of the elderly. Juzen-taiho-to was shown to modulate antigen-specific T-cell responses toward balanced Th1 (cellular-mediated immunity)/Th2 (humoral immunity)-type responses in old BALB/c mice, which have a preferential Th2-type cytokine response pattern (Lijima et al., 1999). Such effects may help prevent the development of diseases associated with immunodysregulation, such as some forms of cancer, and may also contribute to lessen cancer-related fatigue. To this end, future development on the application and mechanistic studies of juzen-taiho-to has potential importance in basic and clinical research of the traditional Chinese therapeutic approach of toning the blood and strengthening Qi (vital energy) in cancer immunotherapy (Zee-Cheng, 1992).

Lentinan

Pursuing the hypothesis that the low-grade fever and fatigue in low natural killer syndrome (LNKS) (see Chapter 3) (Aoki, Usuda, and Miyakoshi, 1987; Aoki et al., 1993) might be abrogated by interventions that normalize natural killer cell function, one group has tested the effects of immunopotentiators in patients diagnosed with LNKS. They found in single-blind trials (contents of medication were not revealed to patients) that while the administration of antipyrectics, nonsteroidal anti-inflammatory drugs, or antibiotics had no detectable effects on fever, lentinan, a glucon extracted from Japanese mushrooms, improved clinical symptoms and increased natural killer cell cytotoxicity and antibody-dependent cellular cytotoxicity in patients with LNKS (Miyakoshi, Aoki, and Mizukoshi, 1984). Although preliminary, this is one of the only studies to document parallel improvements in fatigue and natural killer cell function following an experimental manipulation. Studies on cancer-related fatigue, particularly that associated with immunodysregulation, are warranted.

Lentinan and other beta-glucans, such as schizophyllan and PSK/PSP, also have antitumor effects (Arinaga, Karimine, Takamuku, Nanbara, Inoue, et al., 1992; Arinaga, Karimine, Takamuku, Nanbara, Nagamatsu, et al., 1992; Matsouka et al., 1997; Taguchi, 1987; Tanabe, Imai, and Takechi, 1990; Tari et al., 1994; Wakui et al., 1986; Yoshino et al., 1989). As reviewed by Pelley and Strickland (2000), several papers have begun to tender plausible mechanisms to explain the antitumor action of beta-glucans (Xia and Ross, 1999; Xia et al., 1999; Yan et al., 1999). These papers, all by the same research group, tie together beta-glucans, the macrophage/NK cell CD11b/CD18 carbohydrate receptor (leukocyte complement receptor type 3), and cancer surveillance. A common finding in cancer is the existence of circulating low-affinity antibody to tumor cells. These antibodies are unfortunately not cytolytic (possibly because they have insufficient affinity). However, they have sufficient avidity to trigger a low-level attack by the classical pathway of the complement system (again insufficient to cause lysis). Thus when tumors are removed from patients they are frequently found to be coated with low levels of immunoglobulin and iC3b. CD11b/ CD18 is the high-affinity receptor for β-1-3-glucopyranosyl polysaccharides on neutrophils, NK cells, and monocytes. Xia and colleagues (1999) showed that macrophages and NK cells in the basal state fail to lyse cells with iC3b on their surface but that incubation of these effector cells with as little as 1 µg of β-1-3-glucan "primed" them to lyse iC3b+ target cells. The target cells were not lysed unless they were coated with small amounts of antibody (and iC3b). The priming reaction could be blocked if the macrophages or NK cells had been previously treated with antibody that blocked the CD11b/CD18 receptor, and the priming reaction did not occur in mice that genetically lacked CD11b/ CD18. This priming for cytotoxicity was greater with NK cells than it was for macrophages, and it lasted for about twelve to twenty-four hours.

Yan and colleagues (1999) demonstrated that as mice of several common strains grew from weaning to full adulthood, they developed IgG and IgM antibodies that could bind to several types of common (breast, sarcoma, bladder) murine cancers. When these cancers were implanted in young mice, the tumors grew. If the tumors were harvested several weeks later, immunoglobulin and iC3b were detected on the surfaces of malignant cells. Thus, immune surveillance fails even though antitumor antibody is being made by the animals, the antibody is binding to the tumors, and complement is being activated and deposited on the cancer cells. The NK cells and macrophages of the immune surveillance system were not receiving the second signal to bring them to full activity. In adult mice, this second signal could be supplied by daily injections of beta-glucan resulting in average tumor weights 60 to 90 percent lower than in mice given control injections. In young mice, the amount of antitumor antibody was so low that priming by beta-glucans produced only a 50 percent inhibition of tumor growth.

As pointed out by Yan and colleagues (1999), the form of tumor immunity they described is not equally effective against all types of neoplasms; it does not provide sterilizing immunity with the elimination of every tumor cell but rather decrease in tumor bulk and slowing of tumor growth; and it may be fooled by escape by selection for tumor antigen-negative antitumor response.

Panax ginseng

The ginsengs consist of the dried root of several species of the genus *Panax* of the family Araliaceae. Asian or Oriental ginseng is *Panax ginseng* C.A. Meyer and it is the most commonly used species. The German Commission E monograph suggests the use of ginseng as a tonic to counteract weakness and fatigue, as a restorative for declining stamina, as a remedy for impaired concentration, and as an aid to convalescence (Schulz, Hänsel, and Tyler, 1998). Of the thirty-seven clinical studies on ginseng published between 1968 and 1990, only fifteen were controlled and eight double-blinded. Seventeen showed improvement in physical performance, eleven improvement in intellectual performance, and thirteen an improvement in mood. However, quality of design and statistical analysis in many of the studies are questionable (Foster and Tyler, 1992).

In the treatment of functional fatigue, a multicenter, comparative, double-blind, clinical study in a total of 232 patients showed that 40 mg of ginseng extract plus multivitamins and minerals taken over forty-two days improved the complaints experienced by patients suffering from fatigue, with tolerability comparable to that of placebo (Le Gal, Cathebras, and Strüby, 1996). One should mention, however, that a flaw in the study was the lack of vitamins and minerals in the placebo. In a more recent study (See et al., 1997), an extract of *Panax ginseng* was evaluated for its capacity to stimulate cellular immune function by peripheral blood mononuclear cells from normal individuals and patients with chronic fatigue syndrome. PBMCs isolated on a Ficoll-Hypaque density gradient were tested in the presence or absence of varying concentrations of the extract for natural killer cell cytotoxic activity directed against K562 cell targets and for antibody-dependent cellular cytotoxicity directed against human herpesvirus 6-infected H9 cells. Ginseng, at concentrations greater than or equal to 10 micrograms/Kg, significantly enhanced NK cell function in both groups. Similarly, the addition of the herb significantly increased ADCC of PBMCs from the subject groups. Thus, an extract of *Panax ginseng* enhances cellular immune function of PBMCs from normal individuals as well as from patients with depressed cellular immunity and chronic fatigue syndrome (See et al., 1997). In line with these observations, in another study ginseng treatment was found to lead to an activation of neutrophils and modulation of the immunoglobulin G response to *Pseudomonas aeruginosa,* thereby enhancing the clearance and reducing the formation of immune complexes, effects that resulted in a milder lung pathology in chronic *Pseudomonas aeruginosa* lung infection in cystic fibrosis patients. The therapeutic effects of ginseng may be related to activation of a Th1-type cytokine response and down-regulation of humoral immunity (Song et al., 1998).

Although ginseng is generally well tolerated, it has been implicated as a cause of decreased response to warfarin and may interfere with either digoxin pharmacodynamically or with digoxin monitoring (Cupp, 1999; McRae, 1996; Miller LG, 1998). Nevertheless, some authors claim no relationship between cardiac glycosides and glycosides in ginseng and attribute the interaction with digoxin on contaminants (Awang, 1996; Wong, 1999). In addition, ginseng may cause headache, tremulousness, and manic episodes in patients treated with phenelzine sulfate. Ginseng also should not be used with estrogens or corticosteroids because of possible additive effects. Ginseng may affect blood glucose levels and should not be used by patients with diabetes mellitus (Miller LG, 1998).

Tinospora cordifolia

The active principles of *Tinospora cordifolia,* a traditional Indian plant, possess anticomplementary and immunomodulatory activities (Kapil and Sharma, 1997). Syringin (TC-4) and cordiol (TC-7) inhibited the in vitro immunohemolysis of antibody-coated sheep erythrocytes by guinea pig serum. The reduced immunohemodialysis was found to be secondary to inhibition of the C3-convertase of the classical component pathway. However, higher concentrations showed constant inhibitory effects. The compounds also gave rise to significant increases in immunoglobulin G antibodies in serum. Humoral and cell-mediated immunity were also dose-dependently enhanced. Macrophage activation was reported for cordioside (TC-2), cordiofolioside A (TC-5), and cordiol (TC-7), and this activation was more pronounced with increasing incubation times (Kapil and Sharma, 1997).

Rhodiola rosea

As reviewed by Kelly (2001), *Rhodiola rosea* is a popular plant in traditional medical systems in Eastern Europe and Asia, with a reputation for stimulating the nervous system, decreasing depression, enhancing work performance, eliminating fatigue, and preventing high-altitude sickness. *Rhodiola rosea* has been categorized as an adaptogen by Russian researchers due to its observed ability to increase resistance to a variety of chemical, biological, and physical stressors. Its claimed benefits include antidepressant, anticancer, cardioprotective, and central nervous system enhancement. Research also indicates great utility in asthenic conditions (decline in work performance, sleep difficulties, poor appetite, irritability, hypertension, headaches, and fatigue) developing subsequent to intense physical or intellectual strain. The adaptogenic, cardiopulmonary protective, and central nervous system activities of *Rhodiola rosea* have been attributed primarily to its ability to influence levels and activity of monoamines and opioid peptides such as beta-endorphins (Kelly, 2001).

Kavosporal forte

Neuhaus and colleagues (2000) examined the anxiolytic effect of the herbal preparation Kavosporal forte in twenty patients with situationally induced anxiety. The degree of anxiety was acute in that the patients were waiting for the results of a histopathological diagnosis, carried out on account of suspect mammary findings, and therefore feared they were suffering from a mammary carcinoma. A significant reduction of anxiety compared with the placebo control was seen after a week's treatment with Kavosporal forte, levels of anxiety being measured a priori from the combined scores of two self-rating scales and one observer-rated scale. In addition, a significant increase was noted in alertness, as well as lessening of fatigue, introverted behavior, and excitability, and a reduction in levels of depression under the real therapeutic agent over the observation period. In none of the cases examined did any undesirable side effects occur, and the overall tolerance was also consistently good (Neuhaus et al., 2000).

Astragalus membranaceus

Astragalus membranaceus, a Chinese herb composed mainly of crude saponin and astragaloside, has immunopotentiating activities in rats (Zheng et al., 1998) and as other botanicals (e.g., *Crataegus oxyacantha, Terminalia arjuna,* and *Inula racemosa*) has therapeutic benefit for the treatment of cardiovascular disease (Miller AL, 1998). *Astragalus membranaceus* is often used as a "Qi tonifier" and has been studied for its therapeutic benefit in the treatment of ischemic heart disease, myocardial infarction, heart failure, and relief of anginal pain. Clinical studies have indicated that its in vitro antioxidant activity is the mechanism by which it affords its cardioprotective benefit (Miller AL, 1998).

Limitations and Precautions with Herbal Medicines

Clinical studies on several herbal medicine products have methodological weaknesses, including heterogeneity of the products used, lack of disease definition, and lack of validity and reliability of outcome measures. For instance, it is frequently recognized that traditional Chinese medicines, currently sold in the United States as dietary supplements—as defined by the Dietary Supplement Health and Education Act of 1995 (Chang, 1999)—are an amalgamation of several herbs that generate the putative clinical effects. Because of this historical multiherb approach, the reliance on retrospective data to support the potential health benefits of a single herb extract has severe limitations. Moreover, the polyvalent nature of these products poses a challenge to designing appropriate clinical studies that can provide data for "structure and function" claim substantiation.

Despite the limitations mentioned, herbalists claim that the polypharmacy of botanical remedies provides two advantages over single-ingredient drugs: primary active ingredients in herbs are synergized by secondary compounds, and secondary compounds mitigate the side effects caused by primary active ingredients (Chang, 1999). Moreover, traditional preparation procedures are purported to enhance the therapeutic value of plant derivatives, while at the same time reducing their potential toxicity (Halberstein, 1997). However, the safety and efficacy of herbal products, as well as the validity and generalizability of clinical studies of phytotherapy, will be enhanced by the identification of the pharmacological active component(s) of herbal medicines or by the development of standardized herbal extracts (Chang, 1999).

Herbal products on the market differ in their biochemical composition because of the use of different plant species, plant parts, and extraction methods. For instance, significant heterogeneity has been reported in the oil content of *Hyssopus officinalis* L. species (Lamiaceae family), a spice and folk medicine that is used to combat certain respiratory diseases in Hungary and other Central European countries (Varga et al., 1998). The mode of preparation of certain formulations may also affect the final product as exemplified by allinase, which gets significantly altered during the drying process of garlic powder (Krest and Keusgen, 1999). The interpretation of phytotherapy clinical study data may also be affected by heterogeneity in herbal medication metabolism. For instance, after administration of the herbal medication sho-saiko-to, the urine of half of the study subjects contained two types of flavonoids, *S*-dihydrowogonin and *S*-dihydrooroxylin A, an observation that suggests some individuals might be rapid and poor metabolizers of flavonoids (Li, Homma, and Oka, 1998).

Correct plant identification and accurate labeling are of paramount importance to the clinical application of herbal remedies (Awang, 1997; Wong et al., 1999). Simple and accurate methods to detect the adulteration of commercial herbal products have been developed and are particularly relevant because toxicity related to traditional medicines is becoming more widely recognized as these remedies become popular in developed countries (Hurlbut et al., 1998; Huxtable, 1998; Kim, Lee, et al., 1998; Lu et al., 1997; Moss, 1998; Stewart, Steenkamp, and Zuckerman, 1998). Accidental herbal toxicity occurs not only as a result of a lack of quality control in harvesting and preparation but also because herbal remedies are believed to be harmless. In most cases of plant poisoning, treatment continues to be only symptomatic, with few specific antidotes available. It is important that toxicologists in the West be alert to the possibility of encountering poisoning in patients secondary to traditional remedies (Stewart, Steenkamp, and Zuckerman, 1998). For instance, a case of lead poisoning in a Korean man taking Chinese herbal medicine has been reported. The source of lead exposure was hai ge fen (clamshell powder), one of the thirty-six ingredients of a Chinese herbal medicine formulation (Markowitz et al., 1994). The consumption of ba-baw-san, another Chinese herbal medicine, was significantly associated with increased blood lead in children (Cheng et al., 1998). In four reported cases patients developed hepatic injury during administration of herbal medicines for losing weight with wild germander (Mattei et al., 1992). Fulminant hepatic failure has also been associated with the use of other herbal medications (Bagheri et al., 1998).

Although a large amount of data is available documenting the pharmacologically active ingredients of many plants, it is seldom helpful to the toxicologist in an acute situation. Current analytic methods such as high-performance liquid chromatography, gas chromatography, mass spectrometry, and immunoassays can provide identification of the toxin in those few cases in which the history or symptoms give a clear lead, but broad screening methods remain to be developed. To minimize toxicity from Chinese herbal medicines, a method involving the simultaneous extraction and cleanup of thirteen organochlorine pesticides was developed using supercritical fluid extraction followed by gas chromatography-electron capture detection and mass spectrometric confirmation (Ling, Teng, and Cartwright, 1999).

Paltiel and colleagues (2001) performed a survey of 1,027 Israeli oncology patients to examine the extent of their use of complementary therapies and to compare sociodemographic, psychologic, and medical characteristics, attitudes, and quality of life of users and nonusers of complementary medicine. A total of 526 participants (51.2 percent) had used complementary medicine since their diagnosis, and 357 patients (34.9 percent) had used complementary medicine recently (in the past three months). Factors significantly associated with recent complementary medicine use were as follows: female sex; age thirty-five to fifty-nine years; more education; coming to the hospital by private car; advanced disease status; having a close friend or a relative with cancer; and attending support groups or individual counseling. After controlling for these factors, individually examined psychosocial variables associated with recent complementary medicine use included the following: needs unmet by conventional medicine; helplessness; incomplete trust in the doctor; and changed outlook or beliefs since the diagnosis of cancer. Functional quality of life (including physical, emotional, social, and role function) and symptom (fatigue and diarrhea) scores were significantly worse for recent complementary medicine users compared with nonusers, controlling for age, sex, and current disease status. These observations suggest that increased attention to psychosocial needs within oncology settings is warranted (Paltiel et al., 2001).

Because many herbal medicines cause significant pharmacological activity, and thus potential adverse effects and drug interactions, health care professionals must be familiar with this popular therapeutic modality to help patients discern fact from fiction, avoid harm, and derive any benefits that may be available (Cupp, 1999; Glisson, Crawford, and Street, 1999; Klepser and Klepser, 1999). Manufacturers of herbal products currently are not required to submit proof of safety and efficacy to the FDA before marketing; for this reason, the adverse effects and drug interactions associated with herbal remedies are largely unknown (Barrios, 1999; Riddle, 1999; Sibbald, 1999). In Australia, most herbal drugs are classed as "listed drugs," which are required to satisfy less rigorous safety and efficacy criteria than "registered drugs" (Walter and Rey, 1999). The German Commission E, a regulatory body that evaluates the safety and efficacy of herbs on the basis of clinical trials, cases, and other scientific literature, has established indications and dosage recommendations for many herbal therapies (Keller,

1997). The Ministry of Health and Welfare of the Japanese government has also reported side effects of the traditional Japanese kampo medicines (Catania, 1998).

The mainly unregulated over-the-counter availability of herbal medications opens the possibility for their inappropriate use, including overuse, abuse, or suboptimal use. For instance, a study found that even among adults with access to specialty care for asthma, self-treatment with nonprescription products (herbal medicine, coffee, or black tea use) was common and was associated with increased risk of reported hospitalization. This association was not accounted for by illness severity or other disease covariates and likely reflected delay in utilization of more efficacious treatments (Blanc et al., 1997). Herbal products may also have adverse effects in patients who receive certain types of traditional medications, such as anticoagulant or antiplatelet medication (Catania, 1998; Satake, 1998). For instance, profound anticoagulation was caused by interaction between warfarin, a coumarin anticoagulant, and danshen, a widely used Chinese herbal medicine, in a patient who had undergone mitral valve replacement (Izzat, Yim, and El-Zufari, 1998). Simultaneous oral administration to rats of sho-seiryu-to extract powder, another widely used traditional Chinese herbal medicine, delays the oral absorption of carbamazepine, while one week repeated pretreatment with sho-seiryu-to accelerates the metabolism of carbamazepine, without affecting its protein binding (Ohnishi et al., 1999).

The pharmacological activity, chemical components, and microbial content of herbs, as well as their ability to interfere with prescription medications (Adverse Drug Reactions Advisory Committee, 1999; Zhu, Wong, and Li, 1999), make medicinal herbs potentially dangerous to certain populations of patients, such as renal or transplant patients (Crone and Wise, 1997; Foote and Cohen, 1998). Many herbal medications are nephrotoxic (Ng et al., 1998; Nortier, Depierreux, and Vanherweghem, 1999). For instance, a sixty-six-year-old Chinese man presented with hypokalemic paralysis, rhabdomyolysis, and acute renal failure with proximal tubular acidosis and selective glucosuria after administration of mixed Chinese herbs (Lee et al., 1999); and a patient with systemic lupus erythematosus developed acute renal failure secondary to use of "cat's claw" herbal remedy (Hilepo, Bellucci, and Mossey, 1997).

Ma huang, St. John's wort, wild germander, comfrey, and kava are examples of readily available herbs with the potential for negative effects (Tinsley, 1999). Jui, a traditional Chinese herbal medicine, can induce thrombocytopenia (Azuno et al., 1999), and the Japanese herbal medicine sho-saiko-to (TJ-9) can cause drug-induced interstitial pneumonitis and pulmonary edema, especially in Japanese patients with chronic hepatitis C (Miyazaki et al., 1998; Yamashiki et al., 1997). A severe anaphylactic reaction secondary to the ingestion of a pollen compound prepared by an herbalist was reported in an atopic patient (Chivato et al., 1996), and allergic contact dermatitis has been associated with *Centella asiatica* (Gonzalo-Garijo, Revenga-Arraz, and Bobadilla-Gonzalez, 1996). Despite enthusiastic use as a "cure-all" for a variety of skin conditions, from infectious to psoriasis, there have been reports of allergic reactions to tea tree oil, particularly to the sesquiterpenoid fractions of the oil (Rubel, Freeman, and Southwell, 1998). Contact dermatitis has been reported with the use of other herbal medicines (Al-Suwaidan et al., 1998; Goday-Bujan et al., 1998), and a case of Steven-Johnson syndrome was found to be secondary to consumption of a health drink containing ophiopogonis tuber (mai-meu-dong-tang) (Mochitomi et al., 1998).

Yucuyahui (zoapatle, *Montanoa tomentosa*), a wild herb used as a folk oxytocic remedy, can cause cardiorespiratory depression in newborns (Montoya-Cabrera et al., 1998). Profound neonatal congestive heart failure has been associated with maternal consumption of blue cohosh herbal medication (Jones and Lawson, 1998). The use by pregnant women of *Tripterygium wilfordii,* an herbal medication recommended for rheumatoid arthritis, has been associated with development of occipital meningoencephalocele and cerebellar agenesis in their offspring (Takei et al., 1997). Madder root (*Rubia tinctorum* L.), a traditional herbal medicine used against kidney stones, contains lucidin, a hydroxyanthraquinone, which is mutagenic in bacteria and mammalian cells and induces the formation of DNA adducts (Westendorf, Pfau, and Schulte, 1998). High concentrations of St. John's wort, echinacea, and gingko have adverse effects on hamster oocytes, and St. John's wort is mutagenic to sperm cells and potently inhibits sperm motility and viability (Ondrizek et al., 1999a,b; Tinsley, 1999).

Leaf and seed extracts of *Piper guineense* possess, among other pharmacological properties, a depolarizing neuromuscular blocking action similar to decamethonium (Udoh, Lot, and Braide, 1999). A case of opsoclonus-myoclonus occurring in association with transitional herbal medicine consumption has been reported (Adamolekum and Hakim, 1998). A case of sparteine intoxication associated with using a preparation from lupine seeds has been reported in a patient who took the preparation with the belief that it represented a cure for her recently diagnosed diabetes, although no medical or toxicological evidence supports this (Tsiodras et al., 1999). Hypertensive crises have been seen with herbal treatments (Ruck, Shih, and Marcus, 1999).

Physicians must be alert for adverse effects and drug interactions associated with herbal medicines. They should ask all patients about the use of these products, which is particularly common among patients with chronic ailments for which conventional medicine has no effective treatments (Winterholler, Erbguth, and Neundorfer, 1997). Patients with chronic and life-threatening conditions, such as cancer, often use alternative therapies while receiving conventional medical care, and this population is at increased risk for complications and adverse drug interactions secondary to poor health and complex drug regimens (Crone and Wise, 1997). One study in the United Kingdom found that consumers tend to underreport adverse drug reactions associated with herbal remedies as compared to traditional over-the-counter medications (Barnes et al., 1998).

Homeopathy

Homeopathy is one of the most frequently used complementary therapies worldwide (Jonas, Linde, and Ramirez, 2000). Homeopathy, a system of herbal treatment invented in the early nineteenth century, is based on the concept that "like cures like." This vague concept arose from the observation that the herbal cure for malaria, cinchona bark (quinine), causes fever in both patients and healthy persons. A second idea central to homeopathy is the need to dilute the active substance to vanishingly small amounts before administering it.

Thompson (1999) presented a case history illustrating the practical application of the homeopathic method and its success in managing symptoms of fatigue and anxiety. More recently, Thompson and Reilly (2002) assessed the homeopathic approach to fatigue and other symptom control in one hundred consecutive cancer patients (thirty-nine of which had metastatic disease) attending a designated research cancer homeopathic clinic (nine of the patients had refused conventional cancer treatments). Patients were seen for consultation, lasting up to sixty minutes, for baseline assessment and prescription of a homeopathic remedy, and were assessed again at four to six consultations later. The most common symptoms were pain, fatigue, and hot flushes. Symptom scores for fatigue and hot flushes improved significantly over the study period but pain scores did not. Side effects included a transient worsening of symptoms in a few cases, which settled on stopping the remedy. Fifty-two patients completed the study, and in those patients satisfaction was high; 75 percent (thirty-eight individuals) rated the approach as helpful or very helpful for their symptoms. Further research is needed to explore the use of a homeopathic approach to cancer-related fatigue and other fatiguing illnesses.

Massage Therapy

Rexilius and colleagues (2002) examined the effect of two thirty-minute massages or Healing Touch treatments per week for three weeks on anxiety, depression, subjective caregiver burden, and fatigue experienced by thirty-six caregivers of patients undergoing autologous hematopoietic stem cell transplant. Caregivers in the control group received usual nursing care and a ten-minute supportive visit from one of the researchers. Results showed significant declines in anxiety scores, depression, general fatigue, reduced motivation fatigue, and emotional fatigue for individuals in the massage therapy group only. In the Healing Touch group, anxiety and depression scores decreased, and fatigue and subjective burden increased, but these changes did not achieve statistical significance. The authors concluded that caregivers can benefit from massage therapy in the clinic setting (Rexilius et al., 2002).

A randomized controlled trial with twenty individuals with chronic fatigue syndrome of massage therapy as compared with an attention control condition (sham transcutaneous electrical nerve stimulation [TENS]) showed significant improvements in generalized distress, sleep, anxiety, pain, depression, fatigue, and somatic symptoms on self-report measures (Field et al., 1997). The massage group, as compared with the sham TENS condition, also evidenced significant decreases in the stress-related hormone cortisol. The latter observation is consistent with studies which showed that massage therapy reduced depression, anxiety, and stress hormones in depressed adults and children (Field et al., 1992, 1996).

A study by Brattberg (1999) of forty-eight individuals diagnosed with fibromyalgia (twenty-three in the treatment group and twenty-five in the reference group) showed that a series of fifteen treatments with connective tissue massage conveys a pain-relieving effect of 37 percent, reduces depression and the use of analgesics, and positively affects quality of life. The treatment effects appeared gradually during the ten-week treatment period. Three months after the treatment period, about 30 percent of the pain-relieving effect was gone, and six months after the treatment period, pain was back to about 90 percent of the baseline value.

In contrast to these studies, a study on forty-two HIV-infected individuals yielded no significant impact on immune function or quality-of-life measures for short-term (twelve weeks) massage therapy alone or combined with either exercise training or stress management counseling (Birk et al., 1996). However, the study has several limitations including its power based on the sample size enrolled, whether the appropriate massage techniques were employed, whether the appropriate patient population was investigated, and whether the correct immune parameters to monitor were chosen. In this respect, another study (Ironson et al., 1996) documented that massage therapy is associated with enhancement of the immune system's cytotoxic capacity in HIV-infected individuals.

Acupuncture

Acupuncture has been proven useful in cancer supportive care, particularly in the areas of pain, nausea, and vomiting (Shen and Glaspy, 2001). Management of these complications positively influences quality of life and minimizes contributing factors to cancer-related fatigue. Various acupuncture techniques and methods may be employed, including dry needling, electroacupuncture, acupuncture using hypodermic needles, and injecting various solutions into the acupuncture sites (reviewed in Ridgway, 1999).

Several review and meta-analysis papers on clinical trials (Berman et al., 1999; Berman, Swyers, and Ezzo, 2000; Koenig and Stevermer, 1999; Lee, 2000; Muller et al., 2000; Offenbächer and Stucki, 2000; Ridgway, 1999; White, 1995) as well as National Institutes of Health Consensus Conferences (NIH Consensus Development Panel, 1997; NIH Consensus Conference, 1998) have found that although acupuncture as a therapeutic intervention is widely practiced in the United States and there have been numerous studies regarding its potential usefulness, many of these studies provide equivocal results because of design limitations, sample size, and other factors. The matter is further complicated by inherent difficulties in the use of appropriate controls, such as placebos and sham acupuncture groups.

Despite the limitations described, promising results have emerged, for example, showing efficacy of acupuncture as treatment for adult postoperative and chemotherapy nausea and vomiting and for postoperative dental pain. In other situations, such as addiction, stroke rehabilitation, headache, menstrual cramps, tennis elbow, fibromyalgia, myofascial pain, osteoarthritis, lower back pain, carpal tunnel syndrome, and asthma, acupuncture may be useful as an adjunct treatment or as an acceptable alternative; or it may be included in a comprehensive management program.

Basic science research has demonstrated convincingly that, at least in the context of acute pain, acupuncture's effects are related to the release of a variety of natural opioids. For instance, in a study of twenty-nine fibromyalgia patients, Sprott and colleagues (1998) reported that acupuncture treatment was associated with decreased pain levels, fewer positive tender points, decreased serotonin concentration in platelets, an increase of the serum levels of the pain-modulating substances serotonin and substance P, and improved microcirculation in tender points.

Ridgway (1999) also reported that acupuncture is effective for the treatment of a type of chronic back pain that is possibly associated with a radicullopathically induced, hypersensitivity myofascial syndrome that presents as a fibromyalgia-like syndrome. A high-quality study found that real acupuncture is more effective than sham acupuncture for relieving pain, increasing pain thresholds, improving global ratings, and reducing morning stiffness of fibromyalgia (reviewed in Berman et al., 1999). Electroacupuncture may also be useful in the treatment of fibromyalgia (White, 1995). However, it should be noted that for some fibromyalgia patients, acupuncture can exacerbate symptoms, further complicating its application for this condition (Berman and Swyers, 1999).

Melatonin

Although one study (Payne, 2002) provided evidence for melatonin level changes in cancer patients, the role of exogenous melatonin administration as a therapeutic strategy for cancer-related fatigue remains to be studied and evidence from other fatiguing illnesses is controversial (Citera et al., 2000; Korszun et al., 1999; Press et al., 1998; Webb, 1998; Wikner et al., 1998). It should also be pointed out that the results of a study in which female CBA mice were given melatonin with their drinking water for five consecutive days every month from the age of six months until their natural deaths, showed that the consumption of melatonin did not influence physical strength or the presence of fatigue; it decreased locomotor activity and body temperature; it inhibited free radical processes in serum, brain, and liver; and it increased spontaneous tumor incidence in mice (Anisimov et al., 2001). As pointed out in Chapter 3, the evidence on melatonin seems to lean against its use for cancer-related fatigue.

Neurofeedback

Electroencephalograph neurofeedback has been identified as a potential diagnostic and treatment protocol for CFS symptoms. Test results and clinical findings of EEG neurofeedback in a CFS patient revealed improvements in cognitive abilities, functional skill level, and quality of life (James and Folen, 1996).

IMMUNOTHERAPY

Therapies That Shift Cytokine Expression Patterns

Several therapies have been proposed and are being preliminarily tested for the treatment of fatiguing illnesses based on the premise that immunological changes are at the core of fatigue, in particular, a predominance of a humoral immunity cytokine expression pattern (also known as Th2-type pattern) over a cell-mediated immunity pattern (or Th1-type pattern) (Bosse and Ades, 1989; see Chapter 3). The following subsections summarize several therapeutic regimens aimed at inducing a systemic cell-mediated (Th1-type) immunity pattern predominance, some based on the use of certain vaccines, which are being tested particularly in subpopulations of patients with cancer, chronic fatigue syndrome, and/or with other diseases with documented immune abnormalities. Two such interventions, namely those with *Panax ginseng* and juzen-taiho-to, were already addressed previously under herbal therapy.

As discussed in Chapter 3, several types of cancer can shift the cytokine expression pattern predominance, a change that favors growth of the particular tumors, and these therapies may help treat both the cancer and the cancer-related fatigue. In some models, successful immunotherapy of an established tumor is associated with a change in the balance of T-cell subsets from a Th2- to Th1-type phenotype predominance (Gabrilovich et al., 1996). For instance, tumor-derived tumor growth factor-beta can induce overproduction of interleukin-10, stimulating suppression of antitumor responses; conversely, in vivo administration of antitumor growth factor-beta resulted in prevention of Th2 dominance, reversed immunosuppression, and reconstituted a Th1-type response (Maeda and Shiraishi, 1996). Immunotherapy of cancer and cancer-related fatigue holds promise and is an area of intense research that is being fed by a plethora of sources from herbal medicine, vaccines, and cell therapy to small molecules. Although the mechanisms whereby alterations in the immune system lead to changes in cognitive and functional status remain to be elucidated, the results of the different trials reinforce the need to integrate immunological, endocrinological, and psychological approaches to the understanding of the different manifestations of cancer and cancer-related fatigue. Some of the clinical trials also emphasize the importance of appropriately categorizing patients for interventions and outcome assessments.

Lymph Node Cell-Based Immunotherapy

Adoptive immunotherapy has been investigated in the treatment of cancer and of fatigue (Canevari et al., 1995; Paciucci et al., 1989; Rosenberg, 1984, 1985; Rosenberg and Terry, 1977; Sobol et al., 1999). One modality involves the transfer to tumor-bearing hosts of cells that have antitumor reactivity and are capable of mediating antitumor effects in the body (Dempsey et al., 1982; Fauci et al., 1987). At the beginning, one major roadblock toward broader implementation of such therapy was the inability of humans to produce sufficient quantities of these cells for their adoptive transfer to cancer patients. This deficiency was circumvented by Rosenberg and colleagues (Grimm et al., 1982; Lotze et al., 1981; Rosenstein et al., 1984; Yron et al., 1980), who successfully developed a method for the generation of both murine and human lymphocytes (lymphokine-activated killer cells) that can recognize and lyse fresh cancer cell preparations. LAK cells are usually generated by incubation with interleukin-2, and when transferred in conjunction with interleukin-2 they caused regression of established murine lung and liver metastases in a number of animal tumor models (immuno-genic and nonimmunogenic sarcomas, melanomas, and colonic adenocar-cinoma (Mazumder and Rosenberg, 1984; Mulé, Shu, and Rosenberg, 1984; Mulé et al., 1984; Yano et al., 1991).

Immunotherapies involving the adoptive transfer of interleukin-2 and tumor-infiltrating lymphocytes have also been developed to treat advanced cancer in humans. Kimoto and colleagues (Kimoto, 1992; Kimoto et al., 1994) reported that adoptive immunotherapy of patients bearing malignant diseases using human leukocyte antigen (HLA)-mismatched allogeneic lymphokine-activated killer cells was feasible and effective when auto-logous cells could not be procured. In general, toxic effects were chilliness, fever, and general fatigue which were reversible. Dendritic cells exposed to antigen ex vivo can also induce antigen-specific cellular immunity in pros-tate cancer patients (Burch et al., 2000).

More recent therapeutic interventions are based on stem cells (Margolin et al., 1999; Van Besien et al., 1997) or lymph node cells. Lymph nodes are an attractive source of cells for immune modulation and adoptive therapy. They contain all the critical elements to develop an immune response, in-cluding antigen-presenting cells. Also, the yield of immunologically active cells can be orders of magnitude greater than that from the peripheral blood. Lymph nodes often sequester cancer cells and cancer-specific cytotoxic T lymphocytes in an efficient system designed to eliminate or control cancer spread. The expression of specific adhesion molecules and the locomotor capability of lymph node lymphocytes, and thus the ability to traffic, may also be superior to that of the peripheral blood mononuclear cells (Tedla et al., 1999).

A safety and feasibility study was conduced at the University of Miami using lymph node extraction, ex vivo cell culture in the presence of the Th1-type cytokine interleukin-2, followed by autologous cell reinfusion as a treatment strategy to favor a Th2- to Th1-type cytokine expression shift in selected CFS patients (Klimas and Fletcher, 1999; Klimas et al., 2000; Patarca-Montero, Klimas, and Fletcher, 2000). Lymph nodes were obtained from patients who met the current case definition for chronic fatigue syn-drome and the following inclusion criteria: a history of acute onset; a Karnofsky score less than 80; evidence of immune dysfunction in three or more of the following: greater than one standard deviation above controls for elevated soluble TNF receptor type I (sTNF-RI) levels in serum, or elevated sTNF-RI production in phytohemagglutinin (PHA)-stimulated blood culture; lymphocyte activation (CD2+CD26+ cells greater than 50 percent); or low natural killer cell cytotoxic activity (less than 20 percent). The lymph node cells were cultured for ten to twelve days with anti-CD3 and interleukin-2. These cells were then reinfused into the donor who was monitored for safety and possible clinical benefit. No adverse events were noted in this phase I clinical trial. Of thirteen subjects, two had palpable lymph nodes that proved fibrotic with no viable cells. Of the remaining eleven subjects, all successfully underwent expansion and reinfusion of their lymph node cells. In some of the patients, there was an elevation in the expression of interleukin-2 receptor on CD4+ T cells in the weeks following reinfusion. There was a significant decrease in interleukin-5 (a Th2 cytokine) expression by PHA-stimulated blood cultures observed at one week, which persisted for several weeks postinfusion. Levels of PHA-induced interferon-gamma (a Th1 cytokine) production did not change. There was a trend toward an increase in the ratio of interferon-gamma/interleukin-5 starting at week one and persisting at least twelve weeks postinfusion. Of the eleven subjects in the trial who had cells reinfused, none had significant cognitive improvement. There was a trend toward significant change in speed of visual scanning (Trailmaking Test A). A significant increase was seen in the patients' ability to mentally track and rapidly shift cognitive set, as measured in Trailmaking Test B. Other measures of severity of illness also trended toward improvement. Karnofsky and Symptom Impact profile scores increased significantly. A significant association between clinical improvement and interferon-gamma/interleukin-5 (Th1/Th2) ratio increase was noted. Six patients showed both clinical improvement and Th1/Th2 ratios; four showed neither clinical improvement nor increased Th1/Th2 ratios; and only one patient had a significant clinical improvement and no change in the Th1/Th2 ratio. The lack of adverse effects from this experimental approach to immunomodulation in chronic fatigue syndrome and the favorable clinical and immunologic results observed in the small number of patients studied suggest that further clinical trials are warranted. However, this approach is time-consuming, onerous, and more invasive than other approaches being tested.

These studies on CFS patients were preceded by studies of adoptive CD8+ T-cell immunotherapy of AIDS patients with Kaposi's sarcoma (Klimas, 1992; Klimas et al., 1993; Klimas, Patarca, Maher, et al., 1994; Klimas, Patarca, Walling, et al., 1994; Patarca, Klimas, Walling, et al., 1994, 1995). The research group used a device developed to selectively capture CD8+ T cells for ex vivo culture and instituted basic science and clinical evaluations of the consequences of the infusion, with recombinant interleukin-2, of autologous, activated, and polyclonally expanded CD8+ T cells in AIDS patients with Kaposi's sarcoma and oral hairy leukoplakia. Phase I and II trials showed safety and suggested efficacy in the treatment of these AIDS-associated conditions. The intervention affected the patterns of cytokine expression of CD8+ T lymphocytes and favored a restoration of a strong type 1 response (Patarca, Klimas, Walling, et al., 1995). Studies with plasma exchange in cancer patients also suggest that altering the balance of soluble mediators may have a positive effect for cancer treatment and for fatigue management. For instance, plasma exchange in patients with recurrent colon cancer with evaluable liver metastasis or abdominal tumor with dissemination was associated with, albeit short-lived, improvement of clinical parameters and disappearance of general fatigue (Azuma et al., 1984).

Mycobacterium vaccae

As described in internationally published patent number WO-09826790 by Rook, Stamford, and Zumla, preparations of killed *Mycobacterium vaccae* are able to effect a nonspecific systemic cell-mediated immunity (Th1-type) bias, in particular by down-regulation of humoral immunity Th2-type activity without necessarily concomitant up-regulation of the Th1-type activity. The latter feature is similar to the effect on the Th1/Th2- type proportions of the lymph node cell-based immunotherapy described in the previous subsection.

In cancer patients, the effect of *M. vaccae* injection has been demonstrated by the appearance in the peripheral blood of lymphocytes that spontaneously secrete interleukin-2 (a characteristic Th1-type cytokine) and a decrease in numbers of T cells that secrete interleukin-4 (a characteristic Th2-type cytokine) after in vitro stimulation with phorbol myristate acetate and calcium ionophore. The percentage of lymphocytes showing this activated Th1-type phenotype increases progressively after each successive injection of *M. vaccae,* reaching a plateau in many individuals after three to five injections of 10^9 organisms (days zero, fifteen, thirty, and then monthly).

In experimental animals, a nonspecific systemic bias away from Th2-type activity on administration of *M. vaccae* can be seen as a reduction in the titer of an interleukin-4 (Th2)-dependent antibody response to ovalbumin (an allergen unrelated to *Mycobacterium vaccae* itself), in mice preimmunized so as to establish a Th2-type response predominance. A single injection of *M. vaccae* is able to cause this effect and further injections can enhance it. The effect is nonspecific because it does not require the presence of any component of ovalbumin in the injected preparation.

Briefly, BALB/c mice six to eight weeks old were immunized with 50 μg ovalbumin emulsified in oil (incomplete Freund's adjuvant) on days zero and twenty-four. This is known to evoke a strong Th2-type pattern of response accompanied by immunoglobulin E production and priming for release of two Th2-type cytokines, interleukin-4 and interleukin-5. Animals then received saline or 10^7 autoclaved *M. vaccae* on days fifty-three and eighty-one by subcutaneous injection. Injections of *M. vaccae* reduced the rise in immunoglobulin E levels caused by immunization with ovalbumin. The reduction caused by treatment with *M. vaccae* was significant at all time points tested. Similarly, spleen cells from the immunized animals failed to release interleukin-5 in vitro in response to ovalbumin if the donor animals had been treated with *M. vaccae,* in contrast to spleen cells from immunized animals treated with saline that released large quantities of interleukin-5 in response to ovalbumin. The data show that *M. vaccae* will reduce a Th2-type pattern of response, even when given after immunization with a potent allergen, and without epitopes of the Th2-inducing molecule. There is therefore a nonspecific systemic down-regulation of the Th2-type pattern of response, not dependent upon a direct adjuvant effect on the allergen itself.

The *M. vaccae* used in animals and humans is grown on a solid medium including modified Sauton's medium solidified with 1.3 percent agar. The medium is inoculated with the microorganisms and incubated aerobically for ten days at 32°C to enable growth of the microorganism. The microorganisms are then harvested, weighed, and suspended in diluent to give 100 mg of microorganisms/mL of diluent. The suspension is then further diluted with buffered saline to give a suspension containing 10 mg wet weight (about 10^{10} cells) of microorganisms/mL of diluent and then dispensed into 5 mL multidose vials. The vials containing the live microorganisms are then autoclaved (115 to 125°C) for ten minutes at 69 kPa to kill the microorganisms. The therapeutic agent produced is stored at 4°C before use. Then 0.1 mL of the suspension, containing 1 mg wet weight (about 10^9 cells) of *Mycobacterium vaccae,* is shaken vigorously immediately before being administered by intradermal injection over the left deltoid muscle.

In the same patent publication, Rook, Stamford, and Zumla describe their experience with CFS patients treated with *M. vaccae*. For instance, a CFS patient reported improvement after two injections of a *M. vaccae* preparation. A second one reported that since she had been receiving a *M. vaccae* preparation at two-month intervals, her CFS symptoms and food allergy had improved considerably; she continues to feel very well as long as she continues with her regular injections.

It is worth noting that a relative of *Mycobacterium vaccae,* the tuberculosis vaccine bacillus Calmette-Guérin (BCG) is approved by the FDA for intravesical treatment of carcinoma in situ of the bladder. The mechanism of action of BCG appears to be through immune stimulation, primarily by Th1-type cell-mediated cytotoxicity. Immunization with GM2 and bacillus Calmette-Guérin reduced the risk of relapse in stage III melanoma patients who were free of disease after surgical resection and who had no preexisting anti-GM2 antibodies (Chapman et al., 2000). First reported in 1976, the value of BCG for this application has been demonstrated by a host of studies that have shown decreasing numbers of recurrences as well as evidence of preventing invasion of muscle (Brosman, 1985; Catalona et al., 1987; Herr et al., 1986; Lamm, 1985; Sarosdy and Lamm, 1989). Unfortunately, most patients have at least mild toxicity, and 1 to 2 percent can become septic with bacillus since the vaccine is a live, attenuated one (Lamm et al., 1985). At least ten patients have died as a direct result of BCG use, all within a relatively short time span after the more widespread usage of BCG that followed FDA approval of the drug (Rawls et al., 1990). This is not a problem with the *Mycobacterium vaccae* treatment discussed previously because the bacterium is inactivated before use.

Schult (1984) reported that the main side effects of BCG vaccination by scarification in 511 patients with malignant melanoma since 1974 have been fatigue and exhaustion, swelling of the lymph nodes, influenza-like symptoms, nausea, and dizziness. In only eight patients were the side effects more severe, requiring the cessation of treatment in some of them. One patient developed granulomatous hepatitis and another experienced a reactivation of pulmonary tuberculosis. Allergic reactions occurred in two patients. Another patient developed recurrent erysipelas in the draining areas of the scarification. In two patients the author observed continuous severe joint troubles that were not secondary to metastatic disease. The eighth patient developed keloids at the vaccination sites on the upper arms. One third of the patients had no side effects. Altogether vaccinations were tolerated well by most of the patients. Nearly all of them were able to work normally (Schult, 1984).

It has been proposed that childhood exposure to certain infections and vaccinations, such as BCG, that induce Th1-type immune responses may protect against atopic (allergic) diseases, which are characterized by predominant Th2-type cytokine expression (Marchant et al., 1999; Martinez, 1994; Pershagen, 2000). An indirect support for this theory comes from the observation that the incidence of allergy has increased in most Western countries where BCG vaccination had been stopped (Grüber, Nilsson, and Bjorksten, 2001). However, results from the few epidemiological studies that have addressed the hypothesized association between BCG vaccination and allergic diseases are conflicting (Aaby et al., 2000; Alm et al., 1997; Grüber et al., 2001, 2002; Strannegård et al., 1998) and possibly distorted by selection bias, because they have been carried out in countries where BCG vaccination is either a part of the routine vaccination program or given only to high-risk subjects. In fact, a recent large cross-sectional study by Krause and colleagues (2003) found that BCG-vaccinated children in Greenland have the same risk of atopy as unvaccinated children. Furthermore, no significant differences in the risk of atopy were found according to age at BCG vaccination. As reviewed by Krause and colleagues (2003), five previous studies addressed the hypothesis that BCG vaccination protects against allergic diseases in BCG-vaccinated and unvaccinated children. Strannegård and colleagues (1998) found no protective effect of BCG vaccination on allergic diseases in Swedish four- to nine-year-old children, while a nonsignificant effect was observed among foreigners. Similarly, Alm and colleagues (1997) found no association with BCG vaccination and atopy or allergic diseases in two- to seven-year-old children with atopic heredity. However, a potential protective effect of BCG vaccination may have been masked by the strong genetic predisposition to atopy in children. Furthermore, in Sweden BCG vaccination is given only to children at high risk of tuberculosis, resulting in a BCG vaccination rate of 4 percent (Romanus, Svensson, and Hallander, 1992), a likely source of selection bias. In a study conducted in Africa, Aaby and colleagues (2000) reported that BCG-vaccinated children had a lower prevalence of atopy compared with unvaccinated children, particularly when the vaccine has been administered in the first week after birth. Grüber and colleagues (2001) found no effect of BCG vaccination given before age six months on development of atopy or allergic manifestations at age seven years in a cohort study; in this study, 13 percent of the children at high risk of tuberculosis were vaccinated with BCG, and children born outside of Germany were overrepresented in the BCG-vaccinated group. In another German cross-sectional study among pre-school children, a weak protective effect of BCG vaccination against asthma was observed in German children, whereas a stronger protection effect on atopic manifestations was observed in children of non-German ethnicity (Grüber et al., 2002). Therefore, the jury is still out on whether BCG vaccination may protect against Th2-type immune predominant diseases in populations with particular genetic constitutions (Alm et al., 2002).

Staphylococcal Vaccine

In international published patent number WO-09829133 by Goteborg University Science Invest AB, Carl-Gergard Gottfries and Bjoern Regland describe the use of staphylococcal vaccine to favor Th1-type cell-mediated immunity predominance. These authors also found that variables such as smoking and nickel sensitivity adversely affect the outcome of this form of therapy (Andersson et al., 1998). The treatment is conducted as a series of administrations with increasing doses during a specific period. Preferably, the vaccine is administered in eight to ten increasing doses during four to twelve weeks, preferably for eight to ten weeks. The reason for the increasing doses is that during the first week or weeks, the patient will probably suffer from side effects, and it is therefore advantageous to start with a low dose. The side effects will diminish over time. The first series of administrations is followed by repeated administrations given approximately once a week for five to fifteen weeks, preferably for ten weeks. To prevent recurrence, the repeated administrations are then followed by a maintenance treatment with administrations approximately once a month, which preferably are continued for approximately five years. The doses in the repeated administrations of the maintenance treatment are preferably constant and relatively high. Vitamin B_{12} and/or folacin are preferably administered simultaneously or in parallel with the staphylococcal preparation.

If the known staphylococcal vaccine Staphypan Berna (SB) from the Serum and Vaccine Institute, Bern, Switzerland, is used, a typical treatment schedule may be as follows: eight to ten administrations are made during a period of four to twelve weeks, preferably eight to ten weeks, wherein the dose of the staphylococcal preparation is gradually increased from 0.1 to 1 mL of the pure vaccine. The increase depends on the response from the patient. It may be, for example, 0.1, 0.2, 0.3, 0.4, 0.5, 0.6, 0.7, 0.8, 0.9, and 1.0 mL, respectively. If the patient shows a strong local reaction, it is possible to repeat a dose before increasing it. The dose of staphylococcal preparation in the repeated administration and in maintenance treatment is 1 mL.

As described in the published patent, after a pilot study comprising eight patients was made, a double-blind, placebo-controlled study was performed, comprising a group of twenty-four female adult patients fulfilling the criteria for both fibromyalgia and chronic fatigue syndrome. Seven of the thirteen patients who received the staphylococcal preparation were assessed as being minimally improved, three as being much improved, and the remaining three as unchanged. In the placebo group, three patients were minimally improved and the remaining eight were unchanged. The improvement in the group with the active treatment was statistically significant compared to the improvement in the placebo group. Following the controlled study, twenty-four patients chose to continue with the treatment and twenty of these have been treated for between one and two years. Nineteen of these patients were on the disabled list or received sickness pension prior to the start of the treatment, and one patient was employed part-time. At a one year follow-up after the completed study, nine of the twenty patients were in full- or part-time paid employment; one patient was taking part in a work experience program; and one was at the middle of a two-year training to become a nurse. The treatment strategy used in this study was a series of administrations of staphylococcal preparations given approximately once a week during a period of some months, for example, three months, and thereafter long-term treatment with monthly administrations.

Further studies conducted by this Swedish group have confirmed the findings published in the patent (Zachrisson, Regland, Jahreskog, Jonsson, et al., 2002). In the larger more recently published study, one hundred patients fulfilling the American College of Rheumatology criteria for fibromyalgia and the 1994 CDC criteria for chronic fatigue syndrome were randomized to receive staphylococcus toxoid preparation Staphypan Berna or placebo during six months. Treatment included weekly injections containing 0.1, 0.2, 0.3, 0.4, 0.6, 0.8, 0.9 and 1.0 mL SB or colored sterile water, followed by booster doses given four-weekly until the end point. Main outcome measures were the proportion of responders according to global ratings and the proportion of patients with a symptom reduction of 50 percent or more on a fifteen-item subscale derived from the comprehensive psychopathological rating scale (CPRS). The treatment was well tolerated. Intention-to-treat analysis showed 32/49 (65 percent) responders in the SB group compared to 9/49 (18 percent) in the placebo group, a statistically significant difference. Sixteen patients (33 percent) in the SB group reduced their CPRS scores by at least 50 percent compared to five patients (10 percent) in the placebo group, also a statistically significant difference. Mean change on the CPRS was 10.0 in the SB group and 3.9 in the placebo group, a statistically significant difference. An increase in CPRS symptoms at withdrawal of therapy was noted in the SB group. The authors therefore concluded that treatment with staphylococcus toxoid injections over six months led to significant improvement in patients with fibromyalgia and chronic fatigue syndrome. However, maintenance treatment is required to prevent relapse (Zachrisson, Regland, Jahreskog, Jonsson, et al., 2002).

Sizofiran

Sizofiran, an immunostimulant extracted from suehirotake mushroom *(Schizophyllum commune)* cultured fluid, is under development by Fidia Farmaceutici Italiani Deriviate Industriali e Affini for the potential treatment of cancer and hepatitis B. Sizofiran is licensed by Kaken Pharmaceutical Co., Ltd., Japan. Trials were under way for the treatment of gastric and lung tumor; phase III trials are under way for the treatment of hepatitis B; and the compound is in phase II trials for chronic fatigue syndrome. By August 1999, Kaken was preparing its New Drug Application filing for hepatitis B, but no information is yet available regarding its status.

Sizofiran induces significant rises in the secretion of the Th1-type cytokines interferon-gamma and interleukin-2 into culture media of phytohemmaglutinin or concanavalin A-stimulated human peripheral blood cells in culture. Further reports on sizofiran should become available in the near future.

Cytokine Antagonists

Cytokine antagonists may be exploitable in combating chronic fatiguing illnesses, including the components of cancer-related fatigue, and may inhibit tumor growth as well. The role of anticytokine factors in modulating symptom severity in several diseases, including those that would benefit from immune reconstitution, such as melanoma, renal cell carcinoma, and AIDS, remains to be determined (Redrizzani et al., 1991). In this respect, drugs that decrease tumor necrosis factor production, such as pentoxifylline [Trental; 3,7-dimethyl-1-(5-oxohexyl) xanthine], chlorpromazine, and thalidomide, have shown some efficacy in vitro, in animal models, and in patients with cancer and other ailments such as AIDS and septic shock (Escudier et al., 2002; Fazely et al., 1991; Figg, Arlen, et al., 2001; Figg, Dahut, et al., 2001; Makonkawkeyoon et al., 1993; Moreira et al., 1993; Netea et al., 1995; Paterson et al., 1995; Rajkumar, 2000, 2001a,b; Rajkumar and Witzig, 2000; Sampaio et al., 1991, 1993; Singhal and Mehta, 2001; Singhal et al., 1999; Steins et al., 2002; Strupp et al., 2002; Tuckey, Parry, and McCall, 1993; Weglicki et al., 1993; Zorat and Pozzato, 2002).

The possible usefulness of these agents in the treatment of chronic fatiguing illnesses and cancer-related fatigue remains to be investigated, and cytokine inhibitors are actively being sought and tested (Abraham et al., 1995; Dinarello, Gelfand, and Wolff, 1993; Fisher et al., 1994). However, a pilot study of thalidomide, as an antiangiogenic factor, in nineteen patients with progressive metastatic renal cell carcinoma revealed that fatigue, along with somnolence and constipation, were among the most common but reversible toxicities (Daliani et al., 2002; Singhal and Mehta, 2002). A phase II trial of thalidomide in the treatment of recurrent glioblastoma multiforme revealed that thalidomide had some biological activity and was well tolerated, with the most common toxicity being fatigue (Marx et al., 2001). Thalidomide is relatively successful in the treatment of myeloma and is being investigated in other plasma cell dyscrasias, myelodysplastic syndromes, gliomas, Kaposi's sarcoma, renal cell carcinoma, advanced breast cancer, and colon cancer (Singhal and Mehta, 2001, 2002; Singhal et al., 1999). A study by Neben and colleagues (2001) indicated that high pretreatment plasma basic fibroblast growth factor levels in patients with progressive multiple myeloma are associated with unfavorable parameters of response and survival but nevertheless predict for response to thalidomide therapy. A phase II evaluation by Baidas and colleagues (2000) revealed that single-agent thalidomide has little or no activity in patients with heavily pretreated breast cancer and its use is associated with somnolence and fatigue among other side effects.

It should also be pointed out that reports of lymphoma development after treatment with commercially available antitumor necrosis factor antibodies have been a major concern (Rutgeerts et al., 1999). However, only five of 771 patients who had received infliximab for various disorders in controlled trials have subsequently developed lymphoma (Bickston et al., 1999). One patient was being treated for Crohn's disease, three for rheumatoid arthritis, and one for AIDS; the latter two conditions carry a disease-related increased risk of lymphoma, whereas the lymphoma risk in Crohn's disease remains controversial.

Many anticytokine approaches examined have been undermined by

1. redundancy of function within the immune mediator network as documented in mice with deletions of particular soluble mediator genes (Dalton et al., 1993; Erickson et al., 1994; Huang et al., 1993; Kuhn, Rakewski, and Muller, 1991; Kundig et al., 1993; Oettgen et al., 1994);
2. multiplicity of cytokines produced in a disease process that forestalls the prospect of a rational therapy based on the use of specific antagonists of any single cytokine;
3. use of multiple receptor systems by one cytokine as illustrated by the tumor necrosis factor lectin- and peptide-binding receptors (Lucas et al., 1994) and by the interleukin-1 type I functional receptor and the type II decoy receptor (Colotta et al., 1993);
4. inability to appropriately deal with bioavailability issues;
5. inability to extrapolate results from one animal species to another; and
6. differences in the local and systemic effects of immune mediators (Akira et al., 1990).

As an example of the last limitation, interleukin-1 produced locally by macrophages is a co-stimulatory signal for activation of T lymphocytes (Lowenthal and MacDonald, 1987), while the consequences of high systemic levels of interleukin-1 are fever, leukopenia, intravascular coagulation, and shock, among others (Dinarello and Wolff, 1993; Krueger and

Majde, 1994). Local increased levels of cytokines may also be difficult to interpret clinically, as happens with elevated plasma and synovial fluid levels of the proinflammatory cytokine interleukin-1beta in rheumatoid arthritis that may be secondary to elevated levels of interleukin-1 receptor antagonist, an anti-inflammatory cytokine that competitively binds to receptors of interleukin-1 beta on tissue cells (Dinarello, 1991).

ANTIMICROBIAL THERAPIES

As mentioned in Chapter 3, microbes have been proposed as causative or perpetuating factors in chronic fatiguing illnesses. Based on the postulates of microbial and autoimmune etiologies of chronic fatigue syndrome and other chronic fatiguing illnesses, several interventions have been designed and tested and are covered in this section. These interventions have become possible because of the growing armamentarium of antiviral agents in molecular medicine and their widespread use in clinical practice—changes which have, in turn, arisen thanks to a confluence of novel approaches and a fresh look at past clinical wisdom. It is therefore instructive to review the historical background of the current developments in antiviral and antimicrobial therapy.

Historical Background

The dawn of the twenty-first century is brightened by the growing frequency of use and discovery of antiviral agents, the first fruits of the expanding genomics revolution. This new antiviral era, which flourished from the knowledge provided by the molecular biological characterization of the genetic makeup of viruses, is engendering new chemical and biological agents that are able to treat and not just prevent viral diseases. Hypotheses have also been rekindled that challenge conventional wisdom to expand the realm of diseases of viral etiologies to include pathological processes, such as atherosclerosis and autoimmune disease, that would not have been previously thought to be secondary to infectious processes (Atkinson et al., 1994; Banki et al., 1992; Blick et al., 1990; Ciampolillo et al., 1989; Dang et al., 1991; Gama Sosa et al., 1997; Garry et al., 1990; Jones and Armstrong, 1995; Lagaye et al., 1992; Perl et al., 1991; Silvestris, Williams, and Dammacco, 1995; Talal, Dauphinée, et al., 1990; Talal, Garry, et al., 1990; Tian, Lehmann, and Kaufman, 1994; Trujillo et al., 1993). Regardless of whether the hypotheses prove to be correct, the experience that is being garnered in this antiviral revolution also serves, in the light of the information now available on the genetic makeup of human beings, as an encouraging paradigm for the development of drugs to treat all kinds of human diseases.

The current antiviral drug revolution can trace its first roots to the contributions of scientists such as Spallanzani, who compellingly challenged the theory of spontaneous generation supported by the Roman Catholic Church and revealed the existence of a biological microcosm invisible to the naked eye that could account for many occurrences which were until then shrouded by a cloud of mystical religious beliefs, from the growth of mold on a wet surface to the transmission of certain diseases. Although Girolamo Fracastoro taught, in 1530, that syphilis was a contagious disease spread by "seed," and in 1683 Antony van Leeuwenhoek observed bacteria by using a crude microscope, it was the nineteenth century, with the contributions of scientists such as Louis Pasteur and Robert Koch, that saw the consolidation of the germ theory of diseases and the flourishing of microbiology thanks to the definitive isolation of infectious organisms and the demonstration of their association with disease (Lederberg, 2000). Around that time, Dmitri Ivanowski and Martinus Beijerinck described viruses as small infectious agents that could pass through bacteria-stopping filters.

Following the identification of infectious organisms, immunology was born as a discipline aimed at unraveling the mechanisms used by the body to control and defeat them. Shortly thereafter, modern infectious disease medicine was inaugurated with the discovery of antibiotics in the early part of the twentieth century, an accomplishment based on the observation that fungi produced substances that were able to kill bacteria. The isolation and medical use of penicillin and other naturally occurring antibiotics, as well as the development of their synthetic derivatives, has allowed humankind to control the spread and severity of bacterial epidemics, such as the bubonic plague caused by the bacteria *Yersinia pestis* which killed a large portion of the human population in the Middle Ages.

Unlike the case with bacteria, viruses have no known natural enemies from which to isolate antibiotic-like substances and, until the mid-1980s, viral infections were thought to be inherently preventable in some cases but generally untreatable. Many viral epidemics, such as polio, yellow fever, whooping cough, AIDS, and viral hepatitis, have received worldwide attention in the past and during the twenty-first century. As summarized in Chapter 1, there are also many historical accounts of chronic fatiguing diseases of presumed viral etiology, including George Reinhold Forster's description of the Tapanui flu and the documentation of Akureyri or Iceland disease.

Viral scourges continue to exact a huge toll (Osterholm, 2000). The disastrous AIDS pandemic is merely the most well known. Complications of hepatitis B and C kill approximately one million people each year, and measles continues to be the leading cause of deaths among children even though effective vaccines exist for measles and hepatitis B. Rotavirus, which causes diarrhea, takes the lives of hundreds of thousands, mainly children. Other viral diseases seem to be restricted to specific areas. Ross River virus disease causes acute illness in parts of Australia, and the deadly Ebola and hantavirus occasionally emerge to wreak bloody havoc in Africa and the American South. West Nile virus has terrorized several areas of the United States.

The first half of the twentieth century witnessed the first successful approach to control the spread of several viral infections: the development and worldwide use of vaccines. The concept of vaccination was originally developed by Jenner in eighteenth-century England based on the observation that milkmaids exposed to cows with cowpox were protected from smallpox. In this case, a subclinical infection with one virus was protective of an infection with a related one. The concept was also extended to the treatment of various infectious diseases. Although in many cases the treatment was worse than the disease, the therapeutic approach was somehow useful with particular combinations of infectious agents.

Outstanding triumphs of worldwide vaccination programs have been the eradication of smallpox and soon of poliomyelitis (Marwick, 2000). After smallpox was eliminated as an infectious disease in Great Britain in 1962, two outbreaks occurred, one in 1973 and one in 1978, when smallpox virus under study in laboratories infected susceptible individuals. In both incidents, deaths resulted (Marwick, 2000). With the eradication of poliomyelitis throughout the world soon to be accomplished, steps are being taken to prevent polioviruses that remain in laboratories from escaping into the community and causing disease. These examples stress the need for universal availability of vaccines to effectively eradicate the disease they cause. Unfortunately, we do not have vaccines against all viruses; even in the cases for which we do have vaccines, the vaccine is not universally available. The dramatic success in immunizing children against childhood diseases stands in stark contrast to the much lower percentages of adults who are adequately immunized against common adult diseases. In the case of the flu vaccine, the influenza virus keeps changing; the vaccine has to be updated every year, and it is therefore not fully protective against all viral strains.

One alternative to vaccines has been the use of injections of immunoglobulins, the natural bullets that the body produces to kill foreign invaders. Several decades ago, physicians advocated the use of immunoglobulin injections as a way to "boost" the body's immune defenses and heighten resistance against microbes. The reasoning was perhaps again reflective of the old wisdom of using one infection to protect against another, with the added refinement of using the natural mediators of the body's attack machinery against infections instead of the infectious agent itself.

The limitations of antibodies as antiviral therapeutic agents still leave us with having to treat viral infections and, unlike the case with bacteria, we do not know the natural enemies of viruses from which to isolate antibiotic-like substances. The Nobel laureate Paul Ehrlich preached in the early twentieth century about the usefulness of discovering chemical substances that would act as "magic bullets" against infectious agents with little or no untoward effects to humans. Although the magic bullets studied in Ehrlich's days were too toxic, Ehrlich's vision inspired the pharmaceutical industry's search for therapeutic small molecules, a task that has now been rekindled with the help of modern biology.

Viruses were the first microorganisms whose complete genetic makeup was characterized. The information on viral genes and their protein products has allowed the development of a series of chemicals with targeted antiviral activity. The advent of the AIDS pandemic in the second half of the twentieth century became the largest challenge to infectious disease medicine of the modern era. The discovery and characterization of the first human pathogenic retrovirus, the human T-cell leukemia/lymphoma virus type I (HTLV-I) (Haseltine et al., 1984; Josephs et al., 1984; Sodroski, Patarca, et al., 1984; Sodroski, Trus, et al., 1984), facilitated the discovery of the etiological agent of AIDS, the human immunodeficiency virus type 1 (HIV-1). Determination of the primary structure of HIV-1, first known as HTLV-III or LAV (lymphadenopathy virus) and computerized analysis of the amino acid sequence of the gene products it encodes provided the targets and, at the same time, the reagents to develop rapid and sensitive assay systems for testing potential therapeutic agents with anti-HIV activity (Patarca, Heath, et al., 1987; Ratner et al., 1985; Sodroski et al., 1985). Therefore, anti-HIV therapeutic medicines were born from the marriage between molecular and cellular biology, traditional therapeutic small molecule screening, and the then-incipient discipline of bioinformatics, a marriage that also fueled the resurgence of genomics research (De Clercq, 1995, 1997; Elfassi, Patarca, and Haseltine, 1986; Haseltine and Patarca, 1986; Hirsch and Kaplan, 1987; Johnson and Hoth, 1993; Mitsuya and Broder, 1987; Mitsuya, Yarchoan, and Broder, 1990; Patarca and Haseltine, 1984, 1985, 1986, 1987; Patarca, Dorta, and Ramirez, 1982; Patarca, Haseltine, et al., 1987; Patarca, Heath, et al., 1987; Webster et al., 1989; Yarchoan et al., 1991).

The first databases of nucleic acid and protein sequences were created in the late 1970s. The computerization of algorithms for primary structure comparisons and secondary structure predictions (hydrophilicity and folding structures) and their use to analyze the genetic makeup of the AIDS virus in the framework of the knowledge garnered over decades for other known viruses quickly provided the targets for the development of anti-HIV agents. It is therefore the case that although nonprimate viruses were the first microorganisms whose complete genetic makeup was characterized, it was not until the complete sequence of the AIDS virus became available in an unprecedented record time, thanks in part to the strong public pressure for basic and clinical research, that the information on viral genes and their protein products triggered an exponential growth in the development of chemicals with targeted antiviral activity.

Before the AIDS epidemic, the only antiviral agent that had been widely introduced to clinical practice with modest acceptance was acyclovir. The drug acyclovir, which is used to treat infections by herpes simplex viruses, the causative agents of the most feared venereal disease before the AIDS era, inhibits the viral DNA polymerase, a protein that is needed for the virus to replicate. The drug, after chemical modification by the body, affects mainly the viral DNA polymerase because the latter is sufficiently different from its human cell counterpart. Similar in concept to acyclovir, the first medication introduced for AIDS and diseases related to HIV-1 infection was 3'-azido-2',3'-dideoxy-thymidine (formerly known as azidothymidine [AZT] and currently known as zidovudine [ZDV]), a nucleoside analog that inhibits reverse transcriptase, a critical enzyme for the replication of HIV (De Clercq, 1995, 1997; Hirsch and Kaplan, 1987; Johnson and Hoth, 1993; Mitsuya and Broder, 1987; Mitsuya, Yarchoan, and Broder, 1990; Yarchoan et al., 1991). It is noteworthy that the discovery of reverse transcriptase several decades before the characterization of the AIDS virus had demolished the dogma in molecular biology that genetic information could flow only from DNA to RNA to protein by demonstrating that information could also flow from RNA to DNA, as was exemplified by the life cycle of retroviruses.

The initial success of AZT opened the door for the development of other antiretroviral agents, and no doubt exists today that antiretroviral chemotherapy can bring about reduction of viral load and clinical benefits to HIV-infected individuals. Besides AZT, a variety of 2',3'-dideoxynucleosides have been added to the anti-HIV armamentarium, among them ddI or didanosine, ddC or zalcitabine, d4T or stavudine, and 3TC or lamivudine. Many more are undergoing clinical or preclinical testing. Nonnucleoside reverse transcriptase inhibitors, including navirapine and delavirdine, have also become available and more will emerge in the near future. The high mutation rate of HIV has allowed the selection of viral strains resistant to antiretrovirals, a feature that has fed a constant need for new viral therapeutic targets. As the first clinical application of what has been termed pharmacogenomics, the genomics era has also provided the intermediate- and high-throughput tools to genotype AIDS virus strains from patients to determine their drug-resistance patterns. Changes in antiretroviral therapy choice based on the viral resistance patterns allow better control of viral load and disease progression.

A virus that has approximately fifteen genes, such as HIV, presents a much more limited drug target repertoire than bacteria such as the gut-dwelling *Escherichia coli,* with approximately 1,500 different proteins. The limitation in target variety has rendered the traditional random screening efforts for anti-HIV agents disappointing for the most part, a hurdle that has been the inspiration for the introduction of different drug development approaches. Approximately one decade after the introduction of AZT, the inhibitors of another viral enzyme, protease, were hailed on their way into clinics as the long-awaited panacea for AIDS. The viral protease is needed to cleave the original synthesis products of the virus to generate building blocks required for assembly of new viral particles. The successful development of HIV protease inhibitors is arguably the greatest achievement to date for the relatively new method of structure-based drug design (Erickson et al., 1990; Erickson and Fesik, 1992; Robins, 1986; Tummino et al., 1996; Wlodawer and Erickson, 1993). This design is possible when the structure of the molecular target has been determined by X-ray crystallography, nuclear magnetic resonance (NMR), or remodeling. Unbeknown to many clinicians, the presence in the viral genome and the start point for the generation of the protease gene had been originally predicted in the early 1980s with accuracy down to one amino acid in the first round of analysis of the HIV sequence. But it was not until the structure of this enzyme was determined that the first design studies with HIV-1 began with HIV protease in the early 1990s. Many protease inhibitors are currently available on the market (saquinavir, ritonavir, indinavir, nelfinavir, lopinavir/ritonavir), and another large group is in clinical and preclinical development.

The initial experience with anti-HIV therapy has evinced the greater efficacy, as compared to monotherapy, of appropriately combining multiple classes of antiviral agents in patients with HIV infection. As structure-based drug design methods improve, new therapeutic agents will be effectively developed against novel antiviral targets for HIV-1 therapy. The X-ray crystallography and NMR structures of several HIV-1-encoded proteins have been determined, including the reverse transcriptase, RNase H, integrase, matrix, capsid, nucleocapsid, tat protein, and a domain of gp41. In addition, the structures of the cell surface proteins with which the envelope proteins of HIV interact have also been characterized, i.e., the envelope binding domains of CD4 and those of certain chemokine receptors, such as CCR5. The need to continue to search for and develop drugs against novel antiviral targets for HIV therapy should not be underestimated, because the prevalence of new drug-resistant variants of HIV that are insensitive to even the best current regimens of triple and quadruple combination therapy is rising at an alarming rate, especially in the context of patient nonadherence secondary to the complexity or financial burden of combined regimens.

The discovery of protease inhibitors also illustrates another important strength of the genomics approach to drug discovery. The characterization of the genetic makeup of HIV allowed the development of target-based screens to identify novel lead compounds for specific targets that would otherwise have gone unidentified in cell culture–based assays. In this respect, high-throughput protease assays were responsible for identifying nonpeptidic lead compounds that were subsequently developed into potent protease inhibitors with anti-HIV activity, even though the initial lead compounds had no measurable antiviral activity in tissue culture assays. Conversely, compounds that exhibit antiviral activity in a cell culture–based screen can now be subjected to a battery of mechanism-based tests to profile their mode of action.

The characterization of the genetic makeup of the AIDS virus is also helping to fine-tune the development of AIDS vaccines aimed not only at triggering, as most conventional viral vaccines do, the production of antibodies, the natural bullets that cells of the body's immunological defense system produce to kill foreign invading agents, but also at stimulating cellular immunity, i.e., bringing into action other cells of the body's defense system that can directly kill the virus or the virus-infected cells. Again, in this front, the high mutation rate of the virus and the presence of different variants or clades of HIV in the major geographical areas affected by the epidemic has posed a formidable obstacle to the development of vaccines (Esparza, 1998).

The development of vaccines as well as the preclinical testing of drugs and therapeutic biologicals with anti-HIV activity have found a strong ally in the availability of several naturally derived or man-made animal models, most prominent among which are simian immunodeficiency virus (SIV)-infected macaques; mice with genetically determined severe combined immunodeficiency engrafted with human hematolymphoid cells from fetal liver, thymus, and lymph node (SCID-hu mice); and SCID mice reconstituted with human peripheral blood leukocytes (hu-PBL-SCID mice) (McCune et al., 1990; Mosier et al., 1991). The search for and generation of appropriate animal models for drug and vaccine testing is crucial to the success of the genomics approach for the discovery of new pharmaceuticals and is proving to be a major bottleneck for the pharmaceutical industry.

In theory, antiviral drugs exert their effects by interacting with viral structural components, virally encoded enzymes, viral genomes, or specific host proteins such as cellular receptors, enzymes, or other factors required for viral replication. In principle, any virus-specific step in the viral replicative cycle that differs from that in normal host cell function can serve as a potential target for the development of antiviral therapy. The final litmus test of this approach to drug development takes place at the clinic or the bedside, a process that involves demonstration of both safety and efficacy of a medication, as well as a learning curve for the health care professional in the use of a new therapeutic agent or modality.

The battle against the AIDS virus, despite its limitations, has habituated clinicians to the concept of treating viral infections with drugs, and agents similar in concept to those used for the AIDS virus are now being aimed against the hepatitis viruses. Interestingly, the initial analysis of the HIV primary sequence and its comparison to that of other viruses also put in evidence the existence of a reverse transcriptase gene in hepatitis B virus. Until then, the hepatitis B virus had been believed to be a double-stranded DNA virus, and now it is known that, similar to retroviruses, it replicates through an RNA intermediate. Based on this realization, the nucleoside analog lamivudine is being used for the treatment of chronic hepatitis B virus, while the nucleoside analog ribavirin (1-beta-D-ribofuranozyl-1,2,4-triazole-3-carboxamide) is part of the therapeutic arsenal for combating chronic infection with hepatitis C, an RNA virus. Ribavirin has also shown activity in vitro against dengue virus (Koff, Elm, and Halstead, 1982).

The current use of nucleoside inhibitors extends to other viruses. For instance, ribavirin can be used for treatment of respiratory syncytial virus infection, the leading cause of lower respiratory tract infection (pneumonia and bronchiolitis) in normal infants and children (De Vincenzo, 1997). In the latter indication, ribavirin is delivered by a small particle aerosol generator and, to be effective, must be started as early as possible. Although ribavirin aerosol has also been successfully used for the treatment of severe parainfluenza virus disease in some children with severe immunodeficiency, studies are thus far inadequate to establish efficacy. On the other hand, intravenous ribavirin has been used with successful responses in some cases of adenoviral infection. These experiences demonstrate another important area in the effective clinical use of the new drugs developed from the genomics revolution, namely their adequate delivery by several routes for different indications. In this respect, the genomics-based drug revolution has also fueled an exponential growth rate in the research on drug delivery systems, and many more innovative breakthroughs are on the horizon.

The influence of using antiviral agents to control HIV infection extends further to the battle against the flu (Gubareva, Kaiser, and Hayden, 2000; Monto et al., 1999). Although two important proteins of influenza viruses were known for many years before the AIDS epidemic, it was not until recently that effective drugs that would target these enzymes were developed.

Following the 1942 discovery of an enzyme on the influenza virus surface that removed virus receptors from erythrocytes, the prediction was put forth that an inhibitor of said enzyme might be an active antiviral agent by eliminating the viral cleaning mechanism mediated by red blood cells. Although the first inhibitors of this viral enzyme, known as neuraminidase, were developed in 1969, it was not until 1993, after the crystal structure of the enzyme and improved understanding of the mechanism of catalysis had been achieved, that zanamivir was introduced as a potent and highly specific inhibitor of influenza neuraminidase activity. Inhaled zanamivir (Relenza; Glaxo Wellcome, Inc.) entered clinical trials in 1994 and is now licensed in Australia, Europe, and North America. The first orally active inhibitor, oseltamivir, was described in 1997. It has been approved in Switzerland, Canada, and the United States. A second oral agent has been introduced into the market.

The influenza neuraminidase inhibitors represent a significant advance over the hemagglutinin inhibitors amantadine (Symmetrel; DuPont) and rimantadine (Flumadine; Forest Pharmaceuticals, Inc.) that were available for many years but rarely used in influenza therapy. Amantadine or rimantadine may be given orally early in the course for influenza type-A infections but are not effective for influenza type B. Ribavirin aerosol use has led to the reduction of symptoms in some patients with influenza, types A and B, infections. Amantadine, rimantadine, or zanamivir can also be used prophylactically in immunocompromised patients exposed to influenza-A virus infection. For those exposed to influenza B, only zanamivir is recommended, using one dose daily during the exposure period (Monto et al., 1999). The neuraminidase as compared to the hemagglutinin inhibitors have a broader spectrum of antiviral activity (both influenza A and B as opposed to only A), less potential for emergence of clinically important resistance, better tolerability, and proven efficacy in reducing respiratory events leading to antibiotic use after influenza.

One alternative approach for prophylaxis of influenza and respiratory syncytial virus (RSV) infections has been the use of immunoglobulins, in particular preparations enriched in those directed specifically at certain viruses. RSV is the leading cause of lower respiratory tract infection (pneumonia and bronchiolitis) in normal infants and children. For example, seasonal prophylaxis of RSV infection, in the form of monthly infusions of RSV-polyclonal antibody or the injection of RSV humanized monoclonal antibody (Palivizumab), has been effective in small infants with profound immunodeficiency, pulmonary compromise, and/or bone marrow transplant recipients. A series of antibodies against specific viral targets are being tested at the time and more will be developed as target display libraries continue to allow the selection of effective antibodies among samples with diversity in the thousands.

Many other antiviral agents are in the market and different categories of antiviral agents are at various stages of drug development. For instance, the broad-spectrum capsid-binding agent Pleconaril (VP63843) shows promise for the treatment of rhinovirus infection, the virus causing the common cold, but the drug is available on a compassionate protocol use. Pleconaril may also have therapeutic efficacy in enteroviral aseptic meningoencephalitis. An antiviral drug that could hardly have been conceived of before the advent of genomics is based on the principle of "antisense": the drug, formivirsen, consists of nucleic acid sequences that bind to and neutralize a crucial component of the reproducing virus. It is approved in the United States for the treatment of cytomegalovirus retinitis. One drug being tested in patients with hepatitis C consists of a ribozyme: an RNA molecule that cuts specific viral RNA sequences.

Besides the traditional viral infections, the antiviral agents being developed may also help in the control of diseases where the body loses its balanced control of internal processes. For instance, some viruses become part of our genetic makeup, the so-called endogenous viruses, and their expression serves some functions that are being unraveled. The body appears to keep the expression of endogenous viruses in check, and it has been noted that the unregulated expression of endogenous viruses may play a role in some autoimmune diseases, maladies in which the body attacks itself by making antibodies against its own tissues. One example of such a disease is Sjögren's syndrome, a malady in which the body makes antibodies against the salivary and lacrimal glands and the person suffers dry eyes and mouth. Overexpression of the endogenous viruses called intracisternal A particles have been associated with Sjögren's syndrome.

The realm of antiviral therapy may soon extend to diseases that are not traditionally thought of as viral in origin. For instance, results from several studies in animals and humans have suggested that atherosclerosis, the clogging of blood vessels that can lead to heart attacks or strokes, may be influenced by microbial organisms including viruses such as cytomegalovirus, a herpesvirus family member, and bacteria, such as *Chlamydia, Mycoplasma,* and *Helicobacter pylori* (Benitez, 1999; Buja, 1996; Danesh, Collins, and Peto, 1997; Fabricant et al., 1978; Frothingham, 1911; Kullo, Gau, and Tajik, 2000; Libby, Egan, and Skarlatos, 1997; Ophüls, 1921). The hypothesis is in line with the change in pathogenetical thinking brought about by the link of a bacterium, *Helicobacter pylori,* to peptic ulcer disease and lymphoma associated with the gastrointestinal mucosa (Blaser, 1999). Therefore, antibiotics have joined antacids in the treatment of some forms of peptic ulcer disease.

The recent molecular biology endeavors that have characterized most of the expressed genes in the human body are opening the doors for using natural proteins with antiviral activity, or even chemical substances directed at the proteins in the body that are the portals of invasion of viruses, as the new weapons in our continuing battle against these microbes. A revisit to old tradition brings to mind some useful paradigms. Many cultures around the world discovered that rubbing a frog on an infected wound would help clear the infection and heal the wound. The small proteins responsible for this antibacterial activity in the frog's skin were characterized in the twentieth century. Later, similar proteins were discovered in human beings, some of which also have antiviral activity. Since the genetic makeups and expressed proteins of many different organisms are being deciphered around the world, it is likely that they will continue to discover other natural substances with antiviral activities and maybe even discover those elusive natural enemies of viruses. For instance, one bacterial organism, *Mycoplasma,* has been shown to help the AIDS virus, an observation which supports the hope that there might be another organism that may help kill or control it. In this line of thought, some scientists have proposed that certain populations of people that have proven to be particularly resistant to viral infections despite high-risk behavior may be infected with another organism that confers such protection.

The characterizations of viral genetic makeups, of the proteins that they encode, and of the effects of the latter on cells have also helped to create testing systems for substances present in plants, and it is possible that new chemicals will be derived from the knowledge garnered over centuries in the field of herbal medicine. For instance, Louis Pasteur noted garlic's antibiotic activity in 1858, and, more recently, the sulfur-containing component of garlic, allicin, has been shown to kill all viruses thus far tested in the laboratory (Hadley and Petry, 1999). Plant proteins with antiviral activities may also provide templates for the computational biochemistry search for homologous proteins in humans, a task that may help unravel new natural antiviral agents. In fact, over half of the top twenty-five prescription drugs in the market are derived from plants.

Regardless of the source of the drugs, whether naturally occurring or synthetic, the antiviral drug era will continue to open new doors for novel approaches to viral and nonviral diseases. The determination of the sequence of the genome of viruses and of the protein products that they encode has created the targets for a booming pharmaceutical enterprise and represents the first success story of the genomics revolution. Antiviral drugs provide the first glimpse of the exciting new era of molecular medicine, a discipline that welcomes the twenty-first century as an infant for whom we have great expectations. One can only fathom by extrapolation that if the limited number of viral targets so far worked out has generated a number of potential medications that is in the realm of two orders of magnitude the number of targets, at least 1.2 million medications should in the near future be under investigation for the close to 12,000 genes that express secretory proteins in humans. These medications will allow us to regenerate failing or aging organs, restore deficient or quell excessive bodily functions, and help combat old and new challenges to human health.

The following subsections summarize the different antiviral therapies thus far tested for chronic fatigue syndrome, and they address their rationale despite lack of clear evidence for a direct or indirect viral etiology of chronic fatigue syndrome.

Acyclovir and Related Antiherpetic Drugs

In international published patent number US-058872123, A. M. Lerner reports an approach to alleviate the symptoms of chronic fatigue syndrome with a therapeutically effective amount of one or more pharmaceutically acceptable antiviral agents selected from the group consisting of acyclovir, ganciclovir, valacyclovir, famciclovir, cidofovir, and pharmaceutically acceptable derivatives and mixtures thereof.

Lerner's premise is that, in general, the clinical symptoms and signs of chronic fatigue syndrome resemble those of infectious mononucleosis. Symptoms common to both illnesses include low-grade fever, chills, sore throat, painful anterior or posterior cervical or axillary lymph nodes, muscle weakness, myalgia, generalized headaches, migratory arthralgia, vague neuropsychological complaints, and disturbances of sleep without known medical cause. As with mononucleosis, a CFS patient's attempt to exercise at levels previously tolerable results in a prolonged and more severe manifestation of the fatigue.

Although chronic fatigue syndrome and infectious mononucleosis have several similarities, patients with chronic fatigue syndrome do not have the severe dysphagia and gray exudative pharyngitis often accompanied by submandibular adenopathy, which is associated with infectious mononucleosis and its etiologic agent Epstein-Barr virus. Lerner's research had found in chronic fatigue sufferers the existence of Epstein-Barr virus multiplication, purportedly within epithelial cells of the pharynx and circulating B lymphocytes of the blood. The beta herpesvirus, human cytomegalovirus (HCMV), is also believed to cause infectious mononucleosis-type symptoms, without the exudative pharyngitis.

Lerner points out that chronic fatigue syndrome also includes unique symptoms, such as light-headedness or wooziness of varying severity and duration without antecedent cause; a vague, dull, pressure-like chest ache, generally in the substernal region and sometimes including the left shoulder, which is exhibited with increasing fatigue at the end of the day; and palpitations. There is also often a fourth symptom, tachycardia or rapid heart action, even with minimal or no exertion by the sufferer. Based on the symptoms unique to chronic fatigue syndrome, Lerner further hypothesized that chronic fatigue syndrome is essentially cardiac in origin and that this cardiac basis unlocks the key to the disorder.

In the patent publication, Lerner proposed that the majority of CFS cases constitute a continuing primary herpesvirus infection, specifically Epstein-Barr virus and/or human cytomegalovirus or, alternatively, a reactivation infection with latent Epstein-Barr virus and/or latent human cytomegalovirus. In some lesser number of cases, herpesvirus 6 (HHV-6) or other viruses, such as enteroviruses, may be involved. Seroepidemiologic studies have documented the presence of EBV and/or HCMV in a significant number of CFS sufferers. Lerner's research has further indicated the existence of IgM antibodies to the EBV viral capsid antigen (VCA) or EBV antibodies to early antigen (EA), the latter depicting EBV DNA polymerase activity, which is an indicator of current virus multiplication. In CFS sufferers, there may be additionally or alternatively a significant IgG to HCMV response, as detected by enzyme-linked immunosorbent assay (ELISA), with or without an IgM (ELISA) antibody titer to HCMV.

Lerner points out that the understood virologic cause of chronic fatigue syndrome thus verifies that previous seroepidemiologic studies, attempting to show a singular virologic causation to chronic fatigue syndrome including singular searches for EBV or HCMV antibodies, would have naturally yielded uniformly negative results. At least fifteen different viruses, bacteria, and parasites have been suspected as singular etiologic agents of chronic fatigue syndrome. However, there has been, to date, no clear serologic association with any human virus. Lerner proposes that the previous studies were designed in a way that actually masked the possibility of finding a major two-virus causality.

The two major causative herpesviruses proposed by Lerner, EBV and HCMV, are characterized by latent, nonpermissive, persistent infections. In a nonpermissive infection, a complete infectious virus is not produced. Intracellular infection produces a metabolically altered host cell; however, no progeny capable of infecting a new susceptible cell are created. Instead, the extrachromosomal herpesvirus episome persists for the life of the chronically infected cells. The latent persistent infection and recrudescent infection characteristic of the herpesvirus is common in EBV and HCMV and is consistent with the chronic recrudescent illness of chronic fatigue syndrome.

Productive whole-virus, herpesvirus EBV or HCMV infection is accompanied by lysis of infected cells. In latent infection, complete infectious virus is not produced, and host cell survival continues. With persistent infection, varying levels of infectious virus, latent virus, and reactivation may occur simultaneously. Productive infection is also associated with cellular necrosis and a subsequent inflammatory response. Latency may be associated with little inflammation or morphological changes but may lead only to aberrant biochemical and degenerative cellular functions.

Lerner goes on to point out that existing evidence supports the theory that both HCMV and EBV are cardiotropic, i.e., they have a preference for infecting the heart muscle cells, the so-called human myocytes. Based on Lerner's research, the human cardiac myofiber, similar to the B lymphocyte for EBV and the mononuclear progenitor cell for HCMV, is a site of non-infectious episome-mediated persistent infection. This is different from the human epithelial cell of the pharynx that produced mainly whole infectious EBV virus. HCMV immediate early gene transcripts have been detected in the heart by in situ hybridization techniques in patients with HIV-associated cardiomyopathy. Likewise, the EBV genome was detected by polymerase chain reaction (PCR) amplification of DNA extracted from the heart at autopsy. However, PCR for enteroviruses and cardiac viral cultures were negative. An intense mononuclear cell infiltrate in the myocardium consisted essentially of T cells without identifiable B cells.

Accordingly, Lerner's research has suggested that chronic fatigue syndrome is a nonpermissive, persistent herpesvirus infection of the heart, wherein EBV and/or HCMV nucleic acids are present in the hearts of CFS patients. This hypothesis was generated based in part upon endomyocardial biopsies of patients with chronic fatigue syndrome. The research conducted revealed that all CFS patients have abnormal oscillating T-wave flattenings and T-wave inversions detectable from twenty-four-hour electrocardiographic (Holter) monitoring. An initial twenty-four-hour electrocardiographic T-wave study compared CFS patients to random non-CFS patients from an internal medicine practice, wherein both patient groups were restricted to an age less than fifty years old to minimize the occurrence of chronic diseases in both populations. Notably, chronic diseases such as hypertensive vascular disease, electrolyte abnormalities, and coronary artery disease may produce similar oscillating abnormal T-waves. However, since people suffering from chronic fatigue syndrome are generally young, such chronic diseases rarely afflict CFS sufferers and can thus be excluded as the causative agent. Oscillating T-wave abnormalities described also occur in about 5 percent of normal patients when they assume an upright position. For these same patients, in resting twelve-lead standard ECG, T-waves describing left ventricular depolarization are upright, and the resultant ECG is normal. The 2-D echocardiogram also generally is normal, but the twenty-four-hour ECG recordings (Holter monitoring) are abnormal with oscillating T-wave flattenings or T-wave inversions characteristically incident with the onset of sinus tachycardias and subsequently reverting to normal T-wave configurations with the return of normal sinus rhythms. Although these abnormal T-waves are not specific to chronic fatigue syndrome, and they occur similarly with diverse conditions such as coronary artery disease, hypertensive vascular disease, and electrolyte abnormalities, the abnormal T-waves detected via Holter monitoring were seen much more frequently in twenty-four random CFS patients than in 116 time-, place-, and age-matched random non-CFS patients. Based on Lerner's analysis, the abnormal T-waves at twenty-four-hour recordings in CFS patients are not artifacts and are a significant sign of chronic fatigue syndrome. Lerner purports that the abnormal Holter monitoring in CFS patients is evidence that chronic fatigue syndrome is a cardiomyopathy. Moreover, Lerner has found that the additional symptoms of a dull chest ache coming on at the end of the day not related to exercise, light-headedness or wooziness, and palpitations are CFS symptoms attributable to cardiac involvement of these viruses.

An initial group of CFS patients also demonstrated abnormal left ventricular dynamics characterized by a decreased or falling ejection fraction, abnormal wall motion, or dilatation by radionuclide stress multiple gated acquisition (MUGA) studies. Furthermore, consecutive case series of CFS patients from a single referral center in Birmingham, Michigan, during the years 1987 to 1993 demonstrated abnormal left ventricular dynamic function in 24.1 percent of eighty-seven patients undergoing radionuclide ventriculography by the radioisotopic gated-pool method.

Lerner also reports that, in an effort to diagnose chronic fatigue syndrome using electron microscopy, cardiomyopathic changes including myofiber hypertrophy, myofiber disarray, and degenerative change in myofibers have been seen. On rare occasions, inflammatory myocarditis is evident. Infectious HCMV is not found in the heart, peripheral blood, or urine of the HCMV-infected chronic fatigue syndrome subset of patients. Based on evidence gathered, Lerner conclusively believes that chronic fatigue syndrome is a major newly discovered cardiomyopathy. Lerner has also observed that patients with acute primary EBV infectious mononucleosis who recover rapidly have normal Holter monitoring throughout their illnesses. Lerner also argues that just like chronic fatigue syndrome, herpes simplex virus encephalitis boggled the medical community because etiologic identification based on rising antibodies in serum may or may not be present at a particular time. Diagnosis of this form of encephalitis required isolation of herpes simplex type 1 (HSV-1) from the brains of patients with encephalitis.

Because the herpesviruses are intracellular parasites that use multiple biochemical pathways of the infected host cell, initially problems were associated with achieving clinically useful antiviral activity without adversely affecting normal host cell metabolism and causing toxicity. Therefore, as pointed out in the previous subsection, selective inhibition of herpes simplex virus multiplication by acyclovir represented an important advance in antiviral therapy. Acyclovir was synthesized in 1974 by Beauchamp and Schaeffer of Burroughs-Welcome Company. Acyclovir, 9-([2-hydroxyethoxy]methyl) guanine E, demonstrated significant in vitro antiviral activity against herpesviruses, specifically HSV, varicella zoster virus (VZV), and EBV.

Acyclovir is an acyclic analog of guanosine. The inhibitory activity of acyclovir is highly selective. The enzyme thymidine kinase (TK) of normal uninfected cells does not effectively use acyclovir as a substrate. However, TK encoded by the herpes simplex virus converts acyclovir into acyclovir monophosphate, a nucleotide analog. The monophosphate is further converted into diphosphate by cellular guanylate kinase and into triphosphate by a number of cellular enzymes. Acyclovir triphosphate interferes with herpes simplex virus DNA polymerase and inhibits viral replication. Acyclovir is preferentially taken up and selectively converted to the active triphosphate form by herpesvirus-infected cells. Acyclovir triphosphate binds viral DNA polymerase, acting as a DNA chain terminator. Because acyclovir is taken up selectively by virus-infected cells, the concentration of acyclovir triphosphate is forty to 100 times higher in infected cells than in uninfected cells. Furthermore, viral DNA polymerase exhibits a ten- to thirtyfold greater affinity for acyclovir triphosphate than do cellular DNA polymerases. The higher concentration of the active triphosphate metabolite in infected cells plus the affinity for viral polymerases result in the very low toxicity of acyclovir for normal host cells.

Although EBV and HCMV do not have virus-specific TKs, replication of the EBV and HCMV DNA is significantly impaired. Acyclovir's in vitro antiviral activity is considerably greater in HSV than HCMV. More recently, Boroughs Wellcome has introduced Valtrex (valacyclovir hydrochloride), the hydrochloride salt of the L-valyl ester of acyclovir. Valacyclovir is preferred because of its high bioavailability. As a result of valacyclovir's increased absorption, as compared to acyclovir, for example, less frequent dosages of valacyclovir are required to reach effective antiherpetic levels. Another antiviral agent, ganciclovir, or 9-(1,3-dihydroxy-2-propoxymethyl) guanine, has increased in vitro activity against all herpesviruses as compared to acyclovir, including an eight to twenty times greater activity against HCMV. However, toxicity concerns prevent the use of gancyclovir for a relatively benign HCMV infection.

Another effective antiviral agent is Vistide, or cidofovir, 1-[(s)-3-hydroxy-2-(phosphomethoxy) propyl]cytosine dihydrate. Cidofovir also suppresses replication of the herpesviruses by selective inhibition of viral DNA synthesis. Cidofovir is incorporated into the growing viral DNA chain, a process that results in reductions in the rate of viral DNA synthesis.

Famvir, famciclovir, the 6-deoxy analog of the active antiviral compound penciclovir, is also believed to have antiviral activity against HSV-1 and VZV. Several additional compounds have demonstrated activity against herpesviruses. For instance, foscarnet sodium (trisodium phosphonoformate), a pyrophosphate analog of phosphonoacetic acid, has potent in vitro and in vivo activity against herpesviruses. Foscarnet inhibits the DNA polymerase of all human herpesviruses by blocking the pyrophosphate binding site that prevents chain elongation. Bromovinyl arabinosyl uracil has also exhibited significant inhibition of HSV-1, EBV, and VZV. Fluoroiodo-arabinosyl cytosine and its related compounds offer another potent inhibitor of herpesviruses. Similar to acyclovir, its activity depends on phosphorylation by herpesvirus TK. However, this antiviral agent and its analogs appear to have greater activity than acyclovir and significant activity against VZV and HCMV. (S)-1-((3-hydroxy-2-phosphonyl methoxy) propyl)adenine (HPMPA) is yet another antiviral agent which includes a new class of nucleotide analogs with in vitro activity against HSV-1 and -2, HCMV, VZV, and EBV.

Lerner recommends valacyclovir and ganciclovir as the preferred antiviral agents for chronic fatigue syndrome treatment because the etiologic agents are proposed to be EBV or HCMV. In his studies in the published patent, ten CFS patients, in whom singular EBV persistent infection was demonstrated, were treated with an oral dose of valacyclovir at 10 mg/Kg every six hours and studied over a three-month period. EBV active infection was demonstrated by EBV VCA IgM antibodies and/or elevated EBV EA antibody titers. Each patient's functional status was recorded as a statistically validated energy index (EI). A patient with a 0 EI is bedridden; with an energy index of 1 or 2, any activity by the patient leads to overwhelming, incapacitating fatigue; patients with an energy index between 3 and 5 can, with great effort, be out of bed for several hours each day doing nonphysical activities; patients with an energy index between 6 and 9 can assume normal activities and maintain a forty-hour workweek and, with pacing, maintain a household; and patients with an energy index of 10 have normal energy levels, stamina, and a sense of well-being. The mean baseline EI for the ten CFS patients with EBV was 4.6, and the EI range was 3.5 to 5.5. At the completion of therapy, the same CFS patients had a mean EI of 7.5, a median EI of 7, and a range between 6 and 10. Prior to therapy, five of the ten patients continued to have these symptoms. At the beginning of the trial, five of the ten patients had palpitations, while at the completion of the trial, three of the ten patients had palpitations. At the completion of the trial, eight of the ten patients continued to have positive EA antibody titers.

Another study was conducted to assess the possible efficacy of ganciclovir treatment on a subset of CFS patients with high HCMV IgG ELISA antibody titers; minimal/no serologic evidence of concurrent EBV multiplication; and oscillating ECG abnormalities at Holter monitoring. From March 1993 through June 1994, three men and fifteen women with mean age of 39.7 +/– 7.7 years, with chronic fatigue syndrome, were recruited from a single infectious diseases referral center in Birmingham, Michigan. The eighteen CFS patients had a duration of overwhelming fatigue of more than two years and with oscillating or repetitively abnormal aberrant T-waves at twenty-four-hour ECG recordings using Holter monitoring. In these eighteen CFS patients, baseline standard twelve-lead ECG, 2-D echocardiogram, rest-stress myocardial perfusion (thallium 201 or Tc-99 cardiolyte), and rest-stress multiple gated acquisitions (MUGA) studies as well as coronary angiography excluded coronary artery disease. After placement of a peripheral inserted central catheter or a Groshong catheter, ganciclovir was given intravenously in a dose of 5 mg/Kg at twelve-hour intervals for thirty days. After thirty days, patients were seen at intervals of four to six weeks and evaluated at each of these times. Of the eighteen patients, thirteen improved and resumed their normal pre-CFS activity levels. The mean duration of fatigue prior to therapy was longer in the five patients who did not improve (2.8 years) than in the fifteen who did improve (mean of 1.6). Prior to receiving intravenous ganciclovir, patients who improved, as well as those who did not, experienced marked worsening fatigue with exercise, myalgia, light-headedness, and dull, nonspecific, left-sided chest aches not related to activity. After treatment with ganciclovir, three of the fifteen patients who improved with previously abnormal myocardial dynamics reverted to normal, and in three others, results of MUGA tests improved with lesser degrees of tardokinesis, hypokinesis, or left ventricular dilatation. Right ventricular endomyocardial biopsies showing varying degrees of cardiomyopathic changes characterized by myofiber disarray, myofiber dissolution, myofiber drop out with fibrous replacement, and occasioned myofiber hypertrophy were evident in seven of the fourteen patients. No adverse events or symptoms were attributable to ganciclovir. In an initial test, a single patient had a transient increase in serum creatinine, but upon recalculation of dosage based upon lean body mass in a repeated test, the serum creatinine level reverted to normal.

Lerner also presented a case report in his patent filing. A fifty-one-year-old millwright, who enjoyed excellent health and whose only risk factor for coronary artery disease was cigarette smoking, suddenly experienced overwhelming, progressive fatigue forcing him to stop work. As a result of this fatigue, he was essentially bedridden and slight exertion further worsened his fatigue. He suffered from light-headedness, generalized muscle aches, intermittent sore throat, and an inability to think clearly. The physical exam, chest X-ray, HDL cholesterol levels, and urinalysis were normal. A resting twelve-lead ECG showed an inverted T-wave in standard lead III but was otherwise normal. An IgM antibody titer to HCMV was positive, while Epstein-Bar virus antibody tests were negative. Holter monitoring showed oscillating abnormal flat or inverted T-waves appearing with the onset of sinus tachycardias, and alternating with the reappearance of normal upright T-waves when tachycardias resolved. A myocardial sestamibi perfusion rest/stress showed reversible ischemia of the anterior, apical, and inferior walls, but at cardiac catheterization, the coronary arteries were patent. A stress MUGA study revealed abnormal left ventricular function with a resting ejection fraction of 40 percent (normal greater than 50 percent).

This patient was given daily intravenous ganciclovir treatment at 5 mg/Kg every twelve hours for thirty days. Five months later, the stress MUGA test was repeated and, at this time, the resting ejection fraction had increased 14 percent, from 40 to 54 percent, a normal level. Five months later, the patient's maximal cardiac ejection fraction increased from 54 to 68 percent. At this time, repeat myocardial perfusion studies during exercise were normal. Left ventricular dysfunction was no longer present, and the patient's fatigue had disappeared. Subsequently, the patient resumed work as a millwright and, after a 2.5 year follow-up, remains well with normal left ventricular function.

Based on the results described, Lerner concludes that CFS patients with a significant IgG HCMV antibody titer greater than 120 units, with or without the presence of an IgM HCMV ELISA antibody titer plus an absence of EBV VCA IgM antibody titer, along with an EBV EA antibody titer less than 40, described a group of chronic fatigue syndrome patients that should benefit from ganciclovir treatment.

Ampligen

Ampligen, a form of mismatched double-stranded RNA (dsRNA) with immunostimulatory and antiviral activity, is under development by HEMISPHERx BIOPHARMA, INC., primarily for the potential treatment of chronic fatigue syndrome or myalgic encephalomyelitis. It has been in phase III trials in the United States for this indication. HEMISPHERx and its licensing partner, Bioclone, initiated in 2003 the use of Ampligen for severe chronic fatigue syndrome on a named-patient, cost-recovery basis in

South Africa. It is also under study for other viral infections including hepatitis B virus (HBV), hepatitis C virus (HCV), and HIV.

Based on the premise that the clinical symptoms of chronic fatigue syndrome could be explained by a persistent viral infection, some researchers have reasoned that alterations in the 2',5'-oligoadenylate (2-5) synthetase/RNase L antiviral pathways may underlie chronic fatigue syndrome (Suhadolnik et al., 1999; Vojdani and Lapp, 1999). This dsRNA-dependent, interferon-inducible pathway is part of the antiviral defense mechanism of mammalian cells which also regulates cell growth and differentiation (Lengyel, 1982; Sen and Ransohoff, 1993; Player and Torrence, 1998; Wells and Mallucci, 1985). When activated by dsRNA, 2-5A synthetase converts ATP to 2',5'-linked oligoadenylates. These biologically active 2-5A molecules bind to and activate a latent endoribonuclease (RNase L) to hydrolyze single-stranded viral and cellular RNA, thus inhibiting protein synthesis.

Various studies have demonstrated that several key components of the 2-5A synthetase/RNase L pathway are significantly dysregulated in chronic fatigue syndrome (Suhadolnik, Reichenbach, Hitzges, Adelson, et al., 1994; Suhadolnik, Reichenbach, Hitzges, Sobol, et al., 1994). In chronic fatigue syndrome, 2-5A synthetase is predominantly in its activated form (Suhadolnik, Reichenbach, Hitzges, Adelson, et al., 1994; Suhadolnik, Reichenbach, Hitzges, Sobol, et al., 1994). In addition, bioactive 2-5A levels are significantly elevated and RNase L activity is up-regulated compared to healthy controls (Suhadolnik, Reichenbach, Hitzges, Adelson, et al., 1994; Suhadolnik, Reichenbach, Hitzges, Sobol, et al., 1994). A report has also documented 80, 42, and 37 kDa 2-5A binding proteins that possess 2-5-A-dependent RNase L enzyme activity in extracts of peripheral blood mononuclear cells from individuals with chronic fatigue syndrome (Suhadolnik et al., 1997). These 2-5A binding proteins have been identified by photo affinity labeling with an azido 2-5A photoprobe, immunoprecipitation with a highly purified, recombinant, human 80 kDa RNase L-specific polyclonal antibody, and PhosphorImager analysis of sodium dodecyl sulfate-polyacrylamide gel electrophoresis (SDS-PAGE) under denaturing conditions. The 80 kDa RNase L and the 37 kDa low molecular weight (LMW) RNase L proteins bind 2-5A and have 2-5-A-dependent RNase L enzyme activity following fractionation by analytical gel permeation high-performance liquid chromatography (HPLC) under native (nondenaturing) conditions (Suhadolnik et al., 1997).

Suhadolnik and colleagues (1999) reported that both RNase L activity and bioactive 2-5A concentration are negatively correlated with Karnofsky performance score in CFS fatigue syndrome patients. RNase L activity also positively correlated with a second clinical measure, the Metabolic Screening Questionnaire (MSQ), an observation which suggests that the up-regulation of the 2-5A synthetase/RNase L pathways is an indication of a lower state of general health. A strong correlation between interferon-alpha and LMW RNase L in a subset of the highest 100 interferon-alpha values from all study subjects is consistent with a viral etiology of chronic fatigue syndrome (Suhadolnik et al., 1999).

A highly significant correlation between the 80 kDa RNase L and the LMW RNase L may be derived from the 80 kDa RNase L. Several lines of biochemical evidence are consistent with the possibility that a cellular or virus-encoded protease may be involved in the origin of the LMW RNase L (Suhadolnik et al., 1999). Numerous proteases have been demonstrated to have a functional impact in normal and virus-infected cells. One such example is PKR, which is hydrolyzed by a protease encoded by the poliovirus genome (Vojdani and Lapp, 1999). A second instance is exemplified in the report that proteins in muscle extracts (i.e., actin and myosin) are degraded via ubiquitin-dependent pathways (Solomon, Leckert, and Goldberg, 1998). This degradative process provides amino acids for hepatic gluconeogenesis. For proteins implicated in the control of cell growth and differentiation, such as RNase L, proteolytic degradation in a ubiquitin-dependent manner would protect the cell from formation of abnormal proteins. A third example is proteolytic degradation occurring via the proinflammatory cytokines, interferon-alpha and tumor necrosis factor-alpha. Tumor necrosis factor-alpha levels have been reported to be elevated in individuals with chronic fatigue syndrome compared to controls (Borish et al., 1998; Chao et al., 1991; Patarca, Lutgendorf, et al., 1994; Patarca, Klimas, Sandler, et al., 1995). Interferon-alpha and TNF-alpha together induce the activity of 2-5A synthetase which ultimately results in the selective degradation of 28S ribosomal RNA, a substrate for RNase L (Chapekar and Glazer, 1988). Tumor necrosis factor-alpha may facilitate formation of the LMW RNase L from the 80 kDa RNase L to augment the inhibition of protein synthesis by hydrolyzing RNA.

Through the mechanisms described, the mismatched double-stranded RNA in Ampligen stimulates the production of tumor necrosis factor, interferons, and other lymphokines and has anticancer effects, as does matched double-stranded RNA, but the mismatched version does not share many of the toxic effects of the matched version. Ampligen crosses the blood-brain barrier, shows no rebound effects after withdrawal, and has greater antiviral activity than the interferons, one of the cell's natural antiviral signaling systems. Nevertheless, an initial application to the FDA by HEM Pharmaceuticals, the predecessor to HEMISPHERx, for expanded distribution of Ampligen for treatment of chronic fatigue syndrome was suspended because of cited life-threatening side effects, including hepatic toxicity, severe abdominal pain, and irregular heartbeat.

In 1998, HEMISPHERx received authorization from the FDA to commence a confirmatory placebo-controlled, multicentered, phase III study of Ampligen in chronic fatigue syndrome patients. This confirmatory study commenced in August 1998, with patients enrolled at an investigational site in San Diego, California. The protocol was for a twenty-four-week period in a placebo-controlled, double-blinded trial involving 230 patients. Contractual agreements with additional sites in October 1998, January 1999, and May 1999 brought the total number of sites participating in the phase III trial to eight.

After an encouraging open-label trial, a placebo-controlled, double-blind, multicenter trial, involving ninety-two subjects, was conducted. After twenty-four weeks of Ampligen treatment, significant improvements were noted in physical performance as measured by the primary end point, the Karnofsky performance score, which increased by 43 percent from fifty-three to seventy-six. Secondary end points, which were also met, included reduced cognitive deficit (as assessed by the cognitive subscale of SCL 90-R or neuropsychological function tests); enhanced capacity to perform activities of everyday living; and improvements on treadmill testing (oxygen uptake increased from 1.16 L/min to 1.48 L/min). Notably, significant reductions in the need for other medications and for extended hospital stays were also observed.

HEMISPHERx reviewed physical performance, cognition, and quality-of-life improvements derived from Ampligen treatment in four separate clinical studies at the October 10, 1998, session of the American Association for Chronic Fatigue Syndrome Research Conference. The clinical trials reviewed in the presentation included three open-label studies and one placebo-controlled study. These studies indicated that Ampligen has a favorable safety profile and is well tolerated in primates. In addition, long-term Ampligen patients did not reveal any cardiac abnormalities attributable to the drug; adverse effects occurred in 15 percent of patients, most of which involved occasional skin flushing and dry skin. Beyond this, the number of adverse effects reported by Ampligen patients was not significantly different from those receiving placebo.

In September 1999, HEMISPHERx announced the results of a pharmacoeconomic study that showed considerable cost benefits of using Ampligen, in particular, a reduction in the doses used of other medicines and in the number of days spent in the hospital. Results from a separate study showed that the duration of Ampligen's positive results remained constant for forty-two months after the start of therapy.

A full new drug application to the European Medical Evaluation Agency (EMEA) was submitted in December 1998, with enrollment for a confirmatory phase II European trial for chronic fatigue syndrome to support U.S.

data, and was expected to begin the first quarter of 1999. In February 1999, the company's European marketing application for the treatment of chronic fatigue syndrome cleared the first stage of regulatory review by being designated as complete by the EMEA. The European Union marketing application was withdrawn in April 2000 following HEMISPHERx's signing of a more economically viable manufacturing agreement for the drug. The company expects to file again.

2CVV

In October 1995, Milkhaus Laboratory, Inc., initiated a phase I/II clinical trial of 2CVV for the treatment of chronic fatigue syndrome at the Rhode Island Hospital and the Roger Williams Hospital (Brown University affiliates). The trial was completed and 2CVV is available to patients under a compassionate use program. The compound is also in preclinical evaluation for potential treatment of herpes and cystic fibrosis. No published scientific information is available on this compound and Milkhaus is seeking codevelopment partners worldwide.

Epstein-Barr Virus Vaccine

Aviron and GlaxoSmithKline reported their collaboration on the development of an Epstein-Barr virus vaccine using Aviron's subunit vaccine technology and GlaxoSmithKline's adjuvant technology. The vaccine was expected to have potential in chronic fatigue syndrome and infectious mononucleosis. A phase I trial, with two intramuscular injectable formulations, commenced in December 1977 in Belgium. The randomized, double-blind trial in sixty-seven subjects showed the vaccine to be safe and well tolerated. Laboratory tests showed evidence of immune response in the vaccine recipients. No further reports on this vaccine are available.

Imunovir (Inosine Pranobex)

A pilot study of the clinical impact of the synthetic purine derivative imunovir in sixteen CFS patients revealed enhanced natural killer cell activity and clinical improvement in 60 percent of the patients studied. Ardern Healthcare's Imunovir has immunomodulating and antiviral properties and is currently registered for the treatment of acute and chronic viral infections including herpes and measles. Although the product has also been in development for preventing and delaying progression of AIDS in patients at the early stages of the disease, the efficacy for this indication was questioned and the application for European Union approval was withdrawn in 1991. Besides chronic fatigue syndrome, Imunovir is being studied for the treatment of hepatitis C and infections caused by human papillomavirus.

Influenza Virus Vaccine Alone or in Combination with Other Vaccines

The use of the influenza virus vaccine and the rubella virus vaccine both separately and together have been reported for the treatment of herpesvirus (Epstein-Barr virus) infections. Lieberman (1990) reported the use of influenza virus vaccine given together with histamine and the immune enhancer Staphage Lysate for the treatment of patients suffering from Epstein-Barr virus infection. Patients were also successfully treated with the latter mixture in combination with rubella virus vaccine and with rubella virus vaccine alone.

McMichael (U.S. patent no. 4,880,626)reported relief of lesion pain and lesion enlargement upon treatment of patients with recurrent herpes simplex virus type II infection with compositions including histamine, measles inactivated, attenuated virus, and influenza vaccine (killed) virus. In published patent number U.S. 4,880,626, McMichael presents a composition for alleviating the symptoms of AIDS comprising human chorionic gonadotropin, Staphage Lysate, an influenza virus vaccine, such as Fluogen, and fractionated inactivated HIV virus. McMichael later reported that the thimerosal preservative in influenza vaccine preparations can mediate the antiherpetic activity of the latter composition.

Thimerosal

Thimerosal is a preservative in commercially available influenza virus vaccines (Fluogen, Parke-Davis, Morris Plains, NJ; Fluzone, Connaught Laboratories, Swiftwater, PA; Flu-Immune, Lederle, Wayne, NJ). Studies included in international published patent number WO 98/05350 (Inventor: John McMichael; applicant: Milkhaus Laboratory, Inc., Delanson, New York) provide evidence that thimerosal has antiviral activity and may be useful for the treatment of chronic fatigue syndrome.

In a first study, a phase I/II double-blind human clinical trial was conducted using thimerosal-containing compositions for the treatment of chronic fatigue syndrome. Thirty-six patients suffering from documented chronic fatigue syndrome were studied, of whom thirty-three completed the study. Of the subjects who completed the study, seventeen were treated with placebo and sixteen were treated by sublingual administration six times daily of one drop (0.05 mL) of a composition comprising 2 µL of influenza vaccine containing 0.01 percent (0.2 µg) thimerosal, 0.4 µL rubella virus vaccine, and 576 µL saline. After ten weeks of treatment, the subjects were evaluated and were taken off either drug or placebo and were evaluated further after an additional four weeks of no treatment.

The subjects were evaluated by means of two primary efficacy parameters: a visual analog scale for subjective evaluation of fatigue and a fatigue impact scale comprising thirty-six questions related to cognitive, psychological, and social disorders. Analysis of the results using the visual analog scale showed no statistically significant difference at the 95 percent confidence level between the therapy and the control groups. Although analysis of the results using the fatigue impact scale also failed to demonstrate a statistically significant difference at the 95 percent confidence level between the therapy and placebo groups, the results indicated a trend in favor of the therapy over the placebo, indicative of a therapeutic effect.

McMichael went on to perform several experiments and patient treatments with thimerosal-containing fractions of filtrated influenza virus vaccines. Antiherpes activity of thimerosal with and without influenza vaccine was confirmed with in vitro studies and in seven patients. Specifically, a filter centrifugation technique was used to isolate a 30 kDa fraction of commercially available influenza virus vaccines (FluViron and Fluzone), wherein the vaccine was loaded onto an Ultrafree low-binding spin-filter unit with a 30,000 nominal molecular weight limit and centrifuged in a microfuge until all of the fluid had passed through the filter. In vitro assays with the 30 kDa filtrate fractions (which contained thimerosal present at a concentration of 0.01 percent as a preservative in the commercial vaccine) saw complete inhibition of herpesvirus in a cell culture assay utilizing HSV-1 and HSV-2 infection of A549 (human lung carcinoma) cells.

The fraction obtained was also used in place of dilute influenza virus vaccine in human subjects and was found to improve the clinical response to chronic fatigue syndrome having produced lethargy, a history of mental fogginess, and poor quality of life. Two drops of the thimerosal-containing 30 kDa influenza virus fraction were administered to the subject sublingually, and the subject reported improvement in excess of 70 percent with an increase in energy and mental clarity for the first time in several years. After three weeks, the subject continued to do well with administration of two drops of the composition daily.

A second double-blind study was carried out on sixteen subjects suffering from chronic fatigue syndrome who were given one of three compositions, designated A, B, and C, administered over the course of one month as daily sublingual drops. Each subject was treated by sublingual administration of one drop (0.05 mL) four to six times daily. Composition A comprised 0.0004 percent weight per volume thimerosal (0.2 µg per drop) and 3.2×10^{-7} units neuraminidase per drop in saline. Composition B comprised 0.0004 percent weight per volume thimerosal (0.2 µg per drop) in combination with 0.32 µL rubella virus vaccine (Meruvac, Merck and Co.) in saline. Composition C comprised 0.0004 percent weight per volume thimerosal (0.2 µg per drop) alone in saline. The following parameters were measured by patients' self-reported scores: overall level of fatigue; overall level of pain; severity of flare-ups; muscle cramps; headaches; mental alertness and memory; and overall or average sleep. According to evaluation of these parameters, compositions A and B exhibited significant improvements in the severity of CFS symptoms. Moreover, if the results of one subject treated with composition B are omitted (because physical therapy starting and ending about the same time as the therapy may have adversely affected the results for that subject), the remaining subjects treated with composition B comprising the combination of thimerosal and rubella virus vaccine exhibited the greatest decrease in the severity of CFS symptoms.

Preferred dosages of thimerosal for treatment of subjects suffering from herpesvirus infections range from about 0.05 to 500 µg thimerosal, with about 0.5 to 50 µg thimerosal being preferred and about 5 µg thimerosal being particularly preferred. McMichael also isolated a 5 kDa fraction from the Fluvirin influenza vaccine by further filtration. This fraction, which also contained thimerosal, was effective at inhibiting growth of the herpesvirus in the cell culture experiment described and appeared to be clinically superior in administration in vivo to the 30 kDa fraction. The mechanism of action of thimerosal remains to be documented.

Stealth Virus Vaccine

Incomplete forms of herpesviruses may contribute to a newly defined grouping of atypically structured viruses that cause persistent active infection in the absence of significant viral inflammation (DeGreef et al., 1999; Rettig et al., 1997; Said et al., 1997). Designated "stealth viruses," these agents can induce a vacuolating cytopathic effect (CPE) in human and animal cells. The appearance, progression, and wide host range characteristics of the CPE distinguish stealth viruses from conventional human cytopathic viruses, including human herpesviruses, enteroviruses, and adenoviruses. Electron microscopy, serology, and molecular-based assays can be used to further differentiate stealth viruses from conventional viruses.

In published U.S. patent number WO-09960101, W. J. Martin advances the thesis that chronic fatigue syndrome is but one of many different manifestations of a persistent stealth viral infection within the brain. Martin states that the involvement of the brain in chronic fatigue syndrome is implied by the historical use of terms such as neurasthenia, myalgic encephalomyelitis, epidemic diencephalomyelitis, and limbic encephalopathy. In more recent years, however, several investigators have argued that the disordered brain function is a secondary phenomenon, resulting, for example, from the overproduction of neuromodulatory cytokines from an activated immune system that may be responding excessively to a multitude of normally tolerated ubiquitous microorganisms, such as Epstein-Barr virus, human herpesvirus-6, *Candida albicans, Mycoplasma fermentans, Chlamydia pneumoniae,* etc. Attention has also been given to possible brain damage resulting from exposure to environmental neurotoxins, including the potential release into the circulation of neurotoxic bacterial products from a damaged gastrointestinal tract.

Martin goes on to argue that the shift away from a primary infectious process within the brain has occurred in spite of numerous epidemic outbreaks of CFS-like illnesses. Reasons for this neglect include the failure of established CFS investigators to isolate viruses from CFS patients and by the lack of correlation of disease with conventional antiviral serology. Published studies using PCR to test for evidence of retroviruses, enterovirus, and *Mycoplasma* infections were also flawed by erroneous assumptions concerning the specificity of PCR assays when performed under low stringency conditions. The imposition of a restrictive clinical definition of chronic fatigue syndrome has particularly hindered the capacity to validate any suggested new assay, since it required that only patients with fatigue should test positive. This demand has also obscured epidemiological studies for potential disease transmission within families or communities.

Martin described that a stealth virus isolated from a CFS patient induced an acute illness with prominent neurobehavioral changes in cats. Noninflammatory cellular damage was evident in the brain and throughout all of the animal tissues examined. Cellular damage was also present in the offspring of a virus-inoculated pregnant cat. Heat-inactivated virus material did not induce illness when inoculated into a cat. Moreover, this cat did not develop symptoms when subsequently injected with a virus isolated from a different CFS patient. Although stealth viruses may lack antigens required for cellular immunity, they can retain antigens able to evoke circulating antibodies. The presence of stealth virus-reactive antibodies may, in fact, act as a barrier to the bloodborne spread of infection into the brain. The molecular heterogeneity of stealth viruses, however, poses a limitation with using a single antigen for possible immunization.

Immunization designed to elicit protective antibodies can potentially provide protection against an initial infection. The source of antigen can be from a stealth virus or from a conventional virus with antigen structurally related to those on a particular stealth virus isolate.

SPV-30

Arkopharma SA (France) carried out clinical trials on the tree (boxwood) extract SPV-30 as a natural health product with potential for the treatment of AIDS or chronic fatigue syndrome. SPV-30 is a reverse transcriptase inhibitor and TNF-alpha antagonist. Although SPV-30 use was reported to be safe and to be associated with improvements in CD4 and CD8 cells, energy levels, appetite, memory, weight, and viral load, and a phase III clinical trial of SPV-30 was completed in 1996, the company has not carried out further trials and plans no further developments.

Transfer Factors Against Herpesviruses

Transfer factors (TF) with specific activity against herpesviruses have been documented in chronic fatigue syndrome. With some studies suggesting that persistent viral activity may play a role in perpetuation of chronic fatigue syndrome symptoms, there appears to be a rationale for the use of TF in patients with chronic fatigue syndrome, and some reports have suggested that transfer factors may play a beneficial role in this disorder (Ablashi et al., 1996; De Vinci et al., 1996; Hana et al., 1996; Levine, 1996). For instance, specific HHV-6 TF preparation, administered to two CFS patients, inhibited the HHV-6 infection (Ablashi et al., 1996). Prior to treatment, both patients exhibited an activated HHV-6 infection. TF treatment significantly improved the clinical manifestations of chronic fatigue syndrome in one patient who resumed normal duties within weeks, whereas no clinical improvement was observed in the second patient. Of the twenty patients in a placebo-controlled trial of oral TF (De Vinci et al., 1996), improvement was observed in twelve patients, generally within three to six weeks of beginning treatment. However, in this study, herpesvirus serology (EBV and HHV-6) seldom correlated with clinical response. Treatment with TF of a group of 222 patients suffering from cellular immunodeficiency (CID), frequently combined with chronic fatigue syndrome and/or chronic viral infections by EBV and/or CMV (Hana et al., 1996), showed that age but not gender substantially influenced the failure rate of CID treatment using TF. In older people, it is easier to improve the clinical conditions other than CID; this may be related to the diminished number of lymphocytes, but a placebo effect cannot be totally excluded.

References

Aaby P. (1995). Assumptions and contradictions in measles and measles immunization research: Is measles good for something? *Social Sciences Medicine* 41(5): 673-686.

Aaby P, Samb B, Simondon F, Seck AM, Knudsen K, Whittle H. (1995). Nonspecific beneficial effect of measles immunization: Analysis of mortality studies from developing countries. *British Medical Journal* 311(7003):481-485.

Aaby P, Shaheen SO, Heyes CB, Goudiaby A, Hall AJ, Shiell AW, Jewen H, Marchant A. (2000). Early BCG vaccination and reduction in atopy in Guinea-Bissau. *Clinical and Experimental Allergy* 30(5):644-650.

Aamdal S, Wolff I, Kaplan S, Paridaens R, Kerger J, Schachter J, Wanders J, Franklin HR, Verweij J. (1994). Docetaxel (Taxotere) in advanced malignant melanoma: A phase II study of the EORTC Early Clinical Trials Group. *European Journal of Cancer* 30A(8):1061-1064.

Aapro MS, Cella D, Zagari M. (2002). Age, anemia, and fatigue. *Seminars in Oncology* 29(3 Suppl 8):55-59.

Aaron LA, Bradley LA, Alarcon GS, Alexander RW, Triana-Alexander M, Martin MY, Alberts KR. (1996). Psychiatric diagnoses in patients with fibromyalgia are related to health care-seeking behavior rather than to illness. *Arthritis and Rheumatism* 39(3):436-445.

Aaron LA, Buchwald D. (2000). Tobacco use and chronic fatigue syndrome, fibromyalgia, and temporomandibular disorder. *Archives of Internal Medicine* 160(15):2398-2401.

Aaronson NK, Ahmedzai S, Bergman B, Bullinger M, Cull A, Duez NJ, Filiberti A, Flechtner H, Fleishman SB, de Haes JC, et al. (1993). The European Organization for Research and Treatment of Cancer QLQ-C30: A quality-of-life instrument for use in international clinical trials in oncology. *Journal of the National Cancer Institutes* 85(5):365-376.

Aaserud R, Gramvik P, Olsen SR, Jensen J. (1998). Creatine supplementation delays onset of fatigue during repeated bouts of sprint running. *Scandinavian Journal of Medicine and Science in Sports* 8(5 Pt 1):247-251.

Aass N, Fossa SD, Dahl AA, Moe TJ. (1997). Prevalence of anxiety and depression in cancer patients seen at the Norwegian Radium Hospital. *European Journal of Cancer* 33(10):1597-1604.

Aass N, Fossa SD, Dahl AA, Moe TJ. (1998). [Occurrence of anxiety and depression in cancer patients: An investigation at the Norwegian Radium Hospital]. *Tidsskr Nor Laegeforen* 118(5):698-703.

Abasiyanik A, Oran B, Kaymakci A, Yasar C, Caliskan U, Erkul I. (1996). Conn syndrome in a child, caused by adrenal adenoma. *Journal of Pediatric Surgery* 31(3):430-432.

Abbey SE. (1993). Somatization, illness attribution and the sociocultural psychiatry of chronic fatigue syndrome. In *Chronic Fatigue Syndrome,* Bock BR, Whelan J, eds. New York: Wiley, pp. 238-261.

Abdelnoor AM. (1997). Antigen processing/presenting and oncogenesis. *Critical Reviews in Oncogenesis* 8(4):381-393.

Abdelnoor AM, Heneine W. (1985). HLA-A, B and C typing of a selected group of Lebanese: A preliminary report. *Lebanese Medical Journal* 35:246-250.

Abdelnoor M, Abdelnoor AM. (1993). Comparative study of HLA-A, B and C frequencies in Christians and Moslems in Lebanon. *Lebanese Science Bulletin* 6:67-71.

Abdulhay G, Di Saia PJ, Blessing JA, Creasman WT. (1985). Human lymphoblastoid interferon in the treatment of advanced epithelial ovarian malignancies: A Gynecologic Oncology Group study. *American Journal of Obstetrics and Gynecology* 152(4):418-423.

Abe T, Ohguni S, Tanigawa K, Kato Y. (1994). [Effective treatment with constant subcutaneous infusion of octreotide in a patient with acromegaly associated with diabetic pre-coma and diabetes insipidus]. *Nippon Naibunpi Gakkai Zasshi* 70(9):1029-1038.

Ablashi DV, Eastmann HB, Owen CB, Roman MM, Friedman J, Zabriskie JB, Peterson DL, Pearson GR, Whitman JE. (2000). Frequent HHV-6 reactivation in multiple sclerosis (MS) and chronic fatigue syndrome (CFS) patients. *Journal of Clinical Virology* 16(3):179-191.

Ablashi DV, Handy M, Bernbaum J, Chatlynne LG, Lapps W, Kramarsky B, Berneman ZN, Komaroff AL, Whitman JE. (1998). Propagation and characterization of human herpes virus-7 (HHV-7) isolates in a continuous T-lymphoblastoid cell line (SUPT1). *Journal of Virological Methods* 73(2):123-140.

Ablashi DV, Josephs SF, Buchbinder A, Hellman K, Nakamura S, Llana T, Lusso P, Kaplan M, Dahlberg J, Memon S, et al. (1998). Human B-lymphotropic virus (human herpesvirus-6). *Journal of Virological Methods* 21(1-4):29-48.

Ablashi DV, Levine PH, De Vinci C, Whitman JE Jr, Pizza G, Viza D. (1996). The use of anti HHV-6 transfer factor for the treatment of two patients with chronic fatigue syndrome (CFS): Two case reports. *Biotherapy* 9(1-3):81-86.

Aboulafia D, Miles SA, Saks SR, Mitsuyasu RT. (1989). Intravenous recombinant tumor necrosis factor in the treatment of AIDS-related Kaposi's sarcoma. *Journal of Acquired Immune Deficiency Syndromes* 2(1):54-58.

Abraham E, Wunderink R, Silverman H, Perl TM, Nasraway S, Levy H, Bone R, Wenzel RP, Balk R, Allred R, et al. (1995). Efficacy and safety of monoclonal antibody to human necrosis factor α in patients with sepsis syndrome: A randomized, controlled, double-blind, multicenter clinical trial. *JAMA* 273(12): 934-941.

Abraham J, Bakke S, Rutt A, Meadows B, Merino M, Alexander R, Schrump D, Bartlett D, Choyke P, Robey R, et al. (2002). A phase II trial of combination chemotherapy and surgical resection for the treatment of metastatic adrenocortical carcinoma: Continuous infusion doxorubicin, vincristine, and etoposide with daily mitotane as a P-glycoprotein antagonist. *Cancer* 94(9):2333-2343.

Abrahamsen AF, Loge JH, Hannisdal E, Holte H, Kvaloy S. (1998). Socio-medical situation for long-term survivors of Hodgkin's disease: A survey of 459 patients treated at one institution. *European Journal of Cancer* 34(12):1865-1870.

Abrams DI. (1996). Alternative therapies. In *A Clinical Guide to AIDS and HIV,* Abrams DI, ed. Philadelphia: Lippincott-Raven, p. 379.

Acheson S. (1992). The clinical syndrome variously called benign myalgic encephalomyelitis, Iceland disease and epidemic neuromyasthenia (first published in *American Journal of Medicine,* 569-595). In *The Clinical and Scientific Basis of Myalgic Encephalomyelitis/Chronic Fatigue Syndrome,* Hyde BM, Goldstein J, Levine P, eds. Ottawa: Nightingale Research Foundation, pp. 129-158.

Adachi I, Watanabe T, Takashima S, Narabayashi M, Horikoshi N, Aoyama H, Taguchi T. (1996). A late phase II study of RP56976 (docetaxel) in patients with advanced or recurrent breast cancer. *British Journal of Cancer* 73(2):210-216.

Adachi K, Ogawa M, Usui N, Inagaki J, Horikoshi N, Inoue K, Nakada H, Tada A, Yamazaki H, Mukaiyama T. (1985). [Phase I-II study of recombinant interferon gamma]. *Gan To Kagaku Ryoho* 12(6):1331-1338.

Adachi K, Tanaka J, Sato T, Makino S, Hosaka N, Takao M, Yada I, Namikawa S. (2001). [A case of thymoma with pure red cell aplasia]. *Kyobu Geka* 54(13):1153-1155.

Adamolekum B, Hakim JG. (1998). Opsoclonus-myoclonus associated with traditional medicine ingestion: Case report. *East African Medical Journal* 75(2):120-121.

Adams F, Quesada JR, Gutterman JU. (1984). Neuropsychiatric manifestations of human leukocyte interferon therapy in patients with cancer. *JAMA* 252(7):938-941.

Adenis A, Carlier D, Darloy F, Pion JM, Bonneterre J, Demaille A. (1995). Cytarabine and cisplatin as salvage therapy in patients with metastatic colorectal cancer who failed 5-fluorouracil + folinic acid regimen. French Northern Oncology Group. *American Journal of Clinical Oncology* 18(2):158-160.

Adjei AA, Erlichman C, Davis JN, Cutler DL, Sloan JA, Marks RS, Hanson LJ, Svingen PA, Atherton P, Bishop WR, et al. (2000). A phase I trial of the farnesyl transferase inhibitor SCH66336: Evidence for biological and clinical activity. *Cancer Research* 60(7):1871-1877.

Adler GK, Kinsley BT, Hurwitz S, Mossey CJ, Goldenberg DL. (1999). Reduced hypothalamic-pituitary and sympathoadrenal responses to hypoglycemia in women with fibromyalgia syndrome. *American Journal of Medicine* 106(5):534-543.

Adverse Drug Reactions Advisory Committee (1999). An adverse reaction to the herbal medication in milk thistle *(Silybum marianum). Medical Journal of Australia* 170(5):218-219.

Affleck G, Tennen H, Urrows S, Higgins P, Abeles M, Hall C, Karoly P, Newton C. (1998). Fibromyalgia and women's pursuit of personal goals: A daily process analysis. *Health Psychology* 17(1):40-47.

Affleck G, Urrows S, Tennen H, Higgins O, Abeles M. (1996). Sequential daily relations of sleep, pain intensity, and attention to pain among women with fibromyalgia. *Pain* 68:363-368.

Agargun MY, Tekeoglu I, Gunes A, Adak B, Kara H, Ercan M. (1999). Sleep quality and pain threshold in patients with fibromyalgia. *Comprehensive Psychiatry* 40(3):226-228.

Ahles TA, Saykin AJ, Furstenberg CT, Cole B, Mott LA, Skalla K, Whedon MB, Bivens S, Mitchell T, Greenberg ER, et al. (2002). Neuropsychologic impact of standard-dose systemic chemotherapy in long-term survivors of breast cancer and lymphoma. *Journal of Clinical Oncology* 20(2):485-493.

Ahsberg E, Furst CJ. (2001). Dimensions of fatigue during radiotherapy—An application of the Swedish Occupational Fatigue Inventory (SOFI) on cancer patients. *Acta Oncologica* 40(1):37-43.

Aihara T, Kim Y, Takatsuka Y. (2002). Phase II study of weekly docetaxel in patients with metastatic breast cancer. *Annals of Oncology* 13(2):286-292.

Aistars J. (1987). Fatigue in the cancer patient: A conceptual approach to a clinical problem. *Oncology Nursing Forum* 14(6):25-30.

Ajani JA, Baker J, Pisters PW, Ho L, Feig B, Mansfield PF. (2001). Irinotecan plus cisplatin in advanced gastric or gastroesophageal junction carcinoma. *Oncology* 15(3 Suppl 5):52-54.

Ajani JA, Baker J, Pisters PW, Ho L, Mansfield PF, Feig BW, Charnsangavej C. (2002). CPT-11 plus cisplatin in patients with advanced, untreated gastric or gastroesophageal junction carcinoma: Results of a phase II study. *Cancer* 94(3): 641-646.

Akechi T, Kugaya A, Okamura H, Yamawaki S, Uchitomi Y. (1999). Fatigue and its associated factors in ambulatory cancer patients: A preliminary study. *Journal of Pain Symptomatology and Management* 17(1):42-48.

Akira S, Hirano T, Taga T, Kishimoto T. (1990). Biology of the multifunctional cytokines: IL6 and related molecules IL1 and TNF. *Federation of American Societies of Experimental Biology Journal* 4:2860-2867.

Akira S, Taga T, Kishimoto T. (1993). Inteleukin-6 in biology and medicine. *Advances in Immunology* 54:1-78.

Akiyama A, Ohkubo Y, Hokoishi F, Ito T, Tsuchiya A, Kusama H. (1994). [Bladder carcinoma producing granulocyte colony stimulating factor (G-CSF): A case report]. *Nippon Hinyokika Gakkai Zasshi* 85(7):1135-1138.

Akkus S, Delibas N, Tamer MN. (2000). Do sex hormones play a role in fibromyalgia? *Rheumatology* (Oxford) 39(10):1161-1163.

Ako J, Eto M, Kim S, Iijima K, Watanabe T, Ohike Y, Yoshizumi M, Ouchi Y. (2000). Pericardial constriction due to malignant lymphoma. *Japanese Heart Journal* 41(5):673-679.

Alarcon GS. (1997). Arthralgias, myalgias, facial erythema, and a positive ANA: Not necessarily SLE. *Cleveland Clinic Journal of Medicine* 64(7):361-364.

Albain KS, Swinnen LJ, Erickson LC, Stiff PJ, Fisher RI. (1990). Cisplatin preceded by concurrent cytarabine and hydroxyurea: A pilot study based on an in vitro model. *Cancer Chemotherapy Pharmacology* 27(1):33-40.

Albanes D, Blair A, Taylor PR. (1987). Physical activity and risk of cancer in the NHANES I population. *American Journal of Public Health* 79:744-750.

Alberto P, Rozencweig M, Clavel M, Siegenthaler P, Cavalli F, Gundersen S, Bruntsch U, Renard J, Pinedo H. (1986). Phase II study of 5'-deoxy-5-fluor-ouridine (doxifluridine) in advanced malignant melanoma. *Cancer Chemotherapy Pharmacology* 16(1):78-79.

Alberts M, Smets EM, Vercoulen JH, Garssen B, Bleijenberg G. (1997). "Abbreviated fatigue questionnaire": A practical tool in the classification of fatigue. *Nederlands Tijdschrift voor Geneeskunde* 141(31):1526-1530.

Alberts SR, Erlichman C, Reid JM, Sloan JA, Ames MM, Richardson RL, Goldberg RM. (1998). Phase I study of the duocarmycin semisynthetic derivative KW-2189 given daily for five days every six weeks. *Clinical Cancer Research* 4(9):2111-2117.

Alberts SR, Erlichman C, Sloan J, Okuno SH, Burch PA, Rubin J, Pitot HC, Goldberg RM, Adjei AA, Atherton PJ, et al. (2001). Phase I trial of gemcitabine and CPT-11 given weekly for four weeks every six weeks. *Annals of Oncology* 12(5):627-631.

Albus C. (1997). Chronic fatigue syndrome—A disease entity or an unspecific psychosomatic disorder? *Zeitschrift fur Arztliche Fortbildung und Qualitatssicherung* 91(8):717-721.

Alderson LM, Delalle I. (2002). Case records of the Massachusetts General Hospital weekly clinicopathological exercises: Case 10-2002, a 52-year-old woman with recurrent unsteadiness, slurred speech, and fatigue. *New England Journal of Medicine* 346(13):1009-1015.

Aleksandrowicz J, Skotnicki AB. (1982). *Leukemia Ecology: Ecological Prophylaxis of Leukemia,* Nowak E, tr. Springfield, VA: U.S. Department of Commerce, National Technical Information Service.

Alexander GC, Sehgal AR. (1998). Barriers to cadaveric renal transplantation among blacks, women, and the poor. *JAMA* 280:1148-1152.

Alexander RW, Bradley LA, Alarcon GS, Triana-Alexander M, Aaron LA, Alberts KR, Martin MY, Stewart KE. (1998). Sexual and physical abuse in women with fibromyalgia: Association with outpatient health care utilization and pain medication usage. *Arthritis Care Research* 11(2):102-115.

Ali MA, Kraut MJ, Valdivieso M, Herskovic AM, Du W, Kalemkerian GP. (1998). Phase II study of hyperfractionated radiotherapy and concurrent weekly alternating chemotherapy in limited-stage small cell lung cancer. *Lung Cancer* 22(1): 39-44.

Al-Karim HA, Tan KE, Chi KN, Bryce CJ, Murray NR, Coppin C. (2002). Carboplatin and vinblastine for the treatment of metastatic transitional cell carcinoma of the urothelial tract. *American Journal of Clinical Oncology* 25(5):515-519.

Allain TJ, Bearn JA, Coskeran P, Jones J, Checkley A, Butler J, Wessely S, Miell JP. (1997). Changes in growth hormone, insulin, insulin like growth factors (IGFs), and IGF-binding protein-1 in chronic fatigue syndrome. *Biological Psychiatry* 41(5):567-573.

Allal AS, Bieri S, Brundler MA, Soravia C, Gertsch P, Bernier J, Morel P, Roth AD. (2002). Preoperative hyperfractionated radiotherapy for locally advanced rectal cancers: A phase I-II trial. *International Journal of Radiation Oncology, Biology and Physics* 54(4):1076-1081.

Allal AS, Obradovic M, Laurencet F, Roth AD, Spada A, Marti MC, Kurtz JM. (1999). Treatment of anal carcinoma in the elderly: Feasibility and outcome of radical radiotherapy with or without concomitant chemotherapy. *Cancer* 85(1): 26-31.

Allard N. (2000). [Cancer and fatigue]. *Infirmerie Quebec* 7(4):12-13, 45-49.

Allen J, Packer R, Bleyer A, Zeltzer P, Prados M, Nirenberg A. (1991). Recombinant interferon beta: A phase I-II trial in children with recurrent brain tumors. *Journal of Clinical Oncology* 9(5):783-788.

Allison MA, Jones SE, McGuffey P. (1989). Phase II trial of outpatient interleukin-2 in malignant lymphoma, chronic lymphocytic leukemia, and selected solid tumors. *Journal of Clinical Oncology* 7(1):75-80.

Allison PJ. (2002). Alcohol consumption is associated with improved health-related quality of life in head and neck cancer patients. *Oral Oncology* 38(1):81-86.

Allison PJ, Guichard C, Gilain L. (2000). A prospective investigation of dispositional optimism as a predictor of health-related quality of life in head and neck cancer patients. *Quality of Life Research* 9(8):951-960.

Alm JS, Lilja G, Pershagen G, Scheynius A. (1997). Early BCG vaccination and development of atopy. *Lancet* 350:400-403.

Alm JS, Sanjeevi CB, Miller EN, Dabadghao P, Lilja G, Pershagen G, Blackwell JM, Scheynius A. (2002). Atopy in children in relation to BCG vaccination and genetic polymorphisms at SLC11A1 (formerly NRAMP1) and D2S1471. *Genes and Immunity* 3(2):71-77.

Al-Majid S, McCarthy DO. (2001). Cancer-induced fatigue and skeletal muscle wasting: The role of exercise. *Biological Research and Nursing* 2(3):186-197.

Alpert S, Kloide J, Takada S, Engleman EG. (1987). T-cell regulatory disturbances in the rheumatic diseases. *Rheumatic Diseases Clinics of North America* 13(3): 431-435.

Al-Suwaidan SN, Gad el Rab MO, Al-Fakhiry S, Al Hoqail IA, Al-Maziad A, Sherif AB. (1998). Allergic contact dermatitis from myrrh, a topical herbal medicine used to promote healing. *Contact Dermatitis* 38(2):120-121.

Altman C, Larratt K, Golubjatnikov R. (1988). Immunologic markers in the chronic fatigue syndrome. *Clinical Research* 36:845A.

Alvarez-Lario B, Alonso Valdivielso JL, Alegre Lopez J, Martel Soteres C, Viejo Banuelos JL, Maranon Cabello A. (1996). Fibromyalgia syndrome: Overnight falls in arterial oxygen saturation. *American Journal of Medicine* 101(1):54-60.

Alviggi L, Johnson C, Hoskins PJ, Tee DE, Pyke DA, Leslie RD, Vergani D. (1984). Pathogenesis of insulin-dependent diabetes: A role for activated T lymphocytes. *Lancet* 2:4-6.

Amato R, Meyers C, Ellerhorst J, Finn L, Kilbourn R, Sella A, Logothetis C. (1995). A phase I trial of intermittent high-dose alpha-interferon and dexamethasone in metastatic renal cell carcinoma. *Annals of Oncology* 6(9):911-914.

Ambrogetti A, Olson LG, Sutherland DC, Malcolm JA, Bliss D, Gyulay SG. (1998). Daytime sleepiness and REM sleep abnormalities in chronic fatigue: A case series. *Journal of Chronic Fatigue Syndrome* 4(1):23-36.

American Psychiatric Association. (1994). *Diagnostic and Statistical Manual of Mental Disorders* (DSM-IV), Fourth Edition. Washington, DC: American Psychiatric Association.

Ames BN, Gold LS, Willett WC. (1995). The causes and prevention of cancer. *Proceedings of the National Academy of Sciences of the United States of America* 92:5258-5265.

Anch AM, Lue FA, MacLean AW, Moldofsky H. (1991). Sleep physiology and psychological aspects of fibrositis (fibromyalgia) syndrome. *Canadian Journal of Experimental Psychology* 45:179-184.

Ancoli-Israel S, Moore PJ, Jones V. (2001). The relationship between fatigue and sleep in cancer patients: A review. *European Journal of Cancer Care* 10(4):245-255.

Anderberg UM. (1999). [Stress can induce neuroendocrine disorders and pain] Stress kan ge neuroendokina storningar och smarttillstand. *Lakartidningen* 96 (49):5497-5499.

Anderberg UM. (2000a). Comment on Johns and Littlejohn: The role of sex hormones in pain response. *Pain* 87(1):109-111.

Anderberg UM. (2000b). [Fibromyalgia—Probably a result of prolonged stress syndrome] Fibromyalgi—Sannolikt ett resultat av langvarigt stressyndrom. *Lakartidningen* 97(21):2641-2642.

Anderberg UM, Marteinsdottir I, Theorell T, Von Knorring L. (2000). The impact of life events in female patients with fibromyalgia and in female healthy controls. *European Psychiatry* 15(5):295-301.

Anders A, Petry H, Fleming C, Petry K, Brix P, Lüke W, Gröger H, Schneider E, Kiefer J, Anders F. (1994). Increasing melanoma incidence: Putatively explainable by retrotransposons—Experimental contributions of the xiphophorine Gordon-Kosswig melanoma system. *Pigment Cell Research* 7:433-450.

Anderson B. (1994). Quality of life in progressive ovarian cancer. *Gynecological Oncology* 55(3 Pt 2):S151-S155.

Andersson L, Lindholm T. (1967). Less common manifestations of hyperparathyroidism. *Acta Medica Scandinavica* 182(4):411-418.

Andersson M, Bagby JR, Dyrehag LE, Gottfries CG. (1998). Effects of staphylococcal toxoid vaccine on pain and fatigue in patients with fibromyalgia/chronic fatigue syndrome. *European Journal of Pain* 2:133-142.

Andondonskaja-Renz B, Zeitler H. (1984). Pteridines in plasma and in cells of peripheral blood tumor patients. In *Biochemical and Clinical Aspects of Pteridines,* Volume 3, Pfeiderer W, Wachter H, Curtius HC, eds. Berlin and New York: Walter de Gruyter, pp. 295-311.

Andrykowski MA, Curran SL, Lightner R. (1998). Off-treatment fatigue in breast cancer survivors: A controlled comparison. *Journal of Behavioral Medicine* 21(1):1-18.

Ang D, Wilke WS. (1999). Diagnosis, etiology, and therapy of fibromyalgia. *Comprehensive Therapy* 25(4):221-227.

Angell M. (1997). Antipolymer antibodies, silicone breast implants, and fibromyalgia. *Lancet* 348(9059):1171-1171; discussion 1172-1173.

Angevin E, Valteau-Couanet D, Farace F, Dietrich PY, Lecesne A, Triebel F, Escudier B. (1995). Phase I study of prolonged low-dose subcutaneous recombinant interleukin-2 (IL-2) in patients with advanced cancer. *Journal of Immunotherapy with Emphasis on Tumor Immunology* 18(3):188-195.

Anisimov VN, Zavarzina NY, Zabezhinski MA, Popovich IG, Zimina OA, Shtylick AV, Arutjunyan AV, Oparina TI, Prokopenko VM, Mikhalski AI, et al. (2001). Melatonin increases both life span and tumor incidence in female CBA mice. *Journal of Gerontology Biological Science and Medical Science* 56(7):B311-B323.

Anisman H, Baines MG, Berczi I, Bernstein CN, Blennerhassett MG, Gorczynski RM, Greenberg AH, Kisil FT, Mathison RD, Nagy E, et al. (1996). Neuroimmune mechanisms in health and disease: 2. Disease. *Canadian Medical Association Journal* 155(8):1075-1082.

Ankerst J, Faldt R, Nilsson PG, Flodgren P, Sjogren HO. (1984). Complete remission in a patient with acute myelogenous leukemia treated with leukocyte alpha-interferon and cimetidine. *Cancer Immunology and Immunotherapy* 17(1): 69-71.

Anthoney DA, Twelves CJ. (2001). DNA: Still a target worth aiming at? A review of new DNA-interactive agents. *American Journal of Pharmacogenomics* 1(1): 67-81.

Aoki T, Miyakoshi H, Usuda Y, Herberman RB. (1993). Low NK syndrome and its relationship to chronic fatigue syndrome. *Clinical Immunology and Immunopathology* 69(3):253-265.

Aoki T, Usuda Y, Miyakoshi H. (1987). Low natural killer syndrome: Clinical and immunologic features. *Natural Immunology and Growth Regulation* 6(3):116-118.

Aoki Y, Sato T, Tsuneki I, Watanabe M, Kase H, Fujita K, Kurata H, Tanaka K. (2002). Docetaxel in combination with carboplatin for chemo-naive patients with epithelial ovarian cancer. *International Journal of Gynecological Cancer* 12(6):704-709.

Aoyama H, Asaishi K, Abe R, Kajiwara T, Enomoto K, Yoshida M, Ohasi Y, Tominaga T, Abe O. (1994). [Clinical evaluation of CGS16949A in advanced or recurrent breast cancer—A multi-institutional late phase II clinical trial]. *Gan To Kagaku Ryoho* 21(4):477-484.

Aozasa K, Tokuno N, Ikuno H, Mishima Y. (1982). Malignant histiocytosis showing facial involvement. *Laryngoscope* 92(5):577-579.

Apple RJ, Erlich HA, Klitz W, Manos M, Becker R, Wheeler C. (1994). HLA-DR-DQ associations with cervical carcinoma show papilloma virus-type specificity. *Nature Genetics* 6:157-162.

Araki Y, Muto T, Asakura T. (1999). Psychosomatic symptoms of Japanese working women and their need for stress management. *Indian Health* 37(2):253-262.

Archard LC, Bowles NE, Behan PO, Bell EJ, Doyle D. (1988). Post viral fatigue syndrome: Persistence of enterovirus RNA in muscle and elevated creatinine kinase. *Journal of the Royal Society of Medicine* 81:326-329.

Archer TP, Kourlas PJ, Mazzaferri EL. (1998). Fatigue and abdominal fullness in a 36-year-old woman. *Hospital Practice* 33(3):141-142, 145-146.

Ardizzoni A, Hansen H, Dombernowsky P, Gamucci T, Kaplan S, Postmus P, Giaccone G, Schaefer B, Wanders J, Verweij J. (1997). Topotecan, a new active drug in the second-line treatment of small-cell lung cancer: A phase II study in patients with refractory and sensitive disease. The European Organization for Research and Treatment of Cancer Early Clinical Studies Group and New Drug Development Office, and the Lung Cancer Cooperative Group. *Journal of Clinical Oncology* 15(5):2090-2096.

Ardizzoni A, Pennucci MC, Castagneto B, Mariani GL, Cinquegrana A, Magri D, Verna A, Salvati F, Rosso R. (1994). Recombinant interferon alpha-2b in the treatment of diffuse malignant pleural mesothelioma. *American Journal of Clinical Oncology* 17(1):80-82.

Ardizzoni A, Rosso R, Salvati F, Scagliotti G, Soresi E, Ferrara G, Pennucci C, Baldini E, Cruciani AR, Antilli A, et al. (1991). Combination chemotherapy and interferon alpha 2b in the treatment of advanced non-small-cell lung cancer. The Italian Lung Cancer Task Force (FONICAP). *American Journal of Clinical Oncology* 14(2):120-123.

Arendt J. (1989). Melatonin: A new probe in psychiatric investigation? *British Journal of Psychiatry* 155:585-590.

Arinaga S, Karimine N, Takamuku K, Nanbara S, Inoue H, Nagamatsu M, Ueo H, Akiyoshi T. (1992). Enhanced induction of lymphokine-activated killer activity after Lentinan administration in patients with gastric carcinoma. *International Journal of Immunopharmacology* 14:535-539.

Arinaga S, Karimine N, Takamuku K, Nanbara S, Nagamatsu M, Ueo H, Akiyoshi T. (1992). Enhanced production of interleukin-1 and tumor necrosis factor by peripheral monocytes after Lentinan administration in patients with gastric carcinoma. *International Journal of Immunopharmacology* 14:43-47.

Armstrong CL, Corn BW, Ruffer JE, Pruitt AA, Mollman JE, Phillips PC. (2000). Radiotherapeutic effects on brain function: Double dissociation of memory systems. *Neuropsychiatry, Neuropsychology, Behavior, and Neurology* 13(2):101-111.

Armstrong CL, Hunter JV, Ledakis GE, Cohen B, Tallent EM, Goldstein BH, Tochner Z, Lustig R, Judy KD, Pruitt A, et al. (2002). Late cognitive and radiographic changes related to radiotherapy: Initial prospective findings. *Neurology* 59(1):40-48.

Armstrong CL, Mollman J, Corn BW, Alavi J, Grossman M. (1993). Effects of radiation therapy on adult brain behavior: Evidence for a rebound phenomenon in a phase 1 trial. *Neurology* 43(10):1961-1965.

Armstrong R. (2000). Fibromyalgia: Is recovery impeded by the Internet? *Archives of Internal Medicine* 160(7):1039-1040.

Arnason BGW. (1991). Nervous system-immune system communication. *Reviews of Infectious Diseases* 13(1):S134-S137.

Arnold LM, Keck PE Jr, Welge JA. (2000). Antidepressant treatment of fibromyalgia: A meta-analysis and review. *Psychosomatics* 41(2):104-113.

Arzomand ML. (1998). Chronic fatigue syndrome among school children and their special educational needs. *Journal of Chronic Fatigue Syndrome* 4(3):59-70.

Asada Y, Marutsuka K, Mitsukawa T, Kuribayashi T, Taniguchi S, Sumiyoshi A. (1996). Ganglioneuroblastoma of the thymus: An adult case with the syndrome of inappropriate secretion of antidiuretic hormone. *Human Pathology* 27(5): 506-509.

Asai G, Fukuoka M. (1999). [Phase II studies of gemcitabine for non-small cell lung cancer in Japan]. *Gan To Kagaku Ryoho* 26(7):884-889.

Asanuma N, Hagiwara K, Matsumoto I, Matsuda M, Nakamura F, Kouhara H, Miyamoto M, Miyashita Y, Noguchi S, Morimoto Y. (2002). PTHrP-producing tumor: Squamous cell carcinoma of the liver accompanied by humoral hypercalcemia of malignancy, increased IL-6 and leukocytosis. *Internal Medicine* 41(5):371-376.

Asari J, Yamanobe K, Sasaki T, Yamao N, Kodama N. (1987). [A case of prolactinoma associated with craniopharyngioma]. *No Shinkei Geka* 15(12):1313-1318.

Asencio-Marchante JJ, Terriza-García F. (1998). [Myalgia-fasciculation syndrome] Síndrome de mialgia-fasciculación. *Revista Neurológica* 26(149):162.

Ashbury FD, Findlay H, Reynolds B, McKerracher K. (1998). A Canadian survey of cancer patients' experiences: Are their needs being met? *Journal of Pain Symptomatology Management* 16(5):298-306.

Asim M, Turney JH. (1997). The female patient with faints and fatigue: Don't forget Sjögren's syndrome. *Nephrology, Dialysis and Transplantation* 12(7):1516-1517.

Athanasiadis I, Kies MS, Miller M, Ganzenko N, Joob A, Marymont M, Rademaker A, Gradishar WJ. (1995). Phase II study of all-trans-retinoic acid and alpha-interferon in patients with advanced non-small cell lung cancer. *Clinical Cancer Research* 1(9):973-979.

Atherton P. (1998). *Aloë vera:* Magic or medicine? *Nursing Standard* 12(41):49-52.

Atkins JN, Muss HB, Capizzi RL, Cooper MR, Craig J, Cruz JM, Jackson DV Jr, Powell B, Richards F II, Spurr CL, et al. (1985). Phase I study of high-dose cytarabine and cisplatin in patients with advanced malignancy. *Cancer Treatment Reports* 69(7-8):897-899.

Atkins MB, O'Boyle KR, Sosman JA, Weiss GR, Margolin KA, Ernest ML, Kappler K, Mier JW, Sparano JA, Fisher RI, et al. (1994). Multiinstitutional phase II trial of intensive combination chemoimmunotherapy for metastatic melanoma. *Journal of Clinical Oncology* 12(8):1553-1560.

Atkins MB, Robertson MJ, Gordon M, Lotze MT, DeCoste M, DuBois JS, Ritz J, Sandler AB, Edington HD, Garzone PD, et al. (1997). Phase I evaluation of intravenous recombinant human interleukin 12 in patients with advanced malignancies. *Clinical Cancer Research* 3(3):409-417.

Atkins MB, Vachino G, Tilg HJ, Karp DD, Robert NJ, Kappler K, Mier JW. (1992). Phase I evaluation of thrice-daily intravenous bolus interleukin-4 in patients with refractory malignancy. *Journal of Clinical Oncology* 10(11):1802-1809.

Atkinson JH, Ancoli-Israel S, Slater MA, Garfin SR, Gillin JC. (1988). Subjective sleep disturbances in chronic back pain. *Clinical Journal of Pain* 4:225-232.

Atkinson MA, Bowman MA, Campbell L, Darrow BL, Kaufman DL, Maclaren NK. (1994). Cellular immunity to a determinant common in glutamate decarbocylase and coxsackievirus in insulin-dependent diabetes. *Journal of Clinical Investigation* 94(5):2125-2129.

Atzpodien J, Kirchner H, de Mulder P, Bodenstein H, Oliver T, Palmer PA, Franks CR, Poliwoda H. (1993). Subcutaneous recombinant interleukin-2 and alpha-interferon in patients with advanced renal cell carcinoma: Results of a multicenter phase II study. *Cancer Biotherapy* 8(4):289-300.

Avila H, Rivero J, Herrera F, Fraile G. (1997). Cytotoxicity of a low molecular weight fraction from *Aloë vera (Aloë barbadensis* Miller) gel. *Toxicon* 35(9): 1423-1430.

Awang DVC. (1996). Siberian ginseng toxicity may be case of mistaken identity. *Canadian Medical Association Journal* 155:1237.

Awang DVC. (1997). Quality control and good manufacturing practices: Safety and efficacy of commercial herbals. *Food and Drug Law Journal* 52(3):341-344.

Ayanian JZ, Cleary PD, Weissman JS, Epstein AM. (1999). The effect of patients' preferences on racial differences in access to renal transplantation. *New England Journal of Medicine* 341:1661-1669.

Aylward M. (1996). Government's expert group has reached a consensus on prognosis of chronic fatigue syndrome. *British Medical Journal* 313(7061):885.

Ayres JG, Flint N, Smith EG, Tunnicliffe WS, Fletcher TJ, Hammond K, Ward D, Marmion BP. (1998). Post-infection fatigue syndrome following Q fever. *Quarterly Journal of Medicine* 91(2):105-123.

Azuma N, Kamano T, Yuasa S, Tamura J, Katami A, Sato T, Kishino H, Mizukami K, Kidokoro T. (1984). [Clinical trials of plasma exchange therapy in patients with recurrent colon cancer]. *Gan To Kagaku Ryoho* 11(9):1801-1808.

Azuno Y, Yaga K, Sasayama T, Kimoto K. (1999). Thrombocytopenia induced by Jui, a traditional Chinese herbal medicine. *Lancet* 354(9175):304-305.

Bachle T, Ruhl U, Ott G, Walker S. (2001). [Enteropathy-associated T-cell lymphoma: Manifestation as diet-refractory coeliac disease and ulcerating jejunitis]. *Deutsche Medizinische Wochenschrift* 126(51-52):1460-1463.

Bachmann GA. (2001). Epoetin alfa use in gynecology: Past, present and future. *Journal of Reproductive Medicine* 46(5 Suppl):539-544.

Bacoyiannis C, Dimopoulos MA, Kalofonos HP, Nicolaides C, Aravantinos G, Bafaloukos D, Samelis G, Onyenadum A, Kiamouris CH, Skarlos D, et al. (2002). Vinblastine and interferon-gamma combination with and without 13-cis retinoic acid for patients with advanced renal cell carcinoma: Results of two phase II clinical trials. *Oncology* 63(2):130-138.

Baddley JW, Daberkow D, Hilton CW. (1998). Insulinoma masquerading as factitious hypoglycemia. *Southern Medical Journal* 91(11):1067-1069.

Badger TA, Braden CJ, Mishel MH. (2001). Depression burden, self-help interventions, and side effect experience in women receiving treatment for breast cancer. *Oncology Nursing Forum* 28(3):567-574.

Bafaloukos D, Pavlidis N, Fountzilas G, Skarlos D, Klouvas G, Makrantonakis P, Giannakakis T, Tsavaris N, Kosmidis P. (1996). Recombinant interferon ALFA-2A in combination with carboplatin, vinblastine, and bleomycin in the treatment of advanced malignant melanoma. *American Journal of Clinical Oncology* 19(3):296-300.

Bagheri H, Broue P, Lacroix I, Larrey D, Olives JP, Vaysse P, Ghisolfi J, Montastruc JL. (1998). Fulminant hepatic failure after herbal medicine ingestion in children. *Therapie* 53(1):82-83.

Bagust A, Barraza-Llorens M, Philips Z. (2001). Deriving a compound quality of life measure from the EORTC-QLQ-C30/LC13 instrument for use in economic evaluations of lung cancer clinical trials. *European Journal of Cancer* 37(9): 1081-1088.

Baidas SM, Winer EP, Fleming GF, Harris L, Pluda JM, Crawford JG, Yamauchi H, Isaacs C, Hanfelt J, Tefft M, et al. (2000). Phase II evaluation of thalidomide in patients with metastatic breast cancer. *Journal of Clinical Oncology* 18(14): 2710-2717.

Baier-Bitterlich G, Fuchs D, Murr C, Reibnegger G, Werner Felmayer G, Sgonc R, Böck G, Dierich MP, Wachter H. (1995). Effect of neopterin and 7,8-dihydro-neopterin on tumor necrosis factor-alpha induced programmed cell death. *FEBS Letters* 364:234-238.

Bailey HH, Kohler P, Tuttle R, Carbone PP, Hohneker JA, Clendeninn NJ, Wilding G. (1992). Phase I evaluation of 773U82-HCl in a two-hour infusion repeated daily for three days. *Investigative New Drugs* 10(4):279-287.

Bailey HH, Levy D, Harris LS, Schink JC, Foss F, Beatty P, Wadler S. (2002). A phase II trial of daily perillyl alcohol in patients with advanced ovarian cancer: Eastern Cooperative Oncology Group Study E2E96. *Gynecological Oncology* 85(3):464-468.

Bajetta E, Negretti E, Giannotti B, Brogelli L, Brunetti I, Sertoli MR, Bernengo MG, Sofra MC, Maifredi G, Zumiani G, et al. (1990). Phase II study of interferon alpha-2a and dacarbazine in advanced melanoma. *American Journal of Clinical Oncology* 13(5):405-409.

Bajorunas DR. (1990). Clinical manifestations of cancer-related hypercalcemia. *Seminars in Oncology* 17(2 Suppl 5):16-25.

Baker F, Zabora J, Polland A, Wingard J. (1999). Reintegration after bone marrow transplantation. *Cancer Practice* 7(4):190-197.

Bakhshandeh A, Bruns I, Eberhardt K, Wiedemann GJ. (2000). [Chemotherapy in combination with whole-body hyperthermia in advanced malignant pleural mesothelioma]. *Deutsche Medizinishe Wochenschrift* 125(11):317-319.

Baldini E, Ardizzoni A, Prochilo T, Cafferata MA, Boni L, Tibaldi C, Neumaier C, Conte PF, Rosso R; Italian Lung Cancer Task Force. (2001). Gemcitabine, ifosfamide and navelbine (GIN): Activity and safety of a non-platinum-based triplet in advanced non-small-cell lung cancer (NSCLC). *British Journal of Cancer* 85(10):1452-1455.

Balducci L, Extermann M. (2000). Management of the frail person with advanced cancer. *Critical Reviews in Oncology and Hematology* 33(2):143-148.

Balmer CM. (1985). The new alpha interferons. *Drug Intelligence Clinical Pharmacology* 19(12):887-893.

Banki K, Maceda J, Hurley E, Abloczy E, Mattson DH, Szegedy L, Hung C, Perl A. (1992). Human T-cell lymphotropic virus (HTLV)-related endogenous sequence, HRES-1, encodes a 28-kDa protein: A possible autoantigen for HTLV-I gag reactive autoantibodies. *Proceedings of the National Academy of Sciences of the United States of America* 89(5):1939-1943.

Banno S, Hirashima N, Noda T, Nitta M. (1989). [Chromosomal abnormality of trisomy 4 in a patient with acute nonlymphocytic leukemia (FAB: M2)]. *Rinsho Ketsueki* 30(11):1987-1991.

Banno S, Nitta M, Takada K, Hasegawa R, Niimi T, Yamamoto T. (1993). [Non-Hodgkin's lymphoma with pulmonary involvement and various immunological abnormalities in an elderly patient]. *Nippon Ronen Igakkai Zasshi* 30(6):506-510.

Baracos VE. (2001). Management of muscle wasting in cancer-associated cachexia: Understanding gained from experimental studies. *Cancer* 92(6 Suppl):1669-1677.

Baraczka K, Janko Z, Vargha K, Markus H. (1997). [Clinical experiences with the analgesic effects of citalopram] Klinikai tapasztalatok a citalopram fajdalomcsillapito hatasarol. *Orv Hetil* 138(41):2605-2607.

Barak M, Merzbach D, Gruener N. (1989). Neopterin measured in serum and tissue culture supernates by a competitive enzyme-linked immunosorbant assay. *Clinical Chemistry* 35(7):1467-1471.

Baraniuk JN, Clauw DJ, Gaumond E. (1998). Rhinitis symptoms in chronic fatigue syndrome. *Annals of Allergy, Asthma, and Immunology* 81(4):359-365.

Baraniuk JN, Clauw DJ, MacDowell-Carneiro AL, Bellanti J, Pandiri P, Foong S, Ali M. (1998). IgE concentrations in chronic fatigue syndrome. *Journal of Chronic Fatigue Syndrome* 4(1):13-22.

Barendregt PJ, Visser MR, Smets EM, Tulen JH, van den Meiracker AH, Broomsma F, Markusse HM. (1998). Fatigue in primary Sjögren's syndrome. *Annals of Rheumatic Diseases* 57(5):291-295.

Barker E, Fujimura SF, Fadem MB, Landay AL, Levy JA. (1994). Immunologic abnormalities associated with chronic fatigue syndrome. *Clinical Infectious Diseases* 18(Suppl 1):S136-S141.

Barnd DL, Kerr LA, Metzgar RS, Finn OJ. (1988). Human tumor-specific cytotoxic T-cell lines generated from tumor-draining lymph node infiltrate. *Transplantation Proceedings* 20:339-341.

Barnd DL, Lan MS, Metzgar RS, Finn OJ. (1989). Specific major histocompatibility complex-unrestricted recognition of tumor-associated mucins by human cytotoxic T cells. *Proceedings of the National Academy of Sciences of the United States of America* 86:7159-7163.

Barnes EA, Bruera E. (2002). Fatigue in patients with advanced cancer: A review. *International Journal of Gynecological Cancer* 12(5):424-428.

Barnes J, Mills SY, Abbott NC, Willoughby M, Ernst E. (1998). Different standards for reporting ADRs to herbal remedies and conventional OTC medicines: Face-to-face interviews with 515 users of herbal remedies. *British Journal of Clinical Pharmacology* 45(5):496-500.

Barnish L. (1994). Fatigue and the cancer patient. *British Journal of Nursing* 3(16):806-809.

Barofsky I, Legro MW. (1991). Definition and measurement of fatigue. *Reviews of Infectious Diseases* 13:94-97.

Baron F, Sautois B, Baudoux E, Matus G, Fillet G, Beguin Y. (2002). Optimization of recombinant human erythropoietin therapy after allogeneic hematopoietic stem cell transplantation. *Experimental Hematology* 30(6):546-554.

Barral-Netto M, Da Silva JS, Barral A, Reed S. (1995). Up-regulation of T helper 2 and down-regulation of T helper 1 cytokines during murine retrovirus-induced immunodeficiency syndrome enhances susceptibility of a resistant mouse strain to *Leihmania amazonensis*. *American Journal of Pathology* 146(3):635-642.

Barreras L, Vogel CL, Koch G, Marcus SG. (1988). Phase II trial of recombinant beta (IFN-betaser) interferon in the treatment of metastatic breast cancer. *Investigative New Drugs* 6(3):211-215.

Barrett B, Kiefer D, Rabago D. (1999). Assessing the risks and benefits of herbal medicine: An overview of scientific evidence. *Alternative Therapies in Health and Medicine* 5(4):40-49.

Barrios J. (1999). Is herbal therapy helpful or hazardous? *Journal of the American Dietetic Association* 99(5):530.

Barsevick AM, Whitmer K, Sweeney C, Nail LM. (2002). A pilot study examining energy conservation for cancer treatment-related fatigue. *Cancer Nursing* 25(5): 333-341.

Barsevick AM, Whitmer K, Walker L. (2001). In their own words: Using the common sense model to analyze patient descriptions of cancer-related fatigue. *Oncology Nursing Forum* 28(9):1363-1369.

Barsky AJ, Borus JF. (1999). Functional somatic syndromes. *Annals of Internal Medicine* 130(11):910-921.

Barth WF. (1997). Office evaluation of the patient with musculoskeletal complaints. *American Journal of Medicine* 102(1A):3S-10S.

Bartram HP, Wynder EL. (1989). Physical activity and colon cancer risk? Physiological considerations. *American Journal of Gastroenterology* 84:109-112.

Bartsch HH, Nagel GA, Mull R, Flener R, Pfizenmaier K. (1988). Phase I study of recombinant human tumor necrosis factor-alpha in patients with advanced malignancies. *Molecular Biotherapy* 1(1):21-29.

Bartsch HH, Pfizenmaier K, Schroeder M, Nagel GA. (1989). Intralesional application of recombinant human tumor necrosis factor alpha induces local tumor regression in patients with advanced malignancies. *European Journal of Cancer and Clinical Oncology* 25(2):287-291.

Barwich D, Rohl L. (1974). [Pheochromocytoma of the urinary bladder and bilateral cystic kidneys: Report of a case]. *Schweizer Medizinische Wochenschrift* 104(34):1196-1198.

Barzacchi MC, Nobile MT, Sanguineti O, Sertoli MR, Chiara S, Repetto L, Forno G, Lavarello A, Rosso R. (1994). Treatment of metastatic colorectal carcinoma with lymphoblastoid interferon and 5-fluorouracil: Data of a phase II study. *Anticancer Research* 14(5B):2147-2149.

Baschetti R. (1996a). Chronic fatigue syndrome and neurally mediated hypotension. *JAMA* 275(5):359; discussion 360.

Baschetti R. (1996b). High androgen levels in chronic fatigue patients. *Journal of Clinical Endocrinology and Metabolism* 81(7):2752-2753.

Baschetti R. (1997a). Etiology of chronic fatigue syndrome. *American Journal of Medicine* 102(4):422-423.

Baschetti R. (1997b). Lung function test findings in patients with chronic fatigue syndrome (CFS). *Australian and New Zealand Journal of Medicine* 27(3):346.

Baschetti R. (1997c). Similarity of symptoms in chronic fatigue syndrome and Addison's disease. *European Journal of Clinical Investigation* 27(12):1061-1062.

Baschetti R. (1998). Treating chronic fatigue with exercise: Results are contradictory for patients meeting different diagnostic criteria. *British Medical Journal* 317(7158):600.

Baschetti R. (1999a). Cortisol deficiency may account for elevated apoptotic cell population in patients with chronic fatigue syndrome. *Journal of Internal Medicine* 245(4):409-410.

Baschetti R. (1999b). Fibromyalgia, chronic fatigue syndrome, and Addison disease. *Archives of Internal Medicine* 159(20):2481; discussion 2842-2843.

Baschetti R. (1999c). Investigations of hydrocortisone and fludrocortisone in the treatment of chronic fatigue syndrome. *Journal of Endocrinology and Metabolism* 84(6):2263-2264.

Baschetti R. (1999d). Low-dose hydrocortisone for chronic fatigue syndrome. *JAMA* 281(20):1887.

Baschetti R. (1999e). Overlap of chronic fatigue syndrome with primary adrenocortical insufficiency. *Hormone and Metabolism Research* 31(7):439.

Base J, Navratilova J, Cap J. (1993). [Conn's syndrome in tumors of the adrenal cortex]. *Rozhl Chir* 72(7):296-299.

Bash-Babula J, Toppmeyer D, Labassi M, Reidy J, Orlick M, Senzon R, Alli E, Kearney T, August D, Shih W, et al. (2002). A phase I/pilot study of sequential doxorubicin/vinorelbine: Effects on p53 and microtubule-associated protein 4. *Clinical Cancer Research* 8(5):1057-1064.

Bashey A, Sundaram S, Corringham S, Jones V, Lancaster D, Silva-Gietzen J, Law P, Ball ED. (2001). Use of capecitabine as first-line therapy in patients with metastatic breast cancer relapsing after high-dose chemotherapy and autologous stem cell support. *Clinical Oncology* 13(6):434-437.

Basser RL, Lieschke GJ, Sheridan WP, Fox RM, Green MD. (1991). Recombinant alpha-2b interferon in patients with malignant carcinoid tumour. *Australian and New Zealand Journal of Medicine* 21(6):875-878.

Bassetti S. (1996). [A case from practice: Fibromyalgia] Der Fall aus der Praxis: Fibromyalgie. *Schweizer Rundschift Medizin Praxis* 85(22):730-731.

Basso AM, Depiante-Depaoli M, Molina VA. (1992). Chronic variable stress facilitates tumoral growth: Reversal by imipramine administration. *Life Sciences* 50(23):1789-1796.

Bates DW, Buchwald D, Lee J, Kith P, Doolittle T, Rutherford C, Churchill WH, Schur PH, Werner M, Wybenga D, et al. (1995). Clinical laboratory test findings in patients with chronic fatigue syndrome. *Archives of Internal Medicine* 155: 97-103.

Bauer M, Muha C, Pytel J. (1976). A facial fatigability test: A method for detecting "latent" facial motor lesions by fatigability. *Clinical Otolaryngology* 1(3):233-240.

Baumann R, Tauber MG, Opravil M, Hirschel B, Kinloch S, Chave JP, Pletscher M, Luthy R. (1991). Combined treatment with zidovudine and lymphoblast interferon-alpha in patients with HIV-related Kaposi's sarcoma. *Klinische Wochenschrift* 69(8):360-367.

Baxter JD, Tyrell JB. (1981). The adrenal cortex. In *Endocrinology and Metabolism,* Felig P, Baxter JD, Broadus AE, Frohman LA, eds. New York: McGraw-Hill, pp. 1ff.

Bazelmans E, Bleijenberg G, Vercoulen JH, Van der Meer JW, Folgering H. (1997). The chronic fatigue syndrome and hyperventilation. *Journal of Psychosomatic Research* 43(4):371-377.

Bazelmans E, Vercoulen JH, Galama JM, Van Weel C, Van der Meer JW, Bleijenberg G. (1997). Prevalence of chronic fatigue syndrome and primary fibromyalgia syndrome in the Netherlands. *Tidschrift voor Geneeskunde* 141(31): 1520-1523.

Bazzi MN, Kellogg C. (1991). Weakness, fatigue, and hyponatremia. *Hospital Practice* 26(11):43-44.

Beach P, Siebeneck B, Buderer NF, Ferner T. (2001). Relationship between fatigue and nutritional status in patients receiving radiation therapy to treat lung cancer. *Oncology Nursing Forum* 28(6):1027-1031.

Beal MW. (1998). Women's use of complementary and alternative therapies in reproductive health care. *Journal of Nurse-Midwifery* 43(3):224-234.

Beard CJ, Propert KJ, Rieker PP, Clark JA, Kaplan I, Kantoff PW, Talcott JA. (1997). Complications after treatment with external-beam irradiation in early-stage prostate cancer patients: A prospective multiinstitutional outcomes study. *Journal of Clinical Oncology* 15(1):223-229.

Beard GM. (1869). Neurasthenia, or nervous exhaustion. *Boston Medical and Surgical Journal* 3:217-221.

Beard TC. (1996). Chronic fatigue syndrome and neurally mediated hypotension. *JAMA* 275(5):359, discussion 360.

Beck-Friis J, Ljunggren J, Thoren M, Von Rosen D, Kjellman BF, Wetterberg L. (1985). Melatonin, cortisol and ACTH in patients with major depressive disorder and healthy humans with special reference to the outcome of the dexamethasone suppression test. *Psychoneuroendocrinology* 10:173-186.

Becque Y, Blok S. (1997). [Patients with breast cancer experience fatigue at home: Fatigue under chemotherapy (2)]. *TVZ* 107(21):638-640.

Bedikian AY, Legha SS, Eton O, Buzaid AC, Papadopoulos N, Coates S, Simmons T, Neefe J, von Roemeling R. (1997). Phase II trial of tirapazamine combined with cisplatin in chemotherapy of advanced malignant melanoma. *Annals of Oncology* 8(4):363-367.

Bedikian AY, Legha SS, Eton O, Buzaid AC, Papadopoulos N, Plager C, McIntyre S, Viallet J. (1999). Phase II trial of escalated dose of tirapazamine combined with cisplatin in advanced malignant melanoma. *Anticancer Drugs* 10(8):735-739.

Beh HC. (1997). Effect of noise stress on chronic fatigue syndrome patients. *Journal of Nervous and Mental Disease* 185(1):55-58.

Behan PO, Behan WHM, Bell EJ. (1985). The postviral fatigue syndrome—An analysis of the findings in 50 cases. *Journal of Infection* 10:211-222.

Beisecker A, Cook MR, Ashworth J, Hayes J, Brecheisen M, Helmig L, Hyland S, Selenke D. (1997). Side effects of adjuvant chemotherapy: Perceptions of node-negative breast cancer patients. *Psychooncology* 6(2):85-93.

Bekenbosch F, Van Oers J, Del Rey A, Tilders F, Besedovsky H. (1987). Cortico-tropin-releasing factor-producing neurons in the RT activated by interleukin-1. *Science* 238:524-526.

Belanger K, Jolivet J, Maroun J, Stewart D, Grillo-Lopez A, Whitfield L, Wainman N, Eisenhauer E. (1993). Phase I pharmacokinetic study of DUP-937, a new anthrapyrazole. *Investigative New Drugs* 11(4):301-308.

Belani CP, Aisner J, Hiponia D, Ramanathan R. (1996). Paclitaxel and carboplatin in metastatic non-small cell lung cancer: Preliminary results of a phase I study. *Seminars in Oncology* 23(5 Suppl 12):19-21.

Belew C. (1999). Herbs and the childbearing woman: Guidelines for midwives. *Journal of Nurse-Midwifery* 44(3):231-252.

Belilos E, Carsons S. (1998). Rheumatologic disorders in women. *Medicine Clinics of North America* 82(1):77-101.

Bell DS, Robinson MZ, Pollard J, Robinson T, Floyd B. (1999). A *Parent's Guide to CFIDS*. Binghamton, NY: The Haworth Medical Press.

Bell IR, Baldwin CM, Schwartz GE. (1998). Illness from low levels of environmental chemicals: Relevance to chronic fatigue syndrome and fibromyalgia. *American Journal of Medicine* 105(3A):74S-82S.

Bellm LA, Epstein JB, Rose-Ped A, Martin P, Fuchs HJ. (2000). Patient reports of complications of bone marrow transplantation. *Support Care Cancer* 8(1):33-39.

Bellometti S, Galzigna L. (1999). Function of the hypothalamic adrenal axis in patients with fibromyalgia syndrome undergoing mud-pack treatment. *International Journal of Clinical Pharmacology Research* 19(1):27-33.

Belza B, Henke C, Yelin E, Epstein W, Gillis C. (1993). Correlates of fatigue in older adults with rheumatoid arthritis. *Nursing Research* 42:93-99.

Benasso M, Merlano M, Blengio F, Cavallari M, Rosso R, Toma S. (1993). Concomitant alpha-interferon and chemotherapy in advanced squamous cell carcinoma of the head and neck. *American Journal of Clinical Oncology* 16(6):465-468.

Benedetti JK, Burris HA III, Balcerzak SP, Macdonald JS. (1997). Phase II trial of topotecan in advanced gastric cancer: A Southwest Oncology Group study. *Investigative New Drugs* 15(3):261-264.

Benedetti Panici P, Scambia G, Baiocchi G, Perrone L, Pintus C, Mancuso S. (1989). Randomized clinical trial comparing systemic interferon with diathermocoagulation in primary multiple and widespread anogenital condyloma. *Obstetrics and Gynecology* 74(3 Pt 1):393-397.

Benedict S. (1989). The suffering associated with lung cancer. *Cancer Nursing* 12(1):34-40.

Benitez M. (1999). Atherosclerosis: An infectious disease? *Hospital Practice* 34:79-90.

Bennett A. (1997). A view of the violence contained in chronic fatigue syndrome. *Journal of Analytical Psychology* 42(2):237-251.

Bennett AL, Mayes DM, Fagioli LR, Guerriero R, Komaroff AL. (1997). Somato-medin C (insulin-like growth factor I) levels in patients with chronic fatigue syndrome. *Journal of Psychiatric Research* 31(1):91-96.

Bennett BK, Hickie IB, Vollmer-Conna US, Quigley B, Brennan CM, Wakefield D, Douglas MP, Hansen GR, Tahminjis AJ, Lloyd AR. (1998). The relationship between fatigue, psychological and immunological variables in acute infectious illness. *Australia and New Zealand Journal of Psychiatry* 32(2):180-186.

Bennett R. (1998). Fibromyalgia, chronic fatigue syndrome, and myofascial pain. *Current Opinions in Rheumatology* 10(2):95-103.

Bennett RM, Cook DM, Clark SR, Burckhardt CS, Campbell SM. (1997). Hypothalamic-pituitary-insulin-like growth factor-I axis dysfunction in patients with fibromyalgia. *Journal of Rheumatology* 24(7):1384-1389.

Benz C, Jakobs R, Spiethoff A, Bohrer MH, Riemann JF. (1999). [A rare cause of iron deficiency anemia: Recurrent hemorrhage from a carcinoid of the jejunum—Diagnosis and therapy with enteroscopy]. *Zeitschrift Gastroenterologie* 37(8):725-729.

Ben-Zion I, Shieber A, Buskila D. (1996). Psychiatric aspects of fibromyalgia syndrome. *Harefuah* 131(3-4):127-129.

Beran M, Jeha S, O'Brien S, Estey E, Vitek L, Zurlo MG, Rios MB, Keating M, Kantarjian H. (1997). Tallimustine, an effective antileukemic agent in a severe combined immunodeficient mouse model of adult myelogenous leukemia, induces remissions in a phase I study. *Clinical Cancer Research* 3(12 Pt 1):2377-2384.

Berent R, Hartl P, Rossoll M, Punzengruber C. (1998). [Lambl's excrescence as tumorous heart valve mass]. *Deutsche Medizinishe Wochenschrift* 123(14):423-426.

Berg D. (1998). Irinotecan hydrochloride: Drug profile and nursing implications of a topoisomerase I inhibitor in patients with advanced colorectal cancer. *Oncology Nursing Forum* 25(3):535-543.

Bergamaschi R, Romani A, Versino M, Poli R, Cosi V. (1997). Clinical aspects of fatigue in multiple sclerosis. *Functional Neurology* 12(5):247-251.

Berge MV, Snoek WJ, Nijboer EW, Julius AJ, Aalbers R. (1999). A man with upper respiratory tract infections, general weakness and fever. *European Respiratory Journal* 14(2):469-470.

Berger AM. (1998). Patterns of fatigue and activity and rest during adjuvant breast cancer chemotherapy. *Oncology Nursing Forum* 25(1):51-62.

Berger AM, Farr L. (1999). The influence of daytime inactivity and nighttime restlessness on cancer-related fatigue. *Oncology Nursing Forum* 26(10):1663-1671.

Berger AM, Higginbotham P. (2000). Correlates of fatigue during and following adjuvant breast cancer chemotherapy: A pilot study. *Oncology Nursing Forum* 27(9):1443-1448.

Berger AM, VonEssen S, Khun BR, Piper BF, Farr L, Agrawal S, Lynch JC, Higginbotham P. (2002). Feasibility of a sleep intervention during adjuvant breast cancer chemotherapy. *Oncology Nursing Forum* 29(10):1431-1441.

Berghella AM, Pellegrini P, Del Beato T, Maccarone D, Adorno D, Casciani CU. (1996). Prognostic significance of immunological evaluation in colorectal cancer. *Cancer Biotherapy and Radiopharmacology* 11(6):355-361.

Berglund G, Bolund C, Fornander T, Rutqvist LE, Sjoden PO. (1991). Late effects of adjuvant chemotherapy and postoperative radiotherapy on quality of life among breast cancer patients. *European Journal of Cancer* 27(9):1075-1081.

Bergmann L, Fenchel K, Weidmann E, Enzinger HM, Jahn B, Jonas D, Mitrou PS. (1993). Daily alternating administration of high-dose alpha-2b-interferon and interleukin-2 bolus infusion in metastatic renal cell cancer: A phase II study. *Cancer* 72(5):1733-1742.

Bergmans J, De Meirsman J, Rosselle N. (1975). Absence of ischaemic muscular fatigue in the Lambert-Eaton syndrome. *Electromyography and Clinical Neurophysiology* 15(3):285-289.

Berlin JD, Alberti DB, Arzoomanian RZ, Feierabend CA, Simon KJ, Binger KA, Marnocha RM, Wilding G. (1998-1999). A phase I study of gemcitabine, 5-fluorouracil and leucovorin in patients with advanced, recurrent, and/or metastatic solid tumors. *Investigative New Drugs* 16(4):325-330.

Berlin JD, Tutsch KD, Hutson P, Cleary J, Rago RP, Arzoomanian RZ, Alberti D, Feierabend C, Wilding G. (1997). Phase I clinical and pharmacokinetic study of oral carboxyamidotriazole, a signal transduction inhibitor. *Journal of Clinical Oncology* 15(2):781-789.

Berman BM, Ezzo J, Hadhazy V, Swyers JP. (1999). Is acupuncture effective in the treatment of fibromyalgia? *Journal of Family Practice* 48(3):213-218.

Berman BM, Swyers JP. (1999). Complementary medicine treatments for fibromyalgia syndrome. *Baillieres Best Practice Research in Clinical Rheumatology* 13(3):487-492.

Berman BM, Swyers JP, Ezzo J. (2000). The evidence for acupuncture as a treatment for rheumatologic conditions. *Rheumatic Diseases Clinics of North America* 26(1):103-115.

Bernard S, Gill P, Rosen P, Gavigan M, Steagall A, Ellingham E, Morgan T, Janic G, Ozer H. (1991). A phase I trial of alpha-interferon in combination with pentostatin in hematologic malignancies. *Medical Pediatric Oncology* 19(4): 276-282.

Berndt H. (1992). [A case report from general practice (1): Pale appearance and dyspnea]. *Zeitschrift Arztliche Fortbildung* 86(20):1035-1037.

Berner I, Gaubitz M, Jackisch C, Pfleiderer B. (2002). Comparative examination of complaints of patients with breast-cancer with and without silicone implants. *European Journal of Obstetrics, Gynecology and Reproductive Biology* 102(1): 61-66.

Bernhard J, Ganz PA. (1991). Psychosocial issues in lung cancer patients (Part 2). *Chest* 99(2):480-485.

Bernhard J, Hurny C, Bacchi M, Joss RA, Cavalli F, Senn HJ, Leyvraz S, Stahel R, Ludwig C, Alberto P. (1996). Initial prognostic factors in small-cell lung cancer patients predicting quality of life during chemotherapy. Swiss Group for Clinical Cancer Research (SAKK). *British Journal of Cancer* 74(10):1660-1667.

Bernton EW, Beach J, Holaday JW, Smallridge RC, Fein HG. (1987). Release of multiple hormones by a direct action of interleukin-1 on pituitary cells. *Science* 238:519-521.

Bernton E, Hoover D, Galloway R, Popp K. (1995). Adaptation to chronic stress in military trainees: Adrenal androgens, testosterone, glucocorticoids, IGF-1, and immune function. *Annals of the New York Academy of Sciences* 774:217-231.

Berruti A, Bitossi R, Gorzegno G, Bottini A, Alquati P, De Matteis A, Nuzzo F, Giardina G, Danese S, De Lena M, et al. (2002). Time to progression in metastatic breast cancer patients treated with epirubicin is not improved by the addition of either cisplatin or lonidamine: Final results of a phase III study with a factorial design. *Journal of Clinical Oncology* 20(20):4150-4159.

Bertolin JM, Calvo J. (1997). Chronic fatigue syndrome: To be or not to be? *Medicina Clínica* 108(15):577-579.

Berwaerts J, Moorkens G, Abs R. (1998). Review of neuroendocrine disturbances in the chronic fatigue syndrome: Indications for a role of the growth hormone-IGF-1 axis in the pathogenesis. *Journal of Chronic Fatigue Syndrome* 4(4):81-92.

Besedovsky H, Del Rey A, Sorkin E, Dinarello CA. (1986). Immunoregulatory feedback between interleukin-1 and glucocorticoid hormones. *Science* 233:652-654.

Beutler B, Cerami A. (1988). Cachectin (tumor necrosis factor): A macrophage hormone governing cellular metabolism and inflammatory response. *Endocrinological Reviews* 9:57-66.

Bhargava P, Marshall JL, Dahut W, Rizvi N, Trocky N, Williams JI, Hait H, Song S, Holroyd KJ, Hawkins MJ. (2001). A phase I and pharmacokinetic study of squalamine, a novel antiangiogenic agent, in patients with advanced cancers. *Clinical Cancer Research* 7(12):3912-3919.

Bianchi GP, Grossi G, Bargossi AM. (1997). May peripheral and central fatigue be correlated? Can we monitor them by means of clinical laboratory tools? *Journal of Sports Medicine and Physical Fitness* 37(3):194-199.

Bickston SJ, Lichtenstein GR, Arseneau KO, Cohen RB, Cominelli F. (1999). The relationship between infliximab treatment and lymphoma in Crohn's disease. *Gastroenterology* 117:1433-1437.

Bierens de Haan B, Chapuis G. (1972). [Primary hyperparathyroidism, case reports and general observations]. *Helvetica Chirurgica Acta* 39(5):741-750.

Bierman AS, Clancy CM. (2001). Health disparities among older women: Identifying opportunities to improve quality of care and functional health outcomes. *Journal of the American Medical Women's Association* 56:155-159.

Biesiada G, Kalinowska-Nowak A. (1999). [The coexistence of an intracranial tumor and a positive epidemiologic history of Lyme borreliosis as the reason for diagnostic problems—Case report]. *Przegl Lek* 56(10):682-683.

Billeter M, Streit E, Deuel W. (1991). [Swelling of the knee, fatigue]. *Schweize Rundschrift Meditin Prax* 80(34):859-862.

Birk TJ, MacArthur RD, McGrady A, Khuder S. (1996). Lack of effect of 12 weeks of massage therapy on immune function and quality of life in HIV-infected persons. In Abstracts of the XIth International Conference on AIDS, Volume 2, p. 270. Vancouver, Canada, July 7-12.

Bissett D, McLeod HL, Sheedy B, Collier M, Pithavala Y, Paradiso L, Pitsiladis M, Cassidy J. (2001). Phase I dose-escalation and pharmacokinetic study of a novel folate analogue AG2034. *British Journal of Cancer* 84(3):308-312.

Biswas NR, Beri S, Das GK, Mongre PK. (1996). Comparative double blind multicentric randomised placebo controlled clinical trial of a herbal preparation of eye drops in some ocular ailments. *Journal of the Indian Medical Association* 94(3):101-102.

Bjernulf A, Hall K, Sjogren L, Werner I. (1970). Primary hyperparathyroidism in children: Brief review of the literature and a case report. *Acta Paediatrica Scandinavica* 59(3):249-258.

Bjordal K, Kaasa S. (1992). Psychometric validation of the EORTC Core Quality of Life Questionnaire, 30-item version and a diagnosis-specific module for head and neck cancer patients. *Acta Oncologica* 31(3):311-321.

Bjordal K, Kaasa S, Mastekaasa A. (1994). Quality of life in patients treated for head and neck cancer: A follow-up study 7 to 11 years after radiotherapy. *International Journal of Radiation Oncology, Biology and Physics* 28(4):847-856.

Black PM, Zervas NT. (1997). Diagnosis and surgical treatment of pituitary lesions. *Comprehensive Therapeutics* 3(11):8-15.

Black RB, Leong AS, Crowed PA. (1980). Lymphocyte subpopulations in human lymph nodes: A normal range. *Lymphology* 13:86-90.

Blackburn WD Jr, Grotting JC, Everson MP. (1997). Lack of evidence of systemic inflammatory rheumatic disorders in symptomatic women with breast implants. *Plastic and Reconstructive Surgery* 99(4):1054-1060.

Blackwood SK, MacHale SM, Power MJ, Goodwin GM, Lawrie SM. (1998). Effects of exercise on cognitive and motor function in chronic fatigue syndrome and depression. *Journal of Neurology, Neurosurgery and Psychiatry* 65(4):541-546.

Blade J, Kyle RA, Greipp PR. (1996). Presenting features and prognosis in 72 patients with multiple myeloma who were younger than 40 years. *British Journal of Haematology* 93(2):345-351.

Blade J, Lust JA, Kyle RA. (1994). Immunoglobulin D multiple myeloma: Presenting features, response to therapy, and survival in a series of 53 cases. *Journal of Clinical Oncology* 12(11):2398-2404.

Blade J, San Miguel JF, Escudero ML, Fontanillas M, Besalduch J, Gardella S, Arias J, Garcia-Conde J, Carnero M, Marti JM, et al. (1998). Maintenance treatment with interferon alpha-2b in multiple myeloma: A prospective randomized study from PETHEMA (Program for the Study and Treatment of Hematological Malignancies, Spanish Society of Hematology). *Leukemia* 12(7):1144-1148.

Blanc PD, Kuschner WG, Katz PP, Smith S, Yelin EH. (1997). Use of herbal products, coffee or black tea, and over-the-counter medications as self-treatments among adults with asthma. *Journal of Allergy and Clinical Immunology* 100 (6 Pt 1):789-791.

Blaser MJ. (1999). The changing relationships of *Helicobacter pylori* and humans: Implications for health and disease. *Journal of Infectious Diseases* 179:1523-1530.

Blazeby JM, Brookes ST, Alderson D. (2000). Prognostic value of quality of life scores in patients with oesophageal cancer. *British Journal of Surgery* 87(3): 362-373.

Blazeby JM, Williams MH, Brookes ST, Alderson D, Farndon JR. (1995). Quality of life measurement in patients with oesophageal cancer. *Gut* 37(4):505-508.

Blegvad S, Lippert H, Simper LB, Dybdahl H. (1990). Mediastinal tumours: A report of 129 cases. *Scandinavian Journal of Thoracic Cardiovascular Surgery* 24(1):39-42.

Bleijenberg G. (1997). Attributions and chronic fatigue. *Nederlands Tijdschrift voor Geneeskunde* 141(31):1510-1512.

Blesch KS, Paice JA, Wickham R, Harte N, Schnoor DK, Purl S, Rehwalt M, Kopp PL, Manson S, Coveny SB, et al. (1991). Correlates of fatigue in people with breast or lung cancer. *Oncology Nursing Forum* 18(1):81-87.

Blevins LS Jr, Hall GS, Madoff DH, Laws ER Jr, Wand GS. (1992). Case report: Acromegaly and Cushing's disease in a patient with synchronous pituitary adenomas. *American Journal of Medical Sciences* 304(5):294-297.

Blick M, Bresser J, Lepe-Zuniga JL, Goodacre A, Luethke D, Holder WR, Duvic M. (1990). Identification of human immunodeficiency virus hybridizing sequences in the peripheral blood of a patient with systemic lupus erythematosus. *Journal of the American Academy of Dermatology* 23(4 Part 1):641-645.

Bloom JR, Fobair P, Gritz E, Wellisch D, Spiegel D, Varghese A, Hoppe R. (1993). Psychosocial outcomes of cancer: A comparative analysis of Hodgkin's disease and testicular cancer. *Journal of Clinical Oncology* 11(5):979-988.

Blum JL. (1999). Xeloda in the treatment of metastatic breast cancer. *Oncology* 57 (Suppl 1):16-20.

Blum JL, Jones SE, Buzdar AU, LoRusso PM, Kuter I, Vogel C, Osterwalder B, Burger HU, Brown CS, Griffin T. (1999). Multicenter phase II study of capecitabine in paclitaxel-refractory metastatic breast cancer. *Journal of Clinical Oncology* 17(2):485-493.

Boccardo F. (2000). Hormone therapy of prostate cancer: Is there a role for antiandrogen monotherapy? *Critical Reviews in Oncology and Hematology* 35(2):121-132.

Boccardo F, Guarneri D, Pace M, Decensi A, Oneto F, Martorana G. (1992). Phase II study with lonidamine in the treatment of hormone-refractory prostatic cancer patients. *Tumori* 78(2):137-139.

Bode L, Fersyt R, Czech G. (1993). Borna disease virus infection and affective disorders in man. *Archives of Virology* 7:159-167.

Bogdahn U, Fleischer B, Hilfenhaus J, Rothig HJ, Krauseneck P, Mertens HG, Przuntek H. (1985). Interferon-beta in patients with low-grade astrocytomas— A phase I study. *Journal of Neurooncology* 3(2):125-130.

Bohgaki T, Notoya A, Mukai M, Kohno M. (1999). [Acute lymphoblastic leukemia with breast infiltration during the second trimester of pregnancy and followed by successful delivery]. *Rinsho Ketsueki* 40(8):652-657.

Bohgaki T, Notoya A, Mukai M, Kohno M. (2000). [Perforation of small intestine during hematologic recovery in an elderly man after induction therapy for acute lymphoblastic leukemia L3]. *Rinsho Ketsueki* 41(2):146-151.

Bohle W, Ruther U, Bokemeyer C, Jipp P. (1997). [The synchronous occurrence of acute myeloid leukemia and kidney carcinoma]. *Deutsche Medizinische Wochenschrift* 122(23):743-746.

Bois P. (1968). Peripheral vasodilatation and thymic tumors in magnesium deficient rats. In *Endocrine Aspects of Disease Processes,* Jasmin G, ed. St. Louis, MO: WH Greene Publishers, pp. 337-355.

Bois P, Beaulnes A. (1966). Histamine, magnesium deficiency, and thymic tumors in rats. *Canadian Journal of Physiology and Pharmacology* 44:373-377.

Bok RA, Small EJ. (1999). The treatment of advanced prostate cancer with ketoconazole: Safety issues. *Drug Safety* 20(5):451-458.

Bokemeyer C, Hartmann JT, Kuczyk MA, Truss MC, Beyer J, Jonas U, Kanz L. (1996). The role of paclitaxel in chemosensitive urological malignancies: Current strategies in bladder cancer and testicular germ-cell tumors. *World Journal of Urology* 14(6):354-359.

Bokemeyer C, Hartmann JT, Mayer F, Bohlke I, Kanz L, Von Pawel J, Derigs G, Schroder M. (2000). UFT/leucovorin plus weekly paclitaxel in the treatment of solid tumors. *Oncology* 14(10 Suppl 9):63-67.

Bolla M, de Reijke TM, Zurlo A, Collette L. (2002). Adjuvant hormone therapy in locally advanced and localized prostate cancer: Three EORTC trials. *Frontiers in Radiation Therapy in Oncology* 36:81-86.

Bombardier CH, Buchwald D. (1996). Chronic fatigue, chronic fatigue syndrome, and fibromyalgia: Disability and health-care use. *Medical Care* 34(9):924-930.

Bonfil RD. (2001). CT-2584 (Cell therapeutics). *Current Opinions in Investigational Drugs* 2(3):424-427.

Bonnem EM, Oldham RK. (1987). Gamma-interferon: Physiology and speculation on its role in medicine. *Journal of Biological Response Modifiers* 6(3):275-301.

Boon T, Coolie PG, Van den Eynde B. (1997). Tumor antigens recognized by T cells. *Immunology Today* 18:267-268.

Borden EC. (1992a). Interferons—Expanding therapeutic roles. *New England Journal of Medicine* 326(22):1491-1493.

Borden EC. (1992b). Interferons: Pleiotropic cellular modulators. *Clinical Immunology and Immunopathology* 62(1 Pt 2):S18-S24.

Borden EC, Holland JF, Dao TL, Gutterman JU, Wiener L, Chang YC, Patel J. (1982). Leukocyte-derived interferon (alpha) in human breast carcinoma: The American Cancer Society phase II trial. *Annals of Internal Medicine* 97(1):1-6.

Borden EC, Kim K, Ryan L, Blum RH, Shiraki M, Tormey DC, Comis RL, Hahn RG, Parkinson DR. (1992). Phase II trials of interferons-alpha and -beta in advanced sarcomas. *Journal of Interferon Research* 12(6):455-458.

Borenstein D. (1996). Epidemiology, etiology, diagnostic evaluation, and treatment of low back pain. *Current Opinions in Rheumatology* 8(2):124-129.

Borghardt J, Rosien B, Gortelmeyer R, Lindemann S, Hartleb M, Klingmuller M. (2000). Effects of a spleen peptide preparation as supportive therapy in inoperable head and neck cancer patients. *Arzneimittelforschung* 50(2):178-184.

Borish L, Schmaling K, DiClementi JD, Streib J, Negri J, Jones JF. (1998). Chronic fatigue syndrome: Identification of distinct subgroups on the basis of allergy and psychologic variables. *Journal of Allergy and Clinical Immunology* 102(2): 222-230.

Borner M, Castiglione M, Triller J, Baer HU, Soucek M, Blumgart L, Brunner K. (1992). Considerable side effects of chemoembolization for colorectal carcinoma metastatic to the liver. *Annals of Oncology* 3(2):113-115.

Borok G. (1998). Chronic fatigue syndrome: An atopic state. *Journal of Chronic Fatigue Syndrome* 4(3):39-58.

Borysiewicz LK, Haworth SJ, Cohen J, Munin J, Rickinson A, Sissons JG. (1986). Epstein-Barr virus-specific immune defects in patients with persistent symptoms following infectious mononucleosis. *Quarterly Journal of Medicine* 58: 111-121.

Bosnjak S. (2002). Are Central Eastern European countries involved in clinical trials of supportive care? *Support Care in Cancer* 10(4):303-308.

Bosse D, Ades EW. (1989). Immunotherapy and enhanced antibody-dependent cell-mediated cytotoxicity using virally-infected target cells. *Journal of Clinical Laboratory Immunology* 29(3):109-110.

Bottero P. (2000). Role of Rickettsiae and Chlamydiae in the psychopathology of chronic fatigue syndrome (CFS) patients: A diagnostic and therapeutic report. *Journal of Chronic Fatigue Syndrome* 6(3/4):147-161.

Bouchard B, Fuller BB, Vijayasaradhi S, Houghton AN. (1989). Introduction of pigmentation in mouse fibroblasts by expression of human tyrosinase cDNA. *Journal of Experimental Medicine* 169:2029-2042.

Bouffet E, Philip T, Negrier C, Ffrench M, Frappaz D, Gentilhomme O, Gianella-Borradori A, Brunat-Mentigny M, Blay JY. (1997). Phase I study of interleukin-6 in children with solid tumours in relapse. *European Journal of Cancer* 33(10): 1620-1626.

Bouffet E, Zucchinelli V, Blanchard P, Costanzo P, Frappaz D, Roussin G, Mangavel G, Brunat-Mentigny M. (1996). [School at the end of life: What objectives, what hope?]. *Archives of Pediatrics* 3(6):555-560.

Bouffet E, Zucchinelli V, Costanzo P, Blanchard P. (1997). Schooling as a part of palliative care in paediatric oncology. *Palliative Medicine* 11(2):133-139.

Bou-Holaigah I, Calkins H, Flynn JA, Tunin C, Chang HC, Kan JS, Rowe PC. (1997). Provocation of hypotension and pain during upright tilt table testing in adults with fibromyalgia. *Clinical and Experimental Rheumatology* 15(3):239-246.

Bounous G, Molson J. (1999). Competition for glutamine precursors between the immune system and the skeletal muscle: Pathogenesis of chronic fatigue syndrome. *Medical Hypotheses* 53(4):347-349.

Bower B. (1991). Questions of mind over immunity. *Science News* 139:216-217.

Bower JE, Ganz PA, Aziz N, Fahey JL. (2002). Fatigue and proinflammatory cytokine activity in breast cancer survivors. *Psychosomatic Medicine* 64(4):604-611.

Bower JE, Ganz PA, Desmond KA, Rowland JH, Meyerowitz BE, Belin TR. (2000). Fatigue in breast cancer survivors: Occurrence, correlates, and impact on quality of life. *Journal of Clinical Oncology* 18(4):743-753.

Bowman MA, Kirk JK, Michielutte R, Presisser JS. (1997). Use of amantadine for chronic fatigue syndrome. *Archives of Internal Medicine* 157(11):1264-1265.

Boxer RJ, Waisman J, Lieber MM, Mampaso FM, Skinner DG. (1978). Non-metastatic hepatic dysfunction associated with renal carcinoma. *Journal of Urology* 119(4):468-471.

Bozbora A, Erbil Y, Ozbey N, Kapran Y, Ozarmagan S, Berber E, Molvalilar S. (2000). A young female patient with an androgen-secreting tumor: A rare malignant disease. *Tumori* 86(6):487-488.

Bradley LA, Alberts KR. (1999). Psychological and behavioral approaches to pain management for patients with rheumatic disease. *Rheumatic Diseases Clinics of North America* 25(1):215-232.

Bradley LA, McKendree-Smith NL, Alarcon GS. (2000). Pain complaints in patients with fibromyalgia versus chronic fatigue syndrome. *Current Reviews on Pain* 4(2):148-157.

Branco J, Atalaia A, Paiva T. (1994). Sleep cycles and alpha-delta sleep in fibromyalgia syndrome. *Journal of Rheumatology* 21:1113-1117.

Brand R, Capadano M, Tempero M. (1997). A phase I trial of weekly gemcitabine administered as a prolonged infusion in patients with pancreatic cancer and other solid tumors. *Investigative New Drugs* 15(4):331-341.

Brandberg Y, Kock E, Oskar K, af Trampe E, Seregard S. (2000). Psychological reactions and quality of life in patients with posterior uveal melanoma treated with ruthenium plaque therapy or enucleation: A one year follow-up study. *Eye* 14 (Pt 6):839-846.

Brandes LJ, Simons KJ, Bracken SP, Warrington RC. (1994). Results of a clinical trial in humans with refractory cancer of the intracellular histamine antagonist, N,N-diethyl-2-[4-(phenylmethyl)phenoxy]ethanamine-HCl, in combination with various single antineoplastic agents. *Journal of Clinical Oncology* 12(6):1281-1290.

Brasseur F, Marchand M, Vanwijck R, Herin M, Lethe B, Chomez P, Boon T. (1992). Human gene MAGE-1, which codes for a tumor rejection antigen, is expressed by some breast tumors. *International Journal of Cancer* 52:839-841.

Brattberg G. (1999). Connective tissue massage in the treatment of fibromyalgia. *European Journal of Pain* 12(1):35-41.

Braun DK, Dominguez GK, Pellett PE. (1997). Human herpesvirus 6. *Clinical Microbiology Reviews* 10(3):521-567.

Braybrooke JP, O'Byrne KJ, Saunders MP, Propper DJ, Salisbury AJ, Boardman P, Taylor M, Ganesan TS, Talbot DC, Harris AL. (1997). A phase II study of mitomycin C and oral etoposide for advanced adenocarcinoma of the upper gastrointestinal tract. *Annals of Oncology* 8(3):294-296.

Breau LM, McGrath PJ, Lu JH. (1999). Review of juvenile primary fibromyalgia and chronic fatigue syndrome. *Journal of Developmental Behavioral Pediatrics* 20(4):278-288.

Bredart A, Didier F, Robertson C, Scaffidi E, Fonzo D, Costa A, Goldhirsch A, Autier P. (1999). Psychological distress in cancer patients attending the European Institute of Oncology in Milan. *Oncology* 57(4):297-302.

Breitbart W, Bruera E, Chochinov H, Lynch M. (1995). Neuropsychiatric syndromes and psychological symptoms in patients with advanced cancer. *Journal of Pain Symptomatology Management* 10(2):131-141.

Breitbart W, McDonald MV, Rosenfeld B, Monkman ND, Passik S. (1998). Fatigue in ambulatory AIDS patients. *Journal of Pain and Symptom Management* 15(3): 159-167.

Breitbart W, Rosenfeld B, Kaim M, Funesti-Esch J. (2001). A randomized, double-blind, placebo-controlled trial of psychostimulants for the treatment of fatigue in ambulatory patients with human immunodeficiency virus disease. *Archives of Internal Medicine* 161(3):411-420.

Brennan MR. (1997). Uncomplicated starvation vs. cancer cachexia. *Cancer Research* 37:2359-2364.

Bretscher PA, Wei G, Menon JN, Bielefeldt-Ohmann H. (1992). Establishment of stable, cell-mediated immunity that makes "susceptible" mice resistant to *Leishmania major. Science* 257(5069):539-542.

Breuer K, Diehl V, Ruffer U. (2000). [Long-term toxic sequelae of the treatment of Hodgkin's disease]. *Medizinische Klinik* 95(7):378-384.

Briasoulis E, Karavasilis V, Anastasopoulos D, Tzamakou E, Fountzilas G, Rammou D, Kostadima V, Pavlidis N. (1999). Weekly docetaxel in minimally pretreated cancer patients: A dose-escalation study focused on feasibility and cumulative toxicity of long-term administration. *Annals of Oncology* 10(6):701-706.

Brice P. (2002). [Cured from Hodgkin's disease]. *Bulletin de Cancer* 89(7-8):666-670.

Brichard V, Van Pel A, Wolfe T, Wolfel C, De Plaen E, Lethe B, Coulie P, Boon T. (1993). The tyrosinase gene codes for an antigen recognized by autologous cytolytic T lymphocytes on HLA-A2 melanomas. *Journal of Experimental Medicine* 178:489-495.

Bridges AJ, Anderson JD, Burns DE, Kemple K, Kaplan JD, Lorden T. (1996). Autoantibodies in patients with silicone implants. *Current Topics in Microbiology and Immunology* 210:317-322.

Briggs FE. (1997). Fibromyalgia: An important diagnosis to consider. *Nurse Practice* 22(8):27-28.

Briggs NC, Levine PH. (1994). A comparative review of systemic and neurological symptomatology in 12 outbreaks collectively described as chronic fatigue syndrome, epidemic neuromyasthenia and myalgic encephalomyelitis. *Clinical Infectious Diseases* 18(Suppl. 1):S32-S42.

Brinkmann V, Kristofic C. (1995). Regulation of corticosteroids of Th1 and Th2 cytokine production in human CD4+ effector T cells generated from CD45RO- and CD45RO+ subsets. *Journal of Immunology* 155(7):3322-3328.

Britten CD, Rowinsky EK, Soignet S, Patnaik A, Yao SL, Deutsch P, Lee Y, Lobell RB, Mazina KE, McCreery H, et al. (2001). A phase I and pharmacological study of the farnesyl protein transferase inhibitor L-778,123 in patients with solid malignancies. *Clinical Cancer Research* 7(12):3894-3903.

Brodsky I, Strayer DR, Krueger LJ, Carter WA. (1985). Clinical studies with ampligen (mismatched double-stranded RNA). *Journal of Biological Response Modifiers* 4(6):669-675.

Broeckel JA, Jacobsen PB, Horton J, Balducci L, Lyman GH. (1998). Characteristics and correlates of fatigue after adjuvant chemotherapy for breast cancer. *Journal of Clinical Oncology* 16(5):1689-1696.

Brogden JM, Nevidjon B. (1995). Vinorelbine tartrate (Navelbine): Drug profile and nursing implications of a new vinca alkaloid. *Oncology Nursing Forum* 22(4):635-646.

Brooks JA, Kesler KA, Johnson CS, Ciaccia D, Brown JW. (2002). Prospective analysis of quality of life after surgical resection for esophageal cancer: Preliminary results. *Journal of Surgical Oncology* 81(4):185-194.

Brophy LR, Sharp EJ. (1991). Physical symptoms of combination biotherapy: A quality-of-life issue. *Oncology Nursing Forum* 18(1 Suppl):25-30.

Brosman SA. (1985). The use of bacillus Calmette-Guérin in the therapy of bladder carcinoma in situ. *Journal of Urology* 134:36-39.

Brown CR. (1997). Fibromyalgia. *Practice Periodontics and Aesthetic Dentistry* 9(8):878.

Brown SL, Langone JJ, Brinton LA. (1998). Silicone breast implants and auto-immune disease. *Journal of the American Medical Women's Association* 53(1): 21-24.

Brown TJ, Rowe J, Jingwen L, Shoyab M. (1991). Regulation of IL-6 expression by oncostatin M. *Journal of Immunology* 147:2175-2180.

Bruera E. (1992). Clinical management of anorexiai and cachexia in patients with advanced cancer. *Oncology* 49(Suppl 2):35-42.

Bruera E, Brenneis C, Michaud M, Jackson PI, MacDonald RN. (1988). Muscle electrophysiology in patients with advanced breast cancer. *Journal of the National Cancer Institutes* 80(4):282-285.

Bruera E, Ernst S, Hagen N, Spachynski K, Belzile M, Hanson J, Summers N, Brown B, Dulude H, Gallant G. (1998). Effectiveness of megestrol acetate in patients with advanced cancer: A randomized, double-blind, crossover study. *Cancer Prevention and Control* 2(2):74-78.

Bruera E, MacDonald RN. (1988). Overwhelming fatigue in advanced cancer. *American Journal of Nursing* 88(1):99-100.

Bruera E, Schmitz B, Pither J, Neumann CM, Hanson J. (2000). The frequency and correlates of dyspnea in patients with advanced cancer. *Journal of Pain Symptomatology Management* 19(5):357-362.

Brunelli C, Mosconi P, Boeri P, Gangeri L, Pizzetti P, Cerrai F, Schicchi A, Apolone G, Tamburini M. (2000). Evaluation of quality of life in patients with malignant dysphagia. *Tumori* 86(2):134-138.

Brunetti I, Falcone A, Bertuccelli M, Cianci C, Ricci S, Conte PF. (1994). Double 5-fluorouracil modulation with folinic acid and recombinant alpha-2B-interferon: A phase I-II study in metastatic colorectal cancer patients. *American Journal of Clinical Oncology* 17(3):210-214.

Bruno RL. (1998). Abnormal movements in sleep as a post-polio sequelae. *American Journal of Physical Medicine and Rehabilitation* 77(4):339-343.

Bruno RL, Creange SJ, Frick NM. (1998). Parallels between post-polio fatigue and chronic fatigue syndrome: A common pathophysiology? *American Journal of Medicine* 105(3A):66S-73S.

Bruno RL, Creange S, Zimmerman JR, Frick NM. (1998). Elevated plasma prolactin and EEG slow wave power in post-polio fatigue: Implications for a dopamine deficiency underlying post-viral fatigue syndromes. *Journal of Chronic Fatigue Syndrome* 4(2):61-76.

Bruno RL, Zimmerman JR, Creange SJ, Lewis T, Molzen T, Frick NM. (1996). Bromocriptine in the treatment of post-polio fatigue: A pilot study with implications for the pathophysiology of fatigue. *American Journal of Physical Medicine and Rehabilitation* 75(5):340-347.

Brusick D, Mengs U. (1997). Assessment of the genotoxic risk from laxative senna products. *Environmental and Molecular Mutagenesis* 29(1):1-9.

Bryan CF, Eastman J, Conner B, Baier KA, Durham JB. (1993). Clinical utility of a lymph node normal range obtained by flow cytometry. *Annals of the New York Academy of Sciences* 667:404-406.

Buchali A, Feyer P, Groll J, Massenkeil G, Arnold R, Budach V. (2000). Immediate toxicity during fractionated total body irradiation as conditioning for bone marrow transplantation. *Radiotherapy in Oncology* 54(2):157-162.

Buchsel PC, Murphy BJ, Newton SA. (2002). Epoetin alfa: Current and future indications and nursing implications. *Clinical Journal of Oncology Nursing* 6(5): 261-267.

Buchwald D. (1996). Fibromyalgia and chronic fatigue syndrome: Similarities and differences. *Rheumatic Diseases Clinics of North America* 22(2):219-243.

Buchwald D, Ashley RL, Pearlman T, Kith P, Komaroff AL. (1996). Viral serologies in patients with chronic fatigue and chronic fatigue syndrome. *Journal of Medical Virology* 50(1):25-30.

Buchwald D, Komaroff AL. (1991). Review of laboratory findings for patients with chronic fatigue syndrome. *Review of Infectious Diseases* 13(1):S12-S18.

Buchwald D, Pearlman T, Umali J, Schmaling K, Katon W. (1996). Functional status in patients with chronic fatigue syndrome, other fatiguing illnesses, and healthy individuals. *American Journal of Medicine* 101(4):364-370.

Buchwald D, Umali J, Pearlman T, Kith P, Ashley R, Wener M. (1996). Postinfectious chronic fatigue: A distinct syndrome? *Clinical Infectious Diseases* 23(2):385-387.

Buchwald D, Umali J, Stene M. (1996). Insulin-like growth factor-I (somatomedin C) levels in chronic fatigue syndrome and fibromyalgia. *Journal of Rheumatology* 23(4):739-742.

Buchwald D, Wener MH, Pearlman T, Kith P. (1997). Markers of inflammation and immune activation in chronic fatigue and chronic fatigue syndrome. *Journal of Rheumatology* 23(8):1392-1397.

Buchwalter CL, Miller D, Jenison EL. (2001). Hemolytic anemia and benign pelvic tumors: A case report. *Journal of Reproductive Medicine* 46(4):401-404.

Buckelew SP, Conway R, Parker J, Deuser WE, Read J, Witty TE, Hewett JE, Minor M, Johnson JC, Van Male L, et al. (1998). Biofeedback/relaxation training and exercise intervention for fibromyalgia: A prospective trial. *Arthritis Care Research* 11(3):196-209.

Buckingham R, Fitt J, Sitzia J. (1997). Patients' experiences of chemotherapy: Side-effects of carboplatin in the treatment of carcinoma of the ovary. *European Journal of Cancer Care* 6(1):59-71.

Buckner JC, Burch PA, Cascino TL, O'Fallon JR, Scheithauer BW. (1998). Phase II trial of recombinant interferon-alpha-2a and eflornithine in patients with recurrent glioma. *Journal of Neurooncology* 36(1):65-70.

Buckwalter JA, Lappin DR. (2000). The disproportionate impact of chronic arthralgia and arthritis among women. *Clinical Orthopedics* 372:159-168.

Budd GT, Green S, Baker LH, Hersh EP, Weick JK, Osborne CK. (1991). A Southwest Oncology Group phase II trial of recombinant tumor necrosis factor in metastatic breast cancer. *Cancer* 68(8):1694-1695.

Budgett R. (1998). Fatigue and underperformance in athletes: The overtraining syndrome. *British Journal of Sports Medicine* 32(2):107-110.

Budman DR, Igwemezie LN, Kaul S, Behr J, Lichtman S, Schulman P, Vinciguerra V, Allen SL, Kolitz J, Hock K, et al. (1994). Phase I evaluation of a water-soluble etoposide prodrug, etoposide phosphate, given as a 5-minute infusion on days 1, 3, and 5 in patients with solid tumors. *Journal of Clinical Oncology* 12(9):1902-1909.

Budman DR, Weiselberg L, O'Mara V, Buchbinder A, Lichtman SM, Donahue L, Adams LM. (1999). A phase I study of sequential vinorelbine followed by paclitaxel. *Annals of Oncology* 10(7):861-863.

Buja LM. (1996). Does atherosclerosis have an infectious etiology? *Circulation* 94:872-873.

Bujak DI, Weinstein A, Dornbush RL. (1996). Lyme disease: Clinical and neurocognitive features of the post-Lyme syndrome. *The Journal of Rheumatology* 23(8):1392-1397.

Bukowski R, Ernstoff MS, Gore ME, Nemunaitis JJ, Amato R, Gupta SK, Tendler CL. (2002). Pegylated interferon alfa-2b treatment for patients with solid tumors: A phase I/II study. *Journal of Clinical Oncology* 20(18):3841-3849.

Bukowski RM, Sergi JS, Sharfman WJ, Budd GT, Murthy S, Barna B, Medendorp SV, Yen-Lieberman B, Gibson V, Bauer L, et al. (1991). Phase I trial of natural human interferon beta in metastatic malignancy. *Cancer Research* 51(3):836-840.

Bull JM, Lees D, Schuette W, Whang-Peng J, Smith R, Bynum G, Atkinson ER, Gottdiener JS, Gralnick HR, Shawker TH, et al. (1979). Whole body hyperthermia: A phase-I trial of a potential adjuvant to chemotherapy. *Annals of Internal Medicine* 90(3):317-323.

Bull SS, Melian M. (1998). Contraception and culture: The use of yuyos in Paraguay. *Health Care for Women International* 19(1):49-60.

Bunn PA Jr, Ihde DC, Foon KA. (1987). Recombinant interferon alfa-2a, an active agent in advanced cutaneous T-cell lymphomas. *International Journal of Cancer* 1:9-13.

Burch PA, Breen JK, Buckner JC, Gastineau DA, Kaur JA, Laus RL, Padley DJ, Peshwa MV, Pitot HC, Richardson RL, et al. (2000). Priming tissue-specific cellular immunity in a phase I trial of autologous dendritic cells for prostate cancer. *Clinical Cancer Research* 6(6):2175-2182.

Burckhardt CS, Bjelle A. (1996). Perceived control: A comparison of women with fibromyalgia, rheumatoid arthritis, and systemic lupus erythematosus using a Swedish version of the Rheumatology Attitudes Index. *Scandinavian Journal of Rheumatology* 25(5):300-306.

Burge FI. (1993). Dehydration symptoms of palliative care cancer patients. *Journal of Pain Symptomatology Management* 8(7):454-464.

Burks TF. (2001). New agents for the treatment of cancer-related fatigue. *Cancer* 92(6 Suppl):1714-1718.

Burman LG, Lundblad G, Camner P, Fange R, Lundborg M, Soder P. (1991). [Lysozyme—An enzyme of both historical and current interest as a therapeutical agent]. *Lakartidningen* 88(44):3665-3668.

Burris HA III, Awada A, Kuhn JG, Eckardt JR, Cobb PW, Rinaldi DA, Fields S, Smith L, Von Hoff DD. (1994). Phase I and pharmacokinetic studies of topotecan administered as a 72 or 120 h continuous infusion. *Anticancer Drugs* 5(4):394-402.

Burrows M, Dibble SL, Miaskowski C. (1998). Differences in outcomes among patients experiencing different types of cancer-related pain. *Oncology Nursing Forum* 25(4):735-741.

Burski K, Torjussen B, Paulsen AQ, Boman H, Bollerslev J. (2002). Parathyroid adenoma in a subject with familial hypocalciuric hypercalcemia: Coincidence or causality? *Journal of Clinical Endocrinology and Metabolism* 87(3):1015-1016.

Burstein HJ, Manola J, Younger J, Parker LM, Bunnell CA, Scheib R, Matulonis UA, Garber JE, Clarke KD, Shulman LN, et al. (2000). Docetaxel administered on a weekly basis for metastatic breast cancer. *Journal of Clinical Oncology* 18(6):1212-1219.

Busbridge J, Dacombe MJ, Hopkins S. (1989). Acute central effects of interleukin-6 on body temperature, thermogenesis and food intake in the rat. *Proceedings of the Nutrition Society* 38:48A.

Bush NE, Donaldson GW, Haberman MH, Dacanay R, Sullivan KM. (2000). Conditional and unconditional estimation of multidimensional quality of life after hematopoietic stem cell transplantation: A longitudinal follow-up of 415 patients. *Biology, Blood, and Marrow Transplantation* 6(5A):576-591.

Bush NE, Haberman M, Donaldson G, Sullivan KM. (1995). Quality of life of 125 adults surviving 6-18 years after bone marrow transplantation. *Social Sciences and Medicine* 40(4):479-490.

Buskila D. (1996). Fibromyalgia in children—Lessons from assessing nonarticular tenderness. *Journal of Rheumatology* 23(12):2017-2079.

Buskila D. (1999). Fibromyalgia, chronic fatigue syndrome, and myofascial pain syndrome. *Current Opinions in Rheumatology* 11(2):119-126.

Buskila D. (2000). Fibromyalgia, chronic fatigue syndrome, and myofascial pain syndrome. *Current Opinions in Rheumatology* 12(2):113-123.

Buskila D, Neumann L, Alhoashle A, Abu-Shakra M. (2000). Fibromyalgia syndrome in men. *Seminars in Arthritis and Rheumatism* 30(1):47-51.

Buskila D, Neumann L, Sibirski D, Shvartzman P. (1997). Awareness of diagnostic and clinical features of fibromyalgia among family physicians. *Family Practice* 14(3):238-241.

Buskila D, Zaks N, Neumann L, Livneh A, Greenberg S, Pras M, Langevitz P. (1997). Quality of life in patients with familial Mediterranean fever. *Clinical and Experimental Rheumatology* 15(4):355-360.

Butler C, Rollnick S. (1996). Missing the meaning and provoking resistance: A case of myalgic encephalomyelitis. *Family Practice* 13(1):106-109.

Butler L. (1998). Fatigue in cancer care leads the way for nursing education in Nova Scotia. *Canadian Oncology Nursing Journal* 8(S1):S18.

Butler S, Chalder T, Ron M, Wessely S. (1991). Cognitive behavior therapy in chronic fatigue syndrome. *Journal of Neurology, Neurosurgery and Psychiatry* 54:153-158.

Butow P, Coates A, Dunn S, Bernhard J, Hurny C. (1991). On the receiving end: IV. Validation of quality of life indicators. *Annals of Oncology* 2(8):597-603.

Buzaid AC, Murren J, Durivage HJ. (1991). High-dose cisplatin plus WR-2721 in a split course in metastatic malignant melanoma: A phase II study. *American Journal of Clinical Oncology* 14(3):203-207.

Buzdar AU. (2000). Exemestane in advanced breast cancer. *Anticancer Drugs* 11(8): 609-616.

Buzdar AU, Kau S, Hortobagyi GN, Theriault RL, Booser D, Holmes FA, Walters R, Krakoff IH. (1994). Phase I trial of droloxifene in patients with metastatic breast cancer. *Cancer Chemotherapy Pharmacology* 33(4):313-316.

Bye A, Ose T, Kaasa S. (1995). Quality of life during pelvic radiotherapy. *Acta Obstetrica Gynecologica Scandinavica* 74(2):147-152.

Byeon SW, Pelley RP, Ullrich SE, Waller TA, Bucana CD, Strickland FM. (1998). *Aloë barbadensis* extracts reduce the production of interleukin-10 after exposure to ultraviolet radiation. *Journal of Investigative Dermatology* 100(5):811-817.

Caan BJ, Flatt SW, Rock CL, Ritenbaugh C, Newman V, Pierce JP. (2000). Low-energy reporting in women at risk for breast cancer recurrence. Women's Healthy Eating and Living Group. *Cancer Epidemiology, Biomarkers, and Prevention* 9(10):1091-1097.

Cabral DA, Tucker LB. (1999). Malignancies in children who initially present with rheumatic complaints. *Journal of Pediatrics* 134(1):53-57.

Calabrese JR, Kling MA, Gold PA. (1987). Alterations in immunocompetence during stress, bereavement, and depression: Focus on neuroendocrine regulation. *American Journal of Psychiatry* 144:1123-1134.

Calabrese LH. (1990). Exercise, immunity, cancer and infection. In *Exercise, Fitness and Health,* Bouchard C, Shephard R, Stephens T, eds. Champaign, IL: Human Kinetics, pp. 567-590.

Caligiuri M, Murray C, Buchwald D, Levine H, Cheney P, Peterson D, Komaroff AL, Kitz J. (1987). Phenotypic and functional deficiency of natural killer cells in patients with chronic fatigue syndrome. *Journal of Immunology* 139(10):3306-3313.

Callahan LF, Blalock SJ. (1997). Behavioral and social research in rheumatology. *Current Opinions in Rheumatology* 9(2):126-132.

Calvo E, Cortes J, Rodriguez J, Sureda M, Beltran C, Rebollo J, Martinez-Monge R, Berian JM, de Irala J, Brugarolas A. (2001). Fixed higher dose schedule of suramin plus hydrocortisone in patients with hormone refractory prostate carcinoma: A multicenter phase II study. *Cancer* 92(9):2435-2443.

Camilleri-Brennan J, Steele RJ. (2001). Prospective analysis of quality of life and survival following mesorectal excision for rectal cancer. *British Journal of Surgery* 88(12):1617-1622.

Campbell SM, Clark S, Tindall EA, Forehand ME, Bennett RM. (1983). Clinical characteristics of fibrositis: I. A "blinded," controlled study of symptoms and tender points. *Arthritis and Rheumatism* 26:817-824.

Canevari S, Stoter G, Arienti F, Bolis G, Colnaghi MI, Di Re EM, Eggermont AM, Goey SH, Gratama JW, Lamers CH, et al. (1995). Regression of advanced ovarian carcinoma by intraperitoneal treatment with autologous T lymphocytes retargeted by a bispecific monoclonal antibody. *Journal of the National Cancer Institutes* 87(19):1463-1469.

Cannon JG, Angel JB, Abad LW, O'Grady J, Lundgren N, Fagioli L, Komaroff AL. (1998). Hormonal influences on stress-induced neutrophil mobilization in health and chronic fatigue syndrome. *Journal of Clinical Immunology* 18(4):291-298.

Cannon JG, Angel JB, Abad LW, Vannier E, Mileno MD, Fagioli L, Wolff SM, Komaroff AL. (1997). Interleukin-1beta, interleukin-1 receptor antagonist, and soluble interleukin-1 receptor type II secretion in chronic fatigue syndrome. *Journal of Clinical Immunology* 17(3):253-261.

Cannon JG, Angel JB, Ball RW, Abad LW, Fagioli L, Komaroff AL. (1999). Acute phase responses and cytokine secretion in chronic fatigue syndrome. *Journal of Clinical Immunology* 19(6):414-421.

Cannova JV. (1998). Multiple giant cell tumors in a patient with Gulf War syndrome. *Military Medicine* 163(3):184-185.

Canonica GW, Bagnasco M, Corte G, Ferrini S, Ferrini O, Giordano G. (1982). Circulating T lymphocytes in Hashimoto's disease: Imbalance of subsets and presence of activated cells. *Clinical Immunology and Immunopathology* 23:616-625.

Cantor H, Boyse EA. (1977). Regulation of cellular and humoral immune responses by T-cell subclasses. *Cold Spring Harbor Symposia on Quantitative Biology* 41:23-32.

Canver CC, Lajos TZ, Bernstein Z, DuBois DP, Mentzer RM Jr. (1990). Intracavitary melanoma of the left atrium. *Annals of Thoracic Surgery* 49(2):312-313.

Caplan C. (1998). Chronic fatigue syndrome or just plain tired? *Canadian Medical Association Journal* 159(5):519-520.

Capodaglio P, Strada MR, Lodola E, Grilli C, Panigazzi M, Bazzini G, Bernardo G. (1997). Work capacity of the upper limbs after mastectomy. *Giornale Italiano di Medizina dei Lavoro et Ergonomica* 19(4):172-176.

Caponigro F. (2002). Farnesyl transferase inhibitors: A major breakthrough in anticancer therapy? Naples, April 12, 2002. *Anticancer Drugs* 13(8):891-897.

Capuron L, Gumnick JF, Musselman DL, Lawson DH, Reemsnyder A, Nemeroff CB, Miller AH. (2002). Neurobehavioral effects of interferon-alpha in cancer patients: Phenomenology and paroxetine responsiveness of symptom dimensions. *Neuropsychopharmacology* 26(5):643-652.

Caraceni A, Gangeri L, Martini C, Belli F, Brunelli C, Baldini M, Mascheroni L, Lenisa L, Cascinelli N. (1998). Neurotoxicity of interferon-alpha in melanoma therapy: Results from a randomized controlled trial. *Cancer* 83(3):482-489.

Cardoso F, Ferreira Filho AF, Crown J, Dolci S, Paesmans M, Riva A, Di Leo A, Piccart MJ. (2001). Doxorubicin followed by docetaxel versus docetaxel followed by doxorubicin in the adjuvant treatment of node positive breast cancer: Results of a feasibility study. *Anticancer Research* 21(1B):789-795.

Carducci MA, Gilbert J, Bowling MK, Noe D, Eisenberger MA, Sinibaldi V, Zabelina Y, Chen TL, Grochow LB, Donehower RC. (2001). A phase I clinical and pharmacological evaluation of sodium phenylbutyrate on an 120-h infusion schedule. *Clinical Cancer Research* 7(10):3047-3055.

Carelle N, Piotto E, Bellanger A, Germanaud J, Thuillier A, Khayat D. (2002). Changing patient perceptions of the side effects of cancer chemotherapy. *Cancer* 95(1):155-163.

Carenza L, Villani C, Framarino dei Malatesta ML, Porta RP, Millefiorini M, Antonini G, Bolasco P, Bandiera G, Marzetti L. (1986). Peripheral neuropathy and ototoxicity of dichlorodiamineplatinum: Instrumental evaluation, preliminary results. *Gynecological Oncology* 25(2):244-249.

Carlin BW, Dianzumba SB, Wendel C, Joyner CR. (1986). Right ventricular inflow and outflow obstruction due to adrenal cell carcinoma. *Catheterization Cardiovascular Diagnosis* 12(1):51-54.

Carlsson M, Strang P, Bjurstrom C. (2000). Treatment modality affects long-term quality of life in gynaecological cancer. *Anticancer Research* 20(1B):563-568.

Carpano S, Amodio A, Bucher S, Foggi P, Vici P, Rinaldi M, Mariotti S, Del Monte G, Lopez M. (1999). [Chemotherapy of advanced stage melanoma using cisplatin, epirubicin and alpha-interferon]. *Clinica y Terapia* 150(2):109-114.

Carpenter JS, Gautam S, Freedman RR, Andrykowski M. (2001). Circadian rhythm of objectively recorded hot flashes in postmenopausal breast cancer survivors. *Menopause* 8(3):181-188.

Carriere B, Cummins-Mcmanus B. (2001). Vertebral fractures as initial signs for acute lymphoblastic leukemia. *Pediatric Emergency Care* 17(4):258-261.

Carter BD, Kronenberger WG, Edwards JF, Michalczyk L, Marshall GS. (1996). Differential diagnosis of chronic fatigue in children: Behavioral and emotional dimensions. *Journal of Development and Behavioral Pediatrics* 17(1):16-21.

Carter WA, De Clercq E. (1974). Viral infection and host defense. *Science* 186: 1172-1178.

Carver LA, Connallon PF, Flanigan SJ, Crossley-Miller MK. (1994). Epstein-Barr virus infection in Desert Storm reservists. *Military Medicine* 159(8):580-582.

Casale GP, Vennerstrom JL, Bavari S, Wang TL. (1993). Inhibition of interleukin 2 driven proliferation of mouse CTLL2 cells, by selected carbamate and organophosphate insecticides and congeners of carbaryl. *Immunopharmacology and Immunotoxicology* 15(2-3):199-215.

Casali P, Notkins AL. (1989). CD5+ B lymphocytes, polyreactive antibodies and the human B cell repertoire. *Immunology Today* 10:364-368.

Cascinu S, Casadei V, Del Ferro E, Alessandroni P, Catalano G. (1996). Pamidronate in patients with painful bone metastases, who failed initial treatment with hormones and/or chemotherapy. *Support Care in Cancer* 4(1):31-33.

Cascinu S, Gasparini G, Catalano V, Silva RR, Pancera G, Morabito A, Giordani P, Gattuso D, Catalano G. (1999). A phase I-II study of gemcitabine and docetaxel in advanced pancreatic cancer: A report from the Italian Group for the Study of Digestive Tract Cancer (GISCAD). *Annals of Oncology* 10(11):1377-1379.

Cascinu S, Graziano F, Barni S, Labianca R, Comella G, Casaretti R, Frontini L, Catalano V, Baldelli AM, Catalano G. (2001). A phase II study of sequential chemotherapy with docetaxel after the weekly PELF regimen in advanced gastric cancer: A report from the Italian group for the study of digestive tract cancer. *British Journal of Cancer* 84(4):470-474.

Casey LC, Balk RA, Bone RC. (1993). Plasma cytokines and endotoxin levels correlate with survival in patients with sepsis syndrome. *Annals of Internal Medicine* 21:771-778.

Casper ES, Christman KL, Schwartz GK, Johnson B, Brennan MF, Bertino JR. (1993). Edatrexate in patients with soft tissue sarcoma: Activity in malignant fibrous histiocytoma. *Cancer* 72(3):766-770.

Casper ES, Schwartz GK, Sugarman A, Leung D, Brennan MF. (1997). Phase I trial of dose-intense liposome-encapsulated doxorubicin in patients with advanced sarcoma. *Journal of Clinical Oncology* 15(5):2111-2117.

Cassetta RA. (1995). Waging a battle against cancer pain and fatigue. *American Nurse* 27(1):16.

Cassidy JT. (1998). Progress in diagnosis and understanding chronic pain syndromes in children and adolescents. *Adolescent Medicine* 9(1):101-114.

Castellano TJ, Frank MS, Brandt LJ, Mahadevia P. (1981). Metachronous carcinoma complicating Crohn's disease. *Archives of Internal Medicine* 141(8):1074-1075.

Catalona WJ, Hudson MA, Gillen DP, Andriole GL, Ratliff TL. (1987). Risks and benefits of repeated courses of intravesical bacillus Calmette-Guérin therapy for superficial bladder cancer. *Journal of Urology* 137:220.

Catania PN. (1998). Poblems with herbal remedies in anticoagulated home care patients. *Home Care Provider* 3(5):253-255.

Cathebras P. (1997). [What is a disease?] Qu'est-ce qu'une maladie? *Revue Medicine Interne* 18(10):809-813.

Cathebras P. (2000). [Should fibromyalgia survive the century?] La fibromyalgie doit-elle passer le siecle? *Revue Medicine Interne* 21(7):577-579.

Cathebras P, Lauwers A, Rousset H. (1998). [Fibromyalgia: A citical review] La fibromyalgie: Une revue critique. *Annales Medicine Interne* (Paris) 149(7):406-414.

Catimel G, Chabot GG, Guastalla JP, Dumortier A, Cote C, Engel C, Gouyette A, Mathieu-Boue A, Mahjoubi M, Clavel M. (1995). Phase I and pharmacokinetic study of irinotecan (CPT-11) administered daily for three consecutive days every three weeks in patients with advanced solid tumors. *Annals of Oncology* 6(2):133-140.

Catimel G, Vermorken JB, Clavel M, de Mulder P, Judson I, Sessa C, Piccart M, Bruntsch U, Verweij J, Wanders J, et al. (1994). A phase II study of gemcitabine (LY 188011) in patients with advanced squamous cell carcinoma of the head and neck. EORTC Early Clinical Trials Group. *Annals of Oncology* 5(6):543-547.

Caverzasio J, Rizzoli R, Dayer JM. (1987). Interleukin-1 decreases renal sodium reabsorption: Possible mechanisms of endotoxin-induced natriuresis. *American Journal of Physiology* 252:943-946.

Cavestro GM, Mantovani N, Coruzzi P, Nouvenne A, Marcucci F, Franze A, Di Mario F, Okolicsanyi L. (2002). Hypercalcemia due to ectopic secretion of parathyroid related protein from pancreatic carcinoma: A case report. *Acta Biomedica Ateneo Parmense* 73(1-2):37-40.

Celiker R, Borman P, Oktem F, Gokce-Kutsal Y, Basgoze O. (1997). Psychological disturbance in fibromyalgia: Relation to pain severity. *Clinical Rheumatology* 16(2):179-184.

Cella D. (1997). The Functional Assessment of Cancer Therapy-Anemia (FACT-An) Scale: A new tool for the assessment of outcomes in cancer anemia and fatigue. *Seminars in Hematology* 34(3 Suppl 2):13-19.

Cella D. (1998). Factors influencing quality of life in cancer patients: Anemia and fatigue. *Seminars in Oncology* 25(3 Suppl 7):43-46.

Cella D. (2002). The effects of anemia and anemia treatment on the quality of life of people with cancer. *Oncology* 16(9 Suppl 10):125-132.

Cella D, Bron D. (1999). The effect of epoetin alfa on quality of life in anemic cancer patients. *Cancer Practice* 7(4):177-182.

Cella D, Davis K, Breitbart W, Curt G. (2001). Cancer-related fatigue: Prevalence of proposed diagnostic criteria in a United States sample of cancer survivors. *Journal of Clinical Oncology* 19(14):3385-3391.

Cella D, Dineen K, Arnason B, Reder A, Webster KA, Karabatsos G, Chang C, Lloyd S, Steward J, Stefoski D. (1996). Validation of the functional assessment of multiple sclerosis quality of life instrument. *Neurology* 47(1):129-139.

Cella D, Lai JS, Chang CH, Peterman A, Slavin M. (2002). Fatigue in cancer patients compared with fatigue in the general United States population. *Cancer* 94(2):528-538.

Cella D, Peterman A, Passik S, Jacobsen P, Breitbart W. (1998). Progress toward guidelines for the management of fatigue. *Oncology* 12(11A):369-377.

Cella D, Webster K. (1997). Linking outcomes management to quality-of-life measurement. *Oncology* 11(11A):232-235.

Chagpar A. (1996). Chronic fatigue syndrome: A prodrome to psychosis? *Canadian Journal of Psychiatry—Revue Canadienne de Psychiatrie* 41(8):536-537.

Chakravarthy A, Abrams RA, Yeo CJ, Korman LT, Donehower RC, Hruban RH, Zahurek ML, Grochow LB, O'Reilly S, Hurwitz H, et al. (2000). Intensified adjuvant combined modality therapy for resected periampullary adenocarcinoma: Acceptable toxicity and suggestion of improved 1-year disease-free survival. *International Journal of Radiation Oncology, Biology, and Physics* 48(4):1089-1096.

Chalder T, Berelowitz G, Pawlikowska J, Watts L, Wessely D. (1993). Development of a fatigue scale. *Journal of Psychosomatic Research* 37:147-153.

Chalder T, Power MJ, Wessely S. (1996). Chronic fatigue in the community: A question of attribution. *Psychological Medicine* 26(4):791-800.

Chamberlain MC. (2002). A phase II trial of intra-cerebrospinal fluid alpha interferon in the treatment of neoplastic meningitis. *Cancer* 94(10):2675-2680.

Chambers CR. (1997). Fireworks over fibromyalgia, CFS, and IBS. *Postgraduate Medicine* 102(6):43.

Chan CW, Molassiotis A. (2001). The impact of fatigue on Chinese cancer patients in Hong Kong. *Support Care and Cancer* 9(1):18-24.

Chandola A, Young Y, McAllister J, Axford JS. (1999). Use of complementary therapies by patients attending musculoskeletal clinics. *Journal of the Royal Society of Medicine* 92(1):13-16.

Chandran Nair B, DeVico AL, Nakamura S, Copeland TD, Chen Y, Patel A, O'Neil T, Oroszlan S, Gallo RC, Sarngadharan MG. (1992). Identification of a major growth factor for AIDS-Kaposi's sarcoma cells as oncostatin M. *Science* 255:1430-1440.

Chanecka EJ. (1998). Traditional medicine in Belize: The original primary health care. *Nursing Health Care Perspective* 19(4):178-185.

Chang AY, Boros L, Garrow G, Asbury R. (1995). Paclitaxel by 3-hour infusion followed by 96-hour infusion on failure in patients with refractory malignant disease. *Seminars in Oncology* 22(3 Suppl 6):124-127.

Chang AY, Fisher HA, Spiers AS, Boros L. (1986). Toxicities of human recombinant interferon-alpha 2 in patients with advanced prostate carcinoma. *Journal of Interferon Research* 6(6):713-715.

Chang AY, Garrow GC. (1995). Pilot study of vinorelbine (Navelbine) and paclitaxel (Taxol) in patients with refractory breast cancer and lung cancer. *Seminars in Oncology* 22(2 Suppl 5):66-70; discussion 70-71.

Chang AY, Rubins J, Asbury R, Boros L, Hui LF. (2001). Weekly paclitaxel in advanced non-small cell lung cancer. *Seminars in Oncology* 28(4 Suppl 14):10-13.

Chang J. (1999). Scientific evaluation of traditional Chinese medicine under DSHEA: A conundrum. Dietary Supplement Health and Education Act. *Journal of Alternative and Complementary Medicine* 5(2):181-189.

Chang SM, Kuhn JG, Rizzo J, Robins HI, Schold SC Jr, Spence AM, Berger MS, Mehta MP, Bozik ME, Pollack I, et al. (1998). Phase I study of paclitaxel in patients with recurrent malignant glioma: A North American Brain Tumor Consortium report. *Journal of Clinical Oncology* 16(6):2188-2194.

Chang SM, Kuhn JG, Robins HI, Schold SC, Spence AM, Berger MS, Mehta MP, Bozik ME, Pollack I, Schiff D, et al. (1999). Phase II study of phenylacetate in patients with recurrent malignant glioma: A North American Brain Tumor Consortium report. *Journal of Clinical Oncology* 17(3):984-990.

Chang VT, Hwang SS, Feuerman M, Kasimis BS. (2000). Symptom and quality of life survey of medical oncology patients at a veterans affairs medical center: A role for symptom assessment. *Cancer* 88(5):1175-1183.

Chao CC, Gallagher M, Phair J, Peterson PK. (1990). Serum neopterin and interleukin-6 levels in chronic fatigue syndrome. *Journal of Infectious Diseases* 162:1412-1413.

Chao CC, Janof EN, Hu SX, Thomas K, Gallagher M, Tsang M, Peterson PK. (1991). Altered cytokine release in peripheral blood mononuclear cell cultures from patients with chronic fatigue syndrome. *Cytokine* 3(4):292-298.

Chapekar MS, Glazer RI. (1988). The synergistic cytocidal effect produced by immune interferon and tumor necrosis factor in HT-29 cells is associated with inhibition of rRNA processing and (2,5)-oligo(A) activation of RNase L. *Biochemical and Biophysical Research Communications* 151:1180-1187.

Chapman GB, Elstein AS, Kuzel TM, Nadler RB, Sharifi R, Bennett CL. (1999). A multi-attribute model of prostate cancer patients' preferences for health states. *Quality of Life Research* 8(3):171-180.

Chapman KM, Nelson RA. (1994). Loss of appetite: Managing unwanted weight loss in the older patient. *Geriatrics* 49(3):54-59.

Chapman PB, Einhorn LH, Meyers ML, Saxman S, Destro AN, Panageas KS, Begg CB, Agarwala SS, Schuchter LM, Ernstoff MS, et al. (1999). Phase III multicenter randomized trial of the Dartmouth regimen versus dacarbazine in patients with metastatic melanoma. *Journal of Clinical Oncology* 17(9):2745-2751.

Chapman PB, Lester TJ, Casper ES, Gabrilove JL, Wong GY, Kempin SJ, Gold PJ, Welt S, Warren RS, Starnes HF, et al. (1987). Clinical pharmacology of recombinant human tumor necrosis factor in patients with advanced cancer. *Journal of Clinical Oncology* 5(12):1942-1951.

Chapman PB, Morrissey DM, Panageas KS, Hamilton WB, Zhan C, Destro AN, Williams L, Israel RJ, Livingston PO. (2000). Induction of antibodies against GM2 ganglioside by immunizing melanoma patients using GM2-keyhole limpet hemocyanin + QS21 vaccine: A dose-response study. *Clinical Cancer Research* 6(3):874-879.

Chapman R, Kelsen D, Gralla R, Itri L, Casper E, Young C, Golbey R. (1981). Phase II trial of methylglyoxal-bis-(guanylhydrazone) in non-small-cell lung cancer. *Cancer Clinical Trials* 4(4):389-391.

Charlesworth EA, Nathan RG. (1984). *Stress Management: A Comprehensive Guide to Wellness*. New York: Ballantine Books.

Chaturvedi SK, Maguire GP. (1998). Persistent somatization in cancer: A controlled follow-up study. *Journal of Psychosomatic Research* 45(3):249-256.

Chauhan O, Godhwani JL, Khanna NK, Pendse VK. (1998). Anti-inflammatory activity of *Muktashukti bhasma*. *Indian Journal of Experimental Biology* 36(10): 985-989.

Cheeseman SL, Brannan M, McGown A, Khan P, Gardner C, Gumbrell L, Dickens D, Ranson M. (2000). Phase I and pharmacologic study of CT-2584 HMS, a modulator of phosphatidic acid, in adult patients with solid tumours. *British Journal of Cancer* 83(12):1599-1606.

Chelf JH, Agre P, Axelrod A, Cheney L, Cole DD, Conrad K, Hooper S, Liu I, Mercurio A, Stepan K, et al. (2001). Cancer-related patient education: An overview of the last decade of evaluation and research. *Oncology Nursing Forum* 28(7):1139-1147.

Chen JS, Jan YY, Lin YC, Wang HM, Chang WC, Liau CT. (1998). Weekly 24 h infusion of high-dose 5-fluorouracil and leucovorin in patients with biliary tract carcinomas. *Anticancer Drugs* 9(5):393-397.

Chen MN, Nakazawa S, Hori M. (1993). [A case of primary intracranial chorio-carcinoma with a carotid-cavernous fistula]. *No Shinkei Geka* 21(11):1031-1034.

Chen PM, Lin SH, Fan SF, Chiou TJ, Hsieh RK, Yu IT, Liu JH. (1997). Genotypic characterization and multivariate survival analysis of chronic lymphocytic leukemia in Taiwan. *Acta Haematologica* 97(4):196-204.

Chen YM, Perng RP, Yang KY, Liu TW, Tsai CM, Ming-Liu J, Whang-Peng J. (2000). A multicenter phase II trial of vinorelbine plus gemcitabine in previously untreated inoperable (stage IIIB/IV) non-small cell lung cancer. *Chest* 117(6): 1583-1589.

Cheney PR, Dorman SE, Bell DS. (1989). Interleukin-2 and the chronic fatigue syndrome. *Annals of Internal Medicine* 110(4):321.

Cheng TJ, Wong RH, Lin YP, Hwang YH, Horng JJ, Wang JD. (1998). Chinese herbal medicine, sibship, and blood lead in children. *Occupational Environmental Medicine* 55(8):573-576.

Cherin P, Authier FJ, Gherardi RK, Romero N, Laforet P, Eymard B, Herson S, Caillat-Vigneron N. (2000). Gallium-67 scintigraphy in macrophagic myofasciitis. *Arthritis and Rheumatism* 43(7):1520-1526.

Chernecky C. (1999). Temporal differences in coping, mood, and stress with chemotherapy. *Cancer Nursing* 22(4):266-276.

Chester AC. (1997a). Chronic fatigue syndrome criteria in patients with other forms of unexplained chronic fatigue. *Journal of Psychiatric Research* 31(1):45-50.

Chester AC. (1997b). Neurally mediated hypotension, chronic fatigue syndrome and upper aerodigestive tract reflexes. *Integrative Physiological and Behavioral Science* 32(2):160-161.

Chester AC, Levine PH. (1997). The natural history of concurrent sick building syndrome and chronic fatigue syndrome. *Journal of Psychiatric Research* 31(1):51-57.

Cheung F, Lim KM. (1997). Neurasthenia, depression and somatoform disorder in a Chinese-Vietnamese woman migrant. *Culture, Medicine and Psychiatry* 21(2): 247-258.

Cheynier R, Langlade-Demoyen P, Marescot MR, Blanche S, Blondin G, Wain-Hobson S, Griselli C, Vilmer E, Plata F. (1992). Cytotoxic T lymphocyte responses in the peripheral blood of children born to human immunodeficiency virus-1-infected mothers. *European Journal of Immunology* 22(9):2211-2217.

Chi KN, Gleave ME, Klasa R, Murray N, Bryce C, Lopes de Menezes DE, D'Aloisio S, Tolcher AW. (2001). A phase I dose-finding study of combined treatment with an antisense Bcl-2 oligonucleotide (Genasense) and mitoxantrone in patients with metastatic hormone-refractory prostate cancer. *Clinical Cancer Research* 7(12):3920-3927.

Chia JK, Chia LY. (1999). Chronic *Chlamydia pneumoniae* infection: A treatable cause of chronic fatigue syndrome. *Clinical Infectious Diseases* 29(2):452-453.

Chigot JP, Menegaux F, Achrafi H. (1995). Should primary hyperparathyroidism be treated surgically in elderly patients older than 75 years? *Surgery* 117(4):397-401.

Childs HA III, Spencer SA, Raben D, Bonner JA, Newsome J, Robert F. (2000). A phase I study of combined UFT plus leucovorin and radiotherapy for pancreatic cancer. *International Journal of Radiation Oncology, Biology, and Physics* 47(4):939-944.

Chimenti S, Peris K, Di Cristofaro S, Fargnoli MC, Torlone G. (1995). Use of recombinant interferon alfa-2b in the treatment of basal cell carcinoma. *Dermatology* 190(3):214-217.

Chithra P, Sajithlal GB, Chandrakasan G. (1998a). Influence of *Aloë vera* on collagen characteristics in healing dermal wounds in rats. *Molecular and Cellular Biochemistry* 181(1-2):71-76.

Chithra P, Sajithlal GB, Chandrakasan G. (1998b). Influence of *Aloë vera* on collagen turnover in healing of dermal wounds in rats. *Indian Journal of Experimental Biology* 36(9):896-901.

Chithra P, Sajithlal GB, Chandrakasan G. (1998c). Influence of *Aloë vera* on the glycosaminoglycans in the matrix of healing dermal wounds in rats. *Journal of Ethnopharmacology* 59(3):179-186.

Chithra P, Sajithlal GB, Chandrakasan G. (1998d). Influence of *Aloë vera* on the healing of dermal wounds in diabetic rats. *Journal of Ethnopharmacology* 59(3):195-201.

Chiu TY, Hu WY, Chen CY. (2000). Prevalence and severity of symptoms in terminal cancer patients: A study in Taiwan. *Support Care in Cancer* 8(4):311-313.

Chivato T, Juan F, Montoro A, Laguna R. (1996). Anaphylaxis induced by ingestion of a pollen compound. *Journal of Investigational Allergology and Clinical Immunology* 6(3):208-209.

Choppa PC, Vojdani A, Tagle C, Andrin R, Magtoto L. (1998). Multiplex PCR for the detection of *Mycoplasma fermentans, M. hominis* and *M. penetrans* in cell cultures and blood samples of patients with chronic fatigue syndrome. *Molecular and Cellular Probes* 12(5):301-308.

Chopra V, Dinh TV, Hannigan EV. (1998). Circulating serum levels of cytokines and angiogenic factors in patients with cervical cancer. *Cancer Investigation* 16(3):152-159.

Chow E, Fung K, Panzarella T, Bezjak A, Danjoux, C, Tannock I. (2002). A predictive model for survival in metastatic cancer patients attending an outpatient palliative radiotherapy clinic. *International Journal of Radiation Oncology, Biology and Physics* 53(5):1291-1302.

Chow SN, Seear M, Anderson R, Magee F. (1998). Multiple pulmonary chemodectomas in a child: Results of four different therapeutic regimens. *Journal of Pediatric Hematology and Oncology* 20(6):583-586.

Christman NJ, Oakley MG, Cronin SN. (2001). Developing and using preparatory information for women undergoing radiation therapy for cervical or uterine cancer. *Oncology Nursing Forum* 28(1):93-98.

Christodoulou CV, DeLuca J, Lange G, Johnson SK, Sisto SA, Korn L, Natelson BH. (1998). Relation between neuropsychological impairment and functional disability in patients with chronic fatigue syndrome. *Journal of Neurology, Neurosurgery and Psychiatry* 64(4):431-434.

Christodoulou CV, Ferry DR, Fyfe DW, Young A, Doran J, Sheehan TM, Eliopoulos A, Hale K, Baumgart J, Sass G, Kerr DJ. (1998). Phase I trial of weekly scheduling and pharmacokinetics of titanocene dichloride in patients with advanced cancer. *Journal of Clinical Oncology* 16(8):2761-2769.

Chudgar U, Shah RV, Krishnaswamy H, Chandy M. (1991). Hairy cell leukaemia: A review of nine cases. *Indian Journal of Cancer* 28(3):155-161.

Chun HG, Leyland-Jones B, Cheson BD. (1991). Fludarabine phosphate: A synthetic purine antimetabolite with significant activity against lymphoid malignancies. *Journal of Clinical Oncology* 9(1):175-188.

Chung JH, Cheong JC, Lee JY, Roth HK, Cha YN. (1996). Acceleration of the alcohol oxidation rate in rats with aloin, a quinone derivative of aloe. *Biochemical Pharmacology* 52(9):1461-1468.

Chung-Faye G, Palmer D, Anderson D, Clark J, Downes M, Baddeley J, Hussain S, Murray PI, Searle P, Seymour L, et al. (2001). Virus-directed, enzyme prodrug therapy with nitroimidazole reductase: A phase I and pharmacokinetic study of its prodrug, CB1954. *Clinical Cancer Research* 7(9):2662-2668.

Ciampolillo A, Marini V, Mirakian R, Buscema M, Schulz T, Pujol-Borrel R, Bottazzo GF. (1989). Retrovirus-like sequences in Graves disease: Implications for human autoimmunity. *Lancet* 1(8467):1096-1110.

Cianciolo GJ, Kipnis RJ, Snyderman R. (1984). Similarity between p15E of murine and feline leukaemia viruses and p21 of HTLV. *Nature* 311:515.

Ciccarelli O, Welch JP, Kent GG. (1987). Primary malignant tumors of the small bowel: The Hartford Hospital experience, 1969-1983. *American Journal of Surgery* 153(4):350-354.

Cicogna R, Visioli O. (1988). [A new reflex cardiovascular syndrome: Recurrent vasodepressive syncope caused by lesions or tumors of the parapharyngeal space. Etiopathogenesis, clinical picture, differential diagnosis with carotid sinus syndrome and glossopharyngeal neuralgia-asystole syndrome. Therapy by intracranial resection of the ninth cranial nerve]. *Giornale Italiano di Cardioliogia* 18(5):361-368.

Cimprich B. (1992). Attentional fatigue following breast cancer surgery. *Research Nursing and Health* 15(3):199-207.

Cimprich B. (1993). Development of an intervention to restore attention in cancer patients. *Cancer Nursing* 16(2):83-92.

Cimprich B. (1995). Symptom management: Loss of concentration. *Seminars in Oncology Nursing* 11(4):279-288.

Cimprich B. (1998). Age and extent of surgery affect attention in women treated for breast cancer. *Research Nursing and Health* 21(3):229-238.

Cimprich B. (1999). Pretreatment symptom distress in women newly diagnosed with breast cancer. *Cancer Nursing* 22(3):185-194.

Cimprich B, Ronis DL. (2001). Attention and symptom distress in women with and without breast cancer. *Nursing Research* 50(2):86-94.

Cirigliano M, Sun A. (1998). Advising patients about herbal therapies. *JAMA* 280(18):1565-1566.

Citera G, Arias MA, Maldonado-Cocco JA, Lazaro MA, Rosemffet MG, Brusco LI, Scheines EJ, Cardinalli DP. (2000). The effect of melatonin in patients with fibromyalgia: A pilot study. *Clinical Rheumatology* 19(1):9-13.

Citterio A, Sinforiani E, Verri A, Cristina S, Gerosa E, Nappi G. (1998). Neurological symptoms of the sick building syndrome: Analysis of a questionnaire. *Functional Neurology* 13(3):225-230.

Clague JE, Edwards RHT, Jackson MJ. (1992). Intravenous magnesium loading in chronic fatigue syndrome. *Lancet* 340(8811):124-125.

Clark JI, Gaynor ER, Martone B, Budds SC, Manjunath R, Flanigan RC, Waters WB, Sosman JA. (1999). Daily subcutaneous ultra-low-dose interleukin 2 with daily low-dose interferon-alpha in patients with advanced renal cell carcinoma. *Clinical Cancer Research* 5(9):2374-2380.

Clark P, Burgos-Vargas R, Medina-Palma C, Lavielle P, Marina FF. (1998). Prevalence of fibromyalgia in children: A clinical study of Mexican children. *Journal of Rheumatology* 25(10):2009-2014.

Clark PM, Lacasse C. (1998). Cancer-related fatigue: Clinical practice issues. *Clinical Journal of Oncology Nursing* 2(2):45-53.

Clarke-Steffen L. (2001). Cancer-related fatigue in children. *Journal of Pediatric Oncology Nursing* 18(2 Suppl 1):1-2.

Clarke-Steffen L, Hockenberry-Eaton M, Hinds PS, Mock V, Piper B, White A. (2001). Consensus statements: Analyzing a new model to evaluate fatigue in children with cancer. *Journal of Pediatric Oncology Nursing* 18(2 Suppl 1):21-23.

Claustrat B, Chazot G, Brun J, Jordan D, Sassolas G. (1984). A chronobiological study of melatonin and cortisol secretion in depressed subjects: Plasma melatonin, a biochemical markers in major depression. *Biological Psychiatry* 19: 1215-1228.

Clauw DJ. (1995). Fibromyalgia: More than just a musculoskeletal disease. *American Family Physician* 52(3):843-851, 853-854.

Clauw DJ, Blank C, Hiltz R, Katz P, Potolicchio S. (1994). Polysomnography in fibromyalgia patients. *Arthritis and Rheumatism* 37(Suppl. 9):S348.

Clauw DJ, Chrousos GP. (1997). Chronic pain and fatigue syndromes: Overlapping clinical and neuroendocrine features and potential pathogenic mechanisms. *Neuroimmunomodulation* 4(3):134-153.

Cleare AJ, Bearn J, Allain T, McGregor A, Wessely S, Murray RM, O'Keane V. (1995). Contrasting neuroendocrine responses in depression and chronic fatigue syndrome. *Journal of Affective Disorders* 35(4):283-289.

Cleare AJ, Sookdeo SS, Jones J, O'Keane V, Miell JP. (2000). Integrity of the growth hormone/insulin-like growth factor system is maintained in patients with chronic fatigue syndrome. *Journal of Clinical Endocrinology and Metabolism* 85(4):1433-1439.

Cleare AJ, Wessely S. (1996). Chronic fatigue syndrome: A stress disorder? *British Journal of Hospital Medicine* 55(9):571-574.

Cleary JF, Carbone PP. (1997). Palliative medicine in the elderly. *Cancer* 80(7): 1335-1347.

Cleeland CS. (2000). Cancer-related symptoms. *Seminars in Radiation Oncology* 10(3):175-190.

Cleeland CS. (2001). Cancer-related fatigue: New directions for research—Introduction. *Cancer* 92(6 Suppl):1657-1661.

Cleeland CS, Mendoza TR, Wang XS, Chou C, Harle MT, Morrissey M, Engstrom MC. (2000). Assessing symptom distress in cancer patients: The M.D. Anderson Symptom Inventory. *Cancer* 89(7):1634-1646.

Clements A, Sharpe M, Simkin S, Borrill J, Hawton K. (1997). Chronic fatigue syndrome: A qualitative investigation of patients' beliefs about the illness. *Journal of Psychosomatic Research* 42(6):615-624.

Clemett D, Lamb HM. (2000). Exemestane: A review of its use in postmenopausal women with advanced breast cancer. *Drugs* 59(6):1279-1296.

Clerici M, Berzofsky JA, Shearer GM, Tacket CO. (1991). Exposure to human immunodeficiency virus type 1-specific T helper cell responses before detection of infection by polymerase chain reaction and serum antibodies. *Journal of Infectious Diseases* 164:178-182.

Clerici M, Giorgi JV, Chou C-C, Gudeman VK, Zack JA, Gupta P, Ho H-N, Nishanian PG, Berzofsky JA, Shearer GM. (1992). Cell-mediated immune response to human immunodeficiency virus (HIV) type 1 in seronegative homosexual men with recent sexual exposure to HIV-1. *Journal of Infectious Diseases* 165:1012-1019.

Clerici M, Hakim FT, Venzon DJ, Blatt S, Hendrix CW, Wynn TA, Shearer GM. (1993). Changes in interleukin-2 and interleukin-4 production in asymptomatic, human immunodeficiency virus-seropositive individuals. *Journal of Clinical Investigation* 91:759-765.

Clerici M, Lucey DR, Berzofsky JA, Pinto LA, Wynn TA, Blatt SP, Dolan MJ, Hendrix CW, Wolf SF, Shearer GM. (1993). Restoration of HIV-specific cell-mediated immune responses by interleukin-12 in vitro. *Science* 262:1721-1724.

Coackley A, Hutchinson T, Saltmarsh P, Kelly A, Ellershaw JE, Marshall E, Brunston H. (2002). Assessment and management of fatigue in patients with advanced cancer: Developing guidelines. *International Journal of Palliative Nursing* 8(8):381-388.

Coates A, Dillenbeck CF, McNeil DR, Kaye SB, Sims K, Fox RM, Woods RL, Milton GW, Solomon J, Tattersall MH. (1983). On the receiving end—II. Linear analogue self-assessment (LASA) in evaluation of aspects of the quality of life of cancer patients receiving therapy. *European Journal of Cancer and Clinical Oncology* 19(11):1633-1637.

Coates A, Rallings M, Hersey P, Swanson C. (1986). Phase-II study of recombinant alpha 2-interferon in advanced malignant melanoma. *Journal of Interferon Research* 6(1):1-4.

Coats AJ. (2002). Origin of symptoms in patients with cachexia with special reference to weakness and shortness of breath. *International Journal of Cardiology* 85(1):133-139.

Coelho FM, Sawada NO. (1999). [Fatigue in patients with laryngeal cancer]. *Revista Latino Americana do Enfermagem* 7(5):103-107.

Cogan E. (2000). [Clinical approach to inflammatory syndromes in the aged]. *Revue Medicale de Bruxelles* 21(5):417-422.

Cognis D. (1999). [Possibilities and limits of treating fatigue]. *Soins* 635:26-27.

Cohen AM, Meytes D, Many A, Brenner B, Aghai E, Shaklai M, Kaufman S, Shtalrid M, Attias D, Manor Y, et al. (1995). Interferon-alpha-2b with VMCP for induction in multiple myeloma: The Israel Myeloma Cooperative Group experience. *Israeli Journal of Medical Sciences* 31(10):604-610.

Cohen H, Neumann L, Shore M, Amir M, Cassuto Y, Buskila D. (2000). Autonomic dysfunction in patients with fibromyalgia: Applications of power spectral analysis of heart rate variability. *Seminars in Arthritis and Rheumatism* 29(4): 217-227.

Cohen ML. (1999). Is fibromyalgia a distinct clinical entity? The disapproving rheumatologist's evidence. *Baillieres Best Practice Research in Clinical Rheumatology* 13(3):421-425.

Cohen MZ, Kahn DL, Steeves RH. (1998). Beyond body image: The experience of breast cancer. *Oncology Nursing Forum* 25(5):835-841.

Cohen N, Stempel C, Colombe B. (1990). Soluble interleukin-2 receptor: Detection and potential role in organ transplantation. *Clinical Immunology Newsletter* 10(12):175.

Cohen P. (1997). School and the ME generation. *Nursing Times* 93(49):19.

Cohen S, Tyrrell DA, Smith AP. (1991). Psychological stress and susceptibility to the common cold. *New England Journal of Medicine* 325(9):606-612.

Cohen S, Williamson GM. (1991). Stress and disease in humans. *Psychological Bulletin* 109:5-24.

Cohen SJ, Leichman CG, Yeslow G, Beard M, Proefrock A, Roedig B, Damle B, Letrent SP, DeCillis AP, Meropol NJ. (2002). Phase I and pharmacokinetic study of once daily oral administration of S-1 in patients with advanced cancer. *Clinical Cancer Research* 8(7):2116-2122.

Coiffier B. (2000). The impact and management of anaemia in haematological malignancies. *Medical Oncology* 17(Suppl 1):S2-S10.

Coiffier B, Neidhardt-Berard EM, Tilly H, Belanger C, Bouabdallah R, Haioun C, Brice P, Peaud PY, Pico JL, Janvier M, et al. (1999). Fludarabine alone compared to CHVP plus interferon in elderly patients with follicular lymphoma and adverse prognostic parameters: A GELA study. Groupe d'Etudes des Lymphomes de l'Adulte. *Annals of Oncology* 10(10):1191-1197.

Coker WJ. (1996). A review of Gulf War illness. *Journal of the Royal Naval Medical Service* 82(2):141-146.

Colditz GA, Frazier AL. (1995). Models of breast cancer show that risk is set by events of early life: Prevention must shift focus. *Cancer Epidemiology, Biomarkers, and Prevention* 4:567-571.

Cole DR, Pung J, Kim YD, Berman RA, Cole DF. (1979). Systemic thermotherapy (whole body hyperthermia). *International Journal of Clinical Pharmacology and Biopharmacology* 17(8):329-333.

Coleridge JC, Coleridge HM. (1984). Afferent vagal C fiber innervation of the lungs and airways and its functional significance. *Reviews of Physiology, Biochemistry and Pharmacology* 99:1-110.

Colevas AD, Adak S, Amrein PC, Barton JJ, Costello R, Posner MR. (2000). A phase II trial of palliative docetaxel plus 5-fluorouracil for squamous-cell cancer of the head and neck. *Annals of Oncology* 11(5):535-539.

Colevas AD, Amrein PC, Gomolin H, Barton JJ, Read RR, Adak S, Benner S, Costello R, Posner MR. (2001). A phase II study of combined oral uracil and ftorafur with leucovorin for patients with squamous cell carcinoma of the head and neck. *Cancer* 92(2):326-331.

Colevas AD, Posner MR. (1998). Docetaxel in head and neck cancer: A review. *American Journal of Clinical Oncology* 21(5):482-486.

Collichio FA, Amamoo MA, Fogleman J, Griggs J, Graham M. (2002). Phase II study of low-dose infusional 5-fluorouracil and paclitaxel (Taxol) given every 2 weeks in metastatic breast cancer. *American Journal of Clinical Oncology* 25(2):194-197.

Collichio FA, Pandya K. (1998). Interferon alpha-2b and megestrol acetate in the treatment of advanced renal cell carcinoma: A phase II study. *American Journal of Clinical Oncology* 21(2):209-211.

Collins JJ, Byrnes ME, Dunkel IJ, Lapin J, Nadel T, Thaler HT, Polyak T, Rapkin B, Portenoy RK. (2000). The measurement of symptoms in children with cancer. *Journal of Pain Symptomatology and Management* 19(5):363-377.

Colotta F, Re F, Muzio M, Bertini R, Polentarutti N, Sironi M, Giri JG, Dower SK, Sims JE, Mantovani A. (1993). Interleukin-1 type II receptor: A decoy target for IL-1 that is regulated by IL-4. *Science* 261:472-475.

Colovic R, Micev M, Zogovic S, Colovic N, Stojkovic M, Masirevic V. (2000). [Giant epithelioid leiomyosarcoma of the stomach]. *Srp Arh Celok Lek* 128 (3-4):104-109.

Colton CK. (1988). The interleukin hypothesis: A quantitative assessment. *Kidney International* 33:S27-S29.

Comella P, Southern Italy Cooperative Oncology Group. (2001). Phase III trial of cisplatin/gemcitabine with or without vinorelbine or paclitaxel in advanced non-small cell lung cancer. *Seminars in Oncology* 28(2 Suppl 7):7-10.

Compston ND. (1978). An outbreak of encephalomyelitis in the Royal Free Hospital Group, London, in 1955. *Postgraduate Medical Journal* 54:722-724.

Conley BA, Egorin MJ, Tait N, Rosen DM, Sausville EA, Dover G, Fram RJ, Van Echo DA. (1998). Phase I study of the orally administered butyrate prodrug, tributyrin, in patients with solid tumors. *Clinical Cancer Research* 4(3):629-634.

Conley BA, Egorin MJ, Whitacre MY, Carter DC, Zuhowski EG, Van Echo DA. (1993). Phase I and pharmacokinetic trial of liposome-encapsulated doxorubicin. *Cancer Chemotherapy Pharmacology* 33(2):107-112.

Conley BA, O'Shaughnessy J, Prindiville S, Lawrence J, Chow C, Jones E, Merino MJ, Kaiser-Kupfer MI, Caruso RC, Podgor M, et al. (2000). Pilot trial of the safety, tolerability, and retinoid levels of N-(4-hydroxyphenyl) retinamide in combination with tamoxifen in patients at high risk for developing invasive breast cancer. *Journal of Clinical Oncology* 18(2):275-283.

Connors JM, Andiman WA, Howarth CB, Liu E, Merigan TC, Savage ME, Jacobs C. (1985). Treatment of nasopharyngeal carcinoma with human leukocyte interferon. *Journal of Clinical Oncology* 3(6):813-817.

Connors JM, Silver HK. (1984). Phase I study of weekly high-dose human lymphoblastoid interferon. *Cancer Treatment Reports* 68(9):1093-1096.

Conroy T. (2002). Activity of vinorelbine in gastrointestinal cancers. *Critical Reviews in Oncology and Hematology* 42(2):173-178.

Consroe P, Musty R, Rein J, Tillery W, Pertwee R. (1997). The perceived effects of smoked cannabis on patients with mutliple sclerosis. *European Neurology* 38 (1):44-48.

Contasta I, Pellegrini P, Berghella AM, Del Beato T, Canossi A, Di Rocco M, Adorno D, Casciani CU. (1996). Necessity of biotherapeutic treatments inducing TH1 cell functions in colorectal cancer. *Cancer Biotherapy and Radiopharmacology* 11(6):373-383.

Conti F, Magrini L, Priori R, Valesini G, Bonini S. (1996). Eosinophil cationinc protein serum levels and allergy in chronic fatigue syndrome. *Allergy* 51(2):124-127.

Cook NF, Boore JR. (1997). Managing patients suffering from acute and chronic fatigue. *British Journal of Nursing* 6(14):811-815.

Cooper LA, Hill MN, Powe NR. (2002). Designing and evaluating interventions to eliminate racial and ethnic disparities in health care. *Journal of General Internal Medicine* 17:477-486.

Cooper MR, Fefer A, Thompson J, Case DC Jr, Kempf R, Sacher R, Neefe J, Bickers J, Scarffe JH, Spiegel R, et al. (1986). Alpha-2-interferon/melphalan/prednisone in previously untreated patients with multiple myeloma: A phase I-II trial. *Cancer Treatment Reports* 70(4):473-476.

Cope H, David A, Pelosi A, Mann A. (1994). Predictors of chronic "postviral" fatigue. *The Lancet* 344:864-868.

Cope H, Mann A, Pelosi A, David A. (1996). Psychosocial risk factors for chronic fatigue and chronic fatigue syndrome following presumed viral illness: A case-control study. *Psychological Medicine* 26(6):1197-1209.

Cordero DL, Sisto SA, Tapp WN, LaManca JJ, Pareja JG, Natelson BH. (1996). Decreased vagal power during treadmill walking in patients with chronic fatigue syndrome. *Clinical Autonomic Research* 6(6):329-333.

Cornacoff JB, Gossett KA, Barbolt TA, Dean JH. (1992). Preclinical evaluation of recombinant human interleukin-4. *Toxicology Letters* 64-65(Spec No):299-310.

Corsi MM, Bertelli AA, Gaja G, Fulgenzi A, Ferrero ME. (1998). The therapeutic potential of *Aloë vera* in tumor-bearing rats. *International Journal of Tissue Reactions* 20(4):115-118.

Cortes J, Kantarjian H, O'Brien S, Robertson LE, Pierce S, Talpaz M. (1996). Result of interferon-alpha therapy in patients with chronic myelogenous leukemia 60 years of age and older. *American Journal of Medicine* 100(4):452-455.

Costantini M, Mencaglia E, Giulio PD, Cortesi E, Roila F, Ballatori E, Tamburini M, Casali P, Licitra L, Candis DD, et al. (2000). Cancer patients as "experts" in defining quality of life domains: A multicentre survey by the Italian Group for the Evaluation of Outcomes in Oncology (IGEO). *Quality of Life Research* 9(2):151-159.

Côte KA, Moldofsky H. (1997). Sleep, daytime symptoms, and cognitive performance in patients with fibromyalgia. *Journal of Rheumatology* 24(10):2014-2023.

Courau E, Westeel V, Jacoulet P, Depierre A. (1998). [Treatment of the paraneoplastic Lambert-Eaton syndrome]. *Revue Pneumologie Clinique* 54(2):65-70.

Courneya KS, Blanchard CM, Laing DM. (2001). Exercise adherence in breast cancer survivors training for a dragon boat race competition: A preliminary investigation. *Psychooncology* 10(5):444-452.

Courneya KS, Friedenreich CM. (1999). Physical exercise and quality of life following cancer diagnosis: A literature review. *Annals of Behavioral Medicine* 21(2):171-179.

Coward BL. (1999). Clinical snapshot: Fibromyalgia. *American Journal of Nursing* 99(10):42-43.

Cox BD, Blaxter M, Buckle ALJ, Fenner ND, Golding JF, Gore M, Huppert FA, Nickson J, Roth M, Stark J, et al. (1987). *The Health and Lifestyle Survey.* London: Health Promotion Research Trust.

Cox DL. (1999). Chronic fatigue syndrome: An occupational therapy programme. *Occupational Therapy International* 6(1):52-64.

Cox DL. (2000). *Occupational Therapy and Chronic Fatigue Syndrome.* Philadelphia: Whurr Publishers.

Cox DL, Findley LJ. (1998). The management of chronic fatigue syndrome in an inpatient setting: Presentation of an approach and perceived outcome. *British Journal of Occupational Therapy* 61(9):405-409.

Cox IM, Campbell MJ, Dowson D. (1991). Red blood cell magnesium and chronic fatigue syndrome. *Lancet* 337(8744):757-760.

Coyle CP, Santiago MC. (2002). Healthcare utilization among women with physical disabilities. *Medscape Women's Health* 7(4):2.

Craig NM, Putterman AM, Roenigk RK, Wang TD, Roenigk HH. (1996). Multiple periorbital cutaneous myxomas progressing to scleromyxedema. *Journal of the American Academy of Dermatology* 34(5 Pt 2):928-930.

Crang C. (1999). Learning to cope with the fatigue caused by cancer. *Nursing Times* 95(16):53-55.

Crawford J. (2002). Recombinant human erythropoietin in cancer-related anemia: Review of clinical evidence. *Oncology* 16(9 Suppl 10):41-53.

Creagan ET, Ahmann DL, Green SJ, Long HJ, Frytak S, O'Fallon JR, Itri LM. (1984). Phase II study of low-dose recombinant leukocyte A interferon in disseminated malignant melanoma. *Journal of Clinical Oncology* 2(9):1002-1005.

Creagan ET, Ahmann DL, Green SJ, Long HJ, Rubin J, Schutt AJ, Dziewanowski ZE. (1984). Phase II study of recombinant leukocyte A interferon (rIFN-alpha A) in disseminated malignant melanoma. *Cancer* 54(12):2844-2849.

Creagan ET, Ahmann DL, Long HJ, Frytak S, Sherwin SA, Chang MN. (1987). Phase II study of recombinant interferon-gamma in patients with disseminated malignant melanoma. *Cancer Treatment Reports* 71(9):843-844.

Creagan ET, Buckner JC, Hahn RG, Richardson RR, Schaid DJ, Kovach JS. (1988). An evaluation of recombinant leukocyte A interferon with aspirin in patients with metastatic renal cell cancer. *Cancer* 61(9):1787-1791.

Creagan ET, Kovach JS, Long HJ, Richardson RL. (1986). Phase I study of recombinant leukocyte A human interferon combined with BCNU in selected patients with advanced cancer. *Journal of Clinical Oncology* 4(3):408-413.

Creagan ET, Kovach JS, Moertel CG, Frytak S, Kvols LK. (1998). A phase I clinical trial of recombinant human tumor necrosis factor. *Cancer* 62(12):2467-2471.

Creaven PJ, Madajewicz S, Pendyala L, Takita H, Mittelman A, Huben R, Henderson E, Cushman MK. (1987). Phase I clinical trial of 1-(2-[2-(4-pyridyl)-2-imidazoline-1-yl]-ethyl)-3-(4-carboxy-phenyl) urea (CGP 15720A). *Cancer Chemotherapy Pharmacology* 20(2):145-150.

Creaven PJ, Pendyala L, Petrelli NJ. (1993). Evaluation of alpha difluoromethylornithine as a potential chemopreventive agent: Tolerance to daily oral administration in humans. *Cancer Epidemiology, Biomarkers, and Prevention* 2(3):243-247.

Creek J. (1997). The knowledge base of occupational therapy. In *Occupational Therapy and Mental Health,* Second Edition, Creek J, ed. Edinburgh: Churchill Livingston, pp. 1ff.

Creekmore SP, Harris JE, Ellis TM, Braun DP, Cohen II, Bhoopalam N, Jassak PF, Cahill MA, Canzoneri CL, Fisher RI. (1989). A phase I clinical trial of recombinant interleukin-2 by periodic 24-hour intravenous infusions. *Journal of Clinical Oncology* 7(2):276-284.

Creemers GJ, Gerrits CJ, Schellens JH, Planting AS, van der Burg ME, van Beurden VM, de Boer-Dennert M, Harteveld M, Loos W, Hudson I, et al. (1996). Phase II and pharmacologic study of topotecan administered as a 21-day continuous infusion to patients with colorectal cancer. *Journal of Clinical Oncology* 14(9):2540-2545.

Crockett DM, McCabe BF, Lusk RP, Mixon JH. (1987). Side effects and toxicity of interferon in the treatment of recurrent respiratory papillomatosis. *Annals of Otolaryngology, Rhinology and Laryngology* 96(5):601-607.

Crofford LJ. (1998a). The hypothalamic-pituitary-adrenal stress axis in fibromyalgia and chronic fatigue syndrome. *Zeitschrift Rheumatologie* 57(Suppl 2): 67-71.

Crofford LJ. (1998b). Neuroendocrine abnormalities in fibromyalgia and related disorders. *American Journal of Medical Sciences* 315(6):359-366.

Crofford LJ, Demitrack MA. (1996). Evidence that abnormalities of central neurohormonal systems are key to understanding fibromyalgia and chronic fatigue syndrome. *Rheumatic Diseases Clinics of North America* 22(2):267-284.

Crofford LJ, Engleberg NC, Demitrack MA. (1996). Neurohormonal perturbations in fibromyalgia. *Baillieres Clinical Rheumatology* 10(2):365-378.

Croft P, Schollum J, Silman A. (1994). Population study of tender point counts and pain as evidence of fibromyalgia. *British Medical Journal* 309:696-699.

Croghan MK, Booth A, Meyskens FL Jr. (1988). A phase I trial of recombinant interferon-alpha and alpha-difluoromethylornithine in metastatic melanoma. *Journal of Biological Response Modifiers* 7(4):409-415.

Crom DB, Chathaway DK, Tolley EA, Mulhern RK, Hudson MM. (1999). Health status and health-related quality of life in long-term adult survivors of pediatric solid tumors. *International Journal of Cancer* 12:25-31.

Crombleholme TM, Harris BH, Jacir NN, Latchaw LA, Kretschmar CS, Rosenfield CG, Wolfe LC, Cendron M, Trask C, Wolfe HJ. (1993). The desmoplastic round cell tumor: A new solid tumor of childhood. *Journal of Pediatric Surgery* 28(8):1023-1025.

Crone CC, Wise TN. (1997). Survey of alternative medicine use among organ transplant patients. *Journal of Transplant Coordination* 7(3):123-130.

Crul M, De Klerk GJ, Swart M, Van't Veer LJ, De Jong D, Boerrigter L, Palmer PA, Bol CJ, Tan H, De Gast GC, Beijnen JH, Schellens JH. (2002). Phase I clinical and pharmacologic study of chronic oral administration of the farnesyl protein transferase inhibitor R115777 in advanced cancer. *Journal of Clinical Oncology* 20(11):2726-2735.

Crul M, Rosing H, De Klerk GJ, Dubbelman R, Traiser M, Reichert S, Knebel NG, Schellens JH, Beijnen JH, ten Bokkel Huinink WW. (2002). Phase I and pharmacological study of daily oral administration of perifosine (D-21266) in patients with advanced solid tumours. *European Journal of Cancer* 38(12):1615-1621.

Cruz DN, Mahnensmith RL, Perazella MA. (1997). Intradialytic hypotension: Is midodrine beneficial in symptomatic hemodialysis patients? *American Journal of Kidney Disease* 30(6):772-779.

Csef H. (1999). [Similarities of chronic fatigue syndrome, fibromyalgia and multiple chemical sensitivity]. Gemeinsamkeiten con chronic fatigue syndrom, fibromyalgie und multipler chemischer sensitivität. *Deutsche Medizin Wochenschrift* 124(6):163-169.

Cuellar ML, Gluck O, Molina JF, Gutierrez S, Garcia C, Espinoza R. (1995). Silicone breast implant-associated musculoskeletal manifestations. *Clinical Rheumatology* 14(6):667-672.

Cuende JI, Civeira P, Diez N, Prieto J. (1997). High prevalence without reactivation of herpes virus 6 in subjects with chronic fatigue syndrome. *Anales de Medicina Interna* 14(9):441-444.

Culine S, Roch I, Pinguet F, Romieu G, Bressolle F. (1999). Combination paclitaxel and vinorelbine therapy: In vitro cytotoxic interactions and dose-escalation study in breast cancer patients previously exposed to anthracyclines. *International Journal of Oncology* 14(5):999-1006.

Cull A, Hay C, Love SB, Mackie M, Smets E, Stewart M. (1996). What do cancer patients mean when they complain of concentration and memory problems? *British Journal of Cancer* 74(10):1674-1679.

Cunliffe A, Obeid OA, Powell-Tuck J. (1997). Post-prandial changes in measures of fatigue: Effect of a mixed or a pure carbohydrate or pure fat meal. *European Journal of Clinical Nutrition* 51(12):831-838.

Cunliffe A, Obeid OA, Powell-Tuck J. (1998). A placebo-controlled investigation of the effects of tryptophan or placebo on subjective and objective measures of fatigue. *European Journal of Clinical Nutrition* 52(6):425-430.

Cunningham ME. (1996). Becoming familiar with fibromyalgia. *Orthopedic Nursing* 15(2):33-36.

Cupp MJ. (1999). Herbal remedies: Adverse effects and drug interactions. *American Family Physician* 59(5):1239-1245.

Curt GA. (1999). The evolving face of palliative care in cancer medicine. *Oncologist* 4(1):i.

Curt GA. (2000a). The impact of fatigue on patients with cancer: Overview of FATIGUE 1 and 2. *Oncologist* 5(Suppl 2):9-12.

Curt GA. (2000b). Impact of fatigue on quality of life in oncology patients. *Seminars in Hematology* 37(4 Suppl 6):14-17.

Curt GA. (2001a). Fatigue in cancer. *British Medical Journal* 322(7302):1560.

Curt GA. (2001b). [Fatigue syndrome caused by malignant tumor: An increasing priority in patient care]. *Recenti Progressi Medici* 92(6):408-412.

Curt GA, Breitbart W, Cella D, Groopman JE, Horning SJ, Itri LM, Johnson DH, Miaskowski C, Scherr SL, Portenoy RK, et al. (2000). Impact of cancer-related fatigue on the lives of patients: New findings from the Fatigue Coalition. *Oncologist* 5(5):353-360.

Cushman KE. (1986). Symptom management: A comprehensive approach to increasing nutritional status in the cancer patient. *Seminars in Oncology Nursing* 2(1):30-35.

Cyjon A, Neuman-Levin M, Rakowsky E, Greif F, Belinky A, Atar E, Hardoff R, Brenner B, Sulkes A. (2001). Liver metastases from colorectal cancer: Regional intra-arterial treatment following failure of systemic chemotherapy. *British Journal of Cancer* 85(4):504-508.

Dahut W, Harold N, Takimoto C, Allegra C, Chen A, Hamilton JM, Arbuck S, Sorensen M, Grollman F, Nakashima H, et al. (1996). Phase I and pharmacologic study of 9-aminocamptothecin given by 72-hour infusion in adult cancer patients. *Journal of Clinical Oncology* 14(4):1236-1244.

Dalakas MC, Mock V, Hawkins MJ. (1998). Fatigue: Definitions, mechanisms, and paradigms for study. *Seminars in Oncology* 25(1 Suppl 1):48-53.

Daliani DD, Papandreou CN, Thall PF, Wang X, Perez C, Oliva R, Pagliaro L, Amato R. (2002). A pilot study of thalidomide in patients with progressive metastatic renal cell carcinoma. *Cancer* 95(4):758-765.

Dalton DK, Pitts-Meek S, Keshav S, Figai IS, Bradley A, Stewart TA. (1993). Multiple defects of immune cell function in mice with disrupted interferon-gamma genes. *Science* 259:1739-1745.

Dalzell MD. (1999). Health plans and alternative medicine—Where do physicians fit in? *Managed Care* 8(4):14-18.

D'Amato A, Giovannini C, Pronio A, Cristaldi M, Brini C, Monardo F, Montesani C, Ribotta G. (1998). Solid cystic tumor of the head of the pancreas in a young woman. *Hepatogastroenterology* 45(20):541-544.

Danesh J, Collins R, Peto R. (1997). Chronic infections and coronary heart disease: Is there a link? *Lancet* 350:430-436.

Dang H, Dauphinée MJ, Talal N, Garry RF, Seibold JR, Medsger TA Jr, Alexander S, Feghali CA. (1991). Serum antibody to retroviral gag proteins in systemic sclerosis. *Arthritis and Rheumatism* 34(10):1336-1337.

Darko DF, Mitler MM, Miller JC. (1998). Growth hormone, fatigue, poor sleep, and disability in HIV infection. *Neuroendocrinology* 67(5):317-324.

Dashina TA, Krikorova SA. (1999). The modern concepts of phyto-aromatherapy. *Vopr Kurortol Fizioter Lech Fiz Kult* 2(March/April):47-53.

Da Silva FC. (1993a). Quality of life in prostatic cancer patients. *Cancer* 72(12 Suppl): 3803-3806.

Da Silva FC. (1993b). Quality of life in prostatic carcinoma. *European Urology* 24 (Suppl 2):113-117.

Da Silva FC, Fossa SD, Aaronson NK, Serbouti S, Denis L, Casselman J, Whelan P, Hetherington J, Fava C, Richards B, et al. (1996). The quality of life of patients with newly diagnosed M1 prostate cancer: Experience with EORTC clinical trial 30853. *European Journal of Cancer* 32A(1):72-77.

Da Silva FC, Reis E, Costa T, Denis L. (1993). Quality of life in patients with prostatic cancer: A feasibility study. The Members of Quality of Life Committee of the EORTC Genitourinary Group. *Cancer* 71(3 Suppl):1138-1142.

Davidson JR, MacLean AW, Brundage MD, Schulze K. (2002). Sleep disturbance in cancer patients. *Social Science and Medicine* 54(9):1309-1321.

Davidson JR, Waisberg JL, Brundage MD, MacLean AW. (2001). Nonpharmacologic group treatment of insomnia: A preliminary study with cancer survivors. *Psychooncology* 10(5):389-397.

Davidson NG, Chick JB, Perren TJ, Campbell N, Thompson JM, Chan YT. (1996). A phase II study of single agent paclitaxel in patients at first relapse following initial chemotherapy for breast cancer. *Clinical Oncology* 8(6):358-362.

Davidson NG, Davis AS, Woods J, Snooks S, Cheverton PD. (1999). FILM (5-fluorouracil, ifosfamide, leucovorin and mitomycin C), an alternative chemotherapy regimen suitable for the treatment of advanced breast cancer in the "outpatient" setting. *Cancer Chemotherapy Pharmacology* 44(Suppl):S18-S23.

Davies B, Whitsett SF, Bruce A, McCarthy P. (2002). A typology of fatigue in children with cancer. *Journal of Pediatric Oncology Nursing* 19(1):12-21.

Davies SF, McQuaid KR, Iber C, McArthur CD, Path MJ, Beebe DS, Helseth HK. (1987). Extreme dyspnea from unilateral pulmonary venous obstruction: Demonstration of a vagal mechanism and relief by right vagotomy. *American Reviews of Respiratory Diseases* 136:184-188.

Davis JM, Kohut ML, Jackson DA, Colbert LH, Mayer EP, Ghaffar A. (1998). Exercise effects on lung tumor metastases and in vitro alveolar macrophage antitumor cytotoxicity. *American Journal of Physiology* 274(5 Pt 2):R1454-R1459.

Davis JM, Weaver JA, Kohut ML, Colbert LH, Ghaffar A, Mayer EP. (1998). Immune system activation and fatigue during treadmill running: Role of interferon. *Medicine and Science in Sports and Exercise* 30(6):863-868.

Daynes RA, Araneo BA. (1989). Contrasting effects of glucocorticoids on the capacity of T cells to produce the growth factors interleukin 2 and interleukin 4. *European Journal of Immunology* 19(12):2319-2325.

Daynes RA, Araneo BA, Dowell TA, Huang K, Dudley D. (1990). Regulation of murine lymphokine production in vivo: III. The lymphoid tissue microenvironment exerts regulatory influences over T helper cell function. *Journal of Experimental Medicine* 171(4):979-996.

Daynes RA, Araneo BA, Ershler WB, Maloney C, Li GZ, Ryu SY. (1993). Altered regulation of IL-6 production with normal aging: Possible linkage to the age-associated decline in dehydroepiandrosterone and its sulfated derivative. *Journal of Immunology* 150(12):5219-5230.

Daynes RA, Araneo BA, Hennebold J, Enioutina E, Mu HH. (1995). Steroids as regulators of the mammalian immune response. *Journal of Investigative Dermatology* 105:14S-19S.

Daynes RA, Meikle AW, Araneo BA. (1991). Locally active steroid hormones may facilitate compartmentalization of immunity by regulating the types of lymphokines produced by helper T cells. *Research in Immunology* 142(1):40-45.

Deale A, Chalder T, Marks I, Wessely S. (1997). Cognitive behavior therapy for chronic fatigue syndrome: A randomized controlled trial. *American Journal of Psychiatry* 154(3):408-414.

Deale A, Chalder T, Wessely S. (1998). Illness beliefs and treatment outcome in chronic fatigue syndrome. *Journal of Psychosomatic Research* 45(1 Special No):77-83.

Dean GE, Spears L, Ferrell BR, Quan WD, Groshon S, Mitchell MS. (1995). Fatigue in patients with cancer receiving interferon alpha. *Cancer Practice* 3(3): 164-172.

Dean GE, Stahl C. (2002). Increasing the visibility of patient fatigue. *Seminars in Oncology Nursing* 18(1):20-27.

Deatrick JA, Brennan D, Cameron ME. (1998). Mothers with multiple sclerosis and their children: Effects of fatigue and exacerbations on maternal support. *Nursing Research* 47(4):205-210.

De Becker P, De Meirleir K, Joos E, Campine I, Van Steenberge E, Smitz J, Velkeniers B. (1999). Dehydroepiandrosterone (DHEA) response to i.v. ACTH in patients with chronic fatigue syndrome. *Hormone and Metabolism Research* 31(1):18-21.

De Becker P, Dendale P, De Meirleir K, Campine I, Vandenborne K, Hagers Y. (1998). Autonomic testing in patients with chronic fatigue syndrome. *American Journal of Medicine* 105(3A):22S-26S.

De Boer AG, Genovesi PI, Sprangers MA, Van Sandick JW, Obertop H, Van Lanschot JJ. (2000). Quality of life in long-term survivors after curative transhiatal oesophagectomy for oesophageal carcinoma. *British Journal of Surgery* 87(12):1716-1721.

De Boer MF, McCormick LK, Pruyn JF, Ryckman RM, van den Borne BW. (1999). Physical and psychosocial correlates of head and neck cancer: A review of the literature. *Otolaryngology, Head and Neck Surgery* 120(3):427-436.

Decker TW, Cline-Elsen J, Gallagher M. (1992). Relaxation therapy as an adjunct in radiation oncology. *Journal of Clinical Psychology* 48(3):388-393.

De Clercq E. (1995). Antiviral therapy for human immunodeficiency virus infections. *Clinical Microbiology Reviews* 8:200-239.

De Clercq E. (1997). In search of a selective antiviral chemotherapy. *Clinical Microbiology Reviews* 10:674-693.

DeFreitas E, Hilliand B, Cheney P, Bell D, Kiggundu E, Sankey D, Wroblewska Z, Palladino M, Woodward JP, Koprowski H. (1991). Retroviral sequences related to human T-lymphotropic virus type II in patients with chronic fatigue immune dysfunction syndrome. *Proceedings of the National Academy of Sciences of the United States of America* 88(7):2922-2926.

De Gast GC, Klumpen HJ, Vyth-Dreese FA, Kersten MJ, Verra NC, Sein J, Batchelor D, Nooijen WJ, Schornagel JH. (2000). Phase I trial of combined immunotherapy with subcutaneous granulocyte macrophage colony-stimulating factor, low-dose interleukin 2, and interferon alpha in progressive metastatic melanoma and renal cell carcinoma. *Clinical Cancer Research* 6(4):1267-1272.

Degner LF, Sloan JA. (1995). Symptom distress in newly diagnosed ambulatory cancer patients and as a predictor of survival in lung cancer. *Journal of Pain Symptomatology and Management* 10(6):423-431.

De Graeff A, de Leeuw JRJ, Ros WJ, Hordijk GJ, Battermann JJ, Blijham GH, Winnubst JA. (1999). A prospective study on quality of life of laryngeal cancer patients treated with radiotherapy. *Head and Neck* 21(4):291-296.

De Graeff A, de Leeuw JRJ, Ros WJ, Hordijk GJ, Blijham GH, Winnubst JA. (1999). A prospective study on quality of life of patients with cancer of the oral cavity or oropharynx treated with surgery with or without radiotherapy. *Oral Oncology* 35(1):27-32.

De Gramont A, Grosbois B, Michaux JL, Peny AM, Pollet JP, Smadja N, Krulik M, Debray J, Bernard JF, Monconduit M. (1990). [IgM myeloma: 6 cases and a review of the literature]. *Revue de Medecine Interne* 11(1):13-18.

DeGreef C, Van De Voorde W, Bakkus M, Corthals J, Heirman C, Schots R, Lacor P, Van Camp B, Van Riet I. (1999). Kaposi's sarcoma-associated herpesvirus (KSHV/HHV-8) DNA sequences are absent in leukopheresis products and ex vivo expanded CD34+ cells from multiple myeloma patients. *British Journal of Haematology* 106(4):1033-1036.

De Haes JC, van Knippenberg FC, Neijt JP. (1990). Measuring psychological and physical distress in cancer patients: Structure and application of the Rotterdam Symptom Checklist. *British Journal of Cancer* 62(6):1034-1038.

Deichmann M, Thome M, Jackel A, Utermann S, Bock M, Waldmann V, Naher H. (1998). Non-human immunodeficiency virus Kaposi's sarcoma can be effectively treated with low-dose interferon-alpha despite the persistence of herpesvirus-8. *British Journal of Dermatology* 139(6):1052-1054.

Dejana E, Brenario F, Erroi A, Bussolino F, Mussoni L, Gramse M, Pintucci G, Casali B, Dinarello CA, VanDamme J. (1987). Modulation of endothelial cell function by different molecular species of interleukin-1. *Blood* 69:635-699.

De Jesus M. (2000). Fibromyalgia onset. *American Journal of Nursing* 100(1):14.

De Jong LW, Prins JB, Fiselier TJ, Weemaes CM, Meier-van den Bergh EM, Bleijenberg G. (1997). Chronic fatigue syndrome in young persons. *Nederlands Tijdschrift voor Geneeskunde* 141(31):1513-1516.

De Jong N, Courtens AM, Abu-Saad HH, Schouten HC. (2002). Fatigue in patients with breast cancer receiving adjuvant chemotherapy: A review of the literature. *Cancer Nursing* 25(4):283-297.

De Jong RS, Mulder NH, Uges DR, Sleijfer DT, Hoppener FJ, Groen HJ, Willemse PH, van der Graaf WT, de Vries EG. (1997). Randomised comparison of etoposide pharmacokinetics after oral etoposide phosphate and oral etoposide. *British Journal of Cancer* 75(11):1660-1666.

De Jongh F, de Wit R, Verweij J, Sparreboom A, van den Bent M, Stoter G, van der Burg M. (2002). Dose-dense cisplatin/paclitaxel: A well-tolerated and highly effective chemotherapeutic regimen in patients with advanced ovarian cancer. *European Journal of Cancer* 38(15):2005.

De Kernion JB, Sarna G, Figlin R, Lindner A, Smith RB. (1983). The treatment of renal cell carcinoma with human leukocyte alpha-interferon. *Journal of Urology* 130(6):1063-1066.

Delaplace G. (1997). [Fatigue in oncology]. *Soins* 619:35-41.

Delbanco TL, Daley J, Hartman EE. (1998). A 56-year-old woman with chronic fatigue syndrome, 1 year later. *JAMA* 280(4):372.

Del Mastro L, Costantini M, Morasso G, Bonci F, Bergaglio M, Banducci S, Viterbori P, Conte P, Rosso R, Venturini M. (2002). Impact of two different dose-intensity chemotherapy regimens on psychological distress in early breast cancer patients. *European Journal of Cancer* 38(3):359-366.

Del Mastro L, Venturini M, Giannessi PG, Vigani A, Garrone O, Carnino F, Russo P, Galletti P, Rosso R, Conte PF. (1995). Intraperitoneal infusion of recombinant human tumor necrosis factor and mitoxantrone in neoplastic ascites: A feasibility study. *Anticancer Research* 15(5B):2207-2212.

De Loos WS. (1997). Chronic fatigue syndrome: Fatigue of unknown origin. *European Journal of Clinical Investigation* 27(4):268-269.

Delord JP, Raymond E, Chaouche M, Ruffie P, Ducreux M, Faivre S, Boige V, Le Chevalier T, Rixe O, Baudin E, et al. (2000). A dose-finding study of gemcitabine and vinorelbine in advanced previously treated malignancies. *Annals of Oncology* 11(1):73-79.

De Lorenzo F, Hargreaves J, Kakkar VV. (1996a). Lung function in patients with chonic fatigue syndrome (CFS). *Australian and New Zealand Journal of Medicine* 26(4):563-564.

De Lorenzo F, Hargreaves J, Kakkar VV. (1996b). Possible relationship between chronic fatigue and postural tachycardia syndromes. *Clinical Autonomic Research* 6(5):263-264.

De Lorenzo F, Hargreaves J, Kakkar VV. (1997). Pathogenesis and management of delayed orthostatic hypotension in patients with chronic fatigue syndrome. *Clinical Autonomic Research* 7(4):185-190.

De Lorenzo F, Hargreaves J, Kakkar VV. (1998). Phosphate diabetes in patients with chronic fatigue syndrome. *Postgraduate Medicine Journal* 74(870):229-232.

De Lorenzo F, Kakkar VV. (1996). Twenty-four-hour urine analysis in patients with orthostatic hypotension and chronic fatigue syndrome. *Australian and New Zealand Journal of Medicine* 26(6):849-850.

DeLuca J, Johnson SK, Ellis SP, Natelson BH. (1997a). Cognitive functioning is impaired with chronic fatigue syndrome devoid of psychiatric disease. *Journal of Neurology, Neurosurgery and Psychiatry* 62(2):151-155.

DeLuca J, Johnson SK, Ellis SP, Natelson BH. (1997b). Sudden vs. gradual onset of chronic fatigue syndrome differentiates individuals on cognitive and psychiatric measures. *Journal of Psychiatric Research* 31(1):83-90.

De Marinis F, Rinaldi M, Ardizzoni A, Bruzzi P, Pennucci MC, Portalone L, D'Aprile M, Ripanti P, Romano F, Belli M, et al. (1999). The role of vindesine and lonidamine in the treatment of elderly patients with advanced non-small cell lung cancer: A phase III randomized FONICAP trial. Italian Lung Cancer Task Force. *Tumori* 85(3):177-182.

De Meirleir K, Peterson DL, De Becker P, Englebienne P. (2002). From laboratory to patient care. In *Chronic Fatigue Syndrome: A Biological Approach.* Englebienne P, De Meirleir K, eds. Boca Raton, FL: CRC Press, pp. 265-284.

Demetri GD. (2001). Anaemia and its functional consequences in cancer patients: Current challenges in management and prospects for improving therapy. *British Journal of Cancer* 84(Suppl 1):31-37.

Demetri GD, Gabrilove JL, Blasi MV, Hill RJ, Glaspy J. (2002). Benefits of epoetin alfa in anemic breast cancer patients receiving chemotherapy. *Clinical Breast Cancer* 3(1):45-51.

Demetri GD, von Mehren M, Blanke CD, Van den Abbeele AD, Eisenberg B, Roberts PJ, Heinrich MC, Tuveson DA, Singer S, Janicek M, et al. (2002). Efficacy and safety of imatinib mesylate in advanced gastrointestinal stromal tumors. *New England Journal of Medicine* 347(7):472-480.

Demitrack MA. (1997). Neuroendocrine correlates of chronic fatigue syndrome: A brief review. *Journal of Psychiatric Research* 31(1):69-82.

Demitrack MA. (1998). Neuroendocrine aspects of chronic fatigue syndrome: A commentary. *American Journal of Medicine* 105(3A):11S-14S.

Demitrack MA, Crofford LJ. (1998). Evidence for and pathophysiologic implications of hypothalamic-pituitary-adrenal axis dysregulation in fibromyalgia and chronic fatigue syndrome. *Annals of the New York Academy of Sciences* 840: 684-697.

Dempke W, Schmoll HJ. (2001). [Possible new indications for erythropoietin therapy]. *Medizinische Klinik* 96(8):467-474.

Dempsey RA, Dinarello CA, Mier JW, Rosenwasser CJ, Allegretta M, Brown TE, Parkinson DR. (1982). The differential effects of human leukocyte pyrogen/lymphocyte-activating factor, T cell growth factor, and interferon on human natural killer activity. *Journal of Immunology* 129:2504-2510.

Dencker H. (1972). Symptomatology of resectable periampullary carcinoma. *Acta Chirurgica Scandinavica* 138(6):613-619.

Derman W, Schwellnus MP, Lambert MI, Emms M, Sinclair-Smith C, Kirby P, Noakes TD. (1997). The "worn-out athlete": A clinical approach to chronic fatigue in athletes. *Journal of Sport Sciences* 15(3):341-351.

De Palo G, Stefanon B, Rilke F, Pilotti S, Ghione M. (1984). Human fibroblast interferon in cervical and vulvar intraepithelial neoplasia associated with papilloma virus infection. *International Journal of Tissue Reactions* 6(6):523-527.

De Palo G, Stefanon B, Rilke F, Pilotti S, Ghione M. (1985). Human fibroblast interferon in cervical and vulvar intraepithelial neoplasia associated with viral cytopathic effects: A pilot study. *Journal of Reproductive Medicine* 30(5):404-408.

De Portugal Alvarez J, Rivera Berrio L, Gonzalez San Martin F, Sanchez Rodriguez A, De Portugal E, Del Rivero F. (1996). Etiology of isolated general malaise. *Anales de Medicina Interna* 13(10):471-475.

De Rijk AE, Schreurs KM, Bensing JM. (1998). General practitioners' attributions of fatigue. *Social Science and Medicine* 47(4):487-496.

De Smet PA. (1997). The role of plant-derived drugs and herbal medicines in healthcare. *Drugs* 54(6):801-840.

Dessein PH, Shipton EA, Stanwix AE, Joffe BI. (2000). Neuroendocrine deficiency-mediated development and persistence of pain in fibromyalgia: A promising paradigm? *Pain* 86(3):213-215.

Detmar SB, Muller MJ, Wever LD, Schornagel JH, Aaronson NK. (2001). The patient-physician relationship—Patient-physician communication during outpatient palliative treatment visits: An observational study. *JAMA* 285(10):1351-1357.

Deulofeu R, Gascon J, Gimenez N, Corachan M. (1991). Magnesium and chronic fatigue syndrome. *Lancet* 338(8767):641.

Deuster PA. (1996). Exercise in the prevention and treatment of chronic disorders. *Women's Health Issues* 6(6):320-331.

De Vincenzo J. (1997). Prevention and treatment of respiratory syncytial virus infections. *Advances in Pediatric Infectious Diseases* 13:1-47.

De Vinci C, Levine PH, Pizza G, Fudenberg HH, Orens P, Pearson G, Viza D. (1996). Lessons from a pilot study of transfer factor in chronic fatigue syndrome. *Biotherapy* 9(1-3):87-90.

De Wit R, Pawinsky A, Stoter G, van Oosterom AT, Fossa SD, Paridaens R, Svedberg A, de Mulder PH. (1997). EORTC phase II study of daily oral linomide in metastatic renal cell carcinoma patients with good prognostic factors. *European Journal of Cancer* 33(3):493-495.

De Wit R, Raasveld MHM, Ten Berge JM, Van der Wouw PA, Bakker PJM, Veenhof CHN. (1991). Interleukin-6 concentrations in the serum of patients with AIDS-associated Kaposi's sarcoma during treatment with interferon-alpha. *Journal of Internal Medicine* 229:539-542.

Dhingra K, Talpaz M, Dhingra HM, Ajani JA, Rothberg JM, Gutterman JU. (1991). A phase I trial of recombinant alpha-2a interferon (Roferon-A) with weekly cisplatinum. *Investigative New Drugs* 9(1):37-39.

Dhodapkar M, Rubin J, Reid JM, Burch PA, Pitot HC, Buckner JC, Ames MM, Suman VJ. (1997). Phase I trial of temozolomide (NSC 362856) in patients with advanced cancer. *Clinical Cancer Research* 3(7):1093-1100.

Dhodapkar MV, Li CY, Lust JA, Tefferi A, Phyliky RL. (1994). Clinical spectrum of clonal proliferations of T-large granular lymphocytes: A T-cell clonopathy of undetermined significance? *Blood* 84(5):1620-1627.

Dhodapkar MV, Richardson RL, Reid JM, Ames MM. (1994). Pyrazine diazohydroxide (NSC-361456). Phase I clinical and pharmacokinetic studies. *Investigative New Drugs* 12(3):207-216.

Diamantis I. (1996). Chronic fatigue syndrome following Lyme borreliosis. *Schweizerische Rundschau fur Medizin Praxis* 85(9):287-288.

Diamond CA, Matthay KK. (1988). Childhood acute lymphoblastic leukemia. *Pediatric Annals* 17(3):156-161, 164-170.

Di Bartolomeo M, Bajetta E, Zilembo N, de Braud F, Di Leo A, Verusio C, D'Aprile M, Scanni A, Barduagni M, Barduagni A [corrected to Barduagni M, et al.] (1993). Treatment of carcinoid syndrome with recombinant interferon alpha-2a. *Acta Oncologica* 32(2):235-238.

DiCarlo SE, Collins HL, Chen CY. (1994). Vagal afferents reflexly inhibit exercise in conscious rats. *Medical Science, Sports and Exercise* 26:459-462.

Dickinson CJ. (1997). Chronic fatigue syndrome: Aetiological aspects. *European Journal of Clinical Investigation* 27(4):257-267.

Dickson BA, Franks RC. (1988). Aldosterone-producing adenoma presenting with hypokalemic myopathy: Case report and review. *Clinical Pediatrics* 27(7):344-347.

Dieras V, Fumoleau P, Bourgeois H, Misset JL, Azli N, Pouillart P. (1996). Taxoids in combination chemotherapy for metastatic breast cancer. *Anticancer Drugs* 7 (Suppl 2):47-52.

Di Fabio RP, Soderberg J, Choi T, Hansen CR, Shapiro RT. (1998). Extended outpatient rehabilitation: Its influence on symptom frequency, fatigue, and functional status for persons with progressive multiple sclerosis. *Archives of Physical Medicine and Rehabilitation* 79(2):141-146.

Digel W, Zahn G, Heinzel G, Porzsolt F. (1991). Pharmacokinetics and biological activity in subcutaneous long-term administration of recombinant interferon-gamma in cancer patients. *Cancer Immunology and Immunotherapy* 34(3):169-174.

Dijkman GA, Fernandez del Moral P, Bruynseels J, de Porre P, Denis L, Debruyne FM. (1997). Liarozole (R75251) in hormone-resistant prostate cancer patients. *Prostate* 33(1):26-31.

Dikken C, Sitzia J. (1988). Patients' experiences of chemotherapy: Side-effects associated with 5-fluorouracil + folinic acid in the treatment of colorectal cancer. *Journal of Clinical Nursing* 7(4):371-379.

Dilhuydy JM, Dilhuydy MS, Ouhtatou F, Laporte C, Nguyen TV, Vendrely V. (2001). [Fatigue and radiotherapy: Literature review]. *Cancer Radiotherapy* 5 (Suppl 1):131s-138s.

Dillman RO, Soori G, Wiemann MC, Schulof R, Dobbs TW, Ruben RH, DePriest CB, Church C. (2000). Phase II trial of subcutaneous interleukin-2, subcutaneous interferon-alpha, intravenous combination chemotherapy, and oral tamoxifen in the treatment of metastatic melanoma: Final results of Cancer Biotherapy Research Group 94-11. *Cancer Biotherapy and Radiopharmacology* 15(5):487-494.

Dillman RO, Wiemann M, Oldham RK, Soori G, Bury M, Hafer R, Church C, DePriest C. (1995). Interferon alpha-2a and external beam radiotherapy in the initial management of patients with glioma: A pilot study of the National Biotherapy Study Group. *Cancer Biotherapy* 10(4):265-271.

Dimaggio JJ, Warrell RP Jr, Muindi J, Stevens YW, Lee SJ, Lowenthal DA, Haines I, Walsh TD, Baltzer L, Yaldaei S, et al. (1990). Phase I clinical and pharmacological study of merbarone. *Cancer Research* 50(4):1151-1155.

Dimeo FC. (2001). Effects of exercise on cancer-related fatigue. *Cancer* 92(6 Suppl):1689-1693.

Dimeo FC. (2002). Radiotherapy-related fatigue and exercise for cancer patients: A review of the literature and suggestions for future research. *Frontiers in Radiation Therapy Oncology* 37:49-56.

Dimeo FC, Bertz H, Finke J, Fetscher S, Mertelsmann R, Keul J. (1996). An aerobic exercise program for patients with haematological malignancies after bone marrow transplantation. *Bone Marrow Transplantation* 18(6):1157-1160.

Dimeo FC, Rumberger BG, Keul J. (1998). Aerobic exercise as therapy for cancer fatigue. *Medicine and Science in Sports and Exercise* 30(4):475-478.

Dimeo FC, Stieglitz RD, Novelli-Fischer U, Fetscher S, Keul J. (1999). Effects of physical activity on the fatigue and psychologic status of cancer patients during chemotherapy. *Cancer* 85(10):2273-2277.

Dimeo FC, Stieglitz RD, Novelli-Fischer U, Fetscher S, Mertelsmann R, Keul J. (1997). Correlation between physical performance and fatigue in cancer patients. *Annals of Oncology* 8(12):1251-1255.

Dimeo FC, Tilmann MH, Bertz H, Kanz L, Mertelsmann R, Keul J. (1997). Aerobic exercise in the rehabilitation of cancer patients after high dose chemotherapy and autologous peripheral stem cell transplantation. *Cancer* 79(9):1717-1722.

Dinan TG, Majeed T, Lavelle E, Scott LV, Berti C, Behan P. (1997). Blunted serotonin-mediated activation of the hypothalamic-pituitary-adrenal axis in chronic fatigue syndrome. *Psychoneuroendocrinology* 22(4):261-267.

Dinarello CA. (1988). Biology of interleukin-1. *FASEB Journal* 2:108-115.

Dinarello CA. (1991). Interleukin-1 and interleukin-1 antagonism. *Blood* 77:1627-1652.

Dinarello CA. (1992). Interleukin-1 and tumor necrosis factor: Effects of cytokines in autoimmune diseases. *Seminars in Immunology* 4(3):133-145.

Dinarello CA, Gelfand JA, Wolff SM. (1993). Anticytokine strategies in the treatment of systemic inflammatory response syndrome. *JAMA* 269:1829-1835.

Dinarello CA, Wolff SM. (1993). Mechanism of disease: The role of interleukin 1 in disease. *New England Journal of Medicine* 328:106-113.

Dinges DF, Pack F, Williams K, Gillen KA, Powell JW, Ott GE, Aptowicz C, Pack AL. (1997). Cumulative sleepiness, mood disturbance, and psychomotor vigilance performance decrements during a week of sleep restricted to 4-5 hours per night. *Sleep* 20(4):267-277.

DiPino RK, Kane RL. (1996). Neurocognitive functioning in chronic fatigue syndrome. *Neuropsychology Review* 6(1):47-60.

Di Saia PJ, Gillette P. (1991). Human lymphoblastoid interferon (IFN-alpha-N1) plus doxorubicin, cyclophosphamide, and cisplatin in the treatment of advanced epithelial ovarian malignancies: A phase I-II study of the Gynecologic Oncology Group. *American Journal of Clinical Oncology* 14(1):71-74.

Disayavanish C, Disayavanish P. (1998). Introduction of the treatment method of Thai traditional medicine: Its validity and future perspectives. *Psychiatry and Clinical Neurosciences* 52(Suppl):S334-S337.

Djaldetti R, Ziv I, Achiron A, Melamed E. (1996). Fatigue in multiple sclerosis compared with chronic fatigue syndrome: A quantitative assessment. *Neurology* 46(3):632-635.

Doberauer C, Mengelkoch B, Kloke O, Wandl U, Niederle N. (1991). Treatment of metastatic carcinoid tumors and the carcinoid syndrome with recombinant interferon alpha. *Acta Oncologica* 30(5):603-605.

Dodd M. (2000). Cancer-related fatigue. *Cancer Investigation* 18(1):97.

Dodd MJ, Miaskowski C, Paul SM. (2001). Symptom clusters and their effect on the functional status of patients with cancer. *Oncology Nursing Forum* 28(3):465-470.

Dombernowsky P, Giaccone G, Sandler A, Schwartsmann G. (1998). Gemcitabine and paclitaxel combinations in non-small cell lung cancer. *Seminars in Oncology* 25(4 Suppl 9):44-50.

Domenge C, Hill C, Lefebvre JL, De Raucourt D, Rhein B, Wibault P, Marandas P, Coche-Dequeant B, Stromboni-Luboinski M, Sancho-Garnier H, et al. (2000). Randomized trial of neoadjuvant chemotherapy in oropharyngeal carcinoma. French Groupe d'Etude des Tumeurs de la Tete et du Cou (GETTEC). *British Journal of Cancer* 83(12):1594-1598.

Dominick KL, Gullette EC, Babyack MA, Mallow KL, Sherwood A, Waugh R, Chilikuri M, Keefe FJ, Blumenthal JA. (1999). Predicting peak oxygen uptake among older patients with chronic illness. *Journal of Cardiopulmonary Rehabilitation* 19(2):81-89.

Donald F, Esdaile JM, Kimoff JR, Fitzcharles MA. (1996). Musculoskeletal complaints and fibromyalgia in patients attending a respiratory sleep disorders clinic. *Journal of Rheumatology* 23(9):1612-1616.

Donaldson K. (1998). Introduction to the healing herbs. *ORL Head and Neck Nursing* 16(3):9-16.

Donaldson SS, Wesley MN, DeWys WD, Suskind RM, Jaffe N, VanEys J. (1981). A study of the nutritional status of pediatric cancer patients. *American Journal of Diseases of Childhood* 135(12):1107-1112.

Donnelly S, Walsh D. (1995). The symptoms of advanced cancer. *Seminars in Oncology* 22(2 Suppl 3):67-72.

Donnelly S, Walsh D, Rybicki L. (1995). The symptoms of advanced cancer: Identification of clinical and research priorities by assessment of prevalence and severity. *Journal of Palliative Care* 11(1):27-32.

Donskov F, von der Maase H, Henriksson R, Stiemer U, Wersall P, Nellemann H, Hellstrand K, Engman K, Naredi P. (2002). Outpatient treatment with subcutaneous histamine dihydrochloride in combination with interleukin-2 and interferon-alpha in patients with metastatic renal cell carcinoma: Results of an open single-armed multicentre phase II study. *Annals of Oncology* 13(3):441-449.

Donta ST, Clauw DJ, Engel CC Jr, Guarino P, Peduzzi P, Williams DA, Skinner JS, Barkhuizen A, Taylor T, Kazis LE, et al. (2003). Cognitive behavioral therapy and aerobic exercise for Gulf War veterans' illnesses: A randomized controlled trial. *JAMA* 289(11):1396-1404.

Dooley M, Goa KL. (1999). Capecitabine. *Drugs* 58(1):69-76; discussion 77-78.

Doran T, Stuhlmiller H, Kim JA, Martin EW, Triozzi PL. (1997). Oncogene and cytokine expression of human colorectal tumors responding to immunotherapy. *Journal of Immunotherapy* 20:372-376.

Douillard JY, Bennouna J, Vavasseur F, Deporte-Fety R, Thomare P, Giacalone F, Meflah K. (2000). Phase I trial of interleukin-2 and high-dose arginine butyrate in metastatic colorectal cancer. *Cancer Immunology and Immunotherapy* 49(1):56-61.

Doull J. (1996). Specificity and dosimetry of toxicologic responses. *Regulatory Toxicology and Pharmacology* 24(1):S55-S57.

Dow KH, Ferrell BR, Leigh S, Ly J, Gulasekaram P. (1996). An evaluation of the quality of life among long-term survivors of breast cancer. *Breast Cancer Research and Treatment* 39(3):261-273.

Dowell JE, Johnson DH, Rogers JS, Shyr Y, McCullough N, Krozely P, De Vore RF. (2001). A phase II trial of 6-hydroxymethylacylfulvene (MGI-114, irofulven) in patients with advanced non-small cell cancer previously treated with chemotherapy. *Investigative New Drugs* 19(1):85-88.

Dowsett EG, Colby J. (1997). Chronic fatigue syndrome in children: Journal was wrong to criticize study in children. *British Medical Journal* 315(7113):949.

Drancourt M, Levy MG. (1990). Rickettsial infection. Abstracts of the Eighth Congress of the American Rickettsial Society.

Dreisbach AW, Hendrickson T, Beezhold D, Riesenberg LA, Sklar AH. (1998). Elevated levels of tumor necrosis factor-alpha in post-dialysis fatigue. *International Journal of Artificial Organs* 21(2):83-86.

Drewes AM, Gade K, Nielsen KD, Bjerregard K, Taagholt SJ, Svendsen L. (1995). Clustering of sleep electroencepalographic patterns in patients with the fibromyalgia syndrome. *British Journal of Rheumatology* 34(12):1151-1156.

Drewes AM, Nielsen KD, Taagholt SJ, Bjerregard K, Svendsen L, Gade J. (1995). Sleep intensity in fibromyalgia: Focus on the microstructure of the sleep process. *British Journal of Rheumatology* 34(7):629-635.

Drewes AM, Nielsen KD, Taagholt SJ, Svendsen L, Bjerregard K, Nielsson L, Kristensen L. (1996). Ambulatory polysomnography using a new programmable amplifier system with on-line digitization of data: Technical and clinical findings. *Sleep* 19(4):347-354.

Dreyfuss AI, Clark JR, Norris CM, Rossi RM, Lucarini JW, Busse PM, Poulin MD, Thornhill L, Costello R, Posner MR. (1996). Docetaxel: An active drug for squamous cell carcinoma of the head and neck. *Journal of Clinical Oncology* 14(5):1672-1678.

Droge W, Eck HP, Gmunder H, Mihm S. (1991). Modulation of lymphocyte functions and immune responses by cysteine and cysteine derivatives. *American Journal of Medicine* 91(3C):140S-144S.

Droge W, Holm E. (1997). Role of cysteine and glutathione in HIV infection and other diseases associated with muscle wasting and immunological dysfunction. *Federation of American Societies of Experimental Biology Journal* 11(13):1077-1089.

Droller MJ. (1987). Immunotherapy of metastatic renal cell carcinoma with polyinosinic-polycytidylic acid. *Journal of Urology* 137(2):202-206.

Du SF, Shi LY, Zhang HJ. (1997). [Study on the quality of life in patients with prostate cancer]. *Zhonghua Liu Xing Bing Xue Za Zhi* 18(2):95-97.

DuBois E. (1986). Gamma globulin therapy for chronic mononucleosis syndrome. *AIDS Research and Human Retroviruses* 2(1):S191-S195.

Dugan MC, Dergham ST, Kucway R, Singh K, Biernat L, Du W, Vaitkevicius VK, Crisaman JD, Sarkar FH. (1997). HER-2/neu expression in pancreatic adenocarcinoma: Relation to tumor differentiation and survival. *Pancreas* 14(3):229-236.

Duke JA. (1985). *CRC Handbook for Medicinal Herbs.* Boca Raton, FL: CRC Press.

Dulli D, Schutta H. (1996). Fatigue in MS. *Neurology* 47(5):1351.

Dunne FJ, Dunne CA. (1995). Fibomyalgia syndrome and psychiatric disorder. *British Journal of Hospital Medicine* 54(5):194-197.

Dunstan RH, Donohoe M, Taylor W, Roberts TK, Murdoch RN, Watkins JA, McGregor NR. (1996). Chlorinated hydrocarbons and chronic fatigue syndrome. *Medical Journal of Australia* 164(4):251.

Dunstan RH, Roberts TK, Donohoe M, McGregor NR, Hope D, Taylor WG, Watkins JA, Murdoch RN, Butt HL. (1996). Bioaccumulated chlorinated hydrocarbons and red/white blood cell parameters. *Biochemical and Molecular Medicine* 58(1):77-84.

Duprez DA, De Buyzere ML, Drieghe B, Vanhaverbeke F, Taes Y, Michielsen W, Clement DL. (1998). Long- and short-term blood pressure and RR-interval variability and psychosomatic distress in chronic fatigue. *Clinical Science* 94(1): 57-63.

Durie BG, Clouse L, Braich T, Grimm M, Robertone AB. (1986). Interferon alfa-2b-cyclophosphamide combination studies: In vitro and phase I-II clinical results. *Seminars in Oncology* 13(3 Suppl 2):84-88.

Durlach J. (1980). Clinical aspects of chronic magnesium deficiency. In *Magnesium in Health and Disease,* Cantin M, Seelig M, eds. New York: Spectrum, pp. 883-909.

Durlach J. (1988). *Magnesium in Clinical Practice.* London: John Libbey and Co. Publisher.

Durrigl MA, Fatovic-Ferencic S. (1999). Between symbolism and experience: Croatian glagolitic recipes (fourteenth to fifteenth centuries) dealing with ocular diseases. *Collegium Antropologium* 23(1):249-254.

Durstine JL, Painter P, Franklin BA, Morgan D, Pitetti KH, Roberts SO. (2000). Physical activity for the chronically ill and disabled. *Sports Medicine* 30(3):207-219.

Dutcher JP, Fisher RI, Weiss G, Aronson F, Margolin K, Louie A, Mier J, Caliendo G, Sosman JA, Eckardt JR, et al. (1997). Outpatient subcutaneous interleukin-2 and interferon-alpha for metastatic renal cell cancer: Five-year follow-up of the Cytokine Working Group study. *Cancer Journal Scientific American* 3(3):157-162.

Dutcher JP, Logan T, Gordon M, Sosman J, Weiss G, Margolin K, Plasse T, Mier J, Lotze M, Clark J, et al. (2000). Phase II trial of interleukin 2, interferon alpha, and 5-fluorouracil in metastatic renal cell cancer: A Cytokine Working Group study. *Clinical Cancer Research* 6(9):3442-3450.

Dutta SC, Chang SC, Coffey CS, Smith JA, Jack G, Cookson MS. (2002). Health related quality of life assessment after radical cystectomy: Comparison of ileal conduit with continent orthotopic neobladder. *Journal of Urology* 168(1):164-167.

Dyck D, Allen S, Barron J, Marchi J, Price BA, Spavor L, Tateishi S. (1996). Management of chronic fatigue syndrome: Case study. *AAOHN Journal* 44(2):85-92.

Dykman KD, Tone C, Ford C, Dykman RA. (1998). The effects of nutritional supplements on the symptoms of fibromyalgia and chronic fatigue syndrome. *Integrative Physiology and Behavioral Science* 33(1):61-71.

Eadington DW. (1988). Hypoglycaemia and metabolic acidosis in a patient with an acute leukaemia. *Scottish Medical Journal* 33(4):309-310.

Eaton B, Worrall G. (1998). The fatigue of cancer. *Canadian Medical Association Journal* 159(8):921.

Eby NL, Grufferman S, Huang M, Whiteside T, Sumaya C, Saxinger WC, Herberman RB. (1989). Natural killer cell activity in the chronic fatigue-immune dysfunction syndrome. In *Natural Killer Cells and Host Defenses,* Ades EW, Lopez C, eds. Basel: Karger, pp. 141-145.

Eckhardt SG, Baker SD, Britten CD, Hidalgo M, Siu L, Hammond LA, Villalona-Calero MA, Felton S, Drengler R, Kuhn JG, et al. (2000). Phase I and pharmacokinetic study of irofulven, a novel mushroom-derived cytotoxin, administered for five consecutive days every four weeks in patients with advanced solid malignancies. *Journal of Clinical Oncology* 18(24):4086-4097.

Eckhardt SG, Baker SD, Eckardt JR, Burke TG, Warner DL, Kuhn JG, Rodriguez G, Fields S, Thurman A, Smith L, et al. (1998). Phase I and pharmacokinetic study of GI147211, a water-soluble camptothecin analogue, administered for five consecutive days every three weeks. *Clinical Cancer Research* 4(3):595-604.

Edelstein MB, Schellekens H, Laurent T, Gauci L. (1983). A phase I clinical tolerance study of rDNA alpha 2 human interferon in patients with non-reticuloendothelial system malignancies. *European Journal of Cancer and Clinical Oncology* 19(7):891-894.

Edlavitch SA. (1997). Antipolymer antibodies, silicone breast implants, and fibromyalgia. *Lancet* 349(9059):1170.

Edmonson JH, Kovach JS, Buckner JC, Kvols LK, Hahn RG. (1988). Phase I study of difluoromethylornithine in combination with recombinant alpha 2a-interferon. *Cancer Research* 48(22):6584-6586.

Edmonson JH, Long HJ, Frytak S, Smithson WA, Itri LM. (1987). Phase II study of recombinant alfa-2a interferon in patients with advanced bone sarcomas. *Cancer Treatment Reports* 71(7-8):747-748.

Eggermont AM, Weimar W, Marquet RL, Lameris JD, Jeekel J. (1985). Phase II trial of high-dose recombinant leukocyte alpha-2 interferon for metastatic colorectal cancer without previous systemic treatment. *Cancer Treatment Reports* 69(2):185-187.

Eggermont AM, Weimar W, Tank B, Dekkers-Bijma AM, Marquet RL, Lameris JS, Westbroek DL, Jeekel J. (1986). Clinical and immunological evaluation of 20 patients with advanced colorectal cancer treated with high dose recombinant leukocyte interferon-alpha A (rIFN alpha A). *Cancer Immunology and Immunotherapy* 21(1):81-84.

Ehrenreich B, English D. (1989). *For Her Own Good: 150 Years of Experts' Advice to Women.* New York: Anchor Books.

Ehrmann-Feldmann D, Spitzer WO, Del Greco L, Desmeules L. (1987). Perceived discrimination against cured cancer patients in the work force. *Canadian Medical Association Journal* 136(7):719-723.

Eich W, Hartmann M, Muller A, Fischer H. (2000). The role of psychosocial factors in fibromyalgia syndrome. *Scandinavian Journal of Rheumatology* 113:30-31.

Eifel P, Axelson JA, Costa J, Crowley J, Curran WJ Jr, Deshler A, Fulton S, Hendricks CB, Kemeny M, Kornblith AB, et al. (2001). National Institutes of Health Consensus Development Conference Statement: Adjuvant therapy for breast cancer, November 1-3, 2000. *Journal of the National Cancer Institutes* 93(13):979-989.

Einhorn N, Ling P, Einhorn S, Strander H. (1988). A phase II study on escalating interferon doses in advanced ovarian carcinoma. *American Journal of Clinical Oncology* 11(1):3-6.

Einzig AI, Neuberg D, Remick SC, Karp DD, O'Dwyer PJ, Stewart JA, Benson AB III. (1996). Phase II trial of docetaxel (Taxotere) in patients with adenocarcinoma of the upper gastrointestinal tract previously untreated with cytotoxic chemotherapy: The Eastern Cooperative Oncology Group (ECOG) results of protocol E1293. *Medical Oncology* 13(2):87-93.

Einzig AI, Schuchter LM, Recio A, Coatsworth S, Rodriquez R, Wiernik PH. (1996). Phase II trial of docetaxel (Taxotere) in patients with metastatic melanoma previously untreated with cytotoxic chemotherapy. *Medical Oncology* 13(2):111-117.

Eisenberg DM, Davis RB, Ettner SL, Appel S, Wilkey S, Van Rompay M, Kessler RC. (1998). Trends in alternative medicine use in the United States, 1990-1997: Results of a follow-up national survey. *JAMA* 280(18):1569-1575.

Eisenberger MA, Reyno LM, Jodrell DI, Sinibaldi VJ, Tkaczuk KH, Sridhara R, Zuhowski EG, Lowitt MH, Jacobs SC, Egorin MJ. (1993). Suramin, an active drug for prostate cancer: Interim observations in a phase I trial. *Journal of the National Cancer Institutes* 85(8):611-621.

Eisenberger MA, Sinibaldi VJ, Reyno LM, Sridhara R, Jodrell DI, Zuhowski EG, Tkaczuk KH, Lowitt MH, Hemady RK, Jacobs SC, et al. (1995). Phase I and clinical evaluation of a pharmacologically guided regimen of suramin in patients with hormone-refractory prostate cancer. *Journal of Clinical Oncology* 13(9): 2174-2186.

Eisinger J. (1998). Alcohol, thiamine and fibromyalgia. *Journal of the American College of Nutrition* 17(3):300-302.

Elfassi E, Patarca R, Haseltine WA. (1986). Similarities among the pre-S regions of hepatitis B viruses: Analogy with retroviral transmembrane proteins. *Journal of Theoretical Biology* 121:371-374.

Ellenbogen C. (1997). Lyme disease: Shift the paradigm. *Archives of Family Medicine* 6(2):191-195.

Elling D, Krocker J, Kummel S, Blohmer J, Lichtenegger W, Kohls A, Heinrich J, Quass J, Breitbach P, Kohler U. (2000). [Dose intensified adjuvant chemotherapy in high risk breast carcinoma with 4-9 positive lymph nodes]. *Zentralblatt Gynakologie* 122(4):207-216.

Elliot DL, Goldberg L, Loveless MO. (1997). Graded exercise testing and chronic fatigue syndrome. *American Journal of Medicine* 103(1):84-86.

Elliot GR, Eisdorfer C. (1982). *Stress and Human Health.* New York: Springer.

Ellis J. (1984). Malaise and fatigue. *British Journal of Hospital Medicine* 32(6): 312-314.

Ellis TM, Hardt NS, Atkinson MA. (1997). Antipolymer antibodies, silicone breast implants, and fibromyalgia. *Lancet* 349(9059):1173.

Elmberger E, Bolund C, Lutzen K. (2000). Transforming the exhausting to energizing process of being a good parent in the face of cancer. *Health Care Women International* 21(6):485-499.

Elsasser-Beile U, Drees N, Neumann HA, Schopf E. (1987). Phase II trial of recombinant leukocyte A interferon in advanced malignant melanoma. *Journal of Cancer Research and Clinical Oncology* 113(3):273-278.

Emery P, Gentry KC, Mackay IR, Muirden KD, Rowley M. (1987). Deficiency of the suppressor inducer subset of T lymphocytes in rheumatoid arthritis. *Arthritis and Rheumatism* 30:849-856.

Emilie D, Touitou R, Raphael M, Pechmaur M, Devergnee O, Rea D, Coumbraras J, Crevon MC, Edelman L, Joab I, et al. (1992). In vivo production of interleukin-10 by malignant cells in AIDS lymphomas. *European Journal of Immunology* 22:2937-2942.

Enzinger PC, Ilson DH, Saltz LB, Martin LK, Kelsen DP. (1999). Phase II clinical trial of 13-cis-retinoic acid and interferon-alpha-2a in patients with advanced esophageal carcinoma. *Cancer* 85(6):1213-1217.

Epstein JB, Phillips N, Parry J, Epstein MS, Nevill T, Stevenson-Moore P. (2002). Quality of life, taste, olfactory and oral function following high-dose chemotherapy and allogeneic hematopoietic cell transplantation. *Bone Marrow Transplantation* 30(11):785-792.

Epstein SA, Kay G, Clauw D, Heaton R, Klein D, Krupp L, Kuck J, Leslie V, Masur D, Wagner M, et al. (1999). Psychiatric disorders in patients with fibromyalgia: A multicenter investigation. *Psychosomatics* 40(1):57-63.

Erickson J, Neidhart DJ, Van Dri J, Kempf DJ, Wang XC, Norbeck DW, Plattner JJ, Rittenhouse JW, Turon M, Wideburg N, et al. (1990). Design, activity and 2.8 A crystal structure of C_2 symmetric inhibitor complexed to HIV-1 protease. *Science* 249(4968):527-533.

Erickson JW, Fesik SW. (1992). Macromolecular X-ray crystallography and NM as tools for structure-based drug design. *Annual Review of Medicinal Chemistry* 27:271-289.

Erickson SL, De Sauvage FJ, Kikly K, Carver-Moore K, Pitts-Meek S, Gillet N, Sheehan KCF, Schreiber RD, Goeddel DV, Moore MW. (1994). Decreased sensitivity to tumor necrosis factor but normal T-cell development in TNF receptor-2-deficient mice. *Nature* 372:560-563.

Ernst E, Weihmayr T. (1998a). Phytotherapie. Folge 6: Anwendung am Nervensystem. *Fortschrift Medizin* 116(24):37-38.

Ernst E, Weihmayr T. (1998b). Phytotherapie. Folge 7: Einsatz am Urogenitaltrakt. *Fortschrift Medizin* 116(25):40-41.

Ernst E, Weihmayr T. (1998c). Phytotherapie. Folge 8 (Schluss): Varia. *Fortschrift Medizin* 116(27):40-42.

Ernstoff MS, Trautman T, Davis CA, Reich SD, Witman P, Balser J, Rudnick S, Kirkwood JM. (1987). A randomized phase I/II study of continuous versus intermittent intravenous interferon gamma in patients with metastatic melanoma. *Journal of Clinical Oncology* 5(11):1804-1810.

Escalante CP, Grover T, Johnson BA, Harle M, Guo H, Mendoza TR, Rivera E, Ho V, Lee EL, Cleeland CS. (2001). A fatigue clinic in a comprehensive cancer center: Design and experiences. *Cancer* 92(6 Suppl):1708-1713.

Escudier B, Lassau N, Couanet D, Angevin E, Mesrati F, Leborgne S, Garofano A, Leboulaire C, Dupouy N, Laplanche A. (2002). Phase II trial of thalidomide in renal-cell carcinoma. *Annals of Oncology* 13(7):1029-1035.

Eskander ED, Harvey HA, Givant E, Lipton A. (1997). Phase I study combining tumor necrosis factor with interferon-alpha and interleukin-2. *American Journal of Clinical Oncology* 20(5):511-514.

Eskelinen M, Pasanen P, Kosma VM, Alhava E. (1992). Primary malignant schwannoma of the small bowel. *Annals Chirurgica Gynaecologica* 81(3):326-328.

Eskens FA, Greim GA, van Zuylen C, Wolff I, Denis LJ, Planting AS, Muskiet FA, Wanders J, Barbet NC, Choi L, et al. (2000). Phase I and pharmacological study of weekly administration of the polyamine synthesis inhibitor SAM 486A (CGP 48 664) in patients with solid tumors. European Organization for Research and Treatment of Cancer Early Clinical Studies Group. *Clinical Cancer Research* 6(5):1736-1743.

Esparza J. (1998). The role of United Nations HIV/AIDS Porgram (UNAIDS) in the prevention of the viral transmission. *Medicina* 58:69-70.

Espat NJ, Copeland EM, Moldawer LL. (1994). Tumor necrosis factor and cachexia: A current perspective. *Surgical Oncology* 3:255-262.

Esper P, Redman BG. (1999). Supportive care, pain management, and quality of life in advanced prostate cancer. *Urology Clinics of North America* 26(2):375-389.

Esrig D, Ahlering TE, Lieskovsky G, Skinner DG. (1992). Experience with fossa recurrence of renal cell carcinoma. *Journal of Urology* 147(6):1491-1494.

Esteva FJ, Valero V, Booser D, Guerra LT, Murray JL, Pusztai L, Cristofanilli M, Arun B, Esmaeli B, Fritsche HA, et al. (2002). Phase II study of weekly docetaxel and trastuzumab for patients with HER-2-overexpressing metastatic breast cancer. *Journal of Clinical Oncology* 20(7):1800-1808.

Eton O, Talpaz M, Lee KH, Rothberg JM, Brell JM, Benjamin RS. (1996). Phase II trial of recombinant human interleukin-2 and interferon-alpha-2a: Implications for the treatment of patients with metastatic melanoma. *Cancer* 77(5):893-899.

Euga R, Chalder TL, Deale A, Wessely S. (1996). A comparison of the characteristics of chronic fatigue syndrome in primary and tertiary care. *British Journal of Psychiatry* 168(1):121-126.

Evans LM, Itri LM, Campion M, Wyler-Plaut R, Krown SE, Groopman JE, Goldsweig H, Volberding PA, West SB, Mitsuyasu RT, et al. (1991). Interferon-alpha 2a in the treatment of acquired immunodeficiency syndrome-related Kaposi's sarcoma. *Journal of Immunotherapy* 10(1):39-50.

Evans WJ. (2002). Physical function in men and women with cancer: Effects of anemia and conditioning. *Oncology* 16(9 Suppl 10):109-115.

Everson MP, Blackburn WD Jr. (1997). Antipolymer antibodies, silicone breast implants, and fibromyalgia. *Lancet* 349(9059):1171; discussion 1172-1173.

Fabricant CG, Fabricant J, Litrenta MM, Minick CR. (1978). Virus-induced atherosclerosis. *Journal of Experimental Medicine* 148:335-340.

Fahim MS, Wang M. (1996). Zinc acetate and lyophilized *Aloë barbadensis* as vaginal contraceptive. *Contraception* 53(4):231-236.

Fairclough DL, Fetting JH, Cella D, Wonson W, Moinpour CM. (1999). Quality of life and quality adjusted survival for breast cancer patients receiving adjuvant therapy. Eastern Cooperative Oncology Group (ECOG). *Quality of Life Research* 8(8):723-731.

Fairhurst D, Waterman M, Lynch S. (1997). Cognitive slowing in chronic fatigue syndrome. *Psychosomatic Medicine* 59(6):638.

Faithfull S. (1997). Analysis of data over time: A difficult statistical issue. *Journal of Advanced Nursing* 25(4):853-858.

Faithfull S. (1998). Fatigue in patients receiving radiotherapy. *Professional Nurse* 13(7):459-461.

Faithfull S, Brada M. (1998). Somnolence syndrome in adults following cranial irradiation for primary brain tumours. *Clinical Oncology* 10(4):250-254.

Falcone A, Antonuzzo A, Danesi R, Allegrini G, Monica L, Pfanner E, Masi G, Ricci S, Del Tacca M, Conte P. (1999). Suramin in combination with weekly epirubicin for patients with advanced hormone-refractory prostate carcinoma. *Cancer* 86(3):470-476.

Falcone A, Cianci C, Pfanner E, Ricci S, Lencioni M, Brunetti I, Giulianotti PC, Vannucci L, Mosca F, Conte PF. (1996). Treatment of metastatic renal cell carcinoma with constant-rate floxuridine infusion plus recombinant alpha 2b-interferon. *Annals of Oncology* 7(6):601-605.

Falcone A, Cianci C, Ricci S, Brunetti I, Bertuccelli M, Conte PF. (1993). Alpha-2B-interferon plus floxuridine in metastatic renal cell carcinoma: A phase I-II study. *Cancer* 72(2):564-568.

Falcone A, Pfanner E, Cianci C, Danesi R, Brunetti I, Del Tacca M, Conte PF. (1995). Suramin in patients with metastatic colorectal cancer pretreated with fluoropyrimidine-based chemotherapy: A phase II study. *Cancer* 75(2):440-443.

Falk S, Krishnan J, Meis JM. (1993). Primary angiosarcoma of the spleen: A clinicopathologic study of 40 cases. *American Journal of Surgical Pathology* 17(10):959-970.

Falkson CI, Falkson HC. (1996). A randomised study of CGS 16949A (fadrozole) versus tamoxifen in previously untreated postmenopausal patients with metastatic breast cancer. *Annals of Oncology* 7(5):465-469.

Falkson G, Raats JI, Falkson HC. (1992). Fadrozole hydrochloride, a new nontoxic aromatase inhibitor for the treatment of patients with metastatic breast cancer. *Journal of Steroid Biochemistry and Molecular Biology* 43(1-3):161-165.

Fallowfield L, Gagnon D, Zagari M, Cella D, Bresnahan B, Littlewood TJ, McNulty P, Gorzegno G, Freund M; for the Epoetin Alfa Study Group. (2002). Multivariate regression analyses of data from a randomised, double-blind, placebo-controlled study confirm quality of life benefit of epoetin alfa in patients receiving non-platinum chemotherapy. *British Journal of Cancer* 87(12):1341-1353.

Farag SS, George SL, Lee EJ, Baer M, Dodge RK, Becknell B, Fehniger T, Silverman LR, Crawford J, Bloomfield CD, et al. (2002). Postremission therapy with low-dose interleukin 2 with or without intermediate pulse dose interleukin 2 therapy is well tolerated in elderly patients with acute myeloid leukemia: Cancer and Leukemia Group B study 9420. *Clinical Cancer Research* 8(9):2812-2819.

Fauci AS. (1993). Multifactorial nature of human immunodeficiency virus disease: Implications for therapy. *Science* 262:1011-1018.

Fauci AS, Rosenberg SA, Sherwin SA, Dinarello CA, Longo DL, Lane HC. (1987). Immunomodulators in clinical medicine. *Annals of Internal Medicine* 106:421-433.

Fawzy FI, Cousins N, Fawzy NW, Kemeny ME, Elashoff R, Morton D. (1990). A structured psychiatric intervention for cancer patients: I. Changes over time in methods of coping and affective disturbance. *Archives of General Psychiatry* 47(8):720-725.

Fawzy NW. (1995). A psychoeducational nursing intervention to enhance coping and affective state in newly diagnosed malignant melanoma patients. *Cancer Nursing* 18(6):427-438.

Fazely F, Dezube BJ, Allen-Ryan J, Pardee AB, Ruprecht RM. (1991). Pentoxifylline (Trental) decreases the replication of the human immunodeficiency virus type 1 in human peripheral blood mononuclear cells and in cultured T cells. *Blood* 77(8):1653-1656.

Feinberg B, Kurzrock R, Talpaz M, Blick M, Saks S, Gutterman JU. (1988). A phase I trial of intravenously-administered recombinant tumor necrosis factor-alpha in cancer patients. *Journal of Clinical Oncology* 6(8):1328-1334.

Feliu J, Martin G, Lizon J, Chacon JI, Dorta J, de Castro J, Rodriguez A, Sanchez Heras B, Torrego JC, Espinosa E, et al. (2001). Sequential therapy in advanced non-small-cell lung cancer with weekly paclitaxel followed by cisplatin-gemcitabine-vinorelbine: A phase II study. *Annals of Oncology* 12(10):1369-1374.

Feller N, Versantvoort CH, Boven E, Lankelma J, Pinedo HM, Broxterman HJ. (1994). ATP dependence and activity of drug transporters in vivo and in intact tumor cells. *Proceedings of the Annual Meeting of the American Association of Cancer Research* 35:A2076.

Feng F, Xu B, Jiang Z. (1999). [Clinical study of anastrozole in the treatment of postmenopausal women with advanced breast cancer]. *Zhonghua Zhong Liu Za Zhi* 21(5):376-378.

Ferrell BR, Grant M, Funk B, Garcia N, Otis-Green S, Schaffner ML. (1996). Quality of life in breast cancer. *Cancer Practice* 4(6):331-340.

Ferrell BR, Grant MM, Funk BM, Otis-Green SA, Garcia NJ. (1998). Quality of life in breast cancer survivors: Implications for developing support services. *Oncology Nursing Forum* 25(5):887-895.

Feun LG, Blyden G, Yrizarry J, Dorvil M, Waldman S, Benedetto P, Donnelly E, Curtas J, George M, Savaraj N. (1993). Clinical and pharmacological study of intrahepatic artery infusion of thiotepa. *Cancer Biotherapy* 8(1):43-48.

Feun LG, Savaraj N, Benedetto P, Hanlon J, Sridhar KS, Collier M, Richman S, Liao SH, Clendeninn NJ. (1991). Phase I trial of piritrexim capsules using prolonged, low-dose oral administration for the treatment of advanced malignancies. *Journal of the National Cancer Institutes* 83(1):51-55.

Feun LG, Savaraj N, Hung S, Reddy R, Jeffers L, Benedetto P, Livingstone AS, Ardalan B, Levi JU, Parker T, et al. (1994). A phase II trial of recombinant leukocyte interferon plus doxorubicin in patients with hepatocellular carcinoma. *American Journal of Clinical Oncology* 17(5):393-395.

Feun LG, Savaraj N, Hurley J, Marini A, Lai S. (2000). A clinical trial of intravenous vinorelbine tartrate plus tamoxifen in the treatment of patients with advanced malignant melanoma. *Cancer* 88(3):584-588.

Feun LG, Savaraj N, Moffat F, Robinson D, Liebmann A, Hurley J, Raub WA Jr, Richman SP. (1995). Phase II trial of recombinant interferon-alpha with BCNU, cisplatin, DTIC and tamoxifen in advanced malignant melanoma. *Melanoma Research* 5(4):273-276.

Feyer P. (2000). [Fatigue in cancer patients—Pathophysiology and therapeutic strategies]. *Krankenpfl J* 38(4):116-118.

Fibromyalgia (2000). *Health News* 6(2):1-2.

Fiedler N, Kipen HM, DeLuca J, Kelly-McNeil K, Natelson B. (1996). A controlled comparison of multiple chemical sensitivites and chronic fatigue syndrome. *Psychosomatic Medicine* 58(1):38-49.

Fiedler N, Kipen HM, Natelson B, Ottenweller J. (1996). Chemical sensitivities and the Gulf War: Department of Veterans Affairs research center in basic and clinical studies of environmental hazards. *Regulatory Toxicology and Pharmacology* 24(1 Pt 2):S129-S138.

Fiedler R, Neef H, Hennig H, Rosendahl W, Lautenschlager C. (1997). [Quality of life after pneumonectomy for bronchial carcinoma]. *Zentralblatt Chirurgie* 122(5):327-331.

Fiedler R, Neef H, Rosendahl W. (1999). [Functional outcome and quality of life at least 6 months after pneumonectomy—Effect of operation, adjuvant therapy, tumor stage, sex, type of pneumonia and recurrence]. *Pneumologie* 53(1):45-49.

Fiegl M, Strasser-Wozak E, Geley S, Gsur A, Drach J, Kofler R. (1995). Glucocorticoid-mediated immunomodulation: Hydrocortisone enhances immunosuppressive endogenous retroviral protein (p15E) in mouse immune cells. *Clinical and Experimental Immunology* 101:259-264.

Fiegler W, Langer M, Hedde JP, Scheer M, Felix R, Kazner E. (1986). [Comparison of the computed tomographic changes and the clinical course following the irradiation of intracranial tumors and metastases]. *Strahlentherapie und Onkologie* 162(3):145-151.

Field TM, Grizzle N, Scafidi F, Abrams S. (1996). Massage therapy for infants of depressed mothers. *Infant Behavior and Development* 19:107-112.

Field TM, Morrow C, Valdeon C, Larson S, Kuhn C, Schanberg S. (1992). Massage therapy reduces anxiety in child and adolescent psychiatric patients. *Journal of the American Academy of Child and Adolescent Psychology* 31:125-131.

Field TM, Sunshine W, Hernandez-Reif M, Quintino O, Schanberg S, Kuhn C, Burman I. (1997). Massage therapy effects on depression and somatic symptoms in chronic fatigue syndrome. *Journal of Chronic Fatigue Syndrome* 3:43-52.

Fieler VK. (1997). Side effects and quality of life in patients receiving high-dose rate brachytherapy. *Oncology Nursing Forum* 24(3):545-553.

Figg WD, Arlen P, Gulley J, Fernandez P, Noone M, Fedenko K, Hamilton M, Parker C, Kruger EA, Pluda J, et al. (2001). A randomized phase II trial of docetaxel (taxotere) plus thalidomide in androgen-independent prostate cancer. *Seminars in Oncology* 28(4 Suppl 15):62-66.

Figg WD, Dahut W, Duray P, Hamilton M, Tompkins A, Steinberg SM, Jones E, Premkumar A, Linehan WM, Floeter MK, et al. (2001). A randomized phase II trial of thalidomide, an angiogenesis inhibitor, in patients with androgen-independent prostate cancer. *Clinical Cancer Research* 7(7):1888-1893.

Figlin RA, Belldegrun A, Moldawer N, Zeffren J, deKernion J. (1992). Concomitant administration of recombinant human interleukin-2 and recombinant interferon alfa-2A: An active outpatient regimen in metastatic renal cell carcinoma. *Journal of Clinical Oncology* 10(3):414-421.

Figlin RA, Callaghan M, Sarna G. (1983). Phase II trial of alpha (human leukocyte) interferon administered daily in adenocarcinoma of the colon/rectum. *Cancer Treatment Reports* 67(5):493-494.

Filipovich AH, Mathur A, Kamat D, Shapiro RS. (1992). Primary immunodeficiencies: Genetic risk factors for lymphoma. *Cancer Research* 52(19):5465s-5467s.

Findley JC, Kerns R, Weinberg LD, Rosenberg R. (1998). Self-efficacy as a psychological moderator of chronic fatigue syndrome. *Journal of Behavioral Medicine* 21(4):351-362.

Finestone AJ. (1997). A doctor's dilemma: Is a diagnosis disabling or enabling? *Archives of Internal Medicine* 157(5):491-492.

Finestone HM, Stenn P, Davies F, Stalker C, Fry R, Koumanis J. (2000). Chronic pain and health care utilization in women with a history of childhood sexual abuse. *Child Abuse and Neglect* 24(4):547-556.

Finley JP. (2000). Management of cancer cachexia. *AACN Clinical Issues* 11(4):590-603.

Finter NB, Chapman S, Dowd P, Johnston JM, Manna V, Sarantis N, Sheron N, Scott G, Phua S, Tatum PB. (1991). The use of interferon-alpha in virus infections. *Drugs* 42(5):749-765.

Fiore G, Giacovazzo F, Giacovazzo M. (1997). Three cases of dermatomyositis erroneously diagnosed as "chronic fatigue syndrome." *European Reviews of Medical and Pharmacological Sciences* 1(6):193-195.

Firenzouli F, Gori L. (1999). Guidelines in phytotherapy: Phytotherapy in Italy. Associazione Nazionale Medici Fitoterapeuti (ANMFIT). *Journal of Alternative and Complementary Medicine* 5(2):219-220.

Fiscella K, Franks P, Gold MR, Clancy M. (2000). Inequality in quality: Addressing socioeconomic, racial and ethnic disparities in health care. *JAMA* 283:2579-2584.

Fischer JR, Darjes H, Lahm H, Schindel M, Drings P, Krammer PH. (1994). Constitutive secretion of bioactive transforming growth factor beta 1 by small cell lung cancer cell lines. *European Journal of Cancer* 30A(14):2125-2129.

Fischl MA, Finkelstein DM, He W, Powderly WG, Triozzi PL, Steigbigel RT. (1996). A phase II study of recombinant human interferon-alpha 2a and zidovudine in patients with AIDS-related Kaposi's sarcoma. AIDS Clinical Trials Group. *Journal of Acquired Immune Deficiency Syndromes and Human Retrovirology* 11(4):379-384.

Fischler B, Dendale P, Michiels V, Cluydts R, Kaufman L, De Meirleir K. (1997). Physical fatigability and exercise capacity in chronic fatigue syndrome: Association with disability, somatization and psychopathology. *Journal of Psychosomatic Research* 42(4):368-378.

Fischler B, D'Haenen H, Cluydts R, Michiels V, Demets K, Bossuyt A, Kaufman L, De Meirleir K. (1996). Comparison of 99m TcHMPAO SPECT scan between chronic fatigue syndrome, major depression and healthy controls: An exploratory study of clinical correlates of regional cerebral blood flow. *Neuropsychobiology* 34(4):175-183.

Fischler B, Flamen P, Everaert H, Bossuyt A, De Meirleir K. (1998). Physiopathological significance of 99m Tc HMPAO SPECT scan anomalies in chronic fatigue syndrome. *Journal of Chronic Fatigue Syndrome* 4(4):15-30.

Fischler B, Le Bon O, Hoffmann G, Cluydts R, Kaufman L, De Meirleir K. (1997). Sleep anomalies in the chronic fatigue syndrome: A comorbidity study. *Neuropsychobiology* 35(3):115-122.

Fishbain D. (2000). Evidence-based data on pain relief with antidepressants. *Annals of Medicine* 32(5):305-316.

Fisher A, Konig W. (1991). Influence of cytokines and cellular interactions on the glucocorticoid-induced Ig (E, G, A, M) synthesis of peripheral blood mononuclear cells. *Immunology* 74(2):228-233.

Fisher DJ Jr, Slotman GJ, Opal SM, Pribble JP, Bone RC, Emmanuel G, Ng D, Bloedow DC, Catalano MA. (1994). Initial evaluation of human recombinant interleukin 1 receptor antagonist in the treatment of sepsis syndrome: A randomized, open-label, placebo-controlled multicenter trial. The IL1RA Sepsis Syndrome Study Group. *Critical Care Medicine* 22:12-21.

Fisk JD, Ritvo PG, Ross L, Haase DA, Marrie TJ. (1994). Measuring the functional impact of fatigue: Initial validation of the Fatigue Impact Scale. *Clinical Infectious Diseases* 18(Suppl 1):579-583.

Fitch MI, Bakker D, Conlon M. (1999). [Important issues in clinical practice: Perspectives of oncology nurses]. *Canadian Oncology Nursing Journal* 9(4):151-164.

Fitzcharles MA. (1999). Is fibromyalgia a distinct clinical entity? The approving rheumatologist's evidence. *Baillieres Best Practice Research in Clinical Rheumatology* 13(3):437-443.

Fitzcharles MA, Esdaile JM. (1997). The overdiagnosis of fibromyalgia syndrome. *American Journal of Medicine* 103(1):44-50.

Fitzgibbon EJ, Murphy D, O'Shea K, Kelleher C. (1997). Chronic debilitating fatigue in Irish general practice: A survey of general practitioners' experience. *British Journal of General Practice* 47(423):618-622.

Flandrin G, Daniel MT. (1974). [Hairy cell leukemia, a rare and little known variety of malignant hemopathy]. *Nouvelle Presse Medicale* 3(10):581-586.

Flanigan MJ, Morehouse RL, Shapiro CM. (1995). Determination of observer-rated alpha activity during sleep. *Sleep* 18(8):702-706.

Flanigan RC, Saiers JH, Wolf M, Kraut EH, Smith AY, Blumenstein B, Crawford ED. (1994). Phase II evaluation of merbarone in renal cell carcinoma. *Investigative New Drugs* 12(2):147-149.

Flechtner H, Ruffer JU, Henry-Amar M, Mellink WA, Sieber M, Ferme C, Eghbali H, Josting A, Diehl V. (1998). Quality of life assessment in Hodgkin's disease: A new comprehensive approach. First experiences from the EORTC/GELA and GHSG trials. EORTC Lymphoma Cooperative Group. Groupe D'Etude des Lymphomes de L'Adulte and German Hodgkin Study Group. *Annals of Oncology* 9(Suppl 5):S147-S154.

Fletcher MA, Azen S, Adesberg B, Gjerset G, Hassett J, Kaplan J, Niland JC, Odom-Maryon T, Parker JW, Stites DP, et al. (1989). Immunophenotyping in a multicenter study: The transfusion safety experience. *Clinical Immunology and Immunopathology* 52:38-47.

Fletcher MA, Goldstein AL. (1987). Recent advances in the understanding of the biochemistry and clinical pharmacology of interleukin-2. *Lymphkine Research* 1:45-57.

Fletcher MA, Maher K, Patarca-Montero R, Klimas N. (2000). Comparative analysis of lymphocytes in lymph nodes and peripheral blood of patients with chronic fatigue syndrome. *Journal of Chronic Fatigue Syndrome* 7(3):65-75.

Fletcher WS, Daniels DS, Sondak VK, Dana B, Townsend R, Hynes HE, Hutchins LF, Pancoast JR. (1993). Evaluation of cisplatin and DTIC in inoperable stage III and IV melanoma: A Southwest Oncology Group study. *American Journal of Clinical Oncology* 16(4):359-362.

Flitsch J, Spitzner S, Ludecke DK. (2000). Emotional disorders in patients with different types of pituitary adenomas and factors affecting the diagnostic process. *Experimental and Clinical Endocrinolology and Diabetes* 108(7):480-485.

Flynn A, Yen BR. (1981). Mineral deficiency effects on the generation of cytotoxic T cells and T-helper cell factors in vitro. *Journal of Nutrition* 111:907-913.

Fohlman J, Friman G, Tuvemo T. (1997). Enterovirus infections in new disguise. *Lakartidningen* 94(28-29):2555-2560.

Foltz AT, Gaines G, Gullatte M. (1996). Recalled side effects and self-care actions of patients receiving inpatient chemotherapy. *Oncology Nursing Forum* 23(4): 679-683.

Foon KA, Bottino GC, Abrams PG, Fer MF, Longo DL, Schoenberger CS, Oldham RK. (1985). Phase II trial of recombinant leukocyte A interferon in patients with advanced chronic lymphocytic leukemia. *American Journal of Medicine* 78(2): 216-220.

Foon KA, Roth MS, Bunn PA Jr. (1987). Interferon therapy of non-Hodgkin's lymphoma. *Cancer* 59(3 Suppl):601-604.

Foon KA, Sherwin SA, Abrams PG, Stevenson HC, Holmes P, Maluish AE, Oldham RK, Herberman RB. (1985). A phase I trial of recombinant gamma interferon in patients with cancer. *Cancer Immunology and Immunotherapy* 20(3): 193-197.

Foote J, Cohen B. (1998). Medicinal herb use and the renal patient. *Journal of Renal Nutrition* 8(1):40-42.

Forastiere AA, Natale RB, Takasugi BJ, Goren MP, Vogel WC, Kudla-Hatch V. (1987). A phase I-II trial of carboplatin and 5-fluorouracil combination chemotherapy in advanced carcinoma of the head and neck. *Journal of Clinical Oncology* 5(2):190-196.

Forastiere AA, Perry DJ, Wolf GT, Wheeler RH, Natale RB. (1988). Cisplatin and mitoguazone: An induction chemotherapy regimen in advanced head and neck cancer. *Cancer* 62(11):2304-2308.

Ford CV. (1997). Somatization and fashionable diagnoses: Illness as a way of life. *Scandinavian Journal of Work and Environmental Health* 23(Suppl 3):7-16.

Ford H, Trigwell P, Johnson M. (1998). The nature of fatigue in multiple sclerosis. *Journal of Psychosomatic Research* 45:33-38.

Fordyce WE. (2000). Fibromyalgia and related matters. *Clinical Journal of Pain* 16(2):181-182.

Forester B, Kornfeld DS, Fleiss JL. (1985). Psychotherapy during radiotherapy: Effects on emotional and physical distress. *American Journal of Psychiatry* 142 (1):22-27.

Forester B, Kornfeld DS, Fleiss JL, Thompson S. (1993). Group psychotherapy during radiotherapy: Effects on emotional and physical distress. *American Journal of Psychiatry* 150(11):1700-1706.

Forsberg C, Bjorvell H, Cedermark B. (1996). Well-being and its relation to coping ability in patients with colo-rectal and gastric cancer before and after surgery. *Scandinavian Journal of Caring Science* 10(1):35-44.

Forseth KO, Forre O, Gran JT. (1999). A 5.5 year prospective study of self-reported musculoskeletal pain and of fibromyalgia in a female population: Significance and natural history. *Clinical Rheumatology* 18(2):114-121.

Forseth KO, Gran JT, Husby G. (1997). A population study of the incidence of fibromyalgia among women aged 26-55 yr. *British Journal of Rheumatology* 36(12):1318-1323.

Forsyth LM, Preuss HG, MacDowell AL, Chiazze L, Birkmayer GD, Bellanti JA. (1999). Therapeutic effects of oral NADH on the symptoms of patients with chronic fatigue syndrome. *Annals of Allergy, Asthma and Immunology* 82:185-191.

Fortis C, Foppoli M, Gianotti L, Galli L, Citterio G, Consogno G, Gentilini O, Braga, M (1996). Increased interleukin-10 serum levels in patients with solid tumors. *Cancer Letters* 104:1-5.

Fossa SD. (1996). Quality of life in advanced prostate cancer. *Seminars in Oncology* 23(6 Suppl 14):32-34.

Fossa SD, Aaronson N, Calais da Silva F, Denis L, Newling D, Hosbach G, Kaalhus O. (1989). Quality of life in patients with muscle-infiltrating bladder cancer and hormone-resistant prostatic cancer. *European Urology* 16(5):335-339.

Fossa SD, Aaronson N, de Voogt HJ, da Silva FC. (1990). Assessment of quality of life and subjective response criteria in patients with prostatic cancer. *Progress in Clinical Biological Research* 357:199-202.

Fossa SD, Aaronson N, Newling D, van Cangh PJ, Denis L, Kurth KH, de Pauw M. (1990). Quality of life and treatment of hormone resistant metastatic prostatic cancer. The EORTC Genito-Urinary Group. *European Journal of Cancer* 26 (11-12):1133-1136.

Fossa SD, de Garis ST, Heier MS, Flokkmann A, Lien HH, Salveson A, Moe B. (1986). Recombinant interferon alfa-2a with or without vinblastine in metastatic renal cell carcinoma. *Cancer* 57(8 Suppl):1700-1704.

Fossa SD, Martinelli G, Otto U, Schneider G, Wander H, Oberling F, Bauer HW, Achtnicht U, Holdener EE. (1992). Recombinant interferon alfa-2a with or without vinblastine in metastatic renal cell carcinoma: Results of a European multi-center phase III study. *Annals of Oncology* 3(4):301-305.

Fossa SD, Paus E, Lindegaard M, Newling DW. (1992). Prostate-specific antigen and other prognostic factors in patients with hormone-resistant prostatic cancer undergoing experimental treatment. *British Journal of Urology* 69(2):175-179.

Fossa SD, Slee PH, Brausi M, Horenblas S, Hall RR, Hetherington JW, Aaronson N, de Prijck L, Collette L. (2001). Flutamide versus prednisone in patients with prostate cancer symptomatically progressing after androgen-ablative therapy: A phase III study of the European organization for research and treatment of cancer genitourinary group. *Journal of Clinical Oncology* 19(1):62-71.

Fossa SD, Woehre H, Kurth KH, Hetherington J, Bakke H, Rustad DA, Skanvik R. (1997). Influence of urological morbidity on quality of life in patients with prostate cancer. *European Urology* 31(Suppl 3):3-8.

Foster S, Tyler VE. (1992). *Tyler's Honest Herbal: A Sensible Guide to the Use of Herbs and Related Remedies.* Binghamton, NY: The Haworth Press.

Foulds S, Wakefield CH, Giles M, Gillespie J, Dye JF, Guillou PJ. (1993). Expression of a suppressive p15E-related epitope in colorectal and gastric cancer. *British Journal of Cancer* 68:610-616.

Fountzilas G, Nicolaides C, Bafaloukos D, Kalogera-Fountzila A, Kalofonos H, Samelis G, Aravantinos G, Pavlidis N. (2000). Docetaxel and gemcitabine in anthracycline-resistant advanced breast cancer: A Hellenic Cooperative Oncology Group phase II study. *Cancer Investigation* 18(6):503-509.

Fountzilas G, Papadimitriou C, Aravantinos G, Nicolaides C, Stathopoulos G, Bafaloukos D, Kalofonos H, Ekonomopoulos T, Skarlos D, Pavlidis N, et al. (2001). Dose-dense sequential adjuvant chemotherapy with epirubicin, paclitaxel and CMF in high-risk breast cancer. *Oncology* 60(3):214-220.

Fountzilas G, Skarlos D, Pavlidis NA, Makrantonakis P, Tsavaris N, Kalogera-Fountzila A, Giannakakis T, Beer M, Kosmidis P. (1991). High-dose epirubicin as a single agent in the treatment of patients with advanced breast cancer: A Hellenic Co-operative Oncology Group study. *Tumori* 77(3):232-236.

Fountzilas G, Tsavdaridis D, Kalogera-Fountzila A, Christodoulou CH, Timotheadou E, Kalofonos CH, Kosmidis P, Adamou A, Papakostas P, Gogas H, et al. (2001). Weekly paclitaxel as first-line chemotherapy and trastuzumab in patients with advanced breast cancer: A Hellenic Cooperative Oncology Group phase II study. *Annals of Oncology* 12(11):1545-1551.

Fox RI, Luppi M, Pisa P, Kang HI. (1992). Potential role of Epstein-Barr virus in Sjogren's syndrome and rheumatoid arthritis. *Journal of Rheumatology* 32: 18-24.

Francis K. (1996a). Physical activity: Breast and reproductive cancer. *Comprehensive Therapy* 22:94-99.

Francis K. (1996b). Physical activity in prevention and rehabilitation of breast cancer. *Critical Reviews in Physical Rehabilitation Medicine* 8:323-341.

Francis P, Rowinsky E, Schneider J, Hakes T, Hoskins W, Markman M. (1996). Phase I feasibility and pharmacologic study of weekly intraperitoneal paclitaxel: A Gynecologic Oncology Group pilot study. *Journal of Clinical Oncology* 13(12):2961-2967.

Franco E, Kawa-Ha K, Doi S, Yumura K, Murata M, Ishihara S, Tawa A, Yabuuchi H. (1987). Remarkable depression of CD4+2H4+ T cells in severe chronic active Epstein-Barr virus infection. *Scandinavian Journal of Immunology* 26:769-773.

Frangoul HA, Shaw DW, Hawkins D, Park J. (2000). Diabetes insipidus as a presenting symptom of acute myelogenous leukemia. *Journal of Pediatric Hematology Oncology* 22(5):457-459.

Frankel WL, Shapiro P, Weidner N. (2000). Primary anaplastic large cell lymphoma of the adrenal gland. *Annals of Diagnostic Pathology* 4(3):158-164.

Franklin AJ. (1997). Graded exercise in chronic fatigue syndrome: Including patients who rated themselves as a little better would have altered results. *British Medical Journal* 315(7113):947-948.

Fraschini G, Ciociola A, Esparza L, Templeton D, Holmes FA, Walters RS, Hortobagyi GN. (1991). Evaluation of three oral dosages of ondansetron in the prevention of nausea and emesis associated with cyclophosphamide-doxorubicin chemotherapy. *Journal of Clinical Oncology* 9(7):1268-1274.

Frasci G, D'Aiuto G, Comella P, Apicella A, Thomas R, Capasso I, Di Bonito M, Carteni G, Biglietto M, De Lucia L, et al. (1999). Cisplatin-epirubicin-paclitaxel weekly administration in advanced breast cancer: A phase I study of the Southern Italy Cooperative Oncology Group. *Breast Cancer Research and Treatment* 56(3):239-252.

Frasci G, Iaffaioli RV, Comella G, Comella P, Salzano F, Galizia G, Imbriani A, Persico G. (1994). Intraperitoneal adjuvant immunochemotherapy in operable gastric cancer with serosal involvement. *Clinical Oncology* 6(6):364-370.

Frasci G, Nicolella G, Comella P, Carreca I, DeCataldis G, Muci D, Brunetti C, Natale M, Piantedosi F, Russo A, et al. (2001). A weekly regimen of cisplatin, paclitaxel and topotecan with granulocyte-colony stimulating factor support for patients with extensive disease small cell lung cancer: A phase II study. *British Journal of Cancer* 84(9):1166-1171.

Frasci G, Tortoriello A, Facchini G, Conforti S, Cardone A, Persico G, Mastrantonio P, Iaffaioli RV. (1993). Intraperitoneal (ip) cisplatin-mitoxantrone-interferon-alpha 2b in ovarian cancer patients with minimal residual disease. *Gynecological Oncology* 50(1):60-67.

Frasci G, Tortoriello A, Facchini G, Conforti S, Persico G, Mastrantonio P, Cardone A, Iaffaioli RV. (1994). Carboplatin and alpha-2b interferon intraperitoneal combination as first-line treatment of minimal residual ovarian cancer: A pilot study. *European Journal of Cancer* 30A(7):946-950.

Freeman AL, Al-Bussam N, O'Malley JA, Stutzman L, Bjornsson S, Carter WA. (1977). Pharmacologic effects of polyinosinic-polycytidylic acid in man. *Journal of Medical Virology* 1:79-93.

Freeman R, Komaroff AL. (1997). Does the chronic fatigue syndrome involve the autonomic nervous system? *American Journal of Medicine* 102(4):357-364.

Freund M, von Wussow P, Diedrich H, Eisert R, Link H, Wilke H, Buchholz F, LeBlanc S, Fonatsch C, Deicher H, et al. (1989). Recombinant human interferon (IFN) alpha-2b in chronic myelogenous leukaemia: Dose dependency of response and frequency of neutralizing anti-interferon antibodies. *British Journal of Haematology* 72(3):350-356.

Friedberg F, Jason LA. (1998). *Understanding Chronic Fatigue Syndrome: An Empirical Guide to Assessment and Treatment*. Washington, DC: American Psychological Association.

Friedberg F, Krupp LB. (1994). A comparison of cognitive behavioral treatment for chronic fatigue syndrome and primary depression. *Clinical Infectious Diseases* 18(Suppl 1):S105-S110.

Friedman LC, Lehane D, Webb JA, Weinberg AD, Cooper HP. (1994). Anxiety in medical situations and chemotherapy-related problems among cancer patients. *Journal of Cancer Education* 9(1):37-41.

Friendenreich CM, Courneya KS. (1996). Exercise as rehabilitation for cancer patients. *Clinical Journal of Sport Medicine* 6(4):237-244.

Friendenreich CM, Rohan TE. (1995). Physical activity and the risk of breast cancer. *European Journal of Cancer Prevention* 4:145-151.

Friis S, Mellemkjaer L, McLaughlin JK, Breiting V, Kjaer SK, Blot W, Olsen JH. (1997). Connective tissue disease and other rheumatic conditions following breast implants in Denmark. *Annals of Plastic Surgery* 39(1):1-8.

Frothingham C. (1911). The relation between acute infectious diseases and arterial lesions. *Archives of Internal Medicine* 8:153-162.

Fry AM, Martin M. (1996a). Cognitive idiosyncracies among children with the chronic fatigue syndrome: Anomalies in self-reported activity levels. *Journal of Psychosomatic Research* 41(3):213-223.

Fry AM, Martin M. (1996b). Fatigue in the chronic fatigue syndrome: A cognitive phenomenon? *Journal of Psychosomatic Research* 41(5):415-426.

Fu MR, Anderson CM, McDaniel R, Armer J. (2002). Patients' perceptions of fatigue in response to biochemotherapy for metastatic melanoma: A preliminary study. *Oncology Nursing Forum* 29(6):961-966.

Fuchs D, Baier-Bitterlich G, Wachter H. (1995). Nitric oxide and AIDS dementia. *New England Journal of Medicine* 333(8):521-522.

Fuchs D, Hausen A, Reibnegger G, Werner ER, Dierich MP, Wachter H. (1988). Neopterin as a marker for activated cell-mediated immunity. *Immunology Today* 9:150-155.

Fuchs D, Muur C, Reibnegger G, Weiss G, Werner ER, Werner-Felmayer G, Wachter H. (1994). Nitric oxide synthase and antimicrobial armature of human macrophages. *Journal of Infectious Diseases* 169:224.

Fuchs H, Johnson JS, Sergent JS. (1995). Still more on breast implants and connective-tissue diseases. *New England Journal of Medicine* 333(8):526.

Fujisawa S, Motomura S, Fujita H, Fukawa H, Kanamori H, Noguchi T, Matsuzaki M, Mohri H, Ohkubo T. (1992). [Malignant histiocytosis associated with central neurological symptoms and cerebrospinal fluid involvement]. *Rinsho Ketsueki* 33(7):981-985.

Fujiwara M, Zaha M, Odashiro M, Kawamura J, Hayashi I, Mizoguchi H. (1992). [Use of diltiazem in the anesthetic management of epinephrine predominant pheochromocytoma]. *Masui* 41(7):1175-1179.

Fujiyama S, Sato K, Sakai M, Sato T, Tashiro S, Arakawa M. (1990). A case of type Ia glycogen storage disease complicated by hepatic adenoma. *Hepatogastroenterology* 37(4):432-435.

Fukuda K, Dobbins JG, Wilson LJ, Dunn RA, Wilcox K, Smallwood D. (1997). An epidemiologic study of fatigue with relevance for the chronic fatigue syndrome. *Journal of Psychiatric Research* 31(1):19-29.

Fukuoka M, Takada M, Yokoyama A, Kurita Y, Niitani H. (1997). Phase II studies of gemcitabine for non-small cell lung cancer in Japan. *Seminars in Oncology* 24(2 Suppl 7):S7-42-S7-46.

Fukuzawa T, Sasaki H, Kikuchi S, Hamada T, Tashiro K. (1996). Serum carnitine and disabling fatigue in multiple sclerosis. *Psychiatry and Clinical Neuroscience* 50(6):323-325.

Fulcher KY, White PD. (1997). Randomised controlled trial of graded exercise in patients with the chronic fatigue syndrome. *British Medical Journal* 314(7095):1647-1652.

Fulcher KY, White PD. (1998). Chronic fatigue syndrome: A description of graded exercise treatment. *Physiotherapy* 84(5):223-226.

Fuller NS, Morrison RE. (1998). Chronic fatigue syndrome: Helping patients cope with this enigmatic illness. *Postgraduate Medicine* 103(1):175-176, 179-184.

Fulton C, Knowles G. (2000). Cancer fatigue. *European Journal of Cancer Care* 9(3):167-171.

Funabashi H, Igari Y, Kuroda M, Hashimoto C, Ajima H, Nishimaki T, Morito T, Kasukawa R, Yoshida H, Onizawa N, et al. (1989). [An autopsy case of a patient with myasthenia gravis who showed various symptoms of collagen diseases and complicated with malignant thymoma]. *Ryumachi* 29(3):185-191.

Furst CJ. (1996). Radiotherapy for cancer: Quality of life. *Acta Oncologica* 35 (Suppl 7):141-148.

Furst CJ, Ahsberg E. (2001). Dimensions of fatigue during radiotherapy: An application of the Multidimensional Fatigue Inventory. *Support Care Cancer* 9(5):355-360.

Furue H. (1985). [Phase II studies of interferon alpha-2 Sch 30500 in advanced gastrointestinal carcinoma]. *Gan To Kagaku Ryoho* 12(8):1625-1629.

Furue H. (1986). [Phase I study of human lymphoblastoid alpha-interferon on malignant tumor]. *Gan To Kagaku Ryoho* 13(4 Pt 1):977-983.

Furukawa Y, Nishi K, Mizuno Y, Narabayashi H. (1995). Significance of CSF biopterin and neopterin in hereditary progressive dystonia with marker diurnal fluctuation (HPD)—A clue to pathogenesis. *No to Shinkei—Brain and Nerve* 47(3):261-268.

Furuse K. (1985). [A phase II study of etoposide (NK 171) in small cell lung cancer—Comparison of results between intravenous administration and oral administration]. *Gan To Kagaku Ryoho* 12(12):2352-2357.

Furuse K, Kawahara M, Hasegawa K, Kudoh S, Takada M, Sugiura T, Ichinose Y, Fukuoka M, Ohashi Y, Niitani H, S-1 Cooperative Study Group (Lung Cancer Working Group). (2001). Early phase II study of S-1, a new oral fluoropyrimidine, for advanced non-small-cell lung cancer. *International Journal of Clinical Oncology* 6(5):236-241.

Furuse K, Kinuwaki E, Motomiya M, Nishiwaki H, Hasegawa K, Kobayashi K, Kurita Y, Ohta K, Fukuoka M, Nakajima S, et al. (1994). [Late phase II clinical study of KW-2307 in previously untreated patients with non-small cell lung cancer. KW-2307 Study Group (Lung Cancer Group)]. *Gan To Kagaku Ryoho* 21(12):1941-1947.

Furuse K, Ohta M, Fukuoka M, Kurita Y, Kobayashi K, Hasegawa K, Kimura I, Fujii M, Yoshida S, Kitamura S, et al. (1994). [Early phase II clinical study of KW-2307 in patients with lung cancer. Lung Cancer Section in KW-2307 Study Group]. *Gan To Kagaku Ryoho* 21(6):785-793.

Furuya H, Tsuchiyama S, Sato T, Ishibashi R, Notsu K, Takagi C, Yamamoto H, Kato Y. (1992). [Acute myelogenous leukemia transformed from myelodysplastic syndrome with tetraploid chromosome constitution]. *Rinsho Ketsueki* 33(4):494-499.

Fyfe D, Price C, Langley RE, Pagonis C, Houghton J, Osborne L, Woll PJ, Gardner C, Baguley BC, Carmichael J, Cancer Research Campaign Phase I/II Trials Committee. (2001). A phase I trial of amsalog (CI-921) administered by intravenous infusion using a 5-day schedule. *Cancer Chemotherapy Pharmacology* 47(4):333-337.

Gabriel HH, Urhausen A, Valet G, Heidelbach U, Kindermann W. (1998). Overtraining and immune system: A prospective longitudinal study in endurance athletes. *Medical Science in Sports and Exercise* 30(7):1151-1157.

Gabrilove JL, Cleeland CS, Livingston RB, Sarokhan B, Winer E, Einhorn LH. (2001). Clinical evaluation of once-weekly dosing of epoetin alfa in chemotherapy patients: Improvements in hemoglobin and quality of life are similar to three-times-weekly dosing. *Journal of Clinical Oncology* 19(11):2875-2882.

Gabrilovich DI, Nadaf S, Coark J, Berzofsky JA, Carbone DP. (1996). Dendritic cells in antitumor immune responses: II. Dendritic cells grown from bone marrow precursors, but not mature DC from tumor-bearing mice, are effective antigen carriers in the therapy of established tumors. *Cellular Immunology* 170:111-119.

Gahlinger P. (1999). The power of herbs. *Western Journal of Medicine* 170(5):255-256.

Galbraith DN, Nairn C, Clements GB. (1997). Evidence of enteroviral persistence in humans. *Journal of General Virology* 78(Pt. 2):307-312.

Gall H. (1996). The basis of cancer fatigue: Where does it come from? *European Journal of Cancer Care* 5(2 Suppl):31-34.

Gallagher EM, Buchsel PC. (1998). Breast cancer and fatigue. *American Journal of Nursing* 1:17-20.

Galloway SC, Graydon JE. (1996). Uncertainty, symptom distress, and information needs after surgery for cancer of the colon. *Cancer Nursing* 19(2):112-117.

Galton DA, Goldman JM, Wiltshaw E, Catovsky D, Henry K, Goldenberg GJ. (1974). Prolymphocytic leukaemia. *British Journal of Haematology* 27(1):7-23.

Gama Sosa MA, De Gasperi R, Patarca R, Fletcher MA, Kolodny EH. (1997). Antisulfatide IgG antibodies recognize HIV proteins. *Journal of Acquired Immune Deficiency Syndromes and Human Retrovirology* 15:83-90.

Gamez-Nava JI, Gonzalez-Lopez L, Davis P, Suarez-Almazor ME. (1998). Referral and diagnosis of common rheumatic diseases by primary care physicians. *British Journal of Rheumatology* 37(11):1215-1219.

Gammon MD, John EM. (1993). Recent etiologic hypotheses concerning breast cancer. *Epidemiological Reviews* 15:163-168.

Gandevia SC, Butler JE, Taylor JL, Crawford MR. (1998). Absence of viscerosomatic inhibition with injections of lobeline designed to activate human pulmonary C fibers. *Journal of Physiology* 511:289-300.

Ganju V, Edmonson JH, Buckner JC. (1994). Phase I study of combined alpha interferon, alpha difluoromethylornithine (DFMO), and doxorubicin in advanced malignancy. *Investigative New Drugs* 12(1):25-27.

Gantz NM. (1991). Magnesium and chronic fatigue. *Lancet* 338(8758):66.

Garcia-Borreguero D, Dale JK, Rosnethal NE, Chiara A, O'Fallon A, Bartko JJ, Straus SE. (1998). Lack of seasonal variation of symptoms in patients with chronic fatigue syndrome. *Psychiatry Research* 77(2):71-77.

Garfin SR. (1995). A 50-year-old woman with disabling spinal stenosis. *JAMA* 274(24):1949-1954.

Garg M, Bondade S. (1993). Reversal of age-associated decline in immune response to Pnu-immune vaccine by supplementation with the steroid hormone dehydroepiandrosterone. *Infection and Immunity* 61(5):2238-2241.

Garnick JJ, Singh B, Winkley G. (1998). Effectiveness of a medicament containing silicon dioxide, aloe, and allantoin on aphthous stomatitis. *Oral Surgery, Oral Medicine, Oral Pathology, Oral Radiology, and Endodontics* 86(5):550-556.

Garry RF, Fermin CD, Hart DJ, Alexander SS, Donehower LA, Luo-Zhang H. (1990). Detection of a human intracisternal A-type retroviral particle antigenically related to HIV. *Science* 250(4894):1127-1129.

Garwicz S, Aronson S, Elmqvist D, Landberg T. (1975). Postirradiation syndrome and EEG findings in children with acute lymphoblastic leukaemia. *Acta Paediatrica Scandinavica* 64(3):399-403.

Gastmann UA, Lehmann MJ. (1998). Overtraining and the BCAA hypothesis. *Medicine and Science in Sports and Exercise* 30(7):1173-1178.

Gaston-Johansson F, Fall-Dickson JM, Bakos AB, Kennedy MJ. (1999). Fatigue, pain, and depression in pre-autotransplant breast cancer patients. *Cancer Practice* 7(5):240-247.

Gaston-Johansson F, Fall-Dickson JM, Nanda J, Ohly KV, Stillman S, Krumm S, Kennedy MJ. (2000). The effectiveness of the comprehensive coping strategy program on clinical outcomes in breast cancer autologous bone marrow transplantation. *Cancer Nursing* 23(4):277-285.

Gates LK Jr, Cameron AJ, Nagorney DM, Goellner JR, Farley DR. (1995). Primary leiomyosarcoma of the liver mimicking liver abscess. *American Journal of Gastroenterology* 90(4):649-652.

Gauci L. (1987). Management of cancer patients receiving interferon alfa-2a. *International Journal of Cancer* 1:21-30.

Gaudino EA, Coyle PK, Krupp LB. (1997). Post-Lyme syndrome and chronic fatigue syndrome: Neuropsychiatric similarities and differences. *Archives of Neurology* 54(11):1372-1376.

Gause BL, Sharfman WH, Janik JE, Curti BD, Steis RG, Urba WJ, Smith JW II, Alvord WG, Longo DL. (1998). A phase II study of carboplatin, cisplatin, interferon-alpha, and tamoxifen for patients with metastatic melanoma. *Cancer Investigation* 16(6):374-380.

Gause BL, Sznol M, Kopp WC, Janik JE, Smith JW II, Steis RG, Urba WJ, Sharfman W, Fenton RG, Creekmore SP, et al. (1996). Phase I study of subcutaneously administered interleukin-2 in combination with interferon alfa-2a in patients with advanced cancer. *Journal of Clinical Oncology* 14(8):2234-2241.

Gedalia A, Garcia CO, Molina JF, Bradford NJ, Espinoza LR. (2000). Fibromyalgia syndrome: Experience in a pediatric rheumatology clinic. *Clinical and Experimental Rheumatology* 18(3):415-419.

Gedde-Dahl T, Fossum B, Eriksen JA, Thorsby E, Gaudernack G. (1993). T-cell clones specific for p21 ras-derived peptides: Characterization of their fine specificity and HLA restriction. *European Journal of Immunology* 23:754-760.

Geinitz H, Zimmermann FB, Stoll P, Thamm R, Kaffenberger W, Ansorg K, Keller M, Busch R, van Beuningen D, Molls M. (2001). Fatigue, serum cytokine levels, and blood cell counts during radiotherapy of patients with breast cancer. *International Journal of Radiation Oncology, Biology and Physics* 51(3):691-698.

Gelfand EW. (1990). SCID continues to point the way. *New England Journal of Medicine* 322(24):1741-1743.

Gelfand SG. (1998). Fibromyalgia: More questions and implications. *Arthritis and Rheumatism* 41(6):1138-1139.

Gelin J, Moldawer LL, Lonnroth C. (1991). Role of endogenous tumor necrosis factor alfa and interleukin 1 for experimental tumor growth and the development of cancer cachexia. *Cancer Research* 51:415-421.

Gelmon KA. (1995). Biweekly paclitaxel in the treatment of patients with metastatic breast cancer. *Seminars in Oncology* 22(5 Suppl 12):117-122.

Gelmon KA, Eisenhauer E, Bryce C, Tolcher A, Mayer L, Tomlinson E, Zee B, Blackstein M, Tomiak E, Yau J, et al. (1999). Randomized phase II study of high-dose paclitaxel with or without amifostine in patients with metastatic breast cancer. *Journal of Clinical Oncology* 17(10):3038-3047.

Gelmon KA, Tolcher A, Diab AR, Bally MB, Embree L, Hudon N, Dedhar C, Ayers D, Eisen A, Melosky B, et al. (1999). Phase I study of liposomal vincristine. *Journal of Clinical Oncology* 17(2):697-705.

Gelston A, Sheldon H. (1981). Fatigue, weakness, anemia and hypercalcemia in a 63-year-old woman. *Canadian Medical Association Journal* 124(4):391-396.

Genre D, Protiere C, Macquart-Moulin G, Gravis G, Camerlo J, Alzieu C, Maraninchi D, Moatti JP, Viens P. (2002). Quality of life of breast cancer patients receiving high-dose-intensity chemotherapy: Impact of length of cycles. *Support Care and Cancer* 10(3):222-230.

Gentiloni N, Febbraro S, Barone C, Lemmo G, Neri G, Zannoni G, Capelli A, Gasbarrini G. (1997). Peritoneal mesothelioma in recurrent familial peritonitis. *Journal of Clinical Gastroenterology* 24(4):276-279.

George DK, Evans RM, Gunn IR. (1997). Familial chronic fatigue. *Postgraduate Medical Journal* 73(859):311-313.

Georgoulias V, Androulakis N, Dimopoulos AM, Kourousis C, Kakolyris S, Papadakis E, Apostolopoulou F, Papadimitriou C, Vossos A, Agelidou M, et al. (1998). First-line treatment of advanced non-small-cell lung cancer with docetaxel and cisplatin: A multicenter phase II study. *Annals of Oncology* 9(3):331-334.

Georgoulias V, Kourousis C, Androulakis N, Kakolyris S, Dimopoulos MA, Bouros D, Papadimitriou C, Hatzakis K, Heras P, Kalbakis K, et al. (1997). Docetaxel (Taxotere) and gemcitabine in the treatment of non-small cell lung cancer: Preliminary results. *Seminars in Oncology* 24(4 Suppl 14):S14-22-S14-25.

Georgoulias V, Kourousis C, Kakolyris S, Androulakis N, Dimopoulos MA, Papadakis E, Kotsakis T, Vardakis N, Kalbakis K, Merambeliotakis N, et al. (1997). Second-line treatment of advanced non-small cell lung cancer with paclitaxel and gemcitabine: A preliminary report on an active regimen. *Seminars in Oncology* 24(4 Suppl 12):S12-61-S12-66.

Georgoulias V, Scagliotti G, Miller V, Eckardt J, Douillard JY, Manegold C. (2001). Challenging the platinum combinations: Docetaxel (Taxotere) combined with gemcitabine or vinorelbine in non-small cell lung cancer. *Seminars in Oncology* 28(1 Suppl 2):15-21.

Gerard B, Bleiberg H, Van Daele D, Gil T, Hendlisz A, Di Leo A, Fernez B, Brienza S. (1998). Oxaliplatin combined to 5-fluorouracil and folinic acid: An effective therapy in patients with advanced colorectal cancer. *Anticancer Drugs* 9(4):301-305.

Gerber LH. (2001). Cancer rehabilitation into the future. *Cancer* 92(4 Suppl):975-979.

Gerrits CJ, Burris H, Schellens JH, Eckardt JR, Planting AS, van der Burg ME, Rodriguez GI, Loos WJ, van Beurden V, Hudson I, et al. (1998). Oral topotecan given once or twice daily for ten days: A phase I pharmacology study in adult patients with solid tumors. *Clinical Cancer Research* 4(5):1153-1158.

Gerrits CJ, Burris H, Schellens JH, Planting AS, van den Burg ME, Rodriguez GI, van Beurden V, Loos WJ, Hudson I, Fields S, et al. (1998). Five days of oral topotecan (Hycamtin), a phase I and pharmacological study in adult patients with solid tumours. *European Journal of Cancer* 34(7):1030-1035.

Gerrits CJ, Schellens JH, Creemers GJ, Wissel P, Planting AS, Pritchard JF, DePee S, de Boer-Dennert M, Harteveld M, Verweij J. (1997). The bioavailability of oral GI147211 (GG211), a new topoisomerase I inhibitor. *British Journal of Cancer* 76(7):946-951.

Gerster JC. (1999). [Fibromyalgia: Past and present] Fibromyalgie: Le passe, le present. *Revue Medicale Suisse Romande* 119(6):513-516.

Ghobrial MW, George J, Mannam S, Henien SR. (2002). Severe hypercalcemia as an initial presenting manifestation of hepatocellular carcinoma. *Canadian Journal of Gastroenterology* 16(9):607-609.

Giaccone G, Splinter TA, Debruyne C, Kho GS, Lianes P, van Zandwijk N, Pennucci MC, Scagliotti G, van Meerbeeck J, van Hoesel Q, et al. (1998). Randomized study of paclitaxel-cisplatin versus cisplatin-teniposide in patients with advanced non-small-cell lung cancer. The European Organization for Research and Treatment of Cancer Lung Cancer Cooperative Group. *Journal of Clinical Oncology* 16(6):2133-2141.

Giannakakis T, Ziras N, Kakolyris S, Mavroudis D, Androulakis N, Agelaki S, Parashos M, Sarra E, Dimou T, Hatzidaki D, et al. (2000). Docetaxel in combination with carboplatin for the treatment of advanced non-small cell lung carcinoma: A multicentre phase I study. *European Journal of Cancer* 36(6):742-747.

Gianni L, Capri G, Greco M, Villani F, Brambilla C, Luini A, Crippa F, Bonadonna G. (1991). Activity and toxicity of 4'-iodo-4'-deoxydoxorubicin in patients with advanced breast cancer. *Annals of Oncology* 2(10):719-725.

Gianola FJ, Sugarbaker PH, Barofsky I, White DE, Meyers CE. (1986). Toxicity studies of adjuvant intravenous versus intraperitoneal 5-FU in patients with advanced primary colon or rectal cancer. *American Journal of Clinical Oncology* 9(5):403-410.

Gibbons R, Pheby DFH, Richards C, Bray FI. (1998). Severe CFS/ME of juvenile onset—A report from the CHROME database. *Journal of Chronic Fatigue Syndrome* 4(4):67-80.

Gibson PR, Cheavens J, Warren ML. (1998). Social support in persons with self-reported sensitivity to chemicals. *Research in Nursing and Health* 21(2):103-115.

Gilbert J, Baker SD, Bowling MK, Grochow L, Figg WD, Zabelina Y, Donehower RC, Carducci MA. (2001). A phase I dose escalation and bioavailability study of oral sodium phenylbutyrate in patients with refractory solid tumor malignancies. *Clinical Cancer Research* 7(8):2292-2300.

Gilcrease MZ, Sahin M, Perri RT, Nelson FS, Guzman-Paz M. (1998). Fine needle aspiration of signet-ring cell lymphoma: A case report with differential diagnostic considerations. *Acta Cytologica* 42(6):1461-1467.

Giles FJ, Garcia-Manero G, Cortes JE, Baker SD, Miller CB, O'Brien SM, Thomas DA, Andreeff M, Bivins C, Jolivet J, et al. (2002). Phase II study of troxacitabine, a novel dioxolane nucleoside analog, in patients with refractory leukemia. *Journal of Clinical Oncology* 20(3):656-664.

Giles FJ, Worman CP, Jewell AP, Goldstone AH. (1991). Recombinant alpha-interferons, thyroid irradiation and thyroid disease. *Acta Haematologica* 85(3):160-163.

Gill PS, Bernstein-Singer M, Espina BM, Rarick M, Magy F, Montgomery T, Berry MS, Levine A. (1992). Adriamycin, bleomycin and vincristine chemotherapy with recombinant granulocyte-macrophage colony-stimulating factor in the treatment of AIDS-related Kaposi's sarcoma. *AIDS* 6(12):1477-1481.

Gill PS, Espina BM, Muggia F, Cabriales S, Tulpule A, Esplin JA, Liebman HA, Forssen E, Ross ME, Levine AM. (1995). Phase I/II clinical and pharmacokinetic evaluation of liposomal daunorubicin. *Journal of Clinical Oncology* 13(4):996-1003.

Gilleece MH, Scarffe JH, Ghosh A, Heyworth CM, Bonnem E, Testa N, Stern P, Dexter TM. (1992). Recombinant human interleukin 4 (IL-4) given as daily subcutaneous injections—A phase I dose toxicity trial. *British Journal of Cancer* 66(1):204-210.

Gilliam S. (1992). The 1934 Los Angeles County Hospital epidemic. In *The Clinical and Scientific Basis of Myalgic Encephalomyelitis/Chronic Fatigue Syndrome,* Hyde BM, Goldstein J, Levine P, eds. Ottawa: Nightingale Research Foundation, pp. 119-128.

Gillis TA, Cheville AL, Worsowicz GM. (2001). Cardiopulmonary rehabilitation and cancer rehabilitation: 4. Oncologic rehabilitation. *Archives of Physical Medicine and Rehabilitation* 82(3 Suppl 1):S63-S68.

Gilman CP. (1993). *The Yellow Wallpaper.* New Brunswick, NJ: Rutgers University Press.

Gilmore G. (1994). Resistane to murine acquired immunodeficiency syndrome (MAIDS). *Science* 265:264.

Giovarelli M, Musiani P, Modesti A, Dellabona P, Casorati G, Allione A, Consalvo M, Cavallo F, Di Pierro F, De Giovanni C, et al. (1995). Local release of IL-10 by transfected mouse mammary adenocarcinoma cells does not suppress but enhances antitumor reaction and elicits a strong cytotoxic lymphocyte and antibody-dependent immune memory. *Journal of Immunology* 155:3112-3123.

Girdano DA, Everly GS, Dusek DE. (1997). *Controlling Stress and Tension.* Boston: Allyn and Bacon.

Giuliani A, Cestaro B. (1997). Exercise, free radical generation and vitamins. *European Journal of Cancer Prevention* 6(Suppl 1):S55-S67.

Given B, Given C, Azzouz F, Stommel M. (2001). Physical functioning of elderly cancer patients prior to diagnosis and following initial treatment. *Nursing Research* 50(4):222-232.

Given B, Given CW, McCorkle R, Kozachik S, Cimprich B, Rahbar MH, Wojcik C. (2002). Pain and fatigue management: Results of a nursing randomized clinical trial. *Oncology Nursing Forum* 29(6):949-956.

Given CW, Given B, Azzouz F, Kozachik S, Stommel M. (2001). Predictors of pain and fatigue in the year following diagnosis among elderly cancer patients. *Journal of Pain Symptomatology Management* 21(6):456-466.

Given CW, Given B, Azzouz F, Stommel M, Kozachik S. (2000). Comparison of changes in physical functioning of elderly patients with new diagnoses of cancer. *Medical Care* 38(5):482-493.

Glaser R, Kiecolt-Glaser JK. (1998). Stress-associated immune modulation: Relevance to viral infections and chronic fatigue syndrome. *American Journal of Medicine* 105(3A):35S-42S.

Glaser R, Lafuse WP, Bonneau RH, Atkinson C, Kiecolt-Glaser JK. (1993). Stress-associated modulation of proto-oncogene expression in human peripheral blood leukocytes. *Behavioral Neurosciences* 107(3):525-529.

Glaser V. (1999). Billion-dollar market blossoms as botanicals take root. *Nature Biotechnology* 17(1):17-18.

Glaspy J. (2001). Anemia and fatigue in cancer patients. *Cancer* 92(6 Suppl):1719-1724.

Glaus A. (1993a). Assessment of fatigue in cancer and non-cancer patients and in healthy individuals. *Support Care in Cancer* 1(6):305-315.

Glaus A. (1993b). [Pain and fatigue in tumor patients]. *Schweizerische Rundschau fur Medizin Praxis* 82(9):251-254.

Glaus A. (1994). [Fatigue and cancer—indivisible twins? A comparison between cancer patients, patients with diseases other than cancer and healthy people]. *Pflege* 7(3):183-197.

Glaus A. (1998a). Fatigue—An orphan topic in patients with cancer? *European Journal of Cancer* 34(11):1649-1651.

Glaus A. (1998b). Fatigue and cachexia in cancer patients. *Support Care in Cancer* 6(2):77-78.

Glaus A. (1998c). Fatigue in patients with cancer: Analysis and assessment. *Recent Results in Cancer Research* 145:I-XI, 1-172.

Glaus A. (2001). Fatigue in patients with cancer—From an orphan topic to a global concern. *Support Care and Cancer* 9(1):1-3.

Glaus A, Crow R, Hammond S. (1996a). A qualitative study to explore the concept of fatigue/tiredness in cancer patients and in healthy individuals. *Support Care and Cancer* 4(2):82-96.

Glaus A, Crow R, Hammond S. (1996b). A qualitative study to explore the concept of fatigue/tiredness in cancer patients and in healthy individuals. *European Journal of Cancer Care* 5(2 Suppl):8-23.

Glaus A, Crow R, Hammond S. (1999a). [Fatigue in healthy and cancer patients: 1. A qualitative study on conceptual analysis]. *Pflege* 12(1):11-19.

Glaus A, Crow R, Hammond S. (1999b). [Fatigue in the healthy and in cancer patients: II. A qualitative study for conceptual analysis]. *Pflege* 12(2):75-81.

Glaus A, Muller S. (2000). [Hemoglobin and fatigue in cancer patients: Inseparable twins?] *Schweize Medizinische Wochenschrift* 130(13):471-477.

Gledhill J, Bacon M. (2001). [Evaluating and managing fatigue in oncology]. *Soins* 658:28-31.

Gledhill JA, Rodary C, Mahe C, Laizet C. (2002). [French validation of the revised Piper Fatigue Scale]. *Recherche de Soins Infirmiers* 68:50-65.

Glisson BS, Kurie JM, Perez-Soler R, Fox NJ, Murphy WK, Fossella FV, Lee JS, Ross MB, Nyberg DA, Pisters KM, et al. (1999). Cisplatin, etoposide, and paclitaxel in the treatment of patients with extensive small-cell lung carcinoma. *Journal of Clinical Oncology* 17(8):2309-2315.

Glisson J, Crawford R, Street S. (1999). Review, critique, and guidelines for the use of herbs and homeopathy. *Nurse Practice* 24(4):44-46, 53, 60, passim.

Glover J, Dibble SL, Dodd MJ, Miaskowski C. (1995). Mood states of oncology outpatients: Does pain make a difference? *Journal of Pain Symptomatology and Management* 10(2):120-128.

Goday-Bujan JJ, Oleaga-Morante JM, Yanguas-Bayona I, Gonzalez-Guemes M, Soloeta-Arechavala R. (1998). Allergic contact dermatitis from *Krameria triandra* extract. *Contact Dermatitis* 38(2):120-121.

Godfrey RG. (1996). A guide to the understanding and use of tricylcic antidepressants in the overall management of fibromyalgia and other chronic pain syndromes. *Archives of Internal Medicine* 156(10):1047-1052.

Goel S, Jhawer M, Rajdev L, Hopkins U, Fehn K, Baker C, Chun HG, Makower D, Landau L, Hoffman A, et al. (2002). Phase I clinical trial of irinotecan with oral capecitabine in patients with gastrointestinal and other solid malignancies. *American Journal of Clinical Oncology* 25(5):528-534.

Gogos CA, Kalfarentzos FE, Zoumbos NC. (1990). Effect of different types of total parenteral nutrition on T-lymphocyte subpopulations and NK cells. *American Journal of Clinical Nutrition* 51:119-122.

Gohji K, Yasuno H, Matsumoto O, Kamidono S, Itani A, Hamami G, Morishita S, Yamashita C, Okada M, Nakamura K. (1989). [Clinical analysis of renal cell carcinoma with extension into the inferior vena cava]. *Nippon Gan Chiryo Gakkai Shi* 24(6):1266-1276.

Gold D, Bowden R, Sixbey J, Riggs R, Katon WJ, Ashley R, Obrigewitch RM, Corey L. (1990). Chronic fatigue: A prospective clinical and virologic study. *JAMA* 264(1):48-53.

Goldberg DP, Bridges KW. (1988). Somatic presentations of psychiatric illness in primary care settings. *Journal of Psychosomatic Research* 32:137-144.

Goldberg JS, Vargas M, Rosmarin AS, Milowsky MI, Papanicoloau N, Gudas LJ, Shelton G, Feit K, Petrylak D, Nanus DM. (2002). Phase I trial of interferon alpha2b and liposome-encapsulated all-trans retinoic acid in the treatment of patients with advanced renal cell carcinoma. *Cancer* 95(6):1220-1227.

Goldberg RM, Kaufmann SH, Atherton P, Sloan JA, Adjei AA, Pitot HC, Alberts SR, Rubin J, Miller LL, Erlichman C. (2002). A phase I study of sequential irinotecan and 5-fluorouracil/leucovorin. *Annals of Oncology* 13(10):1674-1680.

Goldberg RT, Pachas WN, Keith D. (1999). Relationship between traumatic events in childhood and chronic pain. *Disability and Rehabilitation* 21(1):23-30.

Goldenberg DL. (1996). What is the future of fibromyalgia? *Rheumatic Diseases Clinics of North America* 22(2):393-406.

Goldenberg DL. (1997). Fibromyalgia, chronic fatigue syndrome, and myofascial pain syndrome. *Current Opinions in Rheumatology* 9(2):135-143.

Goldenberg DL. (1999). Fibromyalgia syndrome a decade later: What have we learned? *Archives of Internal Medicine* 159(8):777-785.

Goldhirsch A, Beer M, Sonntag RW, Tschopp L, Cavalli F, Ryssel HJ, Brunner KW. (1980). [Phase-II-study with vindesine (desacetyl-vinblastine-amide-sulfate) in advanced malignant diseases]. *Schweize Medizinische Wochenschrift* 110(27-28):1063-1067.

Golledge C. (1998). Distinguishing between occupation, purposeful activity and activity. Part 1: Review and explanation. *British Journal of Occupational Therapy* 61(3):100-105.

Golomb HM, Jacobs A, Fefer A, Ozer H, Thompson J, Portlock C, Ratain M, Golde D, Vardiman J, Burke JS, et al. (1986). Alpha-2 interferon therapy of hairy-cell leukemia: A multicenter study of 64 patients. *Journal of Clinical Oncology* 4(6):900-905.

Golomb HM, Ratain MJ, Fefer A, Thompson J, Golde DW, Ozer H, Portlock C, Silber R, Rappeport J, Bonnem E, et al. (1988). Randomized study of the duration of treatment with interferon alfa-2B in patients with hairy cell leukemia. *Journal of the National Cancer Institutes* 80(5):369-373.

Golumbek PT, Lazenby AJ, Levitsky HI, Jaffee LM, Karasuyama H, Baker M, Parsoll DM. (1991). Treatment of established renal cancer by tumor cells engineered to secrete interleukin-4. *Science* 254:713-716.

Gompels MM, Spickett GP. (1996). Chronic fatigue, arthralgia, and malaise. *Annals of Rheumatological Diseases* 55(8):502-503.

Gonzalez MB, Cousins JC, Doraiswamy PM. (1996). Neurobiology of chronic fatigue syndrome. *Progress in Neuro-Psyhcopharmacology and Biological Psychiatry* 20(5):749-759.

Gonzalez R, Sanchez A, Ferguson JA, Balmer C, Daniel C, Cohn A, Robinson WA. (1991). Melatonin therapy of advanced human malignant melanoma. *Melanoma Research* 1(4):237-243.

Gonzalo-Garijo MA, Revenga-Arranz F, Bobadilla-Gonzalez P. (1996). Allergic contact dermatitis due to *Centella asiatica:* A new case. *Allergologia et Immunopathologia* 24(3):132-134.

Goodwin SS. (1997). The marital relationship and health in women with chronic fatigue and immune dysfunction syndrome: Views of wives and husbands. *Nursing Research* 46(3):138-146.

Goosens ME, Rutten-van Molken MP, Leidl RM, Bos SG, Vlaeyen JW, Teeken-Gruben NJ. (1996). Cognitive-educational treatment of fibromyalgia: A randomized clinical trial. II. Economic evaluation. *Journal of Rheumatology* 23(7): 1246-1254.

Goosens ME, Rutten-van Molken MP, Vlaeyen JW, Van der Linden SM. (2000). The cost diary: A measure to direct and indirect costs in cost-effectiveness research. *Journal of Clinical Epidemiology* 53(7):688-695.

Gordon DA. (1997). Fibromyalgia—Out of control? *Journal of Rheumatology* 24(7):1247.

Gordon MS, McCaskill-Stevens WJ, Battiato LA, Loewy J, Loesch D, Breeden E, Hoffman R, Beach KJ, Kuca B, Kaye J, et al. (1996). A phase I trial of recombinant human interleukin-11 (neumega rhIL-11 growth factor) in women with breast cancer receiving chemotherapy. *Blood* 87(9):3615-3624.

Gordon S, Morrison C. (1998). Fibromyalgia and its primary care implications. *Medical-Surgical Nursing* 7(4):207-213.

Gore ME, Rustin G, Schuller J, Lane SR, Hearn S, Beckman RA, Ross G. (2001). Topotecan given as a 21-day infusion in the treatment of advanced ovarian cancer. *British Journal of Cancer* 84(8):1043-1046.

Gore ME, Rustin G, Slevin M, Gallagher C, Penson R, Osborne R, Ledermann J, Cameron T, Thompson JM. (1997). Single-agent paclitaxel in patients with previously untreated stage IV epithelial ovarian cancer. London Gynaecological Oncology and North Thames Gynaecological Oncology Groups. *British Journal of Cancer* 75(5):710-714.

Goshorn RK. (1998). Chronic fatigue syndrome: A review for clinicians. *Seminars in Neurology* 18(2):237-242.

Goss G, Muldal A, Lohmann R, Taylor M, Lopez P, Armitage G, Steward WP. (1995). Didemnin B in favourable histology non-Hodgkin's lymphoma: A phase II study of the National Cancer Institute of Canada Clinical Trials Group. *Investigative New Drugs* 13(3):257-260.

Goss PE. (1999). Risks versus benefits in the clinical application of aromatase inhibitors. *Endocrinology Related Cancer* 6(2):325-332.

Goss PE, Reid CL, Bailey D, Dennis JW. (1997). Phase IB clinical trial of the oligosaccharide processing inhibitor swainsonine in patients with advanced malignancies. *Clinical Cancer Research* 3(7):1077-1086.

Goss PE, Stewart AK, Couture F, Klasa R, Gluck S, Kaizer L, Burkes R, Charpentier D, Palmer M, Tye L, et al. (1999). Combined results of two phase II studies of Taxol (paclitaxel) in patients with relapsed or refractory lymphomas. *Leukemia and Lymphoma* 34(3-4):295-304.

Gotoh T, Miki T, Takayama H, Tsukikawa M, Tsujimura A, Sugao H, Takaha M, Takeda M, Kurata A. (1995). [Giant schwannoma in the pelvic cavity presenting as renal failure: A case report]. *Hinyokika Kiyo* 41(8):621-624.

Goudsmit EM. (1997). Graded exercise in chronic fatigue syndrome: Chronic fatigue syndrome is a heterogeneous condition. *British Medical Journal* 315 (7113):948.

Goudsmit EM. (1998). Treating chronic fatigue with exercise: Exercise, and rest, should be tailored to individual needs. *British Medical Journal* 317(7158):599-600.

Gowans SE, DeHueck A, Voss S, Richardson M. (1999). A randomized, controlled trial of exercise and education for individuals with fibromyalgia. *Arthritis Care Research* 12(2):120-128.

Gozdasoglu S, Unal E, Yavuz G, Pamir A, Reisli I, Deda G, Tarcan A, Babacan E, Cavdar AO. (1995). Granulocyte-macrophage colony stimulating factor (rh-GM-CSF) in the treatment of chemotherapy-induced neutropenia. *Journal of Chemotherapy* 7(5):467-469.

Grady C, Anderson R, Chase GA. (1998). Fatigue in HIV-infected men receiving investigational interleukin-2. *Nursing Research* 47(4):227-234.

Graham MV, Jahanzeb M, Dresler CM, Cooper JD, Emami B, Mortimer JE. (1996). Results of a trial with topotecan dose escalation and concurrent thoracic radiation therapy for locally advanced, inoperable nonsmall cell lung cancer. *International Journal of Radiation Oncology, Biology and Physics* 36(5):1215-1220.

Grahame R. (2000). Pain, distress and joint hyperlaxity. *Joint, Bone and Spine* 67(3):157-163.

Grander D, Einhorn S. (1998). Interferon and malignant disease: How does it work and why doesn't it always? *Acta Oncologica* 37:331-338.

Grant M, Anderson P, Ashley M, Dean G, Ferrell B, Kagawa-Singer M, Padilla G, Robinson SB, Sarna L. (1998). Developing a team for multicultural, multi-institutional research on fatigue and quality of life. *Oncology Nursing Forum* 25(8): 1404-1412.

Grant M, Golant M, Rivera L, Dean G, Benjamin H. (2000). Developing a community program on cancer pain and fatigue. *Cancer Practice* 8(4):187-194.

Grant M, Kravits K. (2000). Symptoms and their impact on nutrition. *Seminars in Oncology Nursing* 16(2):113-121.

Grant S, Roberts J, Poplin E, Tombes MB, Kyle B, Welch D, Carr M, Bear HD. (1998). Phase Ib trial of bryostatin 1 in patients with refractory malignancies. *Clinical Cancer Research* 4(3):611-618.

Grantham M, Einstein D, McCarron K, Lichtin A, Vogt D. (1998). Littoral cell angioma of the spleen. *Abdominal Imaging* 23(6):633-635.

Granzow B. (1999). [Mutual features of chronic fatigue syndrome, fibromyalgia and multiple chemical sensitivity] Gemeinsamkeiten von chronic fatigue syndrom, fibromyalgie uns multipler chemischer sensitivität. *Deutsche Medizin Wochenschrift* 124(41):1224.

Gray JB, Bridges AB, McNeill GP. (1992). Atrial myxoma: A rare cause of progressive exertional dyspnoea. *Scottish Medical Journal* 37(6):186-187.

Graydon JE. (1994). Women with breast cancer: Their quality of life following a course of radiation therapy. *Journal of Advanced Nursing* 19(4):617-622.

Graydon JE, Bubela N, Irvine D, Vincent L. (1995). Fatigue-reducing strategies used by patients receiving treatment for cancer. *Cancer Nursing* 18(1):23-28.

Graydon JE, Sidani S, Irvine D, Vincent L, Bubela N, Harrison D. (1998). Literature review on cancer-related fatigue. *Canadian Oncology Nursing Journal* 8(S1):S5.

Graziano F, Bisonni R, Catalano V, Silva R, Rovidati S, Mencarini E, Ferraro B, Canestrari F, Baldelli AM, De Gaetano A, et al. (2002). Potential role of levocarnitine supplementation for the treatment of chemotherapy-induced fatigue in non-anaemic cancer patients. *British Journal of Cancer* 86(12):1854-1857.

Graziosi C, Pantaleo G, Gantt KR, Fortin J-P, Demarest JF, Cohen OJ, Sékaly RP, Fauci AS. (1994). Lack of evidence for the dichotomy of TH1 and TH2 predominance in HIV-infected individuals. *Science* 265:248-252.

Greco A, Tannock C, Brostoff J, Costa DC. (1997). Brain MR in chronic fatigue syndrome. *American Journal of Neuroradiology* 18(7):1265-1269.

Greco FA. (1999). Docetaxel (Taxotere) administered in weekly schedules. *Seminars in Oncology* 26(3 Suppl 11):28-31.

Greco FA, Burris HA III, Erland JB, Gray JR, Kalman LA, Schreeder MT, Hainsworth JD. (2000). Carcinoma of unknown primary site. *Cancer* 89(12):2655-2660.

Green S. (1999). Sleep cycles, TMD, fibromyalgia, and their relationship to orofacial myofunctional disorders. *International Journal of Orofacial Myology* 25:4-14.

Greenberg DB, Gray JL, Mannix CM, Eisenthal S, Carey M. (1993). Treatment-related fatigue and serum interleukin-1 levels in patients during external beam irradiation for prostate cancer. *Journal of Pain Symptomatology and Management* 8(4):196-200.

Greenberg DB, Sawicka J, Eisenthal S, Ross D. (1992). Fatigue syndrome due to localized radiation. *Journal of Pain Symptomatology Management* 7(1):38-45.

Greenberg HE, Ney G, Ravdin L, Scharf SM, Hilton E. (1995). Sleep quality in Lyme disease. *Sleep* 18:912-916.

Greenberg HS, Chandler WF, Diaz RF, Ensminger WD, Junck L, Page MA, Gebarski SS, McKeever P, Hood TW, Stetson PL, et al. (1988). Intra-arterial bromodeoxyuridine radiosensitization and radiation in treatment of malignant astrocytomas. *Journal of Neurosurgery* 69(4):500-505.

Greenblatt MS, Mangalik A, Ferguson J, Elias L. (1995). Phase I evaluation of therapy with four schedules of 5-fluorouracil by continuous infusion combined with recombinant interferon alpha. *Clinical Cancer Research* 1(6):615-620.

Greene D, Nail LM, Fieler VK, Dudgeon D, Jones LS. (1994). A comparison of patient-reported side effects among three chemotherapy regimens for breast cancer. *Cancer Practice* 2(1):57-62.

Greenhaff PL. (1996). Creatine supplementation: Recent developments. *British Journal of Sports Medicine* 30(4):276-277.

Greenleaf JE, Kozlowski S. (1982). Physiological consequences of reduced physical activity during bed rest. *Exercise and Sports Science Review* 10:84-119.

Greenwood B. (1998). Traditional medicine to DNA vaccines: The advance of medical research in West Africa. *Tropical Medicine and International Health* 3(3): 166-176.

Greer S. (1999). Mind-body research in psychooncology. *Advances in Mind Body Medicine* 15(4):236-244.

Greer S. (2000). Fighting spirit. *Advances in Mind Body Medicine* 16(3):157-158.

Greifzu S. (1998). Fighting cancer fatigue. *Registered Nurse* 61(8):41-43.

Grem JL, Harold N, Shapiro J, Bi DQ, Quinn MG, Zentko S, Keith B, Hamilton JM, Monahan BP, Donavan S, et al. (2000). Phase I and pharmacokinetic trial of weekly oral fluorouracil given with eniluracil and low-dose leucovorin to patients with solid tumors. *Journal of Clinical Oncology* 18(23):3952-3963.

Grem JL, Jordan E, Robson ME, Binder RA, Hamilton JM, Steinberg SM, Arbuck SG, Beveridge RA, Kales AN, Miller JA, et al. (1993). Phase II study of fluorouracil, leucovorin, and interferon alfa-2a in metastatic colorectal carcinoma. *Journal of Clinical Oncology* 11(9):1737-1745.

Grem JL, McAtee N, Murphy RF, Balis FM, Cullen E, Chen AP, Hamilton JM, Steinberg SM, Quinn M, Sorensen JM, et al. (1997). A pilot study of gamma-1b-interferon in combination with fluorouracil, leucovorin, and alpha-2a-interferon. *Clinical Cancer Research* 3(7):1125-1134.

Grem JL, Quinn M, Ismail AS, Takimoto CH, Lush R, Liewehr DJ, Steinberg SM, Balis FM, Chen AP, Monahan BP, et al. (2001). Pharmacokinetics and pharmacodynamic effects of 5-fluorouracil given as a one-hour intravenous infusion. *Cancer Chemotherapy Pharmacology* 47(2):117-125.

Gridelli C. (2001). The ELVIS trial: A phase III study of single-agent vinorelbine as first-line treatment in elderly patients with advanced non-small cell lung cancer. Elderly Lung Cancer Vinorelbine Italian Study. *Oncologist* 6(Suppl 1):4-7.

Gridelli C, Frontini L, Barletta E, Rossi A, Barzelloni ML, Scognamiglio F, Guida C, Gatani T, Fiore F, De Bellis M, et al. (2000). Single agent docetaxel plus granulocyte-colony stimulating factor (G-CSF) in previously treated patients with advanced non small cell lung cancer: A phase II study and review of the literature. *Anticancer Research* 20(2B):1077-1084.

Griep EN, Boersma JW, De Kloet ER. (1993). Altered reactivity of the hypothalamic-pituitary-adrenal axis in the primary fibromyalgia syndrome. *Journal of Rheumatology* 20:469-474.

Griep EN, Boersma JW, Lentjes EG, Prins AP, Van der Korst JK, De Kloet ER. (1998). Function of the hypothalamic-pituitary-adrenal axis in patients with fibromyalgia and low back pain. *Journal of Rheumatology* 25(7):1374-1381.

Griffin DE. (1991). Immunologic abnormalities accompanying acute and chronic viral infections. *Reviews of Infectious Diseases* 13(1):S129-S133.

Griffin WST, Stanley LC, Ling C, White L, MacLeod V, Perrot LJ, White CL, Araoz C. (1989). Brain interleukin 1 and S-100 immunoreactivity are elevated in Down's syndrome and Alzheimer's disease. *Proceedings of the National Academy of Sciences of the United States of America* 86:7611-7615.

Griffith KC, Hart LK. (2000). Characteristics of adolescent cancer survivors who pursue postsecondary education. *Cancer Nursing* 23(6):468-476.

Griggs JJ, Blumberg N. (1998). Recombinant erythropoietin and blood transfusions in cancer chemotherapy-induced anemia. *Anticancer Drugs* 9(10):925-932.

Grimm E, Mazumder A, Zhang HZ, Rosenberg SA. (1982). Lymphokine-activated killer cell phenomenon: Lysis of natural killer resistant fresh solid tumor cells by interleukin 2 activated autologous human peripheral blood lymphocytes. *Journal of Experimental Medicine* 155:1823-1841.

Grimm W, Muller HH. (1999). A randomized controlled trial of the effect of fluid extract of *Echinacea purpurea* on the incidence and severity of colds and respiratory infections. *American Journal of Medicine* 106(2):138-143; comment, 259-260.

Grimmond AP, Spencer RP. (1986). Hepatic mass: Functioning metastatic thymoma 22 years after radiation therapy. *Clinical Nuclear Medicine* 11(8):570-571.

Grion AM, Gaion RM, Cordella L, Bano F, Cannada RA, Innamorati G, Berti T. (1994). [Interferon-alpha: Results of a pharmaco-epidemiologic study]. *Clinica Terapia* 144(3):201-211.

Groopman JE. (1998). Fatigue in cancer and HIV/AIDS. *Oncology* 12(3):335-344.

Groopman JE, Itri LM. (1999). Chemotherapy-induced anemia in adults: Incidence and treatment. *Journal of the National Cancer Institutes* 91(19):1616-1634.

Grosh WW, Brenner DE, Jones HW III, Burnett LS, Greco FA. (1983). Phase II study of vinblastine in advanced refractory ovarian carcinoma. *American Journal of Clinical Oncology* 6(5):571-575.

Gruber AJ, Hudson JI, Pope HG Jr. (1996). The management of treatment-resistant depression in disorders on the interface of psychiatry and medicine: Fibromyalgia, chronic fatigue syndrome, migraine, irritable bowel syndrome, atypical facial pain, and premenstrual dysphoric disorder. *Psychiatry Clinics of North America* 19(2):351-369.

Grüber C, Kulig M, Mergmann R, Guggenmoos-Holzman I, Wahn U. (2001). Delayed hypersensitivity to tuberculin, total immunoglobulin E, specific sensitization, and atopic manifestation in longitudinally followed early Bacille Calmette-Guérin-vaccinated and nonvaccinated children. *Pediatrics* 107:E36.

Grüber C, Meinlschmidt G, Bergmann R, Wahn U, Stark K. (2002). Is early BCG vaccination associated with less atopic disease? An epidemiological study in German preschool children with different ethnic backgrounds. *Pediatric Allergy and Immunology* 13:177-181.

Grüber C, Nilsson L, Bjorksten B. (2001). Do early childhood immunizations influence the development of atopy and do they cause allergic reactions? *Pediatric Allergy and Immunology* 12:296-311.

Grufferman S, Eby NL, Huang M, Whiteside T, Sumaya CV, Saxinger WC, Herfkens RJ, Penkower L, Muldoon SB, Herberman RB. (1988). Epidemiologic investigation of an outbreak of chronic fatigue-immune dysfunction syndrome in a defined population. *American Journal of Epidemiology* 128:898.

Grunberg SM, Kempf RA, Itri LM, Venturi CL, Boswell WD Jr, Mitchell MS. (1985). Phase II study of recombinant alpha interferon in the treatment of advanced non-small cell lung carcinoma. *Cancer Treatment Reports* 69(9):1031-1032.

Grundmann J, Wolff T. (2000). [Mediastinal space-occupying lesion of uncertain histology: Difficulties of differential diagnosis]. *Deutsche Medizinische Wochenschrift* 125(41):1227-1231.

Grunfeld E, Mant D, Yudkin P, Adewuyi-Dalton R, Cole D, Stewart J, Fitzpatrick R, Vessey M. (1996). Routine follow up of breast cancer in primary care: Randomised trial. *British Medical Journal* 313(7058):665-669.

Gubareva LV, Kaiser L, Hayden FG. (2000). Influenza virus neuraminidase inhibitor. *Lancet* 355:827-835.

Guida L, O'Hehir RE, Hawrylowicz CM. (1994). Synergy between dexamethasone and interleukin-5 for the induction of major histocompatibility complex class II expression by human peripheral blood eosinophils. *Blood* 84(8):2733-2740.

Guirguis WR. (1998). Oral treatment of erectile dysfunction: From herbal remedies to designer drugs. *Journal of Sex and Marital Therapy* 24(2):69-73.

Gulbrandsen N, Wisloff F, Brinch L, Carlson K, Dahl IM, Gimsing P, Hippe E, Hjorth M, Knudsen LM, Lamvik J, et al. (2001). Health-related quality of life in multiple myeloma patients receiving high-dose chemotherapy with autologous blood stem-cell support. *Medical Oncology* 18(1):65-77.

Gunn W, Komaroff A, Levine S, Connell D. (1997). Multilab retrovirus test results for CFS patients from 3 different geographical areas. *Mortality and Morbidity Weekly Reports.*

Gunning K, Steele P. (1999). Echinacea for the prevention of upper respiratory tract infections. *Journal of Family Practice* 48(2):93.

Gunthert AR, Pilz S, Kuhn W, Emons G, Meden H. (1999). Docetaxel is effective in the treatment of metastatic endometrial cancer. *Anticancer Research* 19(4C):3459-3461.

Gupta S, Aggarwal S, See D, Starr A. (1997). Cytokine production by adherent and non-adherent mononuclear cells in chronic fatigue syndrome. *Journal of Psychiatric Research* 31(1):149-156.

Gupta S, Aggarwal S, Starr A. (1999). Increased production of interleukin-6 by adherent and non-adherent mononuclear cells during "natural fatigue" but not following "experimental fatigue" in patients with chronic fatigue syndrome. *International Journal of Molecular Medicine* 3(2):209-213.

Gupta S, Vayuvegula B. (1991). A comprehensive immunological analysis in chronic fatigue syndrome. *Scandinavian Journal of Immunology* 33(3):319-327.

Gutstein HB. (2001). The biologic basis of fatigue. *Cancer* 92(6 Suppl):1678-1683.

Gutterman JU, Blumenschein GR, Alexanian R, Yap HY, Buzdar AU, Cabanillas F, Hortobagyi GN, Hersh EM, Rasmussen SL, Harmon M, et al. (1980). Leukocyte interferon-induced tumor regression in human metastatic breast cancer, multiple myeloma, and malignant lymphoma. *Annals of Internal Medicine* 93(3):399-406.

Gutterman JU, Fine S, Quesada J, Horning SJ, Levine JF, Alexanian R, Bernhardt L, Kramer M, Spiegel H, Colburn W, et al. (1982). Recombinant leukocyte A interferon: Pharmacokinetics, single-dose tolerance, and biologic effects in cancer patients. *Annals of Internal Medicine* 96(5):549-556.

Haarstad H, Gundersen S, Wist E, Raabe N, Mella O, Kvinnsland S. (1992). Droloxifene—a new anti-estrogen: A phase II study in advanced breast cancer. *Acta Oncologica* 31(4):425-428.

Haas N, Roth B, Garay C, Yeslow G, Entmacher M, Weinstein A, Rogatko A, Babb J, Minnitti C, Flinker D, et al. (2001). Phase I trial of weekly paclitaxel plus oral estramustine phosphate in patients with hormone-refractory prostate cancer. *Urology* 58(1):59-64.

Haavet OR, Grunfeld B. (1997). [Are life experiences of children significant for the development of somatic disease? A literature review] Er bans livserfaringer av betydning for somatisk sykdomsutvikling? En litteraturoversikt. *Tidsskr Nor Laegeforen* 117(25):3644-3647.

Hackney AC. (1996). The male reproductive system and endurance exercise. *Medical Science, Sports, and Exercise* 28:180-189.

Hadler NM. (1996a). If you have to prove you are ill, you can't get well: The object lesson of fibromyalgia. *Spine* 1521(20):2397-2400.

Hadler NM. (1996b). Is fibromyalgia a useful diagnostic label? *Cleveland Clinic Journal of Medicine* 63(2):85-87.

Hadler NM. (1997a). Fibromyalgia, chronic fatigue, and other iatrogenic diagnostic algorithms: Do some labels escalate illness in vulnerable patients? *Postgraduate Medicine* 102(2):161-162, 165-166, 171-172.

Hadler NM. (1997b). Fibromyalgia: La maladie est morte. Vive le malade! *Journal of Rheumatology* 24(7):1250-1251, discussion 1252.

Hadley SK, Petry JJ. (1999). Medicinal herbs: A primer for primary care. *Hospital Practice* 34(6):105-123.

Hagemeijer A, Prins K, Courtens A. (1997). [A closer look at a frequently occurring and fundamental problem: Fatigue under chemotherapy (1)]. *TVZ* 107(21):634-637.

Hagenbaugh A, Sharma S, Dubinett SM, Wei SH, Aranda R, Cheroutre H, Fowell DJ, Binder S, Tsao B, Locksley RM, et al. (1997). Altered immune responses in interleukin 10 transgenic mice. *Journal of Experimental Medicine* 185:2101-2110.

Hainsworth JD, Burris HA III, Erland JB, Morrissey LH, Meluch AA, Kalman LA, Hon JK, Scullin DC Jr, Smith SW, Greco FA. (1999). Phase I/II trial of paclitaxel by 1-hour infusion, carboplatin, and gemcitabine in the treatment of patients with advanced nonsmall cell lung carcinoma. *Cancer* 85(6):1269-1276.

Hainsworth JD, Burris HA III, Erland JB, Thomas M, Greco FA. (1998). Phase I trial of docetaxel administered by weekly infusion in patients with advanced refractory cancer. *Journal of Clinical Oncology* 16(6):2164-2168.

Hainsworth JD, Burris HA III, Greco FA. (1999). Weekly administration of docetaxel (Taxotere): Summary of clinical data. *Seminars in Oncology* 26(3 Suppl 10):19-24.

Hainsworth JD, Burris HA III, Litchy S, Morrissey LH, Barton JH, Bradof JE, Greco FA. (2000). Weekly docetaxel in the treatment of elderly patients with advanced nonsmall cell lung carcinoma: A Minnie Pearl Cancer Research Network phase II trial. *Cancer* 89(2):328-333.

Hainsworth JD, Burris HA III, Yardley DA, Bradof JE, Grimaldi M, Kalman LA, Sullivan T, Baker M, Erland JB, Greco FA. (2001). Weekly docetaxel in the treatment of elderly patients with advanced breast cancer: A Minnie Pearl Cancer Research Network phase II trial. *Journal of Clinical Oncology* 19(15):3500-3505.

Hainsworth JD, Calvert S, Greco FA. (2002). Paclitaxel and mitoxantrone in the treatment of metastatic breast cancer: A phase II trial of the Minnie Pearl Cancer Research Network. *Cancer Investigation* 20(7-8):863-871.

Hainsworth JD, Hande KR, Satterlee WG, Kuttesch J, Johnson DH, Grindey G, Jackson LE, Greco FA. (1989). Phase I clinical study of N-[(4-chlorophenyl) amino]carbonyl-2,3-dihydro-1H-indene-5-sulfonamide (LY186641). *Cancer Research* 49(18):5217-5220.

Hakamies-Blomqvist L, Luoma ML, Sjostrom J, Pluzanska A, Sjodin M, Mouridsen H, Ostenstad B, Mjaaland I, Ottosson-Lonn S, Bergh J, et al. (2000). Quality of life in patients with metastatic breast cancer receiving either docetaxel or sequential methotrexate and 5-fluorouracil: A multicentre randomised phase III trial by the Scandinavian Breast Group. *European Journal of Cancer* 36(11):1411-1417.

Hakamies-Blomqvist L, Luoma ML, Sjostrom J, Pluzanska A, Sjodin M, Mouridsen H, Ostenstad B, Mjaaland I, Ottosson S, Bergh J, et al. (2001). Timing of quality of life (QoL) assessments as a source of error in oncological trials. *Journal of Advanced Nursing* 35(5):709-716.

Hakimi R. (1996). Chronic fatigue syndrome—Also an insurance medicine problem. *Versicherungsmedizin* 48(2):59-61.

Halberstein RA. (1997). Traditional botanical remedies on a small Caribbean island: Middle (Grand) Caicos, West Indies. *Journal of Alternative and Complementary Medicine* 3(3):227-239.

Hall HJ. (1905). The systematic use of work as a remedy in neurasthenia and allied conditions. *Boston Medical and Surgical Journal* 152(2):29-32.

Hallberg LR, Carlsson SG. (1998). Psychosocial vulnerability and maintaining forces related to fibromyalgia: In-depth interviews with twenty-two female patients. *Scandinavian Journal of Caring Sciences* 12(2):95-103.

Hallum AV III, Alberts DS, Lippman SM, Inclan L, Shamdas GJ, Childers JM, Surwit EA, Modiano M, Hatch KD. (1995). Phase II study of 13-cis-retinoic acid plus interferon-alpha 2a in heavily pretreated squamous carcinoma of the cervix. *Gynecological Oncology* 56(3):382-386.

Hamilos DL, Nutter D, Gershtenson J, Redmond DP, Clementi JD, Schmaling KB, Make BJ, Jones JF. (1998). Core body temperature is normal in chronic fatigue syndrome. *Biological Psychiatry* 43(4):293-302.

Hamilton AS, Radka SF, Bernstein L, Gill PS, Gonsalves M, Naemura JR, Ross RK. (1994). Relationship of serum levels of oncostatin M to AIDS-related and classic Kaposi's sarcoma. *Journal of Acquired Immunodeficiency Syndromes* 7:410-414.

Hamilton BP, Daly BD, Furlong M. (2002). A 41-year-old man with fatigue, weight loss, hypercalcemia, and hepatosplenomegaly. *American Journal of Medical Sciences* 324(1):31-36.

Hamilton J, Butler L, Wagenaar H, Sveinson T, Ward KA, McLean L, Grant D, MacLellan F. (2001). The impact and management of cancer-related fatigue on patients and families. *Canadian Oncology Nursing Journal* 11(4):192-198.

Hamilton JA. (1993). Colony stimulating factors, cytokines and monocyte-macrophages—Some controversies. *Immunology Today* 14(1):18-24.

Hamilton SF. (1998). The fibromyalgia problem. *Journal of Rheumatology* 25(5): 1027-1028, discussion 1028-1030.

Hamm JT, Tormey DC, Kohler PC, Haller D, Green M, Shemano I. (1991). Phase I study of toremifene in patients with advanced cancer. *Journal of Clinical Oncology* 9(11):2036-2041.

Han F, Hu J, Xu H. (1997). Effects of some Chinese herbal medicine and green tea antagonizing mutagenesis caused by cigarette tar. *Chung Hua Yu Fang I Hsueh Tsa Chih* 31(2):71-74.

Han JQ, Chen SD, Zhai LM. (1997). Clinical study of combined Chinese herbal medicine with move stripe field radiation in treating primary hepatocellular carcinoma. *Chung Kuo Chung His I Chieh Ho Tsa Chih* 17(8):465-466.

Han SS. (1998). [Effects of a self-help program including stretching exercise on symptom reduction in patients with fibromyalgia]. *Taehan Kanho* 37(1):78-80.

Hana I, Vrubel J, Pekarek J, Cech K. (1996). The influence of age on transfer factor treatment of cellular immunodeficiency, chronic fatigue syndrome and/or chronic viral infections. *Biotherapy* 9(1-3):91-95.

Handa KK, Sra JS, Akhtar M. (1997). Successful treatment of a patient with chronic fatigue using head-up tilt guided therapy. *Wisconsin Medical Journal* 96(3): 40-42.

Handler RP. (1998). The fibromyalgia problem. *Journal of Rheumatology* 25(5): 1025, discussion, 1028-1030.

Hann DM, Denniston MM, Baker F. (2000). Measurement of fatigue in cancer patients: Further validation of the Fatigue Symptom Inventory. *Quality of Life Research* 9(7):847-854.

Hann DM, Garovoy N, Finkelstein B, Jacobsen PB, Azzarello LM, Fields KK. (1999). Fatigue and quality of life in breast cancer patients undergoing autologous stem cell transplantation: A longitudinal comparative study. *Journal of Pain Symptomatology and Management* 17(5):311-319.

Hann DM, Jacobsen PB, Azzarello LM, Martin SC, Curran SL, Fields KK, Greenberg H, Lyman G. (1998). Measurement of fatigue in cancer patients: Development and validation of the Fatigue Symptom Inventory. *Quality of Life Research* 7(4):301-310.

Hann DM, Jacobsen PB, Martin SC, Kronish LE, Azzarello LM, Fields KK. (1997). Fatigue in women treated with bone marrow transplantation for breast cancer: A comparison with women with no history of cancer. *Support Care in Cancer* 5(1):44-52.

Hann DM, Winter K, Jacobsen P. (1999). Measurement of depressive symptoms in cancer patients: Evaluation of the Center for Epidemiological Studies Depression Scale (CES-D). *Journal of Psychosomatic Research* 46(5):437-443.

Hannonen P, Malminiemi K, Yli-Kerttula U, Isomeri R, Roponen P. (1998). A randomized, double-blind, placebo-controlled study of moclobemide and amitriptyline in the treatment of fibromyalgia in females without psychiatric disorder. *British Journal of Rheumatology* 37(12):1279-1286.

Hansen MK, Krueger JM. (1998). Subdiaphragmatic vagotomy does not block sleep deprivation-induced sleep in rats. *Physiology and Behavior* 64:361-365.

Hansen MK, Taishi P, Chen Z, Krueger JM. (1998). Vagotomy blocks the induction of interleukin-1beta (IL-1beta) mRNA in the brain of rats on response to systemic IL-1beta. *Journal of Neurosciences* 18:2247-2253.

Hansen PB, Vogt KC, Skov RL, Pedersen-Bjergaard U, Jacobsen M, Ralfkiaer E. (1998). Primary gastrointestinal non-Hodgkin's lymphoma in adults: A population-based clinical and histopathologic study. *Journal of Internal Medicine* 244(1):71-78.

Hansen RM, Borden EC. (1992). Current status of interferons in the treatment of cancer. *Oncology* 6(11):19-24.

Hanson Frost M, Suman VJ, Rummans TA, Dose AM, Taylor M, Novotny P, Johnson R, Evans RE. (2000). Physical, psychological and social well-being of women with breast cancer: The influence of disease phase. *Psychooncology* 9(3):221-231.

Hansotia P. (1996). Emotional distress, physical symptoms and sleep disorders. *Wisconsin Medical Journal* 95(12):836-837.

Hantzschel H, Boche K. (1999). [Fibromyalgia syndrome] Das fibromyalgie-syndrom. *Fortschrift Medizin* 117(5):26-28, 30-31.

Hapidou EG, Rollman GB. (1998). Menstrual cycle modulation of tender points. *Pain* 77(2):151-161.

Hara H, Nomura E, Watanabe I, Sako S, Otani M, Tanigawa N. (1999). Advanced gallbladder carcinoma with liver metastasis showing a favorable response after intra-arterial infusion chemotherapy: Report of a case. *Surgery Today* 29(10): 1102-1105.

Harada H, Mandai H, Tsurumi T, Yamamoto N, Tomiya Y. (1975). Diagnosis of carcinoma of the papilla of Vater by duodenofiberscopy: Simultaneous attempt on endoscopic observation, aspiration cytology, retrograde pancreatocholangiography and biopsy. *Gastroenterology Japan* 10(1):6-19.

Harada K, Sugita Y, Kawaba T, Tokunaga T, Sigemori M, Anegawa S. (1992). [Brain metastasis of lung cancer with Eaton-Lambert syndrome—Case report]. *No To Shinkei* 44(8):755-759.

Haraguchi S, Good RA, Cianciolo GJ, James-Yarish M, Day NK. (1993). Transcriptional down-regulation of tumor necrosis factor-alpha gene expression by a synthetic peptide homologous to retroviral envelope protein. *Journal of Immunology* 151:2733-2741.

Harden, J, Schafenacker A, Northouse L, Mood D, Smith D, Pienta K, Hussain M, Baranowski K. (2002). Couples' experiences with prostate cancer: Focus group research. *Oncology Nursing Forum* 29(4):701-709.

Harding SM. (1998). Sleep in fibromyalgia patients: Subjective and objective findings. *American Journal of Medical Sciences* 315(6):367-376.

Harlow BL, Signorello LB, Hall JE, Dailey C, Komaroff AL. (1998). Reproductive correlates of chronic fatigue syndrome. *American Journal of Medicine* 105(3A): 94S-99S.

Harmon DL, McMaster D, McCluskey DR, Shields D, Whitehead AS. (1997). A common genetic variant affecting folate metabolism is not over-represented in chronic fatigue syndrome. *Annals of Clinical Biochemistry* 34(Pt 4):427-429.

Harpham WS. (1999). Resolving the frustration of fatigue. *CA Cancer Journal for Clinicians* 49(3):178-189.

Harrell RA, Cianciolo GJ, Copeland TD, Oroszlan S, Snyderman R. (1986). Suppression of the respiratory burst of human monocytes by a synthetic peptide homologous to envelope proteins of human and animal retroviruses. *Journal of Immunology* 136:3517-3518.

Harrigan P. (1998). Controversy continues over chronic fatigue syndrome. *Lancet* 351(9102):574.

Harris KA, Weinberg V, Bok RA, Kakefuda M, Small EJ. (2002). Low dose ketoconazole with replacement doses of hydrocortisone in patients with progressive androgen independent prostate cancer. *Journal of Urology* 168(2):542-545.

Harrison LB, Shasha D, Homel P. (2002). Prevalence of anemia in cancer patients undergoing radiotherapy: Prognostic significance and treatment. *Oncology* 63 (Suppl 2):11-18.

Harrison P. (1998). Herbal medicine takes root in Germany. *Canadian Medical Association Journal* 158(5):637-639; comments 158(13):1689-1690.

Hart FD. (1998). Underlying signs of fibromyalgia. *Practitioner* 242(1586):407-410.

Hart RD, Ohnuma T, Holland JF, Bruckner H. (1982). Methyl-GAG in patients with malignant neoplasms: A phase I re-evaluation. *Cancer Treatment Reports* 66(1): 65-71.

Hartlapp JH, Munch HJ, Illiger HJ, Wolter H, Jensen JC. (1985). Alternatives to CYVADIC-combination therapy of soft tissue sarcomas. *Klinische Wochenschrift* 63(22):1160-1162.

Hartlapp JH, Munch HJ, Illiger HJ, Wolter H, Jensen JC. (1986). Alternatives to CYVADIC combination therapy of soft tissue sarcomas. *Cancer Chemotherapy Pharmacology* 18(Suppl 2):S20-S22.

Hartmann JT, Quietzsch D, Daikeler T, Kollmannsberger C, Mayer F, Kanz L, Bokemeyer C. (1999). Mitomycin C continuous infusion as salvage chemotherapy in pretreated patients with advanced gastric cancer. *Anticancer Drugs* 10(8):729-733.

Hartz AJ, Kuhn EM, Levine PH. (1998). Characteristics of fatigued persons associated with features of chronic fatigue syndrome. *Journal of Chronic Fatigue Syndrome* 4(3):71-97.

Hasegawa Y, Shirai S, Mishina T, Nakata M, Aikawa K, Yoshida K. (2002). [An elderly non-Hodgkin lymphoma patient with a massive tumor of the heart]. *Rinsho Ketsueki* 43(7):538-542.

Haseltine WA, Patarca R. (1986). AIDS virus and scrapie agent share protein. *Nature* 326:115-116.

Haseltine WA, Sodroski JG, Patarca R, Briggs D, Perkins D, Wong-Staal F. (1984). Structure of the 3'-terminal region of type II human T-lymphotropic virus: Evidence for a new coding region. *Science* 225:419-421.

Haskell CM. (1994). A phase I study of ATP in patients with advanced cancer (meeting abstract). *Proceedings of the Annual Meeting of the American Society of Clinical Oncology* 13:A436.

Haskell CM, Lee LY. (1994). Pharmacokinetics of ATP administered as a 96-hour infusion (meeting abstract). *Proceedings of the Annual Meetings of the American Association of Cancer Research* 35:A2414.

Haskell CM, Wong M, Williams A, Lee LY. (1996). Phase I trial of extracellular adenosine 5'-triphosphate in patients with advanced cancer. *Medical Pediatric Oncology* 27:165-173.

Hass GM, Laing GH, Galt RM, McCreary PA. (1981). Recent advances—Immunopathology of magnesium deficiency in rats: Induction of tumors; incidence, transmission and prevention of lymphoma-leukemia. *Magnesium Bulletin* 3:217-228.

Hassan IS, Bannister BA, Akbar A, Weir W, Bofill M. (1998). A study of the immunology of the chronic fatigue syndrome: Correlation of immunologic markers to health dysfunction. *Clinical Immunology and Immunopathology* 87(1):60-67.

Haub MD, Potteiger JA, Nau KL, Webster MJ, Zebas CJ. (1998). Acute L-glutamine ingestion does not improve maximal effort exercise. *Journal of Sports Medicine and Physical Fitness* 38(3):240-244.

Hausen A, Wachter H. (1982). Pteridines in the assessment of neoplasia. *Journal of Clinical Chemistry and Clinical Biochemistry* 20:593-602.

Hausotter W. (1996). Expert assessment of chronic fatigue syndrome. *Versicherungsmedizin* 48(2):57-59.

Hausotter W. (1998). [Fibromyalgia—A dispensable disease term?] Fibromyalgie—ein entbehrlicher Krankheitsbegriff? *Versicherungsmedizin* 50(1):13-17.

Havsteen H, Bertelsen K, Gadeberg CC, Jacobsen A, Kamby C, Sandberg E, Sengelov L. (1996). A phase 2 study with epirubicin as second-line treatment of patients with advanced epithelial ovarian cancer. *Gynecological Oncology* 63 (2):210-215.

Hawkins MJ, Krown SE, Borden EC, Krim M, Real FX, Edwards BS, Anderson SA, Cunningham-Rundles S, Oettgen HF. (1984). American Cancer Society phase I trial of naturally produced beta-interferon. *Cancer Research* 44(12 Pt 1): 5934-5938.

Hawley JA, Reilly T. (1997). Fatigue revisited. *Journal of Sport Sciences* 15(3): 245-246.

Hayashi I, Muto Y, Fujii Y, Katsuda Y. (1983). [Primary amyloidosis associated with early gastric carcinoma(IIb like IIa type) diagnosed by preoperative gastric biopsy—A case report]. *Gan No Rinsho* 29(14):1686-1692.

Hayes JR. (1991). Depression and chronic fatigue in cancer patients. *Primary Care* 18(2):327-339.

Haylock PJ, Hart LK. (1979). Fatigue in patients receiving localized radiation. *Cancer Nursing* 2(6):461-467.

Healey LA. (1996). On fibromyalgia. *Bulletin of Rheumatic Diseases* 45(6):1.

Heath EI, O'Reilly S, Humphrey R, Sundaresan P, Donehower RC, Sartorius S, Kennedy MJ, Armstrong DK, Carducci MA, Sorensen JM, Kumor K, Kennedy S, Grochow LB. (2001). Phase I trial of the matrix metalloproteinase inhibitor BAY12-9566 in patients with advanced solid tumors. *Cancer Chemotherapy Pharmacology* 48(4):269-274.

Heath EI, Urba S, Marshall J, Piantadosi S, Forastiere AA. (2002). Phase II trial of docetaxel chemotherapy in patients with incurable adenocarcinoma of the esophagus. *Investigative New Drugs* 20(1):95-99.

Heber D, Byerley LO, Chi J. (1986). Pathophysiology of malnutrition in the adult cancer patient. *Cancer Research* 58:1867-1873.

Hegarty TJ, Thornton AF, Diaz RF, Chandler WF, Ensminger WD, Junck L, Page MA, Gebarski SS, Hood TW, Stetson PL, et al. (1990). Intra-arterial bromo-deoxyuridine radiosensitization of malignant gliomas. *International Journal of Radiation Oncology, Biology and Physics* 19(2):421-428.

Heggers JP, Elzaim H, Garfield R, Goodheart R, Listengarten D, Zhao J, and Phillips LG. (1997). Effect of the combination of *Aloë vera,* nitroglycerin and L-NAME on wound healing in the rat excisional model. *Journal of Alternative and Complementary Medicine* 3(2):149-153.

Heggers JP, Kucukcelebi A, Listengarten D, Stabenau J, Ko F, Broemeling LD, Robson MC, Winters WD. (1996). Beneficial effect of aloe on wound healing in an excisional wound model. *Journal of Alternative and Complementary Medicine* 2(2):271-277.

Heidenreich A, Hofmann R. (1999). Quality-of-life issues in the treatment of testicular cancer. *World Journal of Urology* 17(4):230-238.

Heilig B, Fiehn C, Brockhaus M, Galleti H, Pezzutto A, Hunstein W. (1993). Evaluation of soluble tumor necrosis factor (TNF) receptors and TNF receptor antibodies in patients with systemic lupus erythematodes, progressive systemic sclerosis and mixed connective tissue disease. *Journal of Clinical Immunology* 13:321-328.

Heilmann P, Wagner P, Nawroth PP, Ziegler R. (2001). [Therapy of the adrenocortical carcinoma with Lysodren (o,p'-DDD): Therapeutic management by monitoring o,p'-DDD blood levels]. *Medizinsche Klinik* 96(7):371-377.

Heim C, Ehlert U, Hellhammer DH. (2000). The potential role of hypocortisolism in the pathophysiology of stress-related bodily disorders. *Psychoneuroendocrinology* 25(1):1-35.

Heinonen H, Volin L, Uutela A, Zevon M, Barrick C, Ruutu T. (2001). Gender-associated differences in the quality of life after allogeneic BMT. *Bone Marrow Transplantation* 28(5):503-509.

Heinrich M, Ankli A, Frei B, Weimann C, Sticher O. (1998). Medicinal plants in Mexico: Healers' consensus and cultural importance. *Social Science Medicine* 47(11):1859-1871.

Held JL. (1994). Managing fatigue. *Nursing* 24(2):26.

Helder L, Wagner S, Keller R, Klimas N, Antoni M. (1998). Markers of immune activation are associated with psychological distress in patients with CFS. Presented at the Fourth International American Association for Chronic Fatigue Syndrome (AACFS) Conference, October 10-12, Cambridge, Massachusetts.

Held-Warmkessel J, Volpe H, Waldman AR. (1998). Symptom management for patients with pancreatic cancer. *Clinical Journal of Oncology Nursing* 2(4):135-139.

Helgesen A, Fuglsig S. (2000). [Villous adenoma of the rectum with electrolyte imbalance: McKittrick-Wheelock syndrome]. *Ugeskr Laeger* 162(32):4272-4273.

Hellinger WC, Smith TF, Van Scoy RE, Spidzor PG, Forgacs P, Edson RS. (1988). Chronic fatigue syndrome and diagnostic utility of antibody to Epstein-Barr virus early antigen. *JAMA* 260:971-973.

Helliwell PS. (1995). The semeiology of arthritis: Discriminating between patients on the basis of their symptoms. *Annals of Rheumatic Diseases* 54(11):924-926.

Hellsten S, Berge T, Wehlin L. (1981). Unrecognized renal cell carcinoma: Clinical and diagnostic aspects. *Scandinavian Journal of Urology and Nephrology* 15(3):269-272.

Hellstrom OW. (1995). Health promotion and clinical dialogue. *Patient Education Counseling* 25(3):247-256.

Hellstrom OW, Bullington J, Karlsson G, Lindqvist P, Mattsson B. (1998). Doctors' attitudes to fibromyalgia: A phenomenological study. *Scandinavian Journal of Social Medicine* 26(3):232-237.

Hemmeter U, Kocher R, Ladewig D, Hatzinger M, Seifritz E, Lauer CJ, Holsboer-Trachsler E. (1995). [Sleep disorders in chronic pain and generalized tendomyopathy] Schlafstorungen bei chronicschen schmerzen un generalisierter tendomyopathie. *Schweize Medizin Wochenschrift* 125(49):2391-2397.

Hench PK. (1996). Sleep and rheumatic diseases. *Bulletin of Rheumatic Diseases* 45:1-6.

Hendriks MG, van Beijsterveldt BC, Schouten HC. (1998). [The quality of life after stem cell transplantation: Problems with fatigue, sexuality, finances and employment]. *Nederlande Tijdschrift Geneeskunde* 142(20):1152-1155.

Hennessy T. (1994). Nightingale's birthday: A comprehensive approach. *Annales Internationales de Medécine* 121:953-959.

Henriksen H, Riis J, Christophersen B, Moe C. (1997). [Distress symptoms in hospice patients]. *Ugeskr Laeger* 159(47):6992-6996.

Henriksson KG. (1999). Is fibromyalgia a distinct clinical entity? Pain mechanisms in fibromyalgia syndrome: A myologist's view. *Baillieres Best Practice Research in Clinical Rheumatology* 13(3):455-461.

Henry DH. (1997). Haematological toxicities associated with dose-intensive chemotherapy, the role for and use of recombinant growth factors. *Annals of Oncology* 8(Suppl 3):S7-S10.

Henry DH. (1998a). Experience with epoetin alfa and acquired immunodeficiency syndrome anemia. *Seminars in Oncology* 25(3 Suppl 7):64-68.

Henry DH. (1998b). Supplemental iron: A key to optimizing the response of cancer-related anemia to rHuEPO? *Oncologist* 3(4):275-278.

Henter JI, Elinder G, Soder O, Hansson M, Andersson B, Andersson U. (1991). Hypercytokinemia in familial hemophagocytic lymphohistiocytosis. *Blood* 78 (11):2918-2922.

Herbelin A, Nguyen AT, Zingraff J, Urena P, Descamps-Latscha B. (1990). Influence of uremia and hemodialysis on circulating interleukin-1 and tumor necrosis factor alpha. *Kidney International* 37:116-125.

Herben VM, Panday VR, Richel DJ, Schellens JH, van der Vange N, Rosing H, Beusenberg FD, Hearn S, Doyle E, Beijnen JH, et al. (1999). Phase I and pharmacologic study of the combination of paclitaxel, cisplatin, and topotecan administered intravenously every 21 days as first-line therapy in patients with advanced ovarian cancer. *Journal of Clinical Oncology* 17(3):747-755.

Herben VM, ten Bokkel Huinink WW, Schot ME, Hudson I, Beijnen JH. (1998). Continuous infusion of low-dose topotecan: Pharmacokinetics and pharmacodynamics during a phase II study in patients with small cell lung cancer. *Anticancer Drugs* 9(5):411-418.

Herben VM, van Gijn R, Schellens JH, Schot M, Lieverst J, Hillebrand MJ, Schoemaker NE, Porro MG, Beijnen JH, ten Bokkel Huinink WW. (1999). Phase I and pharmacokinetic study of a daily times 5 short intravenous infusion schedule of 9-aminocamptothecin in a colloidal dispersion formulation in patients with advanced solid tumors. *Journal of Clinical Oncology* 17(6):1906-1914.

Herberman RB. (1991). Sources of confounding in immunologic data. *Reviews of Infectious Diseases* 13(1):S84-S86.

Herbst RS, Lynch C, Vasconcelles M, Teicher BA, Strauss G, Elias A, Anderson I, Zacarola P, Dang NH, Leong T, et al. (2001). Gemcitabine and vinorelbine in patients with advanced lung cancer: Preclinical studies and report of a phase I trial. *Cancer Chemotherapy Pharmacology* 48(2):151-159.

Hernandez-Pando R, Rook GA. (1994). The role of TNF-alpha in T-cell mediated inflammation depends on the Th1-/Th2 cytokine balance. *Immunology* 82(4): 591-595.

Herndon JE II, Fleishman S, Kornblith AB, Kosty M, Green MR, Holland J. (1999). Is quality of life predictive of the survival of patients with advanced nonsmall cell lung carcinoma? *Cancer* 85(2):333-340.

Herr HW, O'Sullivan M. (2000). Quality of life of asymptomatic men with non-metastatic prostate cancer on androgen deprivation therapy. *Journal of Urology* 163(6):1743-1746.

Herr HW, Pinsky CM, Whitmore WF Jr, Sogani PC, Oettgen HF, Melanmed MR. (1986). Long-term effect of intravesical bacillus Calmette-Guérin on flat carcinoma in situ of the bladder. *Journal of Urology* 35:265-267.

Herr HW, Warrel RP, Burchenal JH. (1986). Phase I trial of alpha-difluoromethyl ornithine (DFMO) and methylglyoxal bis (guanylhydrazone) (MGBG) in patients with advanced prostatic cancer. *Urology* 28(6):508-511.

Herrmann MA, Shankerman RA, Edwards WD, Shub C, Schaff HV. (1992). Primary cardiac angiosarcoma: A clinicopathologic study of six cases. *Journal of Thoracic Cardiovascular Surgery* 103(4):655-664.

Hersey P, Hasic E, MacDonald M, Edwards A, Spurling A, Coates AS, Milton GW, McCarthy WH. (1985). Effects of recombinant leukocyte interferon (rIFN-alpha A) on tumour growth and immune responses in patients with metastatic melanoma. *British Journal of Cancer* 51(6):815-826.

Hersh EM, Murray JL, Hong WK, Rosenblum MG, Reuben JM, Weilbaecher R, Sarwal AN, Bradley EC, Konrad M, Arnett FC. (1989). Phase I study of cancer therapy with recombinant interleukin-2 administered by intravenous bolus injection. *Biotherapy* 1(3):215-226.

Hesketh PJ, Crowley JJ, Burris HA III, Williamson SK, Balcerzak SP, Peereboom D, Goodwin JW, Gross HM, Moore DF Jr, Livingston RB, et al. (1999). Evaluation of docetaxel in previously untreated extensive-stage small cell lung cancer: A Southwest Oncology Group phase II trial. *Cancer Journal Scientific American* 5(4):237-241.

Hettich R, Wagenknecht B, Weinzierl M, Weiss M, Steinbeck G. (1990). [Fatigue, pulmonary coin lesions and liver tumor]. *Internist* 31(8):538-541.

Heyes MP, Saito K, Milstein S, Schiff SJ. (1995). Quinolinic acid in tumors, hemorrhage and bacterial infections of the central nervous system in children. *Journal of Neurological Sciences* 133(1-2):112-118.

Heyll U, Wachauf P, Senger P, Diewitz M. (1997). Definition of "chronic fatigue syndrome" (CFS). *Medizinische Klinik* 92(4):221-227.

Hickie I, Hadzi-Pavlovic D, Ricci C. (1997). Receiving the diagnosis of neurasthenia. *Psychological Medicine* 27(5):989-994.

Hickie I, Lloyd A, Wakefield D, Ricci C. (1996). Is there a postinfection fatigue syndrome? *Australian Family Physician* 25(12):1847-1852.

Hickok JT, Morrow GR, McDonald S, Bellg AJ. (1996). Frequency and correlates of fatigue in lung cancer patients receiving radiation therapy: Implications for management. *Journal of Pain Symptomatology Management* 11(6):370-377.

Hickson RC, Ball KL, Falduto MT. (1989). Adverse effects of anabolic steroids. *Medical Toxicology and Adverse Drug Exposure* 4:254-271.

Higuchi K, Arakawa T, Ando K, Fujiwara Y, Uchida T, Kuroki T. (1999). Eradication of *Helicobacter pylori* with a Chinese herbal medicine without emergence of resistant colonies. *American Journal of Gastroenterology* 94(5):1419-1420.

Hilden J. (1996). [Diagnosis of fibromyalgia: A critical review of the Scandinavian literature] Fibromyalgidiagnosen: En kritisk oversigt over nordisk litteratur. *Nordisk Medizin* 111(9):308-312.

Hilepo JN, Bellucci AG, Mossey RT. (1997). Acute renal failure caused by "cat's claw" herbal remedy in a patient with systemic lupus erythematosus. *Nephron* 77(3):361.

Hilgers A, Frank J, Bolte P. (1998). Prolongation of central motor conduction time in chronic fatigue syndrome. *Journal of Chronic Fatigue Syndrome* 4(2):23-32.

Hill M, Macfarlane V, Moore J, Gore ME. (1997). Taxane/platinum/anthracycline combination therapy in advanced epithelial ovarian cancer. *Seminars in Oncology* 24(1 Suppl 2):S2-34-S2-37.

Hill W, Greither L, Bartl R, Jehn U, Kolb HJ, Wilmanns W. (1991). [Patient with decreased energy, dyspnea on exertion and splenomegaly]. *Internist* 32(3):154-157.

Hill WM. (1996). Are echoviruses still orphans? *British Journal of Biomedical Sciences* 53(3):221-226.

Hilton A, Fitch M, Deane K. (1998). Evaluation of the fatigue workshops. *Canadian Oncology Nursing Journal* 8(S1):S9-S14.

Hinds G, Bell NP, McMaster D, McCluskey DR. (1994). Normal red cell magnesium concentration and magnesium loading tests in patients with chronic fatigue syndrome. *Annals of Clinical Biochemistry* 31(Pt 5):459-461.

Hinds PS, Hockenberry-Eaton M. (2001). Developing a research program on fatigue in children and adolescents diagnosed with cancer. *Journal of Pediatric Oncology Nursing* 18(2 Suppl 1):3-12.

Hinds PS, Hockenberry-Eaton M, Gilger E, Kline N, Burleson C, Bottomley S, Quargnenti A. (1999). Comparing patient, parent, and staff descriptions of fatigue in pediatric oncology patients. *Cancer Nursing* 22(4):277-288.

Hinds PS, Hockenberry-Eaton M, Quargnenti A, May M, Burleson C, Gilger E, Randall E, Brace-Oneill J. (1999). Fatigue in 7- to 12-year-old patients with cancer from the staff perspective: An exploratory study. *Oncology Nursing Forum* 26(1):37-45.

Hinds PS, Quargnenti AG, Wentz TJ. (1992). Measuring symptom distress in adolescents with cancer. *Journal of Pediatric Oncology Nursing* 9(2):84-86.

Hines JF, Jenson AB, Barnes WA. (1995). Human papilloma viruses: Their clinical significance in the management of cervical carcinoma. *Oncology* 9(4):279-285.

Hinton J. (1994). Which patients with terminal cancer are admitted from home care? *Palliative Medicine* 8(3):197-210.

Hinton J. (1996). Services given and help perceived during home care for terminal cancer. *Palliative Medicine* 10(2):125-134.

Hippo Y, Kawana A, Yoshizawa A, Koshino T, Toyota E, Kobayashi N, Kobori O, Arai T, Kudo K, Kabe J. (1997). [Esophagobronchial fistula and empyema resulting from esophageal carcinoma]. *Nihon Kyobu Shikkan Gakkai Zasshi* 35(5):583-587.

Hirai H, Shimura K, Takahashi R, Kikuta T, Ashihara E, Inada T, Fujita N, Shimazaki C, Akasaka T, Ohno H, Nakagawa M. (1999). [CD5 positive B cell leukemic lymphoma associated with BCL6 rearrangement]. *Rinsho Ketsueki* 40(11):1198-1200.

Hirano T, Matsuda T, Turner M, Miyasaka N, Buchan G, Tang B, Sato K, Shimizu M, Maini R, Feldmann M. (1988). Excessive production of interleukin-6/ B-cell stimulatory factor-2 in rheumatoid arthritis. *European Journal of Immunology* 18:1797-1801.

Hirsch M, Carlander B, Verge M, Tafti M, Anaya J-M, Billiard M, Sany J. (1994). Objective and subjective sleep disturbances in patients with rheumatoid arthritis: A reappraisal. *Arthritis and Rheumatism* 37:41-49.

Hirsch MS, Kaplan JC. (1987). Treatment of human immunodeficiency virus infections. *Antimicrobial Agents and Chemotherapy* 31:839-843.

Hirsh M, Lipton A, Harvey H, Givant E, Hopper K, Jones G, Zeffren J, Levitt D. (1990). Phase I study of interleukin-2 and interferon alfa-2a as outpatient therapy for patients with advanced malignancy. *Journal of Clinical Oncology* 8(10): 1657-1663.

Hishii M, Nitta T, Ishida H, Ebato M, Kurosu A, Yagita A, Sato K, Okumura K. (1995). Human glioma-derived interleukin-10 inhibits antitumor immune responses in vitro. *Neurosurgery* 37:1160-1166.

Hishikawa Y, Shimada T, Miura T, Imajyo Y. (1983). Radiation therapy of carcinoma of the extrahepatic bile ducts. *Radiology* 146(3):787-789.

Hjermstad MJ, Evensen SA, Kvaloy SO, Fayers PM, Kaasa S. (1999). Health-related quality of life 1 year after allogeneic or autologous stem-cell transplantation: A prospective study. *Journal of Clinical Oncology* 17(2):706-718.

Hjermstad MJ, Fossa SD, Bjordal K, Kaasa S. (1995). Test/retest study of the European Organization for Research and Treatment of Cancer Core Quality-of-Life Questionnaire. *Journal of Clinical Oncology* 13(5):1249-1254.

Hjermstad MJ, Loge JH, Evensen SA, Kvaloy SO, Fayers PM, Kaasa S. (1999). The course of anxiety and depression during the first year after allogeneic or autologous stem cell transplantation. *Bone Marrow Transplantation* 24(11):1219-1228.

Hocepied AM, Falkson CI, Falkson G. (1996). A phase II trial of fludarabine in patients with previously treated chronic lymphocytic leukaemia. *South African Medical Journal* 86(5):549-550.

Hockenberry-Eaton M, Hinds PS. (2000). Fatigue in children and adolescents with cancer: Evolution of a program of study. *Seminars in Oncology Nursing* 16(4): 261-272.

Hockenberry-Eaton M, Hinds PS, Alcoser P, O'Neill JB, Euell K, Howard V, Gattuso J, Taylor J. (1998). Fatigue in children and adolescents with cancer. *Journal of Pediatric Oncology Nursing* 15(3):172-182.

Hoffman K, Holmes FA, Fraschini G, Esparza L, Frye D, Raber MN, Newman RA, Hortobagyi GN. (1996). Phase I-II study: Triciribine (tricyclic nucleoside phosphate) for metastatic breast cancer. *Cancer Chemotherapy Pharmacology* 37(3): 254-258.

Hoffman-Goetz L. (1994). Exercise, natural immunity, and tumor metastasis. *Medical Science, Sports, and Exercise* 26:157-163.

Hoffman-Goetz L, Husted J. (1994). Exercise and breast cancer: Review and critical analysis of the literature. *Canadian Journal of Applied Physiology* 19:237-252.

Hoffmann A, Linder R, Kroger B, Schnabel A, Kruger GR. (1996). Fibromyalgia syndrome and chronic fatigue syndrome: Similarities and differences. *Deutsche Medizin Wochenschrift* 121(38):1165-1168.

Hofstra LS, Bos AM, de Vries EG, van der Zee AG, Beijnen JH, Rosing H, Mulder NH, Aalders JG, Willemse PH. (2001). A phase I and pharmacokinetic study of intraperitoneal topotecan. *British Journal of Cancer* 85(11):1627-1633.

Hogan CM. (1998). The nurse's role in diarrhea management. *Oncology Nursing Forum* 25(5):879-886.

Holland JC. (2002). History of psycho-oncology: Overcoming attitudinal and conceptual barriers. *Psychosomatic Medicine* 64(2):206-221.

Holland JC, Korzun AH, Tross S, Silberfarb P, Perry M, Comis R, Oster M. (1986). Comparative psychological disturbance in patients with pancreatic and gastric cancer. *American Journal of Psychiatry* 143(8):982-986.

Holland JM. (1973). Proceedings: Cancer of the kidney—natural history and staging. *Cancer* 32(5):1030-1042.

Holland NW, Gonzalez EB. (1998). Soft tissue problems in older adults. *Clinical Geriatric Medicine* 14(3):601-611.

Holland P. (1997). Coniunctio—in bodily and psychic modes: Dissociation, devitalization and integration in a case of chronic fatigue syndrome. *Journal of Analytical Psychology* 42(2):217-236.

Holland SM. (1996). Host defense against nontuberculous mycobacterial infections. *Seminars in Respiratory Infections* 11:217-230.

Hollen PJ, Gralla RJ, Kris MG, Cox C. (1994). Quality of life during clinical trials: Conceptual model for the Lung Cancer Symptom Scale (LCSS). *Support Care and Cancer* 2(4):213-222.

Hollerbach S, Holstege A, Muscholl M, Mohr V, Ruschoff J, Geissler A, Scholmerich J. (1995). [Masked course of Whipple disease with uveitis, infection, endocardial involvement and abdominal lymphomas—Case report and review of the literature]. *Zeitschrift Gastroenterologie* 33(6):362-367.

Holley S. (2000a). Cancer-related fatigue: Suffering a different fatigue. *Cancer Practice* 8(2):87-95.

Holley S. (2000b). Evaluating patient distress from cancer-related fatigue: An instrument development study. *Oncology Nursing Forum* 27(9):1425-1431.

Holley S. (2002c). A look at the problem of falls among people with cancer. *Clinical Journal of Oncology Nursing* 6(4):193-197.

Holley S, Borger D. (2001). Energy for living with cancer: Preliminary findings of a cancer rehabilitation group intervention study. *Oncology Nursing Forum* 28(9):1393-1396.

Holmes GP, Kaplan JE, Gantz NM, Komaroff AL, Schonberger LB, Straus SS, Jones JF, Dubois RE, Cunningham-Rundles C, Pahwa S, et al. (1988). Chronic fatigue syndrome: A working case definition. *Annals of Internal Medicine* 108:387-389.

Holmes MD, Willett WC. (1995). Can breast cancer be prevented by dietary and lifestyle changes? *Annals of Medicine* 27:429-430.

Holmes MJ, Diack DS, Easingwood A, Cross JP, Carlisle B. (1997). Electron microscope immunocytological profiles in chronic fatigue syndrome. *Journal of Psychiatric Research* 31(1):115-122.

Holoweiko M. (1996). Holding the line on elusive ailments. *Business Health* 14(12):30-32, 35-37.

Holtedahl R. (1999). [Spinal diseases and other musculoskeletal problems—Too much of examination and treatment?] Rygglidelser og andre muskel-og skjett-lidelser—for mye utredning og behandling? *Tidsskr Nor Laegeforen* 119(20): 3042.

Holzner B, Kemmler G, Greil R, Kopp M, Zeimet A, Raderer M, Hejna M, Zochbauer S, Krajnik G, Huber H, et al. (2002). The impact of hemoglobin levels on fatigue and quality of life in cancer patients. *Annals of Oncology* 13(6): 965-973.

Homesley HD, Hall DJ, Martin DA, Lewandowski GS, Vaccarello L, Nahhas WA, Suggs CL, Penley RG. (2001). A dose-escalating study of weekly bolus topotecan in previously treated ovarian cancer patients. *Gynecological Oncology* 83(2):394-399.

Homsi J, Nelson KA, Sarhill N, Rybicki L, LeGrand SB, Davis MP, Walsh D. (2001). A phase II study of methylphenidate for depression in advanced cancer. *American Journal of Hospital Palliative Care* 8(6):403-407.

Homsi J, Walsh D, Nelson KA, LeGrand S, Davis M. (2000). Methylphenidate for depression in hospice practice: A case series. *American Journal of Hospital Palliative Care* 17(6):393-398.

Honkoop AH, Hoekman K, Wagstaff J, Boven E, van Groeningen CJ, Giaccone G, Vermorken JB, Pinedo HM. (1996). Dose-intensive chemotherapy with doxorubicin, cyclophosphamide and GM-CSF fails to improve survival of metastatic breast cancer patients. *Annals of Oncology* 7(1):35-39.

Hood MA, Finley RS. (1991). Fludarabine: A review. *DICP* 25(5):518-524.

Hoogendoorn M, den Ottolander GJ, Hogewind BL, Kluin PM, Bieger R. (1997). A 75-year-old woman with fatigue, monocytosis, and hypothyroidism. *Annals of Hematology* 75(4):173-177.

Hopwood P, Stephens RJ. (2000). Depression in patients with lung cancer: Prevalence and risk factors derived from quality-of-life data. *Journal of Clinical Oncology* 18(4):893-903.

Horne JA, Shackeel BS. (1991). Alpha-like EEG activity in non-REM sleep and the fibromyalgia (fibrositis) syndrome. *Electroencephalographic and Clinical Neurophysiology* 79:271-276.

Horning SJ, Levine JF, Meyer M, Merigan TC, Rosenberg SA. (1983). Phase I study of human leukocyte interferon in patients with advanced cancer. *Journal of Biological Response Modifiers* 2(1):47-56.

Horning SJ, Levine JF, Miller RA, Rosenberg SA, Merigan TC. (1982). Clinical and immunologic effects of recombinant leukocyte A interferon in eight patients with advanced cancer. *JAMA* 247(12):1718-1722.

Horning SJ, Merigan TC, Krown SE, Gutterman JU, Louie A, Gallagher J, McCravey J, Abramson J, Cabanillas F, Oettgen H, et al. (1985). Human interferon alpha in malignant lymphoma and Hodgkin's disease: Results of the American Cancer Society trial. *Cancer* 56(6):1305-1310.

Horny HP, Inniger R, Kaiserling E, Busch FW. (1988). Hemophagocytic syndrome: Differential diagnostic aspects in a case of well-differentiated malignant histiocytosis. *Pathology Research and Practice* 183(1):80-87.

Horti J, Figg WD, Weinberger B, Kohler D, Sartor O. (1988). A phase II study of bromocriptine in patients with androgen-independent prostate cancer. *Oncology Reports* 5(4):893-896.

Hortobagyi GN, Hersh EM, Papadopoulos NE, Frye D, Rios A, Reuben JM, Plager C, Rosenblum M, Quesada J. (1986). Initial clinical studies with copovithane. *Journal of Biological Response Modifiers* 5(4):319-329.

Hosaka T, Tokuda Y, Aoki T, Kojoh Y. (1995). Coping styles among Japanese women with breast cancer. *Tokai Journal of Experimental and Clinical Medicine* 20(2):137-141.

Hoskins CN. (1997). Breast cancer treatment-related patterns in side effects, psychological distress, and perceived health status. *Oncology Nursing Forum* 24(9): 1575-1583.

Hossain MS, Takimoto H, Hamano S, Yoshida H, Ninomiya T, Minamishima Y, Kimura G, Nomoto K. (1999). Protective effects of Hocchu-ekki-to, a Chinese herbal medicine against murine cytomegalovirus infection. *Immunopharmacology* 41(3):169-181.

Houde SC, Kampfe-Leacher R. (1997). Chronic fatigue syndrome: An update for clinicians in primary care. *Nurse Practitioner* 22(7):30, 35-36, 39-40.

Hovgaard DJ, Nissen NI. (1992). Effect of recombinant human granulocyte-macrophage colony-stimulating factor in patients with Hodgkin's disease: A phase I/II study. *Journal of Clinical Oncology* 10(3):390-397.

Hovstadius P, Larsson R, Jonsson E, Skov T, Kissmeyer AM, Krasilnikoff K, Bergh J, Karlsson MO, Lonnebo A, Ahlgren J. (2000). A Phase I study of CHS 828 in patients with solid tumor malignancy. *Clinical Cancer Research* 8(9):2843-2850.

Howell D. (1998). A program to develop research and education in cancer-related fatigue. *Canadian Oncology Nursing Journal* 8(S1):S1-S2.

Howell SJ, Radford JA, Smets EM, Shalet SM. (2000). Fatigue, sexual function and mood following treatment for haematological malignancy: The impact of mild Leydig cell dysfunction. *British Journal of Cancer* 82(4):789-793.

Ho-Yen DO, Carrington D, Armstrong AA. (1988). Myalgic encephalomyelitis and alpha-interferon. *Lancet* 1:125.

Huang JJ, Yeo CJ, Sohn TA, Lillemoe KD, Sauter PK, Coleman J, Hruban RH, Cameron JL. (2000). Quality of life and outcomes after pancreaticoduodenectomy. *Annals of Surgery* 231(6):890-898.

Huang M, Wang J, Lee P, Shama S, Mao JT, Maissner H, Uyemura K, Modlin R, Wollman J, Dubinett SM. (1995). Human nonsmall cell lung cancer cells express a type 2 cytokine pattern. *Cancer Research* 55:3847-3853.

Huang ME, Wartella J, Kreutzer J, Broaddus W, Lyckholm L. (2001). Functional outcomes and quality of life in patients with brain tumours: A review of the literature. *Brain Injury* 15(10):843-856.

Huang S, Hendricks W, Althage A, Hemm S, Bluethmann H, Kamijo R, Vilcek J, Zinkernagel RM, Aguet M. (1993). Immune response in mice that lack the interferon-gamma receptor. *Science* 259:1742-1745.

Huberman M, Bering H, Fallon B, Tessitore J, Sonnenborn H, Paul S, Zeffren J, Levitt D, Groopman J. (1991). A phase I study of an outpatient regimen of recombinant human interleukin-2 and alpha-2a-interferon in patients with solid tumors. *Cancer* 68(8):1708-1713.

Hudes G, Haas N, Yeslow G, Gillon T, Gunnarsson PO, Ellman M, Nordle O, Eriksson B, Miller L, Cisar L, Kopreski M, Viaro D, Hartley-Asp B. (2002). Phase I clinical and pharmacologic trial of intravenous estramustine phosphate. *Journal of Clinical Oncology* 20(4):1115-1127.

Hudes GR, LaCreta F, DeLap RJ, Grillo-Lopez AJ, Catalano R, Comis RL. (1989). Phase I clinical and pharmacologic trial of trimetrexate in combination with 5-fluorouracil. *Cancer Chemotherapy Pharmacology* 24(2):117-122.

Hudes GR, Lipsitz S, Grem J, Morrisey M, Weiner L, Kugler JW, Benson A III. (1999). A phase II study of 5-fluorouracil, leucovorin, and interferon-alpha in the treatment of patients with metastatic or recurrent gastric carcinoma: An Eastern Cooperative Oncology Group study (E5292). *Cancer* 85(2):290-294.

Hudes GR, Nathan FE, Khater C, Greenberg R, Gomella L, Stern C, McAleer C. (1995). Paclitaxel plus estramustine in metastatic hormone-refractory prostate cancer. *Seminars in Oncology* 22(5 Suppl 12):41-45.

Hudes GR, Nathan F, Khater C, Haas N, Cornfield M, Giantonio B, Greenberg R, Gomella L, Litwin S, Ross E, Roethke S, McAleer C. (1997). Phase II trial of 96-hour paclitaxel plus oral estramustine phosphate in metastatic hormone-refractory prostate cancer. *Journal of Clinical Oncology* 15(9):3156-3163.

Hudes GR, Szarka CE, Adams A, Ranganathan S, McCauley RA, Weiner LM, Langer CJ, Litwin S, Yeslow G, Halberr T, et al. (2000). Phase I pharmacokinetic trial of perillyl alcohol (NSC 641066) in patients with refractory solid malignancies. *Clinical Cancer Research* 6(8):3071-3080.

Hudson AJ. (1998). The fibromyalgia problem. *Journal of Rheumatology* 25(5): 1025-1026, discussion 1028-1030.

Hudson JI, Pope HG Jr. (1996). The relationship between fibromyalgia and major depressive disorder. *Rheumatic Diseases Clinics of North America* 22(2):285-303.

Huizing MT, van Warmerdam LJ, Rosing H, Schaefers MC, Lai A, Helmerhorst TJ, Veenhof CH, Birkhofer MJ, Rodenhuis S, Beijnen JH, et al. (1997). Phase I and pharmacologic study of the combination paclitaxel and carboplatin as first-line chemotherapy in stage III and IV ovarian cancer. *Journal of Clinical Oncology* 15(5):1953-1964.

Hume M. (1997). Chronic fatigue syndrome in children: All studies must be subjected to rigorous scrutiny. *British Medical Journal* 315(7113):949.

Humerickhouse RA, Dolan ME, Haraf DJ, Brockstein B, Stenson K, Kies M, Sulzen L, Ratain MJ, Vokes EE. (1999). Phase I study of eniluracil, a dihydropyrimidine dehydrogenase inactivator, and oral 5-fluorouracil with radiation therapy in patients with recurrent or advanced head and neck cancer. *Clinical Cancer Research* 5(2):291-298.

Hunt S, Starkebaum G, Thompson CE. (1998). The fibromyalgia problem. *Journal of Rheumatology* 25(5):1023-1024, discussion 1028-1030.

Huntrakoon M, Callaway LA, Vergara GG. (1987). Systemic rhabdomyosarcoma presenting as leukemia: Case report with ultrastructural study and reviews. *Journal of Surgical Oncology* 35(4):259-265.

Hurd DD. (1983). The chronic leukemias: Clinical picture, diagnosis, and management. *Postgraduate Medicine* 73(5):217-219, 222-227, 231.

Hurlbut JA, Carr JR, Singleton ER, Faul KC, Madson MR, Storey JM, Thomas TL. (1998). Solid-phase extraction cleanup and liquid chromatography with ultraviolet detection of ephedrine alkaloids in herbal products. *Journal of AOAC International* 81(6):1121-1127.

Hurny C, Bernhard J, Joss R, Schatzmann E, Cavalli F, Brunner K, Alberto P, Senn HJ, Metzger U. (1993). "Fatigue and malaise" as a quality-of-life indicator in small-cell lung cancer patients. The Swiss Group for Clinical Cancer Research (SAKK). *Support Care and Cancer* 1(6):316-320.

Hurwitz MM. (1970). Medical mistakes: Misdiagnosis of nervous fatigue. *Geriatrics* 25(2):57 passim.

Hutter JA, Salman M, Stavinoha WB, Satsangi N, Williams RF, Streeper RT, Weintraub ST. (1996). Anti-inflammatory C-glucosyl chromone from *Aloë barbadensis*. *Journal of Natural Products* 59(5):541-543.

Huxtable RJ. (1998). Safety of botanicals: Historical perspective. *Proceedings of the Western Pharmacology Society* 41:1-10.

Huyser BA, Parker JC, Thoreson R, Smarr KL, Johnson JC, Hoffman R. (1998). Predictors of subjective fatigue among individuals with rheumatoid arthritis. *Arthritis and Rheumatism* 41(12):2230-2237.

Hwang SS, Chang VT, Cogswell J, Kasimis BS. (2002). Clinical relevance of fatigue levels in cancer patients at a Veterans Administration medical center. *Cancer* 94(9):2481-2489.

Hyams KC. (1998). Lessons derived from evaluating Gulf War syndrome: Suggested guidelines for investigating outbreaks of new diseases. *Psychosomatic Medicine* 60(2):137-139.

Hyde BM. (1992a). Myalgic encephalomyelitis (chronic fatigue syndrome): An historical perspective. In *The Clinical and Scientific Basis of Myalgic Encephalomyelitis/Chronic Fatigue Syndrome,* Hyde BM, Goldstein J, Levine P, eds. Ottawa: Nightingale Research Foundation, pp. 1ff.

Hyde BM. (1992b). The 1934 Los Angeles County Hospital epidemic. In *The Clinical and Scientific Basis of Myalgic Encephalomyelitis/Chronic Fatigue Syndrome,* Hyde BM, Goldstein J, Levine P, eds. Ottawa: Nightingale Research Foundation, pp. 1ff.

Hyyppa MT, Kronholm E. (1995). Nocturnal motor activity in fibromyalgia patients with poor sleep quality. *Journal of Psychosomatic Research* 39:85-91.

Iaffaioli RV, Frasci G, Facchini G, Pagliarulo C, Pacelli R, Scala S, Espinosa A, Bianco AR. (1991). Alpha 2b interferon (IFN) by intraperitoneal administration via temporary catheter in ovarian cancer: Preliminary data. *European Journal of Gynaecological Oncology* 12(1):69-75.

Ibrahim NK, Buzdar AU, Valero V, Dhingra K, Willey J, Hortobagyi GN. (2001). Phase I study of vinorelbine and paclitaxel by 3-hour simultaneous infusion with and without granulocyte colony-stimulating factor support in metastatic breast carcinoma. *Cancer* 91(4):664-671.

Ibrahim NK, Rahman Z, Valero V, Murray JL III, Frye D, Hortobagyi GN. (2002). Phase I study of vinorelbine and docetaxel with granulocyte colony-stimulating factor support in the treatment of metastatic breast cancer. *Cancer Investigation* 20(1):29-37.

Ibrahim NK, Rahman Z, Valero V, Willey J, Theriault RL, Buzdar AU, Murray JL III, Bast R, Hortobagyi GN. (1999). Phase II study of vinorelbine administered by 96-hour infusion in patients with advanced breast carcinoma. *Cancer* 86(7): 1251-1257.

Ibrahim NK, Valero V, Theriault RL, Willey J, Walters RS, Buzdar AU, Booser DJ, Hortobagyi GN. (2000). Phase I study of vinorelbine by 96-hour infusion in advanced metastatic breast cancer. *American Journal of Clinical Oncology* 23(2): 117-121.

Ichiba Y, Nishizaki Y, Tanizaki M. (1992). Cushing's syndrome due to primary pigmented nodular adrenocortical disease with cardiac myxomas and mucocutaneous lentigines. *Acta Paediatrica* 81(1):91-92.

Ichihara A, Mori K. (1969). [Case of multiple myeloma]. *Iryo* 23(6):816-819.

Ichimaru M, Kamihira S, Moriuchi Y, Kuraishi Y, Usui N, Toki H, Okabe K, Niho Y, Shibuya T, Umei T, et al. (1988). [Clinical study on the effect of natural alpha-interferon (HLBI) in the treatment of adult T-cell leukemia]. *Gan To Kagaku Ryoho* 15(10):2975-2981.

Iida H, Yanagida Y, Sasano S, Tahara S, Kei J, Nitta S. (1994). [A case report of primary fibrosarcoma originated in the heart invading adjacent organs]. *Nippon Kyobu Geka Gakkai Zasshi* 42(10):1967-1971.

Iida S, Takeuchi G, Komatsu H, Banno S, Wakita A, Nitta M, Takada K, Mitomo Y, Yamamoto M, Masuoka H, et al. (1991). [Blastic form of acute erythremia: Report of an autopsy case]. *Rinsho Ketsueki* 32(11):1486-1491.

Ikeda M, Noda K, Hiura M, Tamaya T, Ozaki M, Hatae M, Ozawa M, Yamabe T, Tanaka K, Izumi R, et al. (1998). [Late phase II trial of oral etoposide administered for 21 consecutive days in patients with cervical cancer. ETP 21 Study Group—Cervical Cancer Group]. *Gan To Kagaku Ryoho* 25(14):2249-2257.

Ikeda M, Okada S, Tokuuye K, Ueno H, Okusaka T. (2002). A phase I trial of weekly gemcitabine and concurrent radiotherapy in patients with locally advanced pancreatic cancer. *British Journal of Cancer* 86(10):1551-1554.

Ikemoto S, Nakatani T, Sugimura K, Tanaka H, Maekawa M. (1990). Multiple pulmonary metastases from renal cell carcinoma treated effectively by recombinant interleukin-2. *Urology International* 45(1):54-57.

Ikenaga M, Tsuneto S. (2000). [Hospice and palliative care in the outpatient department]. *Gan To Kagaku Ryoho* 27(11):1674-1679.

Ilson DH, Forastiere A, Arquette M, Costa F, Heelan R, Huang Y, Kelsen DP. (2000). A phase II trial of paclitaxel and cisplatin in patients with advanced carcinoma of the esophagus. *Cancer Journal* 6(5):316-323.

Ilson DH, Sirott M, Saltz L, Heelan R, Huang Y, Keresztes R, Kelsen DP. (1995). A phase II trial of interferon alpha-2A, 5-fluorouracil, and cisplatin in patients with advanced esophageal carcinoma. *Cancer* 75(9):2197-2202.

Ilyin SE, Plata-Salaman CR. (1996a). An approach to study molecular mechanisms involved in cytokine-induced anorexia. *Journal of Neurosciences Methods* 70 (1):33-38.

Ilyin SE, Plata-Salaman CR. (1996b). Molecular regulation of the brain interleukin-1 beta system in obese (fa/fa) and lean (Fa/Fa) Zucker rats. *Brain Research and Molecular Brain Research* 43(1-2):209-218.

Im EO, Lee EO, Park YS. (2002). Korean women's breast cancer experience. *West Journal of Nursing Research* 24(7):751-765; discussion 766-771.

Imai S, Kiyozuka Y, Tsubura Y, Yamamoto H, Morohoshi T, Fujimoto M, Tsujii T. (1986). Pancreatic carcinoma in childhood. *Acta Pathologica Japonica* 36(2): 279-284.

Imai S, Sekigawa S, Ohno Y, Yamamoto H, Tsubura Y. (1981). Giant cell carcinoma of the pancreas. *Acta Pathologica Japonica* 31(1):129-133.

Imai S, Sekigawa S, Yamamoto H, Tsubura Y, Miyanaga M, Narita N, Mikami R. (1982). Bronchiolo-alveolar adenocarcinoma with multiple cysts. *Acta Pathologica Japonica* 32(4):677-682.

Imai T, Yokoi H, Noguchi T, Kawarada Y, Mizumoto R. (1991). Fibrolamellar carcinoma of the liver—A case report. *Gastroenterology Japan* 26(3):382-389.

Inaba T, Shimazaki C, Yoneyama S, Hirai H, Kikuta T, Sumikuma T, Sudo Y, Yamagata N, Ashihara E, Goto H, et al. (1996). t(7;11) and trilineage myelodysplasia in acute myelomonocytic leukemia. *Cancer Genetics and Cytogenetics* 86(1):72-75.

Inuyama Y, Kataura A, Togawa K, Saijo S, Satake B, Takeoda S, Konno A, Ebihara S, Sasaki Y, Kida A, et al. (1999). [Late phase II clinical study of RP56976 (docetaxel) in patients with advanced/recurrent head and neck cancer]. *Gan To Kagaku Ryoho* 26(1):107-116.

Invernizzi F, Monti G, Caviglia AG, Meroni P, Zanussi C. (1991). A new case of IgE myeloma. *Acta Haematologica* 85(1):41-44.

Ionnides CG, Fisk B, Fan D, Biddison WE, Wharton JT, O'Brian CA. (1993). Cytotoxic T cells isolated from ovarian malignant ascites recognize a peptide derived from the Her-2/neu proto-oncogene. *Cellular Immunology* 151:225-234.

Iowa Persian Gulf Study Group. (1997). Self-reported illness and health status among Gulf War veterans: A population-based study. *JAMA* 277(3):238-245.

Iriarte J, Carreno M, De Castro P. (1996). Fatigue and functional system involvement in multiple sclerosis. *Neurología* 11(6):210-215.

Irie M, Asami S, Nagata S, Ikeda M, Miyata M, Kasai H. (2001). Psychosocial factors as a potential trigger of oxidative DNA damage in human leukocytes. *Japanese Journal of Cancer Research* 92(3):367-376.

Irie M, Asami S, Nagata S, Miyata M, Kasai H. (2001). Relationships between perceived workload, stress and oxidative DNA damage. *International Archives of Occupational and Environmental Health* 74(2):153-157.

Irle E, Peper M, Wowra B, Kunze S. (1994). Mood changes after surgery for tumors of the cerebral cortex. *Archives of Neurology* 51(2):164-174.

Ironson G, Field T, Scafidi F, Hashimoto M, Kumar M, Kumar A, Patarca R, Fletcher MA, Price A, Goncalves A, et al. (1996). Massage therapy is associated with enhancement of the immune system's cytotoxic capacity. *International Journal of Neuroscience* 84:205-217.

Irvine DM, Vincent L, Bubela N, Thompson L, Graydon J. (1991). A critical appraisal of the research literature investigating fatigue in the individual with cancer. *Cancer Nursing* 14(4):188-199.

Irvine DM, Vincent L, Graydon JE, Bubela N. (1998). Fatigue in women with breast cancer receiving radiation therapy. *Cancer Nursing* 21(2):127-135.

Irvine DM, Vincent L, Graydon JE, Bubela N, Thompson L. (1994). The prevalence and correlates of fatigue in patients receiving treatment with chemotherapy and radiotherapy: A comparison with the fatigue experienced by healthy individuals. *Cancer Nursing* 17(5):367-378.

Irwin ML, Yasui Y, Ulrich CM, Bowen D, Rudolph RE, Schwartz RS, Yukawa M, Aiello E, Potter JD, McTiernan A. (2002). Effect of exercise on total and intra-abdominal body fat in postmenopausal women: A randomized controlled study. *JAMA* 289(3):323-330.

Isaka S, Shimazaki J, Akaza H, Usami M, Kotake T, Kanetake H, Naito S, Hirao Y, Honma Y, Ohashi Y. (1993). [Assessment of the quality of life of prostate cancer patients]. *Nippon Hinyokika Gakkai Zasshi* 84(9):1611-1617.

Ishihara Y, Nukariya N, Kobayashi K, Yoneda S, Matsuda T, Yakushiji M, Yamakido M, Fukuoka M, Niitani H, Furue H. (1996). [The development of a new QOL questionnaire on chemotherapy-induced emesis and vomiting—Investigation of reliability and validity. Group for Investigation of QOL Questionnaire for Anti-Emetics Used in Cancer Chemotherapy. Joint Research Group for Tropisetron Double-Blind Comparative study]. *Gan To Kagaku Ryoho* 23(6):745-755.

Ishihara Y, Sakai H, Nukariya N, Kobayashi K, Yoneda S, Matsuoka R, Hojo N, Nishiwaki Y, Hoshi A, Kuratomi Y, et al. (1995a). [Development of quality of life (QOL) questionnaire for use of lung cancer patients in palliative therapy—Study of validity and reliability. No.1]. *Gan To Kagaku Ryoho* 22(7):895-902.

Ishihara Y, Sakai H, Nukariya N, Kobayashi K, Yoneda S, Matsuoka R, Hojo N, Nishiwaki Y, Hoshi A, Kuratomi Y, et al. (1995b). [Development of quality of life (QOL) questionnaire for use of lung cancer patients in palliative therapy—Study of validity and reliability no. 2, the effects of chemotherapeutics in QOL]. *Gan To Kagaku Ryoho* 22(8):1087-1093.

Ishii E, Hara T, Mizuno Y, Ueda K. (1988). Vincristine-induced fever in children with leukemia and lymphoma. *Cancer* 61(4):660-662.

Ishii E, Matsuzaki A, Ohnishi Y, Kai T, Ueda K. (1996). Successful treatment with ranimustine and carboplatin for recurrent intraocular retinoblastoma with vitreous seeding. *American Journal of Clinical Oncology* 19(6):562-565.

Ishii Y, Takino Y, Toyo'oka T, Tanizawa H. (1998). Studies of aloe: VI. Cathartic effect of isobarbaloin. *Biological and Pharmaceutical Bulletin* 21(11):1226-1227.

Ishikawa K, Horiba M, Suzuki K, Ishikawa H, Akasaka Y. (1995). [Two case reports of retroperitoneal leiomyosarcoma]. *Hinyokika Kiyo* 41(8):603-607.

Ishikawa S, Takei Y, Tokunaga S, Motomura M, Nakao Y, Hanyu N. (2000). [Response to immunoadsorption and steroid therapies in a patient with carcinomatous Lambert-Eaton myasthenia syndrome accompanied by disturbed consciousness]. *Rinsho Shinkeigaku* 40(5):459-463.

Ishikawa T, Shimizu Y, Kimura E, Takanashi S, Nishizawa K, Kaneko K. (1997). [A case of right ventricular myxoma]. *Nippon Kyobu Geka Gakkai Zasshi* 45(4):645-648.

Israel VK, Jiang C, Muggia FM, Tulpule A, Jeffers S, Leichman L, Morrow CP, Roman L, Leichman CG, Chan KK. (1995). Intraperitoneal 5-fluoro-2'-deoxyuridine (FUDR) and (S)-leucovorin for disease predominantly confined to the peritoneal cavity: A pharmacokinetic and toxicity study. *Cancer Chemotherapy Pharmacology* 37(1-2):32-38.

Itoh Y, Hamada H, Imai T, Saki T, Igarashi T, Yuge K, Fukunaga Y, Yamamoto M. (1997). Antinuclear antibodies in children with chronic nonspecific complaints. *Autoimmunity* 25(4):243-250.

Itri LM. (2002). Managing cancer-related anaemia with epoetin alfa. *Nephrology, Dialysis and Transplantation* 17(Suppl 1):73-77.

Iwagaki H, Hizuta A, Tanaka N, Orita K. (1995). Decreased serum tryptophan in patients with cancer cachexia correlated with increased serum neopterin. *Immunological Investigations* 24(3):467-478.

Iyengar S, Levine PH, Ablashi D, Neequaye J, Pearson GR. (1991). Sero-epidemiological investigations on human herpesvirus 6 (HHV-6) infections using a newly developed early antigen assay. *International Journal of Cancer* 49(4):551-557.

Izban KF, Pooley RJ Jr, Selvaggi SM, Alkan S. (2001). Cytologic diagnosis of peripheral T-cell lymphoma manifesting as ascites: A case report. *Acta Cytologica* 45(3):385-392.

Izzat MB, Yim AP, El-Zufari MH. (1998). A taste of Chinese medicine! *Annals of Thoracic Surgery* 66(3):941-942.

Izzo AA, Sautebin L, Borrelli F, Longo R, Capasso F. (1999). The role of nitric oxide in aloe-induced diarrhea in the rat. *European Journal of Pharmacology* 368(1):43-48.

Jackson RA, Haynes BF, Burch WM, Shimizu K, Bowring MA, Eisenbarth GS. (1984). Ia+ T cells in new onset Grave's disease. *Journal of Clinical Endocrinology and Metabolism* 59:187-190.

Jacobs A, Gold P, Weiden P, Aboulafia D, Rudolph R, Picozzi V, Thompson J. (2000). Interferon alpha-2a and 13-cis-retinoic acid in patients with metastatic renal cell cancer. *Cancer Investigation* 18(5):417-421.

Jacobs G. (1997). Chronic fatigue syndrome in children: Patients organizations are denied a voice. *British Medical Journal* 315(7113):949.

Jacobsen PB, Hann DM, Azzarello LM, Horton J, Balducci L, Lyman GH. (1999). Fatigue in women receiving adjuvant chemotherapy for breast cancer: Characteristics, course, and correlates. *Journal of Pain Symptomatology and Management* 18(4):233-242.

Jacobsen PB, Stein K. (1999). Is fatigue a long-term side effect of breast cancer treatment? *Cancer Control* 6(3):256-263.

Jacobsen S. (2000). [Chronic musculoskeletal pain syndromes] Kroniske muskelsmertesyndromer. *Ugeskr Laeger* 162(15):2178-2180.

Jacobson SK, Daly JS, Thorne GM, McIntosh K. (1997). Chronic parvovirus B19 infection resulting in chronic fatigue syndrome: Case history and review. *Clinical Infectious Diseases* 24(6):1048-1051.

Jacobson W, Saich LK, Borysiewicz LK, Behan WMH, Behan PO, Weghitt TG. (1993). Serum folate and chronic fatigue syndrome. *Neurology* 43:2645-2647.

Jadin CL. (1998). The Rickettsial approach of CFS. In *The Clinical and Scientific Basis of CFS,* Roberts TK, ed. Newcastle, Australia: University of Newcastle, pp. 200-213.

Jadin CL. (1999). The Rickettsial approach of CFS. CFS Manly Conference, Manly, Australia, February.

Jadin CL. (2000). Common clinical and biological windows on CFS and Rickettsial diseases. *Journal of Chronic Fatigue Syndrome* 6(3/4):133-145.

Jadin JB. (1953). Origine des maladies Rickettsiennes. *Annales de la Societé Belge de Medécine Tropicale* 3:1-ff.

Jadin JG. (1962). Au sujet des maladies Rickettsiennes. *Annales de la Societé Belge de Medécine Tropicale* 3:321.

Jahn K, Klenke T. (1999). [Web sites on tinnitus, fibromyalgia, chronic fatigue syndrome, etc.: Here your patients seek information] Webseiten uber tinnitus, fibromyalgie, mudigkeitssendrom, etc.: Hier informieren sich Ihre Patienten. *MMW Fortschrift Medizin* 141(51-52):14.

Jakel P. (2002). Patient communication and strategies for managing fatigue. *Oncology* 16(9 Suppl 10):141-145.

Jákó P. (1995). The role of physical activity in the prevention of certain internal diseases. *Orv Hetil* 136:2379-2383.

Jakobsson L, Hallberg IR, Loven L. (1997). Experiences of daily life and life quality in men with prostate cancer: An explorative study, part I. *European Journal of Cancer Care* 6(2):108-116.

Jakubowski AA, Casper ES, Gabrilove JL, Templeton MA, Sherwin SA, Oettgen HF. (1989). Phase I trial of intramuscularly administered tumor necrosis factor in patients with advanced cancer. *Journal of Clinical Oncology* 7(3):298-303.

James LC, Folen RA. (1996). EEG biofeedback as a treatment for chronic fatigue syndrome: A controlled case report. *Behavioral Medicine* 22(2):77-81.

Jamison JR. (1999a). A psychological profile of fibromyalgia patients: A chiropractic case study. *Journal of Manipulative Physiology Therapy* 22(7):454-457.

Jamison JR. (1999b). Stress: The chiropractic patients' self-perceptions. *Journal of Manipulative Physiology Therapy* 22(6):395-398.

Janda M, Gerstner N, Obermair A, Fuerst A, Wachter S, Dieckmann K, Potter R. (2000). Quality of life changes during conformal radiation therapy for prostate carcinoma. *Cancer* 89(6):1322-1328.

Jansen RL, Slingerland R, Goey SH, Franks CR, Bolhuis RL, Stoter G. (1992). Interleukin-2 and interferon-alpha in the treatment of patients with advanced non-small-cell lung cancer. *Journal of Immunotherapy* 12(1):70-73.

Jansen SJ, Stiggelbout AM, Nooij MA, Noordijk EM, Kievit J. (2000). Response shift in quality of life measurement in early-stage breast cancer patients undergoing radiotherapy. *Quality of Life Research* 9(6):603-615.

Janson ET, Kauppinen HL, Oberg K. (1993). Combined alpha- and gamma-interferon therapy for malignant midgut carcinoid tumors: A phase I-II trial. *Acta Oncologica* 32(2):231-233.

Jariwalla RJ, Harakek S. (1992). HIV suppression by ascorbate and its enhancement by glutathione precursor (PO-B-3697). In Abstracts of the Eighth International Conference on AIDS, Volume 2. Amsterdam, the Netherlands, July 19-24, p. B207.

Jason GW, Pajurkova EM, Taenzer PA, Bultz BD. (1997). Acute effects on neuropsychological function and quality of life by high-dose multiple daily fractionated radiotherapy for malignant astrocytomas: Assessing the tolerability of a new radiotherapy regimen. *Psychooncology* 6(2):151-157.

Jason LA, Eisele H, Taylor RR. (2001). Assessing attitudes toward new names for chronic fatigue syndrome. *Evaluation and the Health Professions* 24(4):424-435.

Jason LA, Wagner L, Rosenthal S, Goodlatte J, Lipkin D, Papernik M, Plioplys S, Plioplys V. (1998). Estimating the prevalence of chronic fatigue syndrome among nurses. *American Journal of Medicine* 105(3A):91S-93S.

Jassem J, Krzakowski M, Roszkowski K, Ramlau R, Slominski JM, Szczesna A, Krawczyk K, Mozejko-Pastewka B, Lis J, Miracki K. (2002). A phase II study of gemcitabine plus cisplatin in patients with advanced non-small cell lung cancer: Clinical outcomes and quality of life. *Lung Cancer* 35(1):73-79.

Jay SJ. (2000). Tobacco use and chronic fatigue syndrome, fibromyalgia, and temporomandibular disorder. *Archives of Internal Medicine* 160(15):2398-2401.

Jayson GC, Middleton M, Lee SM, Ashcroft L, Thatcher N. (1998). A randomized phase II trial of interleukin 2 and interleukin 2-interferon alpha in advanced renal cancer. *British Journal of Cancer* 78(3):366-369.

Jeffcoate WJ. (1999). Chronic fatigue syndrome and functional hypoadrenia—Fighting vainly the old ennui. *Lancet* 353(9151):424-425.

Jelkmann W, Wolff M, Fandrey J. (1995). Modulation of the production of erythropoietin by cytokines: In vitro studies and their clinical implications. In *Erythropoietin in the 90s: Contributions in Nephrology*, Volume 87, Shaefer RM, Heidland A, Hörl WH, eds. Basel: Karger, pp. 68-77.

Jencks B. (1977). *Your Body: Biofeedback at Its Best*. Chicago: Nelson-Hall.

Jenkins CA, Schulz M, Hanson J, Bruera E. (2000). Demographic, symptom, and medication profiles of cancer patients seen by a palliative care consult team in a tertiary referral hospital. *Journal of Pain Symptomatology and Management* 19(3):174-184.

Jensen S, Given BA. (1991). Fatigue affecting family caregivers of cancer patients. *Cancer Nursing* 14(4):181-187.

Jereczek-Fossa BA, Marsiglia HR, Orecchia R. (2001). Radiotherapy-related fatigue: How to assess and how to treat the symptom, a commentary. *Tumori* 87(3):147-151.

Jereczek-Fossa BA, Marsiglia HR, Orecchia R. (2002). Radiotherapy-related fatigue. *Critical Reviews in Oncology and Hematology* 41(3):317-325.

Jerome KR, Barnd DL, Bendt KM, Boyer CM, Taylor-Papadimitriou J, McKenzie FC, Bast RC, Finn OJ. (1991). Cytotoxic T lymphocytes derived from patients with breast adenocarcinoma recognize an epitope present on the protein core of a mucin molecule preferentially expressed by malignant cells. *Cancer Research* 51:2908-2916.

Jobst KA. (1999). Herbal medicine legislation and registration and stretching the mind: Mental exercise for health? *Journal of Alternative and Complementary Medicine* 5(2):107-108.

Johansson JE, Wersall P, Brandberg Y, Andersson SO, Nordstrom L, EPO-Study Group. (2001). Efficacy of epoetin beta on hemoglobin, quality of life, and transfusion needs in patients with anemia due to hormone-refractory prostate cancer—A randomized study. *Scandinavian Journal of Urology and Nephrology* 35(4):288-294.

John MR, Wickert H, Zaar K, Jonsson KB, Grauer A, Ruppersberger P, Schmidt-Gayk H, Murer H, Ziegler R, Blind E. (2001). A case of neuroendocrine oncogenic osteomalacia associated with a PHEX and fibroblast growth factor-23 expressing sinusidal malignant schwannoma. *Bone* 29(4):393-402.

John WJ, Neefe JR, Macdonald JS, Cantrell J Jr, Smith M. (1993). 5-fluorouracil and interferon-alpha-2a in advanced colorectal cancer: Results of two treatment schedules. *Cancer* 72(11):3191-3195.

Johnson DH, Paul D, Hande KR. (1997). Paclitaxel, 5-fluorouracil, and folinic acid in metastatic breast cancer: BRE-26, a phase II trial. *Seminars in Oncology* 24 (1 Suppl 3):S22-S25.

Johnson MI, Hoth DF. (1993). Present status and future prospects for HIV therapies. *Science* 260:1286-1293.

Johnson SK, DeLuca J, Diamond BJ, Natelson BH. (1996). Selective impairment of auditory processing in chronic fatigue syndrome: A comparison with multiple sclerosis and healthy controls. *Perceptual and Motor Skills* 83(1):51-62.

Johnson SK, DeLuca J, Natelson BH. (1996a). Depression in fatiguing illness: Comparing patients with chronic fatigue syndrome, multiple sclerosis and depression. *Journal of Affective Disorders* 39(1):21-30.

Johnson SK, DeLuca J, Natelson BH. (1996b). Personality dimensions in the chronic fatigue syndrome: A comparison with multiple sclerosis and depression. *Journal of Psychiatric Research* 30(1):9-20.

Johnson SP. (1997). Fluoxetine and amitriptyline in the treatment of fibromyalgia. *Journal of Family Practice* 44(2):128-130.

Johnston SR, Constenla DO, Moore J, Atkinson H, A'Hern RP, Dadian G, Riches PG, Gore ME. (1998). Randomized phase II trial of BCDT [carmustine (BCNU), cisplatin, dacarbazine (DTIC) and tamoxifen] with or without interferon alpha (IFN-alpha) and interleukin (IL-2) in patients with metastatic melanoma. *British Journal of Cancer* 77(8):1280-1286.

Joly F, Henry-Amar M, Arveux P, Reman O, Tanguy A, Peny AM, Lebailly P, Mace-Lesec'h J, Vie B, Genot JY, et al. (1996). Late psychosocial sequelae in Hodgkin's disease survivors: A French population-based case-control study. *Journal of Clinical Oncology* 14(9):2444-2453.

Jonas WB, Linde K, Ramirez G. (2000). Homeopathy and rheumatic disease. *Rheumatic Diseases Clinics of North America* 26(1):117-123.

Jones DB, Armstrong NW. (1995). Coxsackievirus and diabetes revisited. *Nature Medicine* 1:284.

Jones E, Lund VJ, Howard DJ, Greenberg MP, McCarthy M. (1992). Quality of life of patients treated surgically for head and neck cancer. *Journal of Laryngology and Otolaryngology* 106(3):238-242.

Jones GJ, Itri LM. (1986). Safety and tolerance of recombinant interferon alfa-2a (Roferon-A) in cancer patients. *Cancer* 57(8 Suppl):1709-1715.

Jones J. (1991). Serologic and immunologic responses in chronic fatigue syndrome with emphasis on the Epstein-Barr virus. *Review of Infectious Diseases* 13(1): S26-S31.

Jones JF. (1985). Epstein-Barr virus and unexplained illness. *Annals of Internal Medicine* 102(6):865-866.

Jones JF, Ray G, Minnich LL, Hicks MJ, Kibler R, Lucas DO. (1985). Evidence for active Epstein-Barr virus infection in patients with persistent, unexplained illnesses: Elevated anti-early antigen antibodies. *Annals of Internal Medicine* 102:1-7.

Jones JF, Straus SE. (1987). Chronic Epstein-Barr virus infection. *Annual Review of Medicine* 38:195-209.

Jones RC. (1996). Fibromyalgia: Misdiagnosed, mistreated and misunderstood? *American Family Physician* 53(1):91-92.

Jones SD, Koh WH, Steiner A, Garrett SL, Calin A. (1996). Fatigue in ankylosing spondylitis: Its prevalence and relationship to disease activity, sleep, and other factors. *The Journal of Rheumatology* 23(3):487-490.

Jones TH, Wadler S, Hupart KH. (1998). Endocrine-mediated mechanisms of fatigue during treatment with interferon-alpha. *Seminars in Oncology* 25(1 Suppl 1):54-63.

Jones TK, Lawson BM. (1998). Pofound neonatal congestive heart failure caused by maternal consumption of blue cohosh herbal medication. *Journal of Pediatrics* 132(3 Pt 1):550-552.

Jordan KM, Landis DA, Downey MC, Osterman SL, Thurm AE, Jason LA. (1998). Chronic fatigue syndrome in children and adolescents. *Journal of Adolescent Health* 22(1):4-18.

Josephs SF, Wong-Staal F, Manzari V, Gallo RC, Sodroski JG, Trus M, Perkins D, Patarca R, Haseltine WA. (1984). Long terminal repeat structure of an American isolate of type I human T-cell leukemia virus. *Virology* 139:340-345.

Joss RA, Bacchi M, Hurny C, Bernhard J, Cerny T, Martinelli G, Leyvraz S, Senn HJ, Stahel R, Siegenthaler P, et al. (1995). Early versus late alternating chemotherapy in small-cell lung cancer. Swiss Group for Clinical Cancer Research (SAKK). *Annals of Oncology* 6(2):157-166.

Joyce E, Blumenthal S, Wessely S. (1996). Memory, attention, and executive function in chronic fatigue syndrome. *Journal of Neurology, Neurosurgery and Psychiatry* 60(5):495-503.

Joyce J, Hotopf M, Wessely S. (1997). The prognosis of chronic fatigue and chronic fatigue syndrome: A systematic review. *Quarterly Journal of Medicine* 90(3): 223-233.

Joyce J, Rabe-Hesketh S, Wessely S. (1998). Reviewing the reviews: The example of chronic fatigue syndrome. *JAMA* 280(3):264-266.

Joyce J, Wessely S. (1996). Chronic fatigue syndrome. *Irish Journal of Psychological Medicine* 13(2):46-50.

Juman S, Robinson P, Balkissoon A, Kelly K. (1994). B-cell non-Hodgkin's lymphoma of the paranasal sinuses. *Journal of Laryngology and Otololaryngology* 108(3):263-265.

Jung S, Schluesener HJ. (1991). Human T lymphocytes recognize a peptide of single point-mutated, oncogenic ras proteins. *Journal of Experimental Medicine* 173:273-276.

Kaasa S, Aass N, Mastekaasa A, Lund E, Fossa SD. (1991). Psychosocial well-being in testicular cancer patients. *European Journal of Cancer* 27(9):1091-1095.

Kaasa S, Knobel H, Loge JH, Hjermstad MJ. (1998). Hodgkin's disease: Quality of life in future trials. *Annals of Oncology* 9(Suppl 5):137-145.

Kaasa S, Loge JH, Knobel H, Jordhoy MS, Brenne E. (1999). Fatigue: Measures and relation to pain. *Acta Anaesthesiologica Scandinavica* 43(9):939-947.

Kadar L, Areberg J, Landberg T, Albertsson M, Mattson S. (1998). Body protein as a prognostic instrument for cancer patients? *Applied Radiation Isotherapy* 49 (5-6):639-641.

Kaden M, Bubenzer RH. (1999). [License fee for fibromyalgia? Illness with trademark protection] Lizenzgebuhr fur fibromyalgie? Krankheit mit markenschutz. *MMW Fortschrift Medizin* 141(46):60.

Kaegi E. (1998). Unconventional therapies for cancer: 1. Essiac. The Task Force on Alternative Therapies of the Canadian Breast Cancer Research Initiative. *Canadian Medical Association Journal* 158(7):897-902.

Kakolyris S, Kouroussis C, Kalbakis K, Mavroudis D, Souglakos J, Vardakis N, Kremos S, Georgoulias V. (2000). Salvage treatment of advanced non-small-cell lung cancer previously treated with docetaxel-based front-line chemotherapy with irinotecan (CPT-11) in combination with cisplatin. *Annals of Oncology* 11(6):757-760.

Kakolyris S, Kouroussis C, Souglakos J, Agelaki S, Kalbakis K, Vardakis N, Vamvakas L, Georgoulias V. (2001). Cisplatin and irinotecan (CPT-11) as second-line treatment in patients with advanced non-small cell lung cancer. *Lung Cancer* 34(Suppl 4):S71-S76.

Kakolyris S, Kouroussis C, Souglakos J, Mavroudis D, Agelaki S, Kalbakis K, Androulakis N, Vardakis N, Vamvakas L, Georgoulias V. (2001). A phase I clinical trial of topotecan given every 2 weeks in patients with refractory solid tumors. *Oncology* 61(4):265-270.

Kalebic T, Kinter A, Poli G, Anderson ME, Meister A, Fauci AS (1991). Suppression of human immunodeficiency virus expression in chronically infected monocytic cells by glutathione, glutathione ester and N-acetylcysteine. *Proceedings of the National Academy of Sciences of the United States of America* 88(3):986-990.

Kalia M. (1973). Effects of certain cerebral lesions on the J reflex. *Pflügers Archives* 343:297-308.

Kalinkovich A, Livshits G, Engelmann H, Harpaz N, Burstein R, Kaminsky M, Wallach D, Bentwich Z. (1993). Soluble tumor necrosis factor receptors (sTNF-R) and HIV infection: Correlation to CD8+ lymphocytes. *Clinical and Experimental Immunology* 93:350-355.

Kallich JD, Tchekmedyian NS, Damiano AM, Shi J, Black JT, Erder MH. (2002). Psychological outcomes associated with anemia-related fatigue in cancer patients. *Oncology* 16(9 Suppl 10):117-124.

Kalman D, Villani LJ. (1997). Nutritional aspects of cancer-related fatigue. *Journal of the American Dietetic Association* 97(6):650-654.

Kamihira S, Soda H, Kinoshita K, Ichimaru M. (1983). [Effect of human lymphoblast interferon in adult T-cell leukemia and non-Hodgkin's lymphoma]. *Gan To Kagaku Ryoho* 10(10):2188-2193.

Kamiya T, Honda K, Kizaki M, Maruyama T, Masuda T, Suzuki O, Ookawa H, Kiryu Y, Takahashi S, Yasumura K, et al. (1985). [Clinicopathological studies on disseminated carcinomatosis of the bone marrow occurring through metastasis of gastric carcinoma]. *Gan No Rinsho* 31(7):819-826.

Kamiyama T, Une Y, Satou Y, Sano F, Uchino J, Morita Y, Nojima T. (1990). [A case of non-functioning adrenocortical tumor]. *Gan No Rinsho* 36(7):847-853.

Kanagawa O, Vaupel BA, Gayama S, Koehler G, Kopf M. (1993). Resistance of mice deficient in IL-4 to retrovirus-induced immunodeficiency syndrome (MAIDS). *Science* 262:240-242.

Kanazawa K, Honma S, Yuzawa H, Takeuchi S. (1984). [Clinical effects of human fibroblast interferon in advanced gynecological cancers]. *Gan To Kagaku Ryoho* 11(6):1276-1283.

Kanazawa M, Maruyama T, Suzuki T, Soejima K, Hayashi M, Yamazaki K. (1998). A case of rapidly progressing small cell lung cancer incidentally found during the course of renal failure. *Keio Journal of Medicine* 47(1):45-51.

Kane RL, Gantz NM, DiPino RK. (1997). Neuropsychological and psychological functioning in chronic fatigue syndrome. *Neuropsychiatry, Neuropsychology and Behavioral Neurology* 10(1):25-31.

Kankuri M, Pelliniemi TT, Pyrhonen S, Nikkanen V, Helenius H, Salminen E. (2001). Feasibility of prolonged use of interferon-alpha in metastatic kidney carcinoma: A phase II study. *Cancer* 92(4):761-767.

Kanno H, Kitami K, Senga Y, Takahashi T, Nagashima Y. (1993). [Successful management for advanced renal cell carcinoma under combination therapy with human lymphoblastoid interferon-alpha and UFT (mixture of tegafur and uracil): A case report]. *Hinyokika Kiyo* 39(8):725-729.

Kanou T, Nosou Y, Yoshinaka K, Yanagawa E, Niimoto M, Hattori T, Miura K, Kuramoto J. (1986). [Microangiopathic hemolytic anemia associated with gastric cancer]. *Gan No Rinsho* 32(9):1029-1034.

Kantarjian HM, O'Brien S, Smith TL, Rios MB, Cortes J, Beran M, Koller C, Giles FJ, Andreeff M, Kornblau S, et al. (1999). Treatment of Philadelphia chromosome-positive early chronic phase chronic myelogenous leukemia with daily doses of interferon alpha and low-dose cytarabine. *Journal of Clinical Oncology* 17(1):284-292.

Kantor TV, Whiteside TL, Friberg D, Buckingham RB, Medsger TA Jr. (1992). Lymphokine-activated killer cell and natural killer cell activities in patients with systemic sclerosis. *Arthritis and Rheumatism* 35:694-699.

Kapas L, Hansen MK, Chang HY, Krueger JM. (1998). Vagotomy attenuates but does not prevent the somnogenic and febrile effects of lypopolysaccharide in rats. *American Journal of Physiology* 274:R406-R411.

Kapil A, Sharma S. (1997). Immunopotentiating compounds from *Tinospora cordifolia*. *Journal of Ethnopharmacology* 58(2):89-95.

Karczmar GS, Meyerhoff DJ, Boska MD, Hubesch B, Poole J, Matson GB, Valone F, Weiner MW. (1991). P-31 spectroscopy study of response of superficial human tumors to therapy. *Radiology* 179:149-153.

Karczmar GS, Meyerhoff DJ, Speder A, Valone F, Wilkinson M, Shine N, Boska MD, Weiner MW. (1989). Response of tumors to therapy studied by 31P magnetic resonance spectroscopy. *Investigative Radiology* 24:1020-1023.

Karp JE. (2001). Farnesyl protein transferase inhibitors as targeted therapies for hematologic malignancies. *Seminars in Hematology* 38(3 Suppl 7):16-23.

Karp SE. (1998). Low-dose intravenous bolus interleukin-2 with interferon-alpha therapy for metastatic melanoma and renal cell carcinoma. *Journal of Immunotherapy* 21(1):56-61.

Kasai H. (1994). [A new assessment of quality of life (QOL) for cancer patients]. *Hokkaido Igaku Zasshi* 69(2):282-292.

Kasamatsu T, Ohmi K, Takeuchi S, Takamizawa H, Matsuzawa M, Kawana T, Ueda K, Kubo H, Tsumuji Y, Kawashima Y, et al. (1985). [Clinical study of recombinant interferon alpha-2 (Sch 30500) in advanced gynecological cancers]. *Gan To Kagaku Ryoho* 12(8):1656-1660.

Kashani-Sabet M, Sagebiel RW, Collins HE, Glassberg AB, Allen RE, Leong SP, Small EJ. (1999). Outpatient combination chemoimmunotherapy for patients with metastatic melanoma: Results of a phase I/II trial. *Cancer* 86(10):2160-2165.

Kasl SV, Evans AS, Niederman JC. (1979). Psychosocial risk factors in the development of infectious mononucleosis. *Psychosomatic Medicine* 41:445-466.

Kaslow JE, Rucker L, Onishi R. (1989). Liver extract-folic acid-cyanocobalamin vs. placebo for chronic fatigue syndrome. *Archives of Internal Medicine* 149:2501-2503.

Kasper CE, Sarna LP. (2000). Influence of adjuvant chemotherapy on skeletal muscle and fatigue in women with breast cancer. *Biology Research and Nursing* 2(2):133-139.

Katayama Y, Matsuda H, Katoh Y, Kohri K, Iguchi M, Kurita T, Fujii R. (1989). [Multiple myeloma in a patient with primary hyperparathyroidism]. *Hinyokika Kiyo* 35(8):1369-1372.

Kato M, Liu W, Yi H, Asai N, Hayakawa A, Kozaki K, Takahashi M, Nakashima I. (1998). The herbal medicine Sho-saiko-to inhibits growth and metastasis of malignant melanoma primarily developed in ret-transgenic mice. *Journal of Investigative Dermatology* 111(4):640-644.

Kato T, Niwa M, Saito Y, Ogoshi K, Shimizu K, Nashimoto A, Kato K, Akai S. (1990). [Evaluation of quality of life in arterial infusion chemotherapy of hepatocellular carcinoma]. *Gan To Kagaku Ryoho* 17(8 Pt 2):1623-1628.

Katon W, Russo J. (1992). Chronic fatigue syndrome criteria: A critique of the requirement for multiple physical complaints. *Archives of Internal Medicine* 152:1604-1609.

Katon W, Walker EA. (1993). The relationship of chronic fatigue to psychiatric illness in community, primary care and tertiary care samples. In *Chronic Fatigue Syndrome,* Bock BR, Whelan J, eds. New York: Wiley, pp. 193-211.

Katsumata K, Yamamoto K, Shibata K, Murano A, Kawasaki M, Moriwaki R, Nagakawa Y, Ogata T, Koyanagi Y, Kusama M. (1997). [Efficacy of combination chemotherapy with mitoxantrone, vincristine, doxifluridine and prednisolone for recurrence of breast cancer]. *Gan To Kagaku Ryoho* 24(15):2227-2232.

Katz BZ, Salimi B, Kim S, Nsiah-Kumi P, Wagner-Weiner L. (2001). Epstein-Barr virus burden in adolescents with systemic lupus erythematosus. *Pediatric Infectious Diseases Journal* 20(2):148-153.

Katz JN, Barrett J, Liang MH, Bacon AM, Kaplan H, Kieval RI, Lindsey SM, Roberts WN, Sheff DM, Spencer RT, et al. (1997). Sensitivity and positive predictive value of Medicare Part B physician claims for rheumatologic diagnoses and procedures. *Arthritis and Rheumatism* 40(9):1594-1600.

Katz RS, Kravitz HM. (1996). Fibromyalgia, depression, and alcoholism: A family history study. *Journal of Rheumatology* 23(1):149-154.

Kaur M, Reed E, Sartor O, Dahut W, Figg WD. (2002). Suramin's development: What did we learn? *Investigative New Drugs* 20(2):209-219.

Kavanaugh AF. (1996). Fibromyalgia or multi-organ dysesthesia? *Arthritis and Rheumatism* 39(1):180-181.

Kawabata G, Mizuno Y, Okamoto Y, Nomi M, Hara I, Okada H, Arakawa S, Kamidono S. (1999). [Laparoscopic resection of retroperitoneal tumors: Report of two cases]. *Hinyokika Kiyo* 45(10):691-694.

Kawai K, Sato K, Nishijima Y, Sasaki A, Yamashita J, Ishikawa H, Koiso K. (1990). [Interferon alpha and gamma in the treatment of renal cell carcinoma]. *Nippon Jinzo Gakkai Shi* 32(2):231-236.

Kawanishi H, Aoyama T, Yoshida T, Sasaki M, Itoh T. (2001). [Bladder carcinoma producing granulocyte colony-stimulating factor (G-CSF): A case report]. *Hinyokika Kiyo* 47(6):429-432.

Kawasaki K, Kodama M, Matsushita A. (1983). Caerulein, a cholecystokinin-related peptide, depresses somatic function via the vagal afferent system. *Life Scientist* 33:1045-1050.

Kayitalire L, Thomas F, Le Chevalier T, Toussaint C, Tursz T, Spielmann M. (1992). Phase II study of a combination of elliptinium and vinblastine in metastatic breast cancer. *Investigative New Drugs* 10(4):303-307.

Kazumori H, Sizuku T, Uchida Y, Moritani M, Yamamoto S. (1998). [A case of giant hepatocellular carcinoma effectively treated with UFT]. *Gan To Kagaku Ryoho* 25(8):1213-1216.

Keefe FJ, Caldwell DS. (1997). Cognitive behavioral control of arthritis pain. *Medicine Clinics of North America* 81(1):277-290.

Keel P. (1998). Psychological and psychiatric aspects of fibromyalgia syndrome (FMS). *Zeitschrift Rheumatologie* 57(Suppl. 2):97-100.

Keitel W. (1997). [Backache from the internal medicine-rheumatologic viewpoint] Ruckenschmerz aus internistisch-rheumatologischer sicht. *Zeitschrift Arztliche Fotbildung* (Jena) 90(8):671-676.

Keizer HJ, Ouwerkerk J, Welvaart K, van der Velde CJ, Cleton FJ. (1995). Ifosfamide treatment as a 10-day continuous intravenous infusion. *Journal of Cancer Research and Clinical Oncology* 121(5):297-302.

Kelemen J, Lang E, Balint G, Trocsanyi M, Muller W. (1998). Orthostatic sympathetic derangement of baroreflex in patients with fibromyalgia. *Journal of Rheumatology* 25(4):823-825.

Kelemen J, Muller W. (1998). [Secondary fibromyalgia: Differentiation of primary and secondary fibromyalgia is necessary for successful therapy] Sekundare fibromyalgien: Differenzierung primarer und sekundarer fibromyalgien notwendig fur erfolgreiche therapie. *Fortschritt Medizin* 116(10):44-46.

Keller K. (1997). Besondere Therapierichtungen aus der Sicht des BfArM. *Zeitschrift Arztliche Fortbildung Qualitatssicherheit* 91(7):669-674.

Keller RH, Lane JL, Klimas N, Reiter WM, Fletcher MA, van Riel F, Morgan R. (1994). Association between HLA class II antigens and the chronic fatigue immune dysfunction syndrome. *Clinical Infectious Diseases* 18(Suppl 1):S154-S156.

Kelley DS, Daudu PA, Branch LB, Johnson HL, Taylor PC, Mackey B. (1994). Energy restriction decreases number of circulating natural killer cells and serum levels of immunoglobulins in overweight women. *European Journal of Clinical Nutrition* 48:9-18.

Kellokumpu-Lehtinen P, Nordman E. (1988). Combined interferon and vinblastine treatment of advanced melanoma and renal cell cancer. *Cancer Detection and Prevention* 12(1-6):523-529.

Kellokumpu-Lehtinen P, Nordman E. (1990). Recombinant interferon-alpha 2a and vinblastine in advanced renal cell cancer: A clinical phase I-II study. *Journal of Biological Response Modifiers* 9(4):439-444.

Kellokumpu-Lehtinen P, Nordman E, Toivanen A. (1989). Combined interferon and vinblastine treatment of advanced melanoma: Evaluation of the treatment results and the effects of the treatment on immunological functions. *Cancer Immunology and Immunotherapy* 28(3):213-217.

Kelly GS. (2001). Rhodiola rosea: A possible plant adaptogen. *Alternative Medicine Reviews* 6(3):293-302.

Kelly K, Crowley JJ, Bunn PA Jr, Hazuka MB, Beasley K, Upchurch C, Weiss GR, Hicks WJ, Gandara DR, Rivkin S, et al. (1995). Role of recombinant interferon alfa-2a maintenance in patients with limited-stage small-cell lung cancer responding to concurrent chemoradiation: A Southwest Oncology Group study. *Journal of Clinical Oncology* 13(12):2924-2930.

Kelly K, Lovato L, Bunn PA, Livingston RB, Zangmeister J, Taylor SA, Roychowdhury D, Crowley JJ, Gandara DR. (2001). Cisplatin, etoposide, and paclitaxel with granulocyte colony-stimulating factor in untreated patients with extensive-stage small cell lung cancer: A phase II trial of the Southwest Oncology Group. *Clinical Cancer Research* 7(8):2325-2329.

Kelly MC. (1997). Fibromyalgia syndrome. *Irish Medical Journal* 90(1):14, 16.

Kelly WK, Osman I, Reuter VE, Curley T, Heston WD, Nanus DM, Scher HI. (2000). The development of biologic end points in patients treated with differentiation agents: An experience of retinoids in prostate cancer. *Clinical Cancer Research* 6(3):838-846.

Kelly-Williams S, Zmijewski M, Tomaszewski E. (1989). Lymphocyte subpopulations in "normal" lymph nodes harvested from cadavers. *Laboratory Medicine* 20:487-490.

Kelsen D, Chapman R, Bains M, Heelan R, Dukeman M, Golbey R. (1982). Phase II study of methyl-GAG in the treatment of esophageal carcinoma. *Cancer Treatment Reports* 66(6):1427-1429.

Kelsen D, Lovett D, Wong J, Saltz L, Buckley M, Murray P, Heelan R, Lightdale C. (1992). Interferon alfa-2a and fluorouracil in the treatment of patients with advanced esophageal cancer. *Journal of Clinical Oncology* 10(2):269-274.

Kelsen DP, Yagoda A, Warrell R, Chapman R, Whittes R, Gralla RJ, Casper E, Young CW. (1982). Phase II trials of methylglyoxal-bis (guanylhydrazone). *American Journal of Clinical Oncology* 5(2):221-225.

Kelsey JL, Gammon MD. (1991). The epidemiology of breast cancer. *CA Cancer Journal for Clinicians* 41:146-165.

Kemeny N, Israel K, O'Hehir M. (1990). Phase II trial of 10-Edam in patients with advanced colorectal carcinoma. *American Journal of Clinical Oncology* 13(1): 42-44.

Kempenaers C, Simenon G, Elst MV, Fransolet L, Mingard P, De Maertelaer V, Appelboom T, Mendlewicz J. (1994). Effect of antidencephalon immune serum on pain and sleep in primary fibromyalgia. *Neuropsychobiology* 30:66-72.

Kempf RA, Grunberg SM, Daniels JR, Skinner DG, Venturi CL, Spiegel R, Neri R, Greiner JM, Rudnick S, Mitchell MS. (1986). Recombinant interferon alpha-2 (INTRON A) in a phase II study of renal cell carcinoma. *Journal of Biological Response Modifiers* 5(1):27-35.

Kendler BS. (1997). Melatonin: Media hype or therapeutic breakthrough? *Nursing Practice* 22(2):66-67, 71-72, 77.

Kennedy M, Felson DT. (1996). A prospective long-term study of fibromyalgia syndrome. *Arthritis and Rheumatism* 39(4):682-685.

Kenner C. (1998). Fibromyalgia and chronic fatigue: The holistic perspective. *Holistic Nursing Practice* 12(3):55-63.

Kent-Braun JA, Sharma KR, Weiner MW, Massie B, Miller RG. (1993). Central basis of muscle fatigue in chronic fatigue syndrome. *Neurology* 43:125-131.

Keppel KG, Pearcy JN, Wagener DK. (2000). Trends in racial and ethnic-specific rates for the health status indicators: United States, 1990-98. *Healthy People 2000 Statistical Notes* 23:1-16.

Keren-Rosenberg S, Muggia FM. (1997). Response to estramustine phosphate and paclitaxel in patients with advanced breast cancer: A phase I study. *Seminars in Oncology* 24(1 Suppl 3):S26-S29.

Khayat D, Borel C, Azab M, Paraisot D, Malaurie E, Bouloux C, Weil M. (1992). Phase I study of datelliptium chloride, hydrochloride given by 24-h continuous intravenous infusion. *Cancer Chemotherapy Pharmacology* 30(3):226-228.

Khuri FR, Fossella FV, Lee JS, Murphy WK, Shin DM, Markowitz AB, Glisson BS. (1998). Phase II trial of recombinant IFN-alpha2a with etoposide/cisplatin induction and interferon/megestrol acetate maintenance in extensive small cell lung cancer. *Journal of Interferon and Cytokine Research* 18(4):241-245.

Kibler R, Lucas DO, Hicks MJ, Poulos BT, Jones JF. (1985). Immune function in chronic active Epstein-Barr virus infection. *Journal of Clinical Immunology* 5:46-54.

Kidera Y, Sugimori H, Tanaka M, Jimi S, Watanabe E, Kato Y, Morita T, Shigyo R, Yamashita H, Nishimura A, et al. (1982). [FT-207 maintenance therapy of malignant gynecologic cancer]. *Gan To Kagaku Ryoho* 9(8):1407-1411.

Kiebert GM, Curran D, Aaronson NK, Bolla M, Menten J, Rutten EH, Nordman E, Silvestre ME, Pierart M, Karim AB. (1998). Quality of life after radiation therapy of cerebral low-grade gliomas of the adult: Results of a randomised phase III trial on dose response (EORTC trial 22844). EORTC Radiotherapy Co-operative Group. *European Journal of Cancer* 34(12):1902-1909.

Kiebert GM, Hanneke J, de Haes CJ, Kievit J, van de Velde CJ. (1990). Effect of peri-operative chemotherapy on the quality of life of patients with early breast cancer. *European Journal of Cancer* 26(10):1038-1042.

Kikwilu EN, Hiza JF. (1997). Tooth bud extraction and rubbing of herbs by traditional healers in Tanzania: Prevalence, and sociological and environmental factors influencing in the practices. *International Journal of Paediatric Dentistry* 7(1):19-24.

Kim ES, Lu C, Khuri FR, Tonda M, Glisson BS, Liu D, Jung M, Hong WK, Herbst RS. (2001). A phase II study of STEALTH cisplatin (SPI-77) in patients with advanced non-small cell lung cancer. *Lung Cancer* 34(3):427-432.

Kim HS, Lee BM. (1997). Inhibition of benzo[a]pyrene-DNA adduct formation by *Aloë barbadensis* Miller. *Carcinogenesis* 18(4):771-776.

Kim J, Modlin RL, Moy RL, Dubinett SM, McHugh T, Nickoloff BJ, Uyemura K. (1995). IL-10 production in cutaneous basal and squamous cell carcinomas: A mechanism for evaluating the local T-cell immune response. *Journal of Immunology* 155:2240-2247.

Kim J, Zhi J, Satoh H, Koss-Twardy SG, Passe SM, Patel IH, Pazdur R. (1998). Pharmacokinetics of recombinant human interferon-alpha 2a combined with 5-fluorouracil in patients with advanced colorectal carcinoma. *Anticancer Drugs* 9(8):689-696.

Kim JS, Kim JS, Cho MJ, Song KS, Yoon WH. (2002). Preoperative chemoradiation using oral capecitabine in locally advanced rectal cancer. *International Journal of Radiation Oncology, Biology, and Physics* 54(2):403-408.

Kim KH, Lee JG, Kim DG, Kim MK, Park JH, Shin YG, Lee SK, Jo TH, Oh ST. (1998). The development of a new method to detect the adulteration of commercial aloe gel powders. *Archives of Pharmaceutical Research* 21(5):514-520.

Kim SJ, Maeura Y, Ueda N, Saito M, Matsunaga S. (1999). [A case of hepatic arterial infusion chemotherapy with docetaxel for liver metastasis from breast cancer]. *Gan To Kagaku Ryoho* 26(12):1959-1962.

Kim Y, Roscoe JA, Morrow GR. (2002). The effects of information and negative affect on severity of side effects from radiation therapy for prostate cancer. *Support Care and Cancer* 10(5):416-421.

Kim YH, Kim JS, Choi YH, In KH, Park HS, Hong DS, Jeong TJ, Lee YY, Nam E, Lee SN, et al. (2002). Phase II study of docetaxel and cisplatin combination chemotherapy in metastatic or unresectable localized non-small-cell lung cancer. *International Journal of Clinical Oncology* 7(2):114-119.

Kimoto Y. (1992). Use of human leukocyte antigen-mismatched allogeneic lymphokine-activated killer cells and interleukin-2 in the adoptive immunotherapy of patients with malignancies. *Human Cell* 5(3):226-235.

Kimoto Y, Tanaka T, Tanji Y, Fujiwara A, Taguchi T. (1994). Use of human leukocyte antigen-mismatched allogeneic lymphokine-activated killer cells and interleukin-2 in the adoptive immunotherapy of patients with malignancies. *Biotherapy* 8(1):41-50.

Kimura K. (1984). [A cooperative phase I-II study of HLBI in patients with malignant tumors]. *Gan To Kagaku Ryoho* 11(6):1324-1331.

Kimura K, Suga S, Kano H, Sakakibara K, Hayashi T, Nakai T, Nagano I, Yokoyama Y, Morise K, Hayakawa M, et al. (1986). [Phase II study of epirubicin on gastric cancer—A cooperative study of the Tokai Cancer Chemotherapy Group]. *Gan To Kagaku Ryoho* 13(7):2440-2445.

Kimura K, Yamada K, Yoshida T. (1986). [Phase II study of NK 171 (etoposide) on malignant lymphomas and acute leukemia: A cooperative study group on NK 171 in hematological malignancies]. *Gan To Kagaku Ryoho* 13(3 Pt 1):496-501.

King MT, Dobson AJ, Harnett PR. (1996). A comparison of two quality-of-life questionnaires for cancer clinical trials: The Functional Living Index–Cancer (FLIC) and the Quality of Life Questionnaire Core Module (QLQ-C30). *Journal of Clinical Epidemiology* 49(1):21-29.

Kinney P, Triozzi P, Young D, Drago J, Behrens B, Wise H, Rinehart JJ. (1990). Phase II trial of interferon-beta-serine in metastatic renal cell carcinoma. *Journal of Clinical Oncology* 8(5):881-885.

Kirkwood JM, Bender C, Agarwala S, Tarhini A, Shipe-Spotloe J, Smelko B, Donnelly S, Stover L. (2002). Mechanisms and management of toxicities associated with high-dose interferon alfa-2b therapy. *Journal of Clinical Oncology* 20(17):3703-3718.

Kirkwood JM, Ernstoff MS, Davis CA, Reiss M, Ferraresi R, Rudnick SA. (1985). Comparison of intramuscular and intravenous recombinant alpha-2 interferon in melanoma and other cancers. *Annals of Internal Medicine* 103(1):32-36.

Kirsh KL, Passik S, Holtsclaw E, Donaghy K, Theobald D. (2001). I get tired for no reason: A single item screening for cancer-related fatigue. *Journal of Pain Symptomatology Management* 22(5):931-937.

Kissel W, Mahnig P. (1998). [Fibromyalgia (generalized tendomyopathy) in expert assessment: Analysis of 158 cases] Die fibromyalgie (generalisierte tendomyopathie) in der begutachtungsituation: Analyse von 158 fallen. *Schweize Rundschift Medizin Praxis* 87(16):538-545.

Kitamura K. (1993). [Clinical application of new cytokines]. *Rinsho Byori* 41(4): 390-398.

Kitani T, Kuratsune H, Fuke I, Nakamura Y, Nakaya T, Asahi S, Tobiume M, Yamaguti M, Machii T, Inagi R, Yamanishi K, Ikuta K. (1996). Possible correlation between Borna disease virus infection and Japanese patients with chronic fatigue syndrome. *Microbiology and Immunology* 40(6):459-462.

Kjaergaard J. (1998). [Fibromyalgia] Fibromyalgi. *Ugeskr Laeger* 160(25):3751.

Klepser TB, Klepser ME. (1999). Unsafe and potentially safe herbal therapies. *American Journal of Health System Pharmacy* 56(2):125-138.

Klepstad P, Borchgrevink PC, Kaasa S. (2000). Effects on cancer patients' health-related quality of life after the start of morphine therapy. *Journal of Pain Symptomatology and Management* 20(1):19-26.

Klepstad P, Hilton P, Moen J, Fougner B, Borchgrevink PC, Kaasa S. (2002). Self-reports are not related to objective assessments of cognitive function and sedation in patients with cancer pain admitted to a palliative care unit. *Palliative Medicine* 16(6):513-519.

Klima U, Wimmer-Greinecker G, Harringer W, Mair R, Gross C, Brucke P. (1993). Cardiac angiosarcoma—A diagnostic dilemma. *Cardiovascular Surgery* 1(6): 674-676.

Klimas N. (1998). Pathogenesis of chronic fatigue syndrome and fibromyalgia. *Growth Hormone and IGF Research* 52(Suppl B):123-126.

Klimas N, Salvato F, Morgan R, Fletcher MA. (1990). Immunologic abnormalities in chronic fatigue syndrome. *Journal of Clinical Microbiology* 28(6):1403-1410.

Klimas NG. (1992). Clinical impact of adoptive therapy with purified CD8 cells in HIV infection. *Seminars in Hematology* 29:40-43.

Klimas NG, Fletcher MA. (1999). Alteration of type 1/type 2 cytokine pattern following adoptive immunotherapy of patients with chronic fatigue syndrome (CFS) using autologous ex vivo expanded lymph node cells. Abstract, II International Conference on CFS, Brussels, Belgium, June.

Klimas NG, Fletcher MA, Walling J, Garcia-Morales R, Patarca R, Moody D, Okarma T. (1993). Ex vivo CD8 lymphocyte activation, expansion and re-infusion into donors with rIL-2—A phase I study. In *Septieme Colloque des Cent Gardes: Retroviruses of Human AIDS and Related Animal Disease,* Girard M, Valette L, eds. Paris, France: Fondation Marcel Merieux, pp. 285-290.

Klimas NG, Morgan R, Salvato F, Van Riel F, Millon C, Fletcher MA. (1992). Chronic fatigue syndrome and psychoneuroimmunology. In *Stress and Disease Progression: Perspectives in Behavioral Medicine,* Schneiderman N, McCabe P, Baum A, eds. Hillsdale, NJ: Lawrence Erlbaum, Assoc., pp. 121-137.

Klimas NG, Patarca R, Maher K, Smith M, Jin X-Q, Huang H-S, Walling J, Gamber C, Fletcher MA. (1994). Immunomodulation with autologous, ex vivo manipulated T lymphocytes in HIV-1 disease. *Clinical Immunology Newsletter* 14:101-105.

Klimas NG, Patarca R, Walling J, Garcia R, Mayer V, Albarracin C, Moody D, Okarma T, Fletcher MA. (1994). Changes in the clinical and immunological stati of AIDS patients upon adoptive therapy with activated autologous CD8+ T cells and interleukin-2 infusion. *Journal of Acquired Immune Deficiency Syndromes* 8:1073-1081.

Klimas NG, Patarca-Montero R, Maher K, Smith M, Bathe O, Fletcher MA. (2000). Clinical and immunologic effects of autologous lymph node cell transplant in chronic fatigue syndrome. *Journal of Chronic Fatigue Syndrome* 8(1):39-55.

Klineberg I, McGregor N, Butt H, Dunstan H, Roberts T, Zerves M. (1998). Chronic orofacial muscle pain: A new approach to diagnosis and management. *Alpha Omega* 91(2):25-28.

Klonoff DC. (1996). Chronic fatigue syndrome and neurally mediated hypotension. *JAMA* 275(5):359-360.

Klug GA, McAuley E, Clark S. (1989). Factors influencing the development and maintenance of aerobic fitness: Lessons applicable to the fibrositis syndrome. *Journal of Rheumatology* 16(Suppl 19):30-39.

Knobel H, Havard Loge J, Brit Lund M, Forfang K, Nome O, Kaasa S. (2001). Late medical complications and fatigue in Hodgkin's disease survivors. *Journal of Clinical Oncology* 19(13):3226-3233.

Knobel H, Loge JH, Nordoy T, Kolstad AL, Espevik T, Kvaloy S, Kaasa S. (2000). High level of fatigue in lymphoma patients treated with high dose therapy. *Journal of Pain Symptomatology and Management* 19(6):446-456.

Knobf MT. (1986). Physical and psychologic distress associated with adjuvant chemotherapy in women with breast cancer. *Journal of Clinical Oncology* 4(5):678-684.

Knobf MT. (1990). Symptoms and rehabilitation needs of patients with early stage breast cancer during primary therapy. *Cancer* 66(6 Suppl):1392-1401.

Knop J, Stremer R, Nauman C, DeMaeyer E, Macher M. (1982). Interferon inhibits the suppressor T cell response of delayed hypersensitivity. *Nature* 296:757-759.

Knowles G, Borthwick D, McNamara S, Miller M, Leggot L. (2000). Survey of nurses' assessment of cancer-related fatigue. *European Journal of Cancer Care* 9(2):105-113.

Knuth A, Bernhard H, Klein O, Meyer zum Buschenfelde KH. (1992). Combination fluorouracil, folinic acid, and interferon alfa-2a: An active regimen in advanced pancreatic carcinoma. *Seminars in Oncology* 19(2 Suppl 3):211-214.

Kobashi-Schoot JA, Hanewald GJ, van Dam FS, Bruning PF. (1985). Assessment of malaise in cancer patients treated with radiotherapy. *Cancer Nursing* 8(6): 306-313.

Kobayashi K, Takeda F, Teramukai S, Gotoh I, Sakai H, Yoneda S, Noguchi Y, Ogasawara H, Yoshida K. (1998). A cross-validation of the European Organization for Research and Treatment of Cancer QLQ-C30 (EORTC QLQ-C30) for Japanese with lung cancer. *European Journal of Cancer* 34(6):810-815.

Kobayashi M, Imai K, Kiren H, Nakai K, Saruki K, Umeyama T, Ito Y, Yamanaka H, Makino T, Machida M, et al. (1987). [Therapy of renal cell carcinoma: 3. Interferon therapy]. *Hinyokika Kiyo* 33(4):508-514.

Kobayashi M, Imai K, Yamanaka H, Takahashi H, Mashimo T, Shimizu N, Koya J, Yajima H, Kawashima K, Kitaura K. (1989). [Combination therapy of renal cell carcinoma with interferon-alpha and UFT (or FT-207)]. *Nippon Gan Chiryo Gakkai Shi* 24(7):1437-1446.

Kobayashi Y, Urabe A. (1988). [Gamma interferon therapy of cancer patients]. *Gan To Kagaku Ryoho* 15(4 Pt 2-1):804-809.

Koch H. (2002). [Rehabilitation after surgery for gastrointestinal malignant tumors]. *Zeitschrift Gastroenterologie* 40(Suppl 1):S84-S89.

Koczocik-Przedpelska J, Bombicki K, Bik T. (1994). Electrophysiological studies of nerve and muscle in comparative neoplasia. *Electromyography and Clinical Neurophysiology* 34(4):237-241.

Koda RT, Garcia AA, Chatterjee DJ, Li WY, Parimoo D, Jeffers S, Rogers M, Leichman CG, Leichman L, Wu EY, et al. (1999). Phase I study of AG 331, a novel thymidylate synthase inhibitor, in patients with refractory solid tumors. *Cancer Chemotherapy Pharmacology* 43(6):489-496.

Kodama M, Kodama T, Murakami M. (1996a). The value of dehydroepiandrosterone-annexed vitamin C infusion treatment in the clinical control of chronic fatigue syndrome (CFS): I. A pilot study of the new vitamin C infusion treatment with a volunteer CFS patient. *In Vivo* 10(6):575-584.

Kodama M, Kodama T, Murakami M. (1996b). The value of dehydroepiandrosterone-annexed vitamin C infusion treatment in the clinical control of chronic fatigue syndrome (CFS): II. Characterization of CFS patients with special references to their response to a new vitamin C infusion treatment. *In Vivo* 10(6):585-596.

Koeller JM. (1998). Clinical guidelines for the treatment of cancer-related anemia. *Pharmacotherapy* 18(1):156-169.

Koenig C, Stevermer J. (1999). Acupuncture in the treatment of fibromyalgia. *Journal of Family Practice* 48(7):497.

Koff WC, Elm JL Jr, Halstead SB. (1982). Antiviral effects of ribavirin and 6-mercapto-9-tetrahydro-2-fyrylpurine against dengue viruses in vitro. *Antiviral Research* 21(1-2):69-79.

Kohl HW, LaPorte RA, Blair SN. (1988). Physical activity and cancer: An epidemiological perspective. *Sports Medicine* 6:222-237.

Koide J. (1985). Functional property of Ia-positive T cells in peripheral blood from patients with systemic lupus erythematosus. *Scandinavian Journal of Immunology* 22:577-584.

Koike N, Akaogi E, Fujiwara A, Onizuka M, Yuasa Y, Kinoshita T, Atake S, Mitsui K, Hori M. (1992). [A resected case of thymolipoma]. *Kyobu Geka* 45(6):522-524.

Kolitz JE, Wong GY, Welte K, Merluzzi VJ, Engert A, Bialas T, Polivka A, Bradley EC, Konrad M, Gnecco C, et al. (1988). Phase I trial of recombinant interleukin-2 and cyclophosphamide: Augmentation of cellular immunity and T-cell mitogenic response with long-term administration of rIL-2. *Journal of Biological Response Modifiers* 7(5):457-472.

Kollmannsberger C, Mross K, Jakob A, Kanz L, Bokemeyer C. (1999). Topotecan, a novel topoisomerase I inhibitor: Pharmacology and clinical experience. *Oncology* 56(1):1-12.

Koltyn KF, Robins HI, Schmitt CL, Cohen JD, Morgan WP. (1992). Changes in mood state following whole-body hyperthermia. *International Journal of Hyperthermia* 8(3):305-307.

Komaki R, Janjan NA, Ajani JA, Lynch PM, Fairweather JS, Raijman I, Blumenshein GR, Ho L, Pisters PW, Feig BW, et al. (2000). Phase I study of irinotecan and concurrent radiation therapy for upper GI tumors. *Oncology* 14(12 Suppl 14):34-37.

Komaroff AL. (1997). A 56-year-old woman with chronic fatigue syndrome. *JAMA* 278(14):1179-1185.

Komaroff AL, Buchwald DS. (1998). Chronic fatigue syndrome: An update. *Annual Reviews of Medicine* 49:1-13.

Komaroff AL, Fagioli LR, Doolittle TH, Gandek B, Gleit MA, Guerreiro RT, Kornish RJ II, Ware NC, Ware JE Jr, Bates DW. (1996). Health status in patients with chronic fatigue syndrome and in the general population and disease comparison groups. *American Journal of Medicine* 101(3):281-290.

Komaroff AL, Fagioli LR, Geiger AM, Doolittle TH, Lee J, Kornish RJ, Gleit MA, Guerriero RT. (1996). An examination of the working case definition of chronic fatigue syndrome. *American Journal of Medicine* 100:56-64.

Konstantinov K, von Mikecz A, Buchwald D, Jones J, Gerace L, Tan EM. (1996). Autoantibodies to nuclear antigens in chronic fatigue syndrome. *Journal of Clinical Investigation* 98(8):1888-1896.

Kopp M, Schweigkofler H, Holzner B, Nachbaur D, Niederwieser D, Fleischhacker WW, Sperner-Unterweger B. (1998). Time after bone marrow transplantation as an important variable for quality of life: Results of a cross-sectional investigation using two different instruments for quality-of-life assessment. *Annals of Hematology* 77(1-2):27-32.

Kori-Lindner C. (1999). Pflanzliche Arzneimittel—eine Standortbestimmung: Wirksamkeit und Nutzen der Phytopharmaka. *Fortschrift Medizin* 117(7):38-40.

Korn JH. (1997). Antipolymer antibodies, silicone breast implants, and fibromyalgia. *Lancet* 349(9059):1171.

Kornblith AB, Herndon JE, Silverman LR, Demakos EP, Odchimar-Reissig R, Holland JF, Powell BL, De Castro C, Ellerton J, Larson RA, et al. (2002). Impact of azacytidine on the quality of life of patients with myelodysplastic syndrome treated in a randomized phase III trial: A Cancer and Leukemia Group B study. *Journal of Clinical Oncology* 20(10):2441-2452.

Kornblith AB, Herndon JE II, Zuckerman E, Cella DF, Cherin E, Wolchok S, Weiss RB, Diehl LF, Henderson E, Cooper MR, et al. (1998). Comparison of psychosocial adaptation of advanced stage Hodgkin's disease and acute leukemia survivors. Cancer and Leukemia Group B. *Annals of Oncology* 9(3):297-306.

Kornblith AB, Herr HW, Ofman US, Scher HI, Holland JC. (1994). Quality of life of patients with prostate cancer and their spouses: The value of a data base in clinical care. *Cancer* 73(11):2791-2802.

Kornek GV, Haider K, Kwasny W, Raderer M, Schull B, Payrits T, Depisch D, Kovats E, Lang F, Scheithauer W. (2002). Treatment of advanced breast cancer with docetaxel and gemcitabine with and without human granulocyte colony-stimulating factor. *Clinical Cancer Research* 8(5):1051-1056.

Korszun A, Papadopoulos E, Demitrack M, Engleberg C, Crofford L. (1998). The relationship between temporomandibular disorders and stress-associated syndromes. *Oral Surgery, Oral Medicine, Oral Pathology, Oral Radiology, and Endodontics* 86(4):416-420.

Korszun A, Sackett-Lundeen L, Papadopoulos E, Brucksch C, Masterson L, Engelberg NC, Haus E, Demitrack MA, Crofford L. (1999). Melatonin levels in women with fibromyalgia and chronic fatigue syndrome. *Journal of Rheumatology* 26(12):2675-2680.

Korszun A, Young EA, Engleberg NC, Masterson L, Dawson EC, Spindler K, McClure LA, Brown MB, Crofford LJ. (2000). Follicular phase hypothalamic-pituitary-gonadal axis function in women with fibromyalgia and chronic fatigue syndrome. *Journal of Rheumatology* 27(6):1526-1530.

Koshizuka K, Serizawa M, Mouri N, Muto S, Takano K, Tada Y, Nakagomi H, Hada M. (2001). [Effect of weekly docetaxel in patients with recurrent breast cancer]. *Gan To Kagaku Ryoho* 28(8):1117-1120.

Kosmas C, Agelaki S, Giannakakis T, Mavroudis D, Kouroussis C, Kalbakis K, Papadouris S, Souglakos J, Malamos N, Georgoulias V. (2002). Phase I study of vinorelbine and carboplatin combination in patients with taxane and anthracycline pretreated advanced breast cancer. *Oncology* 62(2):103-109.

Kosmas C, Tsavaris NB, Polyzos A, Malamos NA, Katsikas M, Antonopoulos MJ. (2000). Phase I study of dose-escalated paclitaxel, ifosfamide, and cisplatin (PIC) combination chemotherapy in advanced solid tumours. *British Journal of Cancer* 82(2):300-307.

Kottke MK. (1998). Scientific and regulatory aspects of nutraceutical products in the United States. *Drug Development and Industrial Pharmacy* 24(12):1177-1195.

Kouroussis C, Agelaki S, Mavroudis D, Souglakos J, Kakolyris S, Kalbakis K, Vardakis N, Reppa D, Hatzidaki D, Samonis G, et al. (2000). A dose escalation study of weekly docetaxel in patients with advanced solid tumors. *Cancer Chemotherapy Pharmacology* 46(6):488-492.

Kouroussis C, Androulakis N, Kakolyris S, Souglakos J, Maltezakis G, Metaxaris G, Chalkiadakis G, Samonis G, Vlachonikolis J, Georgoulias V. (1998). First-line treatment of advanced nonsmall cell lung carcinoma with docetaxel and vinorelbine. *Cancer* 83(10):2083-2090.

Kouroussis C, Kakolyris S, Androulakis N, Heras P, Vlachonicolis J, Vamvakas L, Vlata M, Hatzidaki D, Samonis G, Georgoulias V. (1998). Salvage chemotherapy with paclitaxel, vinorelbine, and cisplatin (PVC) in anthracycline-resistant advanced breast cancer. *American Journal of Clinical Oncology* 21(3):226-232.

Kouroussis C, Kakolyris S, Mavroudis D, Androulakis N, Kalbakis K, Agelaki S, Sarra E, Souglakos J, Christodoulakis M, Samonis G, et al. (2001). A dose-finding study of the weekly administration of paclitaxel in patients with advanced solid tumors. *American Journal of Clinical Oncology* 24(4):404-407.

Koyama S, Moriyama Y, Shibata A, Miura Y, Abe T, Asano S, Miyazaki T, Miura A, Kariyone S, Toyama K, et al. (1988). [Clinical studies of natural interferon alpha (HLBI) in chronic myelogenous leukemia—A multi-institutional cooperative study in Japan]. *Gan To Kagaku Ryoho* 15(10):2959-2966.

Kraft K. (1999). Phyopharmaka und Arzneimittelrecht. *Forschung in Komplementarmedizin* 61(1):19-23.

Kramer JA, Curran D, Piccart M, de Haes JC, Bruning P, Klijn J, Van Hoorebeeck I, Paridaens R. (2000). Identification and interpretation of clinical and quality of life prognostic factors for survival and response to treatment in first-line chemotherapy in advanced breast cancer. *European Journal of Cancer* 36(12):1498-1506.

Kramer M, Wells CL. (1996). Does physical activity reduce risk of estrogen-dependent cancer in women? *Medical Science, Sports and Exercise* 28:322-334.

Kramer PA, Oosterhuis WP, van Kammen E, Hazenberg BP, Balhuizen JC, Dinkelaar RB. (1993). A patient with a variant form of hairy cell leukaemia. *Netherlands Journal of Medicine* 43(5-6):262-268.

Krause TG, Hviid A, Koch A, Friborg J, Hjuler T, Wohlfahrt J, Rosing Olsen O, Kristensen B, Melbye M. (2003). BCG vaccination and risk of atopy. *JAMA* 289(8):1012-1015.

Kreis W, Budman D. (1999). Daily oral estramustine and intermittent intravenous docetaxel (Taxotere) as chemotherapeutic treatment for metastatic, hormone-refractory prostate cancer. *Seminars in Oncology* 26(5 Suppl 17):34-38.

Kreis W, Budman DR, Fetten J, Gonzales AL, Barile B, Vinciguerra V. (1999). Phase I trial of the combination of daily estramustine phosphate and intermittent docetaxel in patients with metastatic hormone refractory prostate carcinoma. *Annals of Oncology* 10(1):33-38.

Krest I, Keusgen M. (1999). Quality of herbal remedies from *Allium sativum:* Differences between alliinase from garlic powder and fresh garlic. *Planta Medicina* 65(2):139-143.

Kriegler M, Perez C, DeFay K, Albert I, Lu SD. (1988). A novel form of TNF-cachectin in a cell surface cytotoxic transmembrane protein: Ramification for the complex physiology of TNF. *Cell* 53:45-53.

Kriegmair M, Oberneder R, Hofstetter A. (1995). Interferon alfa and vinblastine versus medroxyprogesterone acetate in the treatment of metastatic renal cell carcinoma. *Urology* 45(5):758-762.

Krigel RL, Padavic-Shaller KA, Rudolph AR, Konrad M, Bradley EC, Comis RL. (1990). Renal cell carcinoma: Treatment with recombinant interleukin-2 plus beta-interferon. *Journal of Clinical Oncology* 8(3):460-467.

Krigel RL, Padavic-Shaller KA, Rudolph AR, Litwin S, Konrad M, Bradley EC, Comis RL. (1988). A phase I study of recombinant interleukin 2 plus recombinant beta-interferon. *Cancer Research* 48(13):3875-3881.

Krilov LR, Fisher M, Friedman SB, Reitman D, Mandel FS. (1998). Course and outcome of chronic fatigue in children and adolescents. *Pediatrics* 102(2 Pt 1):360-366.

Krishnasamy M. (2000). Fatigue in advanced cancer—Meaning before measurement? *International Journal of Nursing Studies* 37(5):401-414.

Kroenke K, Wood DR, Mangelsdroff AD, Meir NJ, Powell JB. (1988). Chronic fatigue in primary care: Prevalence, patient characteristics, and outcome. *JAMA* 260:929-934.

Kroep JR, Peters GJ, van Moorsel CJ, Catik A, Vermorken JB, Pinedo HM, van Groeningen CJ. (1999). Gemcitabine-cisplatin: A schedule finding study. *Annals of Oncology* 10(12):1503-1510.

Kroger MJ, Menzel T, Gschwend JE, Bergmann L. (1999). Life quality of patients with metastatic renal cell carcinoma and chemo-immunotherapy—A pilot study. *Anticancer Research* 19(2C):1553-1555.

Krsnich-Shriwise S. (1997). Fibromyalgia syndrome: An overview. *Physical Therapy* 77(1):68-75.

Krueger JM, Majde JA. (1994). Microbial products and cytokines in sleep and fever regulation. *Critical Reviews in Immunology* 14(3-4):355-379.

Kruit WH, Goey SH, Monson JR, Stahel RA, Calabresi F, Mertelsmann R, Holdener EE, Eggermont AM, Bolhuis RL, de Mulder PH, et al. (1991). Clinical experience with the combined use of recombinant interleukin-2 (IL2) and interferon alfa-2a (IFN alpha) in metastatic melanoma. *British Journal of Haematology* 79(Suppl 1):84-86.

Krumholz HM. (1988). Weight loss, fatigue, and a palpable node. *Hospital Practice* 23(6):267, 272.

Krupp LB, La Rocca NG, Muir-Nash J, Steinberg AD. (1989). The Fatigue Severity Scale: Application to patients with multiple sclerosis and systemic lupus erythematosus. *Archives of Neurology* 46:1121-1123.

Krupp LB, Pollina DA. (1996). Mechanisms and management of fatigue in progressive neurological disorders. *Current Opinions in Neurology* 9(6):456-460.

Krupp PJ, Lee FY, Bohm JW, Nicholls RA, Batson HW. (1975). Therapy of advanced epidermoid carcinoma of vulva: Report of 13 patients, with review of recent literature. *Obstetrics and Gynecology* 46(4):433-438.

Kryeger JM. (1995). Cytokines and sleep. *International Archives of Allergy and Immunology* 106:97-100.

Kryger M, Shapiro CM. (1992). Pain and distress at night. *Sleep Solutions* 5:1-20.

Kudoh S, Sawa T, Kurihara N, Furuse K, Kurita Y, Fukuoka M, Takada M, Takaku F, Ogawa M, Ariyoshi Y. (1996). Phase II study of recombinant human interleukin 3 administration following carboplatin and etoposide chemotherapy in small-cell lung cancer patients. SDZ ILE 964 (IL-3) Study. *Cancer Chemotherapy Pharmacology* 38(Suppl):S89-S95.

Kudoh S, Yamada M. (1998). [Cytokine in cancer chemotherapy—Clinical trials of IL-3, IL-11 and thrombopoietin against thrombocytopenia]. *Gan To Kagaku Ryoho* 25(2):171-176.

Kuehn R, Rajewsky K, Mueller W. (1991). Generation and analysis of interleukin-4 deficient mice. *Science* 254:713-716.

Kuenstner S, Langelotz C, Budach V, Possinger K, Krause B, Sezer O. (2002). The comparability of quality of life scores. a multitrait multimethod analysis of the EORTC QLQ-C30, SF-36 and FLIC questionnaires. *European Journal of Cancer* 38(3):339-348.

Kuhn JG. (2002). Chemotherapy-associated hematopoietic toxicity. *American Journal of Health System and Pharmacy* 59(15 Suppl 4):S4-S7.

Kuhn P. (2000). [Fibromyalgia at the crossroads of rheumatology, psychology and social work] La fibromyalgie au carrefour de la rheumatologie, de la psychologie et des assurances sociales. *R. Darioli et J. Perdrix, RMSR,* 120:471-474.

Kuhn R, Rakewski K, Muller W. (1991). Generation and analysis of interleukin-4-deficient mice. *Science* 254:707-710.

Kujala UM, Taimela S, Viljanen T. (1999). Leisure physical activity and various pain symptoms among adolescents. *British Journal of Sports Medicine* 33(5): 325-328.

Kukita K, Shirakawa T, Kojima A, Yoshida H, Yoshida K, Tokuomi H, Kurano R. (1992). [An autopsy case of pulmonary metastasis of cholangiocellular carcinoma associated with marked fibrotic change of the lungs]. *Nihon Kyobu Shikkan Gakkai Zasshi* 30(9):1738-1742.

Kulig JW. (1991). Chronic fatigue syndrome and fibromyalgia in adolescence. *Adolescent Medicine* 2(3):473-484.

Kullavanijaya P, Kulthanan K. (1990). Malignant histiocytosis with panniculitis— A case report. *Journal of Dermatology* 17(7):435-439.

Kuller LH. (1995). The etiology of breast cancer—From epidemiology to prevention. *Public Health Reviews* 23:157-213.

Kullo IJ, Gau GT, Tajik J. (2000). Novel risk factors for atherosclerosis. *Mayo Clinic Proceedings* 75:369-380.

Kumar VP, Kuttan R, Kuttan G. (1999a). Effect of "rasayanas," a herbal drug preparation on cell-mediated immune responses in tumour bearing mice. *Indian Journal of Experimental Biology* 37(1):23-26.

Kumar VP, Kuttan R, Kuttan G. (1999b). Effect of "rasayanas," a herbal drug preparation on immune responses and its significance in cancer treatment. *Indian Journal of Experimental Biology* 37(1):27-31.

Kumita S, Nishimura T, Hayashida K, Uehara T, Mitani I, Yamagami H, Okizuka H, Imakita M. (1989). [Pericardial fibrosarcoma demonstrated by Ga-67 scintigraphy]. *Kaku Igaku* 26(6):787-792.

Kundig TM, Schorle H, Bachmann MF, Hengartner H, Zinkernagel RM, Horak I. (1993). Immune responses in interleukin-2-deficient mice. *Science* 262:1059-1061.

Kunikane H, Kurita Y, Watanabe K, Yokoyama A, Noda K, Fujita Y, Yoneda S, Nakai Y, Niitani H. (2001). A study of the combination of gemcitabine hydrochloride (LY188011) and cisplatin in non-small-cell lung cancer: 3-week schedule. *International Journal of Clinical Oncology* 6(6):284-290.

Kunkel EJ, Bakker JR, Myers RE, Oyesanmi O, Gomella LG. (2000). Biopsychosocial aspects of prostate cancer. *Psychosomatics* 41(2):85-94.

Kunkel EJ, Myers RE, Lartey PL, Oyesanmi O. (2000). Communicating effectively with the patient and family about treatment options for prostate cancer. *Seminars in Urology and Oncology* 18(3):233-240.

Kurata T, Shimada Y, Tamura T, Yamamoto N, Hyodo I, Saeki T, Takashima S, Fujiwara K, Wakasugi H, Kashimura M. (2000). Phase I and pharmacokinetic study of a new taxoid, RPR 109881A, given as a 1-hour intravenous infusion in patients with advanced solid tumors. *Journal of Clinical Oncology* 18(17):3164-3171.

Kuratsune H, Yamaguti K, Lindh G, Evengard B, Takahashi M, Machii T, Matsumura K, Takaishi J, Kawata S, Langstrom B, et al. (1998). Low levels of serum acylcarnitine in chronic fatigue syndrome and chronic hepatitis type C, but not seen in other diseases. *International Journal of Molecular Medicine* 2(1):51-56.

Kurie JM, Lee JS, Griffin T, Lippman SM, Drum P, Thomas MP, Weber C, Bader M, Massimini G, Hong WK. (1996). Phase I trial of 9-cis retinoic acid in adults with solid tumors. *Clinical Cancer Research* 2(2):287-293.

Kurihara K, Nagai H, Kasahara K, Kawai T, Saito K, Kanazawa K. (2000). Pleomorphic carcinoma of the pancreas with massive lymphocytic stromal infiltration and long-term survival after resection. *International Journal of Pancreatology* 27(3):241-248.

Kurihara M, Izumi T, Denda T, Mahara K, Isomura S, Hanada E. (1990). [Quality of life in gastrointestinal cancer chemotherapy—From the standpoint of cancer chemotherapy]. *Gan To Kagaku Ryoho* 17(4 Pt 2):887-894.

Kurita A, Takashima S, Sakakihara Y, Tsunekawa K, Matsuzaka T. (1993). [Efficacy of FEM (5-fluorouracil, epirubicin, mitomycin C) therapy for resected advanced gastric cancer. Ehime Gastric Cancer Study Meeting]. *Gan To Kagaku Ryoho* 20(15):2319-2324.

Kuriya K, Ono S, Shiba T, Watanabe K. (1996). [QOL after radiotherapy for esophageal cancer]. *Nippon Igaku Hoshasen Gakkai Zasshi* 56(8):564-569.

Kuroda H, Kishimoto T, Yasunaga Y, Takatera H, Fujioka H, Kosugi K, Tsujimoto M. (1992). [Retroperitoneal giant malignant fibrous histiocytoma: Report of a case]. *Hinyokika Kiyo* 38(10):1143-1146.

Kuroda M, Kotake T, Sonoda T, Maekawa M, Okajima E, Okawa T, Ikoma F, Kurita T, Nakamura T, Itatani H, et al. (1985). [The clinical evaluation of hochuekkito for symptoms of malignant neoplasm patients]. *Hinyokika Kiyo* 31(1):173-177.

Kuroi K, Bando H, Nagai S, Tanaka C, Hayashi K, Toi M. (2001). [Efficacy of weekly docetaxel therapy for advanced or recurrent breast cancer]. *Gan To Kagaku Ryoho* 28(6):797-802.

Kurt RA, Park JA, Panell MC, Schluter SF, Marchalonis JJ, Carolus B, Akporiaye ET. (1995). T lymphocytes infiltrating sites of tumor rejection and progression display identical V beta usage but different cytotoxic activities. *Journal of Immunology* 154:3969-3974.

Kurtz ME, Given B, Kurtz JC, Given CW. (1994). The interaction of age, symptoms, and survival status on physical and mental health of patients with cancer and their families. *Cancer* 74(7 Suppl):2071-2078.

Kurtz ME, Kurtz JC, Given CC, Given B. (1996). Concordance of cancer patient and caregiver symptom reports. *Cancer Practice* 4(4):185-190.

Kurtz ME, Kurtz JC, Given CW, Given B. (1993). Loss of physical functioning among patients with cancer: A longitudinal view. *Cancer Practice* 1(4):275-281.

Kurtze N, Gundersen KT, Svebak S. (1998). The role of anxiety and depression in fatigue and patterns of pain among subgroups of fibromyalgia patients. *British Journal of Medical Psychology* 71(Pt 2):185-194.

Kurtze N, Gundersen KT, Svebak S. (1999). Quality of life, functional disability and lifestyle among subgroups of fibromyalgia patients: The significance of anxiety and depression. *British Journal of Medical Psychology* 72(Pt 4):471-484.

Kurzrock R. (2001). The role of cytokines in cancer-related fatigue. *Cancer* 92 (6 Suppl):1684-1688.

Kurzrock R, Feinberg B, Talpaz M, Saks S, Gutterman JU. (1989). Phase I study of a combination of recombinant tumor necrosis factor-alpha and recombinant interferon-gamma in cancer patients. *Journal of Interferon Research* 9(4):435-444.

Kurzrock R, Rosenblum MG, Quesada JR, Sherwin SA, Itri LM, Gutterman JU. (1986). Phase I study of a combination of recombinant interferon-alpha and recombinant interferon-gamma in cancer patients. *Journal of Clinical Oncology* 4(11):1677-1683.

Kurzrock R, Rosenblum MG, Sherwin SA, Rios A, Talpaz M, Quesada JR, Gutterman JU. (1985). Pharmacokinetics, single-dose tolerance, and biological activity of recombinant gamma-interferon in cancer patients. *Cancer Research* 45(6): 2866-2872.

Kuuppelomaki M, Lauri S. (1998). Cancer patients' reported experiences of suffering. *Cancer Nursing* 21(5):364-369.

Kuzel TM, Kies MS, Wu N, Hsieh YC, Rademaker AW. (2002). Phase I trial of oral estramustine and 3-hr infusional paclitaxel for the treatment of hormone refractory prostate cancer. *Cancer Investigation* 20(5-6):634-643.

Kuzmits R, Ludwig H, Legenstein E, Szekeresz T, Kratzik C, Hofbauer J. (1986). Neopterin as tumor marker: Serum and urinary neopterin concentrations in malignant diseases. *Journal of Clinical Chemistry and Clinical Biochemistry* 24: 119-124.

Kuzmits R, Rumpold H, Muller MM, Schopf G. (1986). The use of biolumiscence to evaluate the influence of chemotherapeutic drugs on ATP levels of malignant cell lines. *Journal of Clinical Chemistry and Clinical Biochemistry* 24:293-298.

Kwon BS, Haq AK, Pomerantz SH, Halaban R. (1987). Isolation and sequence of a cDNA for human tyrosinase that maps at the mouse c-albinolocus. *Proceedings of the National Academy of Sciences of the United States of America* 84:7473-7477.

Kyle RA. (1999). Clinical aspects of multiple myeloma and related disorders including amyloidosis. *Pathology and Biology* 47(2):148-157.

Kyle RA, Bayrd ED. (1975). Amyloidosis: Review of 236 cases. *Medicine* 54(4): 271-299.

Kyriaki M, Eleni T, Efi P, Ourania K, Vassilios S, Lambros V. (2001). The EORTC core quality of life questionnaire (QLQ-C30, version 3.0) in terminally ill cancer patients under palliative care: Validity and reliability in a Hellenic sample. *International Journal of Cancer* 94(1):135-139.

LaBan MM, Martin T, Pechur J, Sarnacki S. (1998). Physical and occupational therapy in the treatment of patients with multiple sclerosis. *Physical Medicine and Rehabilitation Clinics of North America* 9(3):603-614.

Labianca R, Pancera G, Tedeschi L, Dallavalle G, Luporini A, Luporini G. (1992). High dose alpha-2b interferon + folinic acid in the modulation of 5-fluorouracil: A phase II study in advanced colorectal cancer with evidence of an unfavourable cost/benefit ratio. *Tumori* 78(1):32-34.

Labots E, Puhlmann G. (1997). Report action on fatigue and its consequences. *Oncologica* 14(2):29-32.

LaChapelle FL, Finlayson MA. (1998). Brain injury and healthy controls. *Brain Injury* 12(8):649-659.

Lagaye S, Vexiau P, Morozov V, Guenebaut-Claudet V, Tobaly-Tapiero J, Canivet M, Cathelineau G, Peries J, Emanoil-Ravier R. (1992). Human spumavirus-related sequences in the DNA of leukocytes from patients with Graves disease. *Proceedings of the National Academy of Sciences of the United States of America* 89(21):10070-10074.

Lahita RG. (1982). Sex hormones and immunity. In *Basic and Clinical Immunology,* Stites DP, Stobo JD, Fudenberg HH, eds. Los Altos, CA: Lange, pp. 293-294.

Lai CL, Lau JY, Wu PC, Ngan H, Chung HT, Mitchell SJ, Corbett TJ, Chow AW, Lin HJ. (1993). Recombinant interferon-alpha in inoperable hepatocellular carcinoma: A randomized controlled trial. *Hepatology* 17(3):389-394.

Lai S, Goldman JA, Child AH, Engel A, Lamm SH. (2000). Fibromyalgia, hypermobility, and breast implants. *Journal of Rheumatology* 27(9):2237-2241.

Lakein DA, Fantie BD, Grafman J, Ross S, O'Fallon A, Dale J, Straus SE. (1997). Patients with chronic fatigue syndrome and accurate feeling-of-knowing judgments. *Journal of Clinical Psychology* 53(7):635-645.

Lakusta CM, Atkinson MJ, Robinson JW, Nation J, Taenzer PA, Campo MG. (2001). Quality of life in ovarian cancer patients receiving chemotherapy. *Gynecological Oncology* 81(3):490-495.

LaManca JJ, Sisto SA, DeLuca J, Johnson SK, Lange G, Pareja J, Cook S, Natelson BH. (1998). Influence of exhaustive treadmill exercise on cognitive functioning in chronic fatigue syndrome. *American Journal of Medicine* 105(3A):59S-65S.

LaManca JJ, Sisto SA, Zhou X, Ottenweller JE, Cook S, Peckerman A, Zhang Q, Denny TN, Gause WC, Natelson BH. (1999). Immunological response in chronic fatigue syndrome following a graded exercise test to exhaustion. *Journal of Clinical Immunology* 19(2):135-142.

Lamb HM, Adkins JC. (1998). Letrozole: A review of its use in postmenopausal women with advanced breast cancer. *Drugs* 56(6):1125-1140.

Lamm DL. (1985). Bacillus Calmette-Guérin immunotherapy for bladder cancer. *Journal of Urology* 134(1):40-47.

Lamm DL, Stogdill VD, Stogdill BJ, Crispen RG. (1985). Complications of bacillus Calmette-Guérin immunotherapy in 1,278 patients with bladder cancer. *Journal of Urology* 135:272.

Lamm SH. (1997). Antipolymer antibodies, silicone breast implants, and fibromyalgia. *Lancet* 349(9059):1170-1171; discussion 1172-1173.

Landay AL, Jessop C, Lennette ET, Levy JA. (1991). Chronic fatigue syndrome: Clinical condition associated with immune activation. *Lancet* 338:707-712.

Lands R, Foust J. (1996). Renal cell carcinoma and autoimmune hemolytic anemia. *Southern Medical Journal* 89(4):444-445.

Lane RJ, Barrett MC, Taylor DJ, Kemp GJ, Lodi R. (1998). Heterogeneity in chronic fatigue syndrome: Evidence from magnetic resonance spectroscopy of muscle. *Neuromuscular Disorders* 8(3-4):204-209.

Lane RJ, Barrett MC, Woodrow D, Moss J, Fletcher R, Archard LC. (1998). Muscle fibre characteristics and lactate responses to exercise in chronic fatigue syndrome. *Journal of Neurology, Neurosurgery and Psychiatry* 64(3):362-367.

Lane TJ, Manu P, Matthews DA. (1988). Prospective diagnostic evaluation of adults with chronic fatigue. *Clinical Research* 36:714A.

Lang B, Vincent A. (1996). Autoimmunity to ion channels and other proteins in paraneoplastic disorders. *Current Opinions in Immunology* 8:865-871.

Lange G, Wang S, DeLuca J, Natelson BH. (1998). Neuroimaging in chronic fatigue syndrome. *American Journal of Medicine* 105(3A):50S-53S.

Langendijk JA, Aaronson NK, De Jong JM, ten Velde GP, Muller MJ, Lamers RJ, Slotman BJ, Wouters EF. (2001). Prospective study on quality of life before and after radical radiotherapy in non-small-cell lung cancer. *Journal of Clinical Oncology* 19(8):2123-2133.

Langendijk JA, Aaronson NK, De Jong JM, ten Velde GP, Muller MJ, Slotman BJ, Wouters EF. (2002). Quality of life after curative radiotherapy in stage I non-small-cell lung cancer. *International Journal of Radiation Oncology, Biology, and Physics* 53(4):847-853.

Langendijk JA, Aaronson NK, ten Velde GP, de Jong JM, Muller MJ, Wouters EF. (2000). Pretreatment quality of life of inoperable non-small cell lung cancer patients referred for primary radiotherapy. *Acta Oncologica* 39(8):949-958.

Langendijk JA, ten Velde GP, Aaronson NK, de Jong JM, Muller MJ, Wouters EF. (2000). Quality of life after palliative radiotherapy in non-small cell lung cancer: A prospective study. *International Journal of Radiation Oncology Biology and Physics* 47(1):149-155.

Langer CJ. (2002). Elderly patients with lung cancer: Biases and evidence. *Current Treatment Options in Oncology* 3(1):85-102.

Langer CJ, Leighton JC, Comis RL, O'Dwyer PJ, McAleer CA, Bonjo CA, Engstrom PF, Litwin S, Johnson S, Ozols RF. (1995). Paclitaxel by 24- or 1-hour infusion in combination with carboplatin in advanced non-small cell lung cancer: The Fox Chase Cancer Center experience. *Seminars in Oncology* 22(4 Suppl 9): 18-29.

Langer CJ, Leighton J, McAleer C, Comis R, O'Dwyer P, Ozols R. (1995). Paclitaxel and carboplatin in the treatment of advanced non-small cell lung cancer. *Seminars in Oncology* 22(3 Suppl 6):64-69.

Langer CJ, Schaebler D, Sauter E, DeMaria D, Johnson C, Reilly DM, Clark J, Leighton J, Aks C, Litwin S, et al. (1998). Phase II study of *N*-phosphonacetyl-L-aspartate, recombinant interferon-alpha, and fluorouracil infusion in advanced squamous cell carcinoma of the head and neck. *Head and Neck* 20(5):385-391.

Langworth S, Stromberg R. (1996). A case of high mercury exposure from dental amalgam. *European Journal of Oral Science* 104(3):320-321.

Lapp CW. (1997). Exercise limits in chronic fatigue syndrome. *American Journal of Medicine* 103(1):83-84.

Lapp CW, Hyman HL. (1997). Diagnosis of chronic fatigue syndrome. *Archives of Internal Medicine* 157(22):2663-2664.

Lappin TR, Maxwell AP, Johnston PG. (2002). EPO's alter ego: Erythropoietin has multiple actions. *Stem Cells* 20(6):485-492.

Laroche M, Tack Y. (1999). Hypophosphoremia secondary to idiopathic moderate phosphate diabetes: A differential diagnosis with primary fibromyalgia. *Clinical and Experimental Rheumatology* 17(5):628.

Larsen B, Otto H, Dorscheid E, Larsen R. (1999). [Effects of long-term opioid therapy on psychomotor function in patients with cancer pain or non-malignant pain]. *Anaesthesist* 48(9):613-624.

Laser T. (1998). [Comment on W. Hausotter: Fibromyalgia—a dispensable disease concept? (letter)] Zu W. Hausotter: Fibromyalgie—ein entbehrlciher krankheitsbegriff? *Versicherungsmedizin* 50(4):154-156.

Latash M, Kalugina E, Nicholas J, Orpett C, Stefoski D, Davis F. (1996). Myogenic and central neurogenic factors in fatigue in multiple sclerosis. *Multiple Sclerosis* 1(4):236-241.

Lauritzen AF, Delsol G, Hansen NE, Horn T, Ersboll J, Hou-Jensen K, Ralfkiaer E. (1994). Histiocytic sarcomas and monoblastic leukemias: A clinical, histologic, and immunophenotypical study. *American Journal of Clinical Pathology* 102 (1):45-54.

Lautenschlager J. (2000). Present state of medication therapy in fibromyalgia syndrome. *Scandinavian Journal of Rheumatology* 113:32-36.

La Verde G, Arienti D. (2002). [Cancer-related fatigue in hematological cancer: Hematologist's and patient's view]. *Recenti Progressi Medizina* 93(9):463-469.

Lavey RS. (1998). Clinical trial experience using erythropoietin during radiation therapy. *Strahlentherapie Onkologie* 174(Suppl 4):24-30.

Lavietes MH, Bergen MT, Natelson BH. (1998). Measurement of CO_2 in chronic fatigue syndrome patients. *Journal of Chronic Fatigue Syndrome* 4(3):3-12.

Lavrenkov K, Man S, Geffen DB, Cohen Y. (2002). Experience of hormonal therapy with anastrozole for previously treated metastatic breast cancer. *Israeli Medical Association Journal* 4(3):176-177.

Lawlor PG, Nekolaichuk C, Gagnon B, Mancini IL, Pereira JL, Bruera ED. (2000). Clinical utility, factor analysis, and further validation of the memorial delirium assessment scale in patients with advanced cancer: Assessing delirium in advanced cancer. *Cancer* 88(12):2859-2867.

Lawrence CC, Gilbert CJ, Peters WP. (1996). Evaluation of symptom distress in a bone marrow transplant outpatient environment. *Annals of Pharmacotherapy* 30(9):941-945.

Lawrence TS, Dworzanin LM, Walker-Andrews SC, Andrews JC, Ten Haken RK, Wollner IS, Lichter AS, Ensminger WD. (1991). Treatment of cancers involving the liver and porta hepatis with external beam irradiation and intraarterial hepatic fluorodeoxyuridine. *International Journal of Radiation Oncology, Biology and Physics* 20(3):555-561.

Laylander JA. (1999a). A nutrient/toxin interaction theory of the etiology and pathogenesis of chronic pain-fatigue syndromes: Part I. *Journal of Chronic Fatigue Syndrome* 4(2):77-108.

Laylander JA. (1999b). A nutrient/toxin interaction theory of the etiology and pathogenesis of chronic pain-fatigue syndromes: Part II. *Journal of Chronic Fatigue Syndrome* 5(1):93-126.

Layzer RB. (1998). Asthenia and the chronic fatigue syndrome. *Muscle and Nerve* 21(12):1609-1611.

Leavitt M, Martinson IM, Liu CY, Armstrong V, Hornberger L, Zhang JQ, Han XP. (1999). Common themes and ethnic differences in family caregiving the first year after diagnosis of childhood cancer: Part II. *Journal of Pediatric Nursing* 14(2):110-122.

Leddy SK. (1997). Healthiness, fatigue, and symptom experience in women with and without breast cancer. *Holistic Nursing Practice* 12(1):48-53.

Lederberg J. (2000). Infectious history. *Science* 288:287-293.

Lee CK, Han SS, Mo YK, Kim RS, Chung MH, Park YI, Lee SK, Kim YS. (1997). Prevention of ultraviolet radiation-induced suppression of accessory cell function of Langerhans cells by *Aloë vera* gel components. *Immunopharmacology* 37(2-3):153-162.

Lee CT, Wu MS, Lu K, Hsu KT. (1999). Renal tubular acidosis, hypokalemic paralysis, rhabdomyolysis, and acute renal failure—A rare presentation of Chinese herbal nephropathy. *Renal Failure* 21(2):227-230.

Lee E, Park KK, Lee JM, Chun KS, Kang JY, Lee SS, Surh YJ. (1998). Suppression of mouse skin tumor promotion and induction in apoptosis in HL-60 cells by *Alpinia oxyphylla* Miquel (Zingiberaceae). *Carcinogenesis* 19(8):1377-1381.

Lee EH. (2001). Fatigue and hope: Relationships to psychosocial adjustment in Korean women with breast cancer. *Applied Nursing Research* 14(2):87-93.

Lee I-M. (1994). Physical activity, fitness and cancer. In *Physical Activity, Fitness and Health,* Bouchard C, Shephard R, Stephens T, eds. Champaign, IL: Human Kinetics, pp. 814-831.

Lee I-M. (1995). Exercise and physical health: Cancer and immune function. *Research Quarterly* 66:286-291.

Lee JE, Lowy AM, Thompson WA, Lu M, Loflin PT, Skibber JM, Evans DB, Curley SA, Mansfield PF, Reveille JD. (1996). Association of gastric adenocarcinoma with HLA class II gene DQB1*0301. *Gastroenterology* 111:426-432.

Lee KA. (2001). Sleep and fatigue. *Annual Reviews of Nursing Research* 19:249-273.

Lee KA, Hicks G, Nino-Murcia G. (1991). Validity and reliability of a scale to assess fatigue. *Psychiatry Research* 36:291-298.

Lee L. (1999). Introducing herbal medicine into conventional health care settings. *Journal of Nurse-Midwifery* 44(3):253-266.

Lee MJ, Lee OH, Yoon SH, Lee SK, Chung MH, Park YI, Sung CK, Choi JS, Kim KW. (1998). In vitro angiogenic activity of *Aloë vera* gel on calf pulmonary artery endothelial (CPAE) cells. *Archives of Pharmeceutical Research* 21(3):260-265.

Lee P. (1998). Recent developments in chronic fatigue syndrome. *American Journal of Medicine* 105(3A):1S.

Lee PP, Zeng D, McCaulay AE, Chen YF, Geiler C, Umetsu DT, Chao NJ. (1997). T helper 2-dominant antilymphoma immune response is associated with fatal outcome. *Blood* 90:1611-1617.

Lee TL. (2000). Acupuncture and chronic pain management. *Annals of the Academy of Medicine of Singapore* 29(1):17-21.

Lee YC, Sutton FJ, Cohen ML, Green DC. (1985). Insidious onset of fatigue, dyspnea, and leg edema. *Archives of Internal Medicine* 145(10):1893-1894.

Le Gal M, Cathebras P, Strüby K. (1996). Pharmaton capsules in the treatment of functional fatigue: A double-blind study versus placebo evaluated by a new methodology. *Phytotherapy Research* 10:49-53.

Leger-Ravet MB, Borgonovo G, Amato A, Lemaigre G, Franco D. (1996). Carcinosarcoma of the liver with mesenchymal differentiation: A case report. *Hepatogastroenterology* 43(7):255-259.

Legha SS, Papadopoulos NE, Plager C, Ring S, Chawla SP, Evans LM, Benjamin RS. (1987). Clinical evaluation of recombinant interferon alfa-2a (Roferon-A) in metastatic melanoma using two different schedules. *Journal of Clinical Oncology* 5(8):1240-1246.

Le Grand SB. (2002). Cancer fatigue—More data, less information? *Current Oncological Reports* 4(4):275-279.

Lehmann M, Foster C, Dickhuth HH, Gastmann U. (1998). Autonomic imbalance hypothesis and overtraining syndrome. *Medical Science in Sports and Exercise* 30(7):1140-1145.

Lehto RH, Cimprich B. (1999). Anxiety and directed attention in women awaiting breast cancer surgery. *Oncology Nursing Forum* 26(4):767-772.

Leiby JM, Unverfurth DV, Neidhart JA. (1986). High-dose mitoxantrone in metastatic breast cancer: A phase I-II trial. *Cancer Treatment Reports* 70(7):899-901.

Leigh TJ, Hindmarch I, Bird HA, Wright V. (1998). Comparison of sleep in osteoarthritis patients and age-sex matched healthy controls. *Annals of Rheumatic Diseases* 47:40-42.

Leitgeb C, Pecherstorfer M, Fritz E, Ludwig H. (1994). Quality of life in chronic anemia of cancer during treatment with recombinant human erythropoietin. *Cancer* 73(10):2535-2542.

Lekander M, Fredrikson M, Wik G. (2000). Neuroimmune relations in patients with fibromyalgia: A positron emission tomography study. *Neurosciences Letters* 282(3):193-196.

LeMoine L. (1997). Essiac: An historical perspective. *Canadian Oncology Nursing Journal* 7(4):216-221.

Lengyel P. (1982). Biochemistry of interferons and their actions. *Annual Reviews of Biochemistry* 51:251-282.

Lentjes EG, Griep EN, Boersma JW, Romijn FP, De Kloet ER. (1997). Glucocorticoid receptors, fibromyalgia and low back pain. *Psychoneuroendocrinology* 22(8):603-614.

Lentz MJ, Landis CA, Rothermel J, Shaver JL. (1999). Effects of selective slow wave sleep disruption on musculoskeletal pain and fatigue in middle aged women. *Journal of Rheumatology* 26(7):1586-1592.

Leonard RC, Cameron DA, Anderson A, Ostrowski J, Howell A. (2000). Idarubicin and cyclophosphamide—An active oral chemotherapy regimen for advanced breast cancer. *Critical Reviews in Oncology and Hematology* 33(1):61-66.

Leonhardt T. (2000). [Fibromyalgia—a new name of an old "malady": Fatigue and pain syndrome with a historical background] Fibromyalgi—nytt namn pa gammal "sjuka": Trotthets-och smartsyndrome med historisk bakgrung. *Lakartidningen* 97(21):2618-2620, 2623-2624.

Leslie M. (1999). Fibromyalgia syndrome: A comprehensive approach to identification and management. *Clinical Excellence in Nurse Practice* 3(3):165-171.

Levenson T, Greenberger PA, Murphy R. (1996). Peripheral blood eosinophilia, hyperimmunoglobulinemia A and fatigue: Possible complications following rupture of silicone breast implants. *Annals of Allergy, Asthma, and Immunology* 77(2):119-122.

Levine MN, Guyatt GH, Gent M, De Pauw S, Goodyear MD, Hryniuk WM, Arnold A, Findlay B, Skillings JR, Bramwell VH, et al. (1988). Quality of life in stage II breast cancer: An instrument for clinical trials. *Journal of Clinical Oncology* 6(12):1798-1810.

Levine P, Clauw DJ, Claman HC, Robertson AD, Ketch L. (2000). Silicone breast implants, chronic fatigue syndrome and fibromyalgia. *Journal of Chronic Fatigue Syndrome* 7(1):53-74.

Levine PH. (1996). The use of transfer factors in chronic fatigue syndrome: Prospects and problems. *Biotherapy* 9(1-3):77-79.

Levine PH. (1997). Epidemiologic advances in chronic fatigue syndrome. *Journal of Psychiatric Research* 31(1):7-18.

Levine PH. (1998). Chronic fatigue syndrome comes of age. *American Journal of Medicine* 105(3A):2S-6S.

Levine PH, Atherton M, Fears T, Hoover R. (1994). An approach to studies of cancer subsequent to clusters of chronic fatigue syndrome: Use of data from the Nevada State Cancer Registry. *Clinical Infectious Diseases* 18(Suppl1):S49-S53.

Levine PH, Fears TR, Cummings P, Hoover RN. (1998). Cancer and a fatiguing illness in Northern Nevada—A causal hypothesis. *Annals of Epidemiology* 8(4):245-249.

Levine PH, Jacobson S, Pocinki AG, Cheny P, Peterson D, Connelly RR, Weil R, Robinson SM, Ablashi DM, Salahuddin SZ. (1992). Clinical, epidemiologic, and virologic studies in four clusters of the chronic fatigue syndrome. *Archives of Internal Medicine* 152(8):1611-1616.

Levine PH, Peterson D, McNamee FL, O'Brien K, Gridley G, Hagerty M, Brady J, Fears T, Atherton M, Hoover R. (1992). Does chronic fatigue syndrome predispose to non-Hodgkin's lymphoma? *Cancer Research* 52(19 Suppl.):5516s-5518s; discussion 5518s-5521s.

Levine PH, Snow PG, Ranum BA, Paul C, Holmes MJ. (1997). Epidemic neuromyasthenia and chronic fatigue syndrome in West Otago, New Zealand: A 10-year follow-up. *Archives of Internal Medicine* 157(7):750-754.

Levine PH, Whiteside TL, Friberg D, Bryant J, Colclough G, Herberman RB. (1998). Dysfunction of natural killer activity in a family with chronic fatigue syndrome. *Clinical Immunology and Immunopathology* 88(1):96-104.

Levine S. (1999). Borna disease virus proteins in patients with CFS. *Journal of Chronic Fatigue Syndrome* 5(3/4):199-206.

Levy JA, Greenspan D, Ferro F, Lennette ET. (1990). Frequent isolation of HHV-6 from saliva and high seroprevalence of the virus in the population. *Lancet* 335:1047-1050.

Levy S, Herberman R, Lippman M, d'Angelo T. (1987). Correlation of stress factors with sustained depression of natural killer cell activity and predicted prognosis in patients with breast cancer. *Journal of Clinical Oncology* 5(3):348-353.

Lewis NL, Scher R, Gallo JM, Engstrom PF, Szarka CE, Litwin S, Adams AL, Kilpatrick D, Brady D, Weiner LM, et al. (2002). Phase I and pharmacokinetic study of irinotecan in combination with raltitrexed. *Cancer Chemotherapy Pharmacology* 50(4):257-265.

Li C, Homma M, Oka K. (1998). Characteristics of delayed excretion of flavonoids in human urine after administration of Shosaiko-to, a herbal medicine. *Biological Pharmacy Bulletin* 21(12):1251-1257.

Li C, Zou G, Bian H, Ju X. (2001). [Summarization of studies on Chinese marine medicinal animal *Syngnthus acus*]. *Zhong Yao Cai* 24(9):686-688.

Li HY, Qian LS, Feng SZ. (1997). Clinical observation on treatment of complications with Chinese medicine according to syndrome differentiation of post-bone marrow transplantation in 22 patients with leukemia. *Chung Kuo Chung His I Chieh Ho Tsa Chih* 17(10):581-583.

Li T, Tamada K, Abe K, Tada H, Onoe Y, Tatsugami K, Harada M, Kubo C, Nomoto K. (1999). The restoration of the antitumor T-cell response from stress-induced suppression using a traditional Chinese herbal medicine Hocchu-ekki-to (TJ-B4:Bu-Zhong-Yi-Qi-Tang). *Immunopharmacology* 43(1):11-21.

Li XH, Gan XJ, Ji JM. (1996). Clinical observation on aplastic anemia treated with Chinese herbal medicine combined with cord blood infusion. *Chung Kuo Chung His I Chieh Ho Tsa Chih* 16(9):522-524.

Li XS. (1997). Progress in modern research on mechanism of Chinese herbal medicine in the treatment of lumbar intervertebral disc prolapse. *Chung Kuo Chung His I Chieh Ho Tsa Chih* 17(2):122-124.

Libbus MK. (1996). Women's beliefs regarding persistent fatigue. *Issues in Mental Health Nursing* 17(6):589-600.

Libby P, Egan D, Skarlatos S. (1997). Roles of infectious agents in atherosclerosis and restenosis: An assessment of the evidence and need for future research. *Circulation* 96:4095-4103.

Libretto SE, Barrett-Lee PJ, Branson K, Gorst DW, Kaczmarski R, McAdam K, Stevenson P, Thomas R. (2001). Improvement in quality of life for cancer patients treated with epoetin alfa. *European Journal of Cancer Care* 10(3):183-191.

Lichstein KL, Means MK, Noe SL, Aguillard RN. (1997). Fatigue and sleep disorders. *Behaviour Research and Therapy* 35(8):733-740.

Lieb K, Dammann G, Berger M, Bauer J. (1996). Chronic fatigue syndrome: Definition, diagnostic measures and therapeutic possibilities. *Nervenartz* 67(9):711-720.

Lieberman PM. (1990). Infleunza virus vaccine and Epstein-Barr virus infection. *Clinical Ecology* 7(3):51.

Liesen H, Uhlenbruck G. (1992). Sports immunology. *Sport Science Review* 1:94-116.

Lijima K, Sun S, Cyong JC, Jyonouchi H. (1999). Juzen-taiho-to, a Japanese herbal medicine, modulates type 1 and type 2 T-cell responses in old BALB/c mice. *American Journal of Chinese Medicine* 27(2):191-203.

Lilenbaum RC, Schwartz MA, Seigel L, Belette F, Blaustein A, Wittlin FN, Davila E. (2001). Phase II trial of weekly docetaxel in second-line therapy for nonsmall cell lung carcinoma. *Cancer* 92(8):2158-2163.

Lilleaas UB. (1997). [Women's health—When the body breaks down (interview by Marianne Monsen)] Kvinnehelse—nar kroppen gar I stykker. *Tidsskr Sykepl* 85(20):42-43.

Lilleby W, Fossa SD, Waehre HR, Olsen DR. (1999). Long-term morbidity and quality of life in patients with localized prostate cancer undergoing definitive radiotherapy or radical prostatectomy. *International Journal of Radiation Oncology, Biology and Physics* 43(4):735-743.

Lin YC, Chen JS, Wang CH, Wang HM, Chang HK, Liaul CT, Yang TS, Liaw CC, Liu HE. (2001). Weekly high-dose 5-fluorouracil (5-FU), leucovorin (LV) and bimonthly cisplatin in patients with advanced gastric cancer. *Japanese Journal of Clinical Oncology* 31(12):605-609.

Lind M, Vernon C, Cruickshank D, Wilkinson P, Littlewood T, Stuart N, Jenkinson C, Grey-Amante P, Doll H, Wild D. (2002). The level of haemoglobin in anaemic cancer patients correlates positively with quality of life. *British Journal of Cancer* 86(8):1243-1249.

Lind P, Langsteger W, Koltringer P, Eber B, Kammerhuber F, Smolle-Juttner F, Eber O. (1990). Localization of mediastinal parathyroid adenoma by T1-201 scintiscan and SPECT. *Klinische Wochenschrift* 68(9):472-475.

Lindal E, Bergmann S, Thorlacius S, Stefansson JG. (1997). Anxiety disorders: A result of long-term chronic fatigue—The psychiatric characteristics of the sufferers of Iceland disease. *Acta Neurologica Scandinavica* 96(3):158-162.

Lindberg NE, Lindberg E. (2000). [Use available knowledge—also when it is not complete. Current example: Chronic fatigue syndrome, fibromyalgia] Anvand befintlig kunskap—aven nar den ar ofullstandig aktuella exempel: Kroniskt trotthetssyndrom, fibromyalgi. *Lakartidningen* 97(21):2651-2652.

Linde A, Andersson B, Svenson SB, Ahrne H, Carlsson M, Forsberg P, Hugo H, Karstop A, Lenkei R, Lindwall A, et al. (1992). Serum levels of lymphokines and soluble cellular receptors in primary EBV infection and in patients with chronic fatigue syndrome. *Journal of Infectious Diseases* 165:994-1000.

Linde K. (1999). Review: Heterogeneous studies show that echinacea may be effective for preventing and treating the common cold. *American College of Physicians Journal Club* 131(1):19.

Lindelman C, Mellstedt H, Biverfeld P. (1983). Blood and lymph node T-lymphocyte subsets in non-Hodgkin lymphomas. *Scandinavian Journal of Hematology* 30:69-78.

Lindley C, Vasa S, Sawyer WT, Winer EP. (1998). Quality of life and preferences for treatment following systemic adjuvant therapy for early-stage breast cancer. *Journal of Clinical Oncology* 16(4):1380-1387.

Lindley CM, Hirsch JD. (1992). Nausea and vomiting and cancer patients' quality of life: A discussion of Professor Selby's paper. *British Journal of Cancer Supplement* 19:S26-S29.

Ling YC, Teng HC, Cartwright C. (1999). Supercritical fluid extraction and cleanup of organochlorine pesticides in Chinese herbal medicine. *Journal of the Chromatography Association* 835(1-2):145-147.

Lipkin DM, Papernik M, Kaan R. (1997). Chronic fatigue. *American Journal of Psychiatry* 154(9):1322.

Lippi G, Guidi G. (2000). Laboratory screening for erythropoietin abuse in sport: An emerging challenge. *Clinical Chemistry and Laboratory Medicine* 38(1):13-19.

Lippman SM, Parkinson DR, Itri LM, Weber RS, Schantz SP, Ota DM, Schusterman MA, Krakoff IH, Gutterman JU, Hong WK. (1992). 13-cis-retinoic acid and interferon alpha-2a: Effective combination therapy for advanced squamous cell carcinoma of the skin. *Journal of the National Cancer Institutes* 84(4):235-241.

Lipton A, Harvey H, Givant E, Hopper K, Lawler J, Matthews Y, Hirsh M, Zeffren J. (1993). Interleukin-2 and interferon-alpha-2a outpatient therapy for metastatic renal cell carcinoma. *Journal of Immunotherapy* 13(2):122-129.

Liska DJ. (1998). The detoxification enzyme systems. *Alternative Medicine Reviews* 3(3):187-198.

Lissoni P, Giani L, Zerbini S, Trabattoni P, Rovelli F. (1998). Biotherapy with the pineal immunomodulating hormone melatonin versus melatonin plus *Aloë vera* in untreatable advanced solid neoplasms. *Natural Immunity* 16(1):27-33.

Littlejohn GO. (1996). Rheumatology: 2. Fibromyalgia syndrome. *Medical Journal of Australia* 165(7):387-391.

Littlewood T, Mandelli F. (2002). The effects of anemia in hematologic malignancies: More than a symptom. *Seminars in Oncology* 29(3 Suppl 8):40-44.

Littlewood TJ. (2001). Erythropoietin for the treatment of anemia associated with hematological malignancy. *Hematology and Oncology* 19(1):19-30.

Littlewood TJ. (2002). Management options for cancer therapy-related anaemia. *Drug Safety* 25(7):525-535.

Littlewood TJ, Bajetta E, Nortier JW, Vercammen E, Rapoport B, Epoetin Alfa Study Group. (2001). Effects of epoetin alfa on hematologic parameters and quality of life in cancer patients receiving nonplatinum chemotherapy: Results of a randomized, double-blind, placebo-controlled trial. *Journal of Clinical Oncology* 19(11):2865-2874.

Littlewood TJ, Cella D, Nortier JW, Epoetin Alfa Study Group. (2002). Erythropoietin improves quality of life. *Lancet Oncology* 3(8):459-460.

Litwin MS, Lubeck DP, Henning JM, Carroll PR. (1998). Differences in urologist and patient assessments of health related quality of life in men with prostate cancer: Results of the CaPSURE database. *Journal of Urology* 159(6):1988-1992.

Liu X, Song S, Guan Z, Wu S, Duan Y, Yu J, Yang L. (2002). [Capecitabine (Xeloda) in the treatment of relapsed and metastatic breast cancer]. *Zhonghua Zhong Liu Za Zhi* 24(1):71-73.

Llewelyn MB. (1996). Assessing the fatigued patient. *British Journal of Hospital Medicine* 55(3):125-129.

Llewellyn-Thomas HA, Thiel EC, McGreal MJ. (1992). Cancer patients' evaluations of their current health states: The influences of expectations, comparisons, actual health status, and mood. *Medical Decision Making* 12(2):115-122.

Lloyd AR. (1998). Chronic fatigue and chronic fatigue syndrome: Shifting boundaries and attributions. *American Journal of Medicine* 105(3A):7S-10S.

Lloyd AR, Gandevia S, Brockman A, Hales J, Wakefield D. (1994). Cytokine production and fatigue in patients with chronic fatigue syndrome and healthy control subjects in response to exercise. *Clinical Infectious Diseases* 18(Suppl 1): S142-S146.

Lloyd AR, Hanna DA, Wakefield D. (1988). Interferon and myalgic encephalomyelitis. *Lancet* 1:471.

Lloyd AR, Hickie I, Brockman A, Hickie C, Wilson A, Dwyer J, Wakefield D. (1993). Immunologic and psychologic therapy for patients with chronic fatigue syndrome: A double-blind, placebo-controlled trial. *American Journal of Medicine* 94(2):197-202.

Lloyd AR, Hickie I, Hickie C, Dwyer J, Wakefield D. (1992). Cell-mediated immunity in patients with chronic fatigue syndrome, healthy controls and patients with major depression. *Clinical and Experimental Immunology* 87(1):76-79.

Lloyd AR, Wakefield D, Boughton CR, Dwyer JM. (1989). Immunological abnormalities in the chronic fatigue syndrome. *Medical Journal of Australia* 151:122-124.

Lodi R, Taylor DJ, Radda GK. (1997). Chronic fatigue syndrome and skeletal muscle mitochondrial function. *Muscle and Nerve* 20(6):765-766.

Loge JH, Abrahamsen AF, Ekeberg O, Kaasa S. (1999). Hodgkin's disease survivors more fatigued than the general population. *Journal of Clinical Oncology* 17(1):253-261.

Loge JH, Abrahamsen AF, Ekeberg O, Kaasa S. (2000). Fatigue and psychiatric morbidity among Hodgkin's disease survivors. *Journal of Pain Symptomatology and Management* 19(2):91-99.

Loge JH, Ekeberg O, Kaasa S. (1998). Fatigue in the general Norwegian population: Normative data and associations. *Journal of Psychosomatic Research* 45:53-65.

Loge JH, Kaasa S. (2000). [Occurrence and diagnosis of psychiatric conditions in palliative medicine]. *Tidsskr Nor Laegeforen* 120(27):3275-3279.

Lohmann K, Prohl A, Schwarz E. (1996). Multiple chemical sensitivity disorder in patients with neurotoxic illnesses. *Gesundheitswesen* 58(6):322-331.

Longman AJ, Braden CJ, Mishel MH. (1996). Side effects burden in women with breast cancer. *Cancer Practice* 4(5):274-280.

Longman AJ, Braden CJ, Mishel MH. (1997). Pattern of association over time of side-effects burden, self-help, and self-care in women with breast cancer. *Oncology Nursing Forum* 24(9):1555-1560.

Longman AJ, Braden CJ, Mishel MH. (1999). Side-effects burden, psychological adjustment, and life quality in women with breast cancer: Pattern of association over time. *Oncology Nursing Forum* 26(5):909-915.

Lopez AM, Ketchum M, Nichols H, Xu MJ, Peng YM, Dorr R, Alberts DS. (2000). A phase I trial of AUC-directed carboplatin with infusional doxorubicin and ifosfamide plus G-CSF in patients with advanced gynecologic malignancies. *Cancer Chemotherapy Pharmacology* 46(5):411-415.

Loprinzi CL, Pisansky TM, Fonseca R, Sloan JA, Zahasky KM, Quella SK, Novotny PJ, Rummans TA, Dumesic DA, Perez EA. (1998). Pilot evaluation of venlafaxine hydrochloride for the therapy of hot flashes in cancer survivors. *Journal of Clinical Oncology* 16(7):2377-2381.

Lotze MT, Grimm E, Mazumder A, Strausser JL, Rosenberg SA. (1981). Lysis of fresh and cultured autologous tumor by human lymphocytes cultured in T-cell growth factor. *Cancer Research* 41:4420-4425.

Louie S, Cai J, Law R, Lin G, Lunardi-Iskandar Y, Jung B, Masood R, Gill P. (1995). Effects of interleukin-1 and interleukin-1 receptor antagonist in AIDS-Kaposi's sarcoma. *Journal of Acquired Immunodeficiency Syndromes* 8:455-460.

Love RR, Vogel VG. (1997). Breast cancer prevention strategies. *Oncology* 11:161-173.

Lovely MP. (1998). Quality of life of brain tumor patients. *Seminars in Oncology Nursing* 14(1):73-80.

Lovely MP, Miaskowski C, Dodd M. (1999). Relationship between fatigue and quality of life in patients with glioblastoma multiformae. *Oncology Nursing Forum* 26(5):921-925.

Lowenthal JW, MacDonald HR. (1987). Binding and internalization of interleukin 1 by T cells: Direct evidence for high- and low-affinity classes of interleukin 1 receptor. *Journal of Experimental Medicine* 164:1060-1074.

Lowes MA, Bishop GA, Crotty K, Barretson RS, Halliday GM. (1997). T helper 1 cytokine mRNA is increased in spontaneously regressing primary melanomas. *Journal of Investigative Dermatology* 108:914-919.

Lu Y, Zheng Q, Wu N, Zhou J, Bao T. (1997). Studies on all-spectrum analysis for X-ray diffraction of Chinese herbal medicine *Calculus bovis. Chung Kuo I Hsueh Ko Hsueh Yuan Hsueh Pao* 19(5):331-336.

Lu YH, Xin CL, Zhou YF, Liu XW, Chi JW, Chang X. (1996). Effect of hedgehog hydnum on the delay of fatigue in mice. *Sheng Li Hsueh Pao—Acta Physiologica Sinica* 48(1):98-101.

Lucas R, Magez S, De Leys R, Fransen L, Scheerlinck J-P, Rampelberg M, Sablon E, De Baetselier P. (1994). Mapping the lectin-like activity of tumor necrosis factor. *Science* 263:814-817.

Ludwig H. (1999). Epoetin in cancer-related anaemia. *Nephrology, Dialysis and Transplantation* 14(Suppl 2):85-92.

Ludwig H. (2002). Anemia of hematologic malignancies: What are the treatment options? *Seminars in Oncology* 29(3 Suppl 8):45-54.

Ludwig H, Cohen AM, Huber H, Nachbaur D, Jungi WF, Senn H, Gunczler P, Schuller J, Eckhardt S, Seewann HL, et al. (1991). Interferon alfa-2b with VMCP compared to VMCP alone for induction and interferon alfa-2b compared to controls for remission maintenance in multiple myeloma: Interim results. *European Journal of Cancer* 27(Suppl 4):S40-S45.

Ludwig H, Fritz E, Leitgeb C, Pecherstorfer M, Samonigg H, Schuster J. (1994). Prediction of response to erythropoietin treatment in chronic anemia of cancer. *Blood* 84(4):1056-1063.

Luebbert K, Dahme B, Hasenbring M. (2001). The effectiveness of relaxation training in reducing treatment-related symptoms and improving emotional adjustment in acute non-surgical cancer treatment: A meta-analytical review. *Psychooncology* 10(6):490-502.

Lugaresi E, Cirignotta F, Zucconi M, Mondini S, Lenzi PL, Coccagna G. (1981). Good and poor sleepers: An epidemiological survey of the San Marino population. In *Sleep/Wake Disorders: Natural history,* Guilleminault C, Lugaresi E, eds. New York: Raven Press, pp. 1-2.

Lumachi F, Zucchetta P, Angelini F, Borsato N, Polistina F, Favia G, D'Amico DF. (2000). Tumors of the parathyroid glands. Changes in clinical features and in noninvasive localization studies sensitivity. *Journal of Experimental and Clinical Cancer Research* 19(1):7-11.

Lundin J, Kimby E, Bergmann L, Karakas T, Mellstedt H, Osterborg A. (2001). Interleukin 4 therapy for patients with chronic lymphocytic leukaemia: A phase I/II study. *British Journal of Haematology* 112(1):155-160.

Lusso P, Salahuddin SZ, Ablashi DV, Gallo RC, Di Marzo Veronese F, Markham PD. (1987). Diverse tropism of HBLV (human herpesvirus 6). *Lancet* 2(8561): 743.

Lustgarten J, Theobald M, Labadie C, Laface D, Peterson P, Disis L, Cheever MA, Sherman LA. (1997). Identification of Her-2/neu CTL epitopes using double transgenic mice expressing HLA-A2.1 and human CD8. *Human Immunology* 52:109-118.

Lutgendorf S, Antoni MH, Ironson G, Fletcher MA, Penendo F, Van Riel F, Baum A, Schneiderman N, Klimas N. (1995). Physical symptoms of chronic fatigue syndrome are exacerbated by the stress of Hurricane Andrew. *Psychosomatic Medicine* 57:310-323.

Lutgendorf S, Klimas N, Antoni M, Brickman A, Fletcher MA. (1995). Relationships of cognitive difficulties to immune measures, depression and illness burden in chronic fatigue syndrome. *Journal of Chronic Fatigue Syndrome* 1:23-41.

Lutgendorf SK, Anderson B, Rothrock N, Buller RE, Sood AK, Sorosky JI. (2000). Quality of life and mood in women receiving extensive chemotherapy for gynecologic cancer. *Cancer* 89(6):1402-1411.

Lutz ST, Huang DT, Ferguson CL, Kavanagh BD, Tercilla OF, Lu J. (1997). A retrospective quality of life analysis using the Lung Cancer Symptom Scale in patients treated with palliative radiotherapy for advanced nonsmall cell lung cancer. *International Journal of Radiation Oncology, Biology and Physics* 37(1):117-122.

Lutz ST, Norrell R, Bertucio C, Kachnic L, Johnson C, Arthur D, Schwarz M, Palardy G. (2001). Symptom frequency and severity in patients with metastatic or locally recurrent lung cancer: A prospective study using the Lung Cancer Symptom Scale in a community hospital. *Journal of Palliative Medicine* 4(2): 157-165.

Luzuriaga K, Koup R, Pikora C, Brettler D, Sullivan J. (1991). Deficient human immunodeficiency virus type-1-specific cytotoxic T cell responses in vertically infected children. *Journal of Pediatrics* 119:230-236.

Lynch G, Kemeny N, Chun H, Martin D, Young C. (1985). Phase I evaluation and pharmacokinetic study of weekly iv thymidine and 5-FU in patients with advanced colorectal carcinoma. *Cancer Treatment Reports* 69(2):179-184.

Lynch JW, Hei DL, Braylan RC, Rimzsa LM, Staab EV, Bewsher CJ, Mendenhall NP, Hudson JK. (2002). Phase II study of fludarabine combined with interferon-alpha-2a followed by maintenance therapy with interferon-alpha-2a in patients with low-grade non-Hodgkin's lymphoma. *American Journal of Clinical Oncology* 25(4):391-397.

Lynch JW, Smith GD, Kaplan GA, House JS. (2000). Income inequality and mortality: Importance to health of individual income, psychosocial environment, or material conditions. *British Medical Journal* 320:1200-1204.

Lynch TJ Jr. (2001). Review of two phase II randomized trials of single-agent docetaxel in previously treated advanced non-small cell lung cancer. *Seminars in Oncology* 28(3 Suppl 9):5-9.

MacAvoy S, Moritz D. (1992). Nursing diagnoses in an oncology population. *Cancer Nursing* 15(4):264-270.

Macbeth FR, Bolger JJ, Hopwood P, Bleehen NM, Cartmell J, Girling DJ, Machin D, Stephens RJ, Bailey AJ. (1996). Randomized trial of palliative two-fraction versus more intensive 13-fraction radiotherapy for patients with inoperable non-small cell lung cancer and good performance status. Medical Research Council Lung Cancer Working Party. *Clinical Oncology* 8(3):167-175.

MacDonald KL, Osterholm MT, LeDell KH, White KE, Schenck CH, Chao CC, Persing DH, Johnson RC, Barker JM, Peterson PK. (1996). A case-control study to assess possible triggers and cofactors in chronic fatigue syndrome. *American Journal of Medicine* 100(5):548-554.

MacFarlane GJ, Croft PR, Schollum J, Silman AJ. (1996). Widespread pain: Is an improved classification possible? *Journal of Rheumatology* 23(9):1628-1632.

MacFarlane GJ, Lowenfels AB. (1994). Physical activity and colon cancer. *European Journal of Cancer Prevention* 3:393-398.

MacFarlane JG, Shahal B, Mously C, Moldofsky H. (1996). Periodic K-alpha sleep EEG activity and periodic limb movements during sleep: Comparisons of clinical features and sleep parameters. *Sleep* 19(3):200-204.

MacHale SM, Cavanaugh JT, Bennie J, Carroll S, Goodwin GM, Lawrie SM. (1998). Diurnal variation of adrenocortical activity in chronic fatigue syndrome. *Neuropsychobiology* 38(4):213-217.

Machida T, Koiso K, Takaku F, Ogawa M. (1987). [Phase II study of recombinant human interferon gamma (S-6810) in renal cell carcinoma. Urological Cooperative Study Group of Recombinant Human Interferon Gamma (S-6810)]. *Gan To Kagaku Ryoho* 14(2):440-445.

Mackay CR. (1992). Migration pathways and immunologic memory among T lymphocytes. *Seminars in Immunology* 4:51-58.

Mackay CR, Martson WL, Dudler L. (1990). Naïve and memory T cells show distinct pathways of lymphocyte recirculation. *Journal of Experimental Medicine* 171:801-817.

Macquart-Moulin G, Viens P, Genre D, Bouscary ML, Resbeut M, Gravis G, Camerlo J, Maraninchi D, Moatti JP. (1999). Concomitant chemoradiotherapy for patients with nonmetastatic breast carcinoma: Side effects, quality of life, and organization. *Cancer* 85(10):2190-2199.

Macquart-Moulin G, Viens P, Palangie T, Bouscary ML, Delozier T, Roche H, Janvier M, Fabbro M, Moatti JP. (2000). High-dose sequential chemotherapy with recombinant granulocyte colony-stimulating factor and repeated stem-cell support for inflammatory breast cancer patients: Does impact on quality of life jeopardize feasibility and acceptability of treatment? *Journal of Clinical Oncology* 18(4):754-764.

Madden T, Tran HT, Beck D, Huie R, Newman RA, Pusztai L, Wright JJ, Abbruzzese JL. (2000). Novel marine-derived anticancer agents: A phase I clinical, pharmacological, and pharmacodynamic study of dolastatin 10 (NSC 376128) in patients with advanced solid tumors. *Clinical Cancer Research* 6(4):1293-1301.

Maeda H, Shiraishi A. (1996). TGF-beta contributes to the shift toward Th2-type responses through direct and IL-10-mediated pathways in tumor-bearing mice. *Journal of Immunology* 156:73-78.

Maehara N, Sasaki T, Watanabe A, Sugimoto Y, Hayashi T, Eri Y, Suzumura H, Asaji K, Furuya E. (1998). Significance of measuring urinary 17-ketosteroid sulfates at the workplace. *Rinsho Byori—Japanese Journal of Clinical Pathology* 46(6):553-559.

Maes M, Libbrecht I, Delmeire L, Lin A, De Clerck L, Scharpe S, Janca A. (1999). Changes in platelet alpha-2-adrenoreceptors in fibromyalgia: Effects of treatment with antidepressants. *Neuropsychobiology* 40(3):129-133.

Maes M, Lin A, Bonaccorso S, Van Hunsel F, Van Gastel A, Delmeire L, Biondi M, Bosmans E, Kenis G, Scharpe S. (1998). Increased 24-hour urinary cortisol excretion in patients with post-traumatic stress disorder and patients with major depression, but not in patients with fibromyalgia. *Acta Psychiatrica Scandinavica* 98(4):328-335.

Maetzel A, Ferraz MB, Bombardier C. (1998). A review of cost-effectiveness analyses in rheumatology and related disciplines. *Current Opinions in Rheumatology* 10(2):136-140.

Maggi E, Giudizi MG, Biagiotti R, Annunziato F, Manetti R, Piccinni M-P, Parronchi P, Sampognaro S, Giannarini L, et al. (1994). Th2-like CD8+ T cells showing B cell helper function and reduced cytolytic activity in human immunodeficiency virus type 1 infection. *Journal of Experimental Medicine* 180:489-495.

Maggi E, Mazzetti M, Ravina A, Annunziato F, De Carli M, Piccinni P, Manetti R, Carbonari M, Pesce AM, Del Prete G, et al. (1994). Ability of HIV to promote a TH1 to TH0 shift and to replicate peferentially in TH2 and TH0 cells. *Science* 265:244-248.

Magnusson AE, Nias DK, White PD. (1996). Is perfectionism associated with fatigue? *Journal of Psychosomatic Research* 41(4):377-383.

Magnusson K, Karlsson E, Palmblad C, Leitner C, Paulson A. (1997). Swedish nurses' estimation of fatigue as a symptom in cancer patients—Report of a questionnaire. *European Journal of Cancer Care* 6(3):186-191.

Magnusson K, Moller A, Ekman T, Wallgren A. (1999). A qualitative study to explore the experience of fatigue in cancer patients. *European Journal of Cancer Care* 8(4):224-232.

Mahmoud HH, Pui CH, Kennedy W, Jaffe HS, Crist WM, Murphy SB. (1992). Phase I study of recombinant human interferon gamma in children with relapsed acute leukemia. *Leukemia* 6(11):1181-1184.

Mahowald MW, Mahowald ML, Bundlie SR, Ytterberg SR. (1989). Sleep fragmentation in rheumatoid arthritis. *Arthritis and Rheumatism* 32:974-983.

Mahrle G, Schulze HJ. (1990). Recombinant interferon-gamma (rIFN-gamma) in dermatology. *Journal of Investigative Dermatology* 95(6 Suppl):132S-137S.

Mai M, Sakata Y, Kanamaru R, Kurihara M, Suminaga M, Ota J, Hirabayashi N, Taguchi T, Furue H. (1999). [A late phase II clinical study of RP56976 (docetaxel) in patients with advanced or recurrent gastric cancer: A cooperative study group trial (group B)]. *Gan To Kagaku Ryoho* 26(4):487-496.

Maidannik VG. (1996). [The diagnosis and treatment of fibromyalgia] Diagnostika I lechenie fibromialgii. *Lik Sprava* (7-9):26-30.

Maier T. (1998). [Fibromyalgia (generalized tendomyopathy) in expert assessment] Die fibromyalgie (generalisierte tendomyopathie) in der begutachtungssituation. *Schweize Rundschrift Medizin Praxis* 87(22):788-789.

Mailis A. (1996). Fibromyalgia 20 years later; what have we really accomplished? *Journal of Rheumatology* 23(1):193; discussion 193-194.

Maini RN, Elliott MJ, Brennan FM, Feldman M. (1995). Beneficial effects of tumor necrosis factor-alpha (TNF-α) blockade in rheumatoid arthritis (RA). *Clinical and Experimental Immunology* 101:207-212.

Maini RN, Elliott MJ, Brennan FM, Williams RO, Chu CQ, Paleolog E, Charles PJ, Taylor PC, Feldmann M. (1995). Monoclonal anti-TNF-α antibody as a probe of pathogenesis and therapy of rheumatoid arthritis. *Immunological Reviews* 144:195-223.

Maisey NR, Norman A, Watson M, Allen MJ, Hill ME, Cunningham D. (2002). Baseline quality of life predicts survival in patients with advanced colorectal cancer. *European Journal of Cancer* 38(10):1351-1357.

Majewski S, Jablonska S. (1997). Human papilloma virus associated tumors of the skin and mucosa. *Journal of the American Academy of Dermatology* 36:659-685.

Major MS, Bumpous JM, Flynn MB, Schill K. (2001). Quality of life after treatment for advanced laryngeal and hypopharyngeal cancer. *Laryngoscope* 111(8):1379-1382.

Majumdar SR, Fletcher RH, Evans AT. (1999). How does colorectal cancer present? Symptoms, duration, and clues to location. *American Journal of Gastroenterology* 94(10):3039-3045.

Makela MO. (1999). Is fibromyalgia a distinct clinical entity? The epidemiologist's evidence. *Baillieres Best Practice Research in Clinical Rheumatology* 13(3): 415-419.

Makonkawkeyoon S, Limson-Pobre RN, Moeira AL, Schauf V, Kaplan G. (1993). Thalidomide inhibits the replication of human immunodeficiency virus type 1. *Proceedings of the National Academy of Sciences of the United States of America* 90(13):5974-5978.

Malak R, Abdelnoor AM. (1997). Human leukocyte antigen frequencies in a selected group of Lebanese Greek Orthodox. *Lebanese Medical Journal* 45:78-83.

Malakhovski S, Small I, Bokk MI. (1990). The mechanism of the neuromotor disorders in the period of the primary reaction to irradiation. *Radiobiologiya* 30:238-242.

Malik UR, Makower DF, Wadler S. (2001). Interferon-mediated fatigue. *Cancer* 92(6 Suppl):1664-1668.

Malkovsky M, Loveland B, North M, Asherton GL, Gao L, Ward P, Fiers W. (1987). Recombinant interleukin-2 directly augments the cytotoxicity of human monocytes. *Nature* 32(6101):262-265.

Malone JD, Paige-Dobson B, Ohl C, DiGiovanni C, Cunnion S, Roy MJ. (1996). Possibilities for unexplained chronic illnesses among reserve units deployed in Operation Desert Shield/Desert Storm. *Southern Medical Journal* 89(12):1147-1155.

Malone JL, Simms TE, Gray GC, Wagner KF, Burge JR, Burke DS. (1990). Sources of variability in repeated T-helper lymphocyte counts from human immunodeficiency virus type 1-infected patients: Total lymphocyte count fluctuations and diurnal cycle are important. *Journal of Acquired Immune Deficiency Syndromes* 3(2):144-151.

Malt UF, Nerdrum P, Oppedal B, Gundersen R, Holte M, Lone J. (1997). Physical and mental problems attributed to dental amalgam fillings: A descriptive study of 99 self-referred patients compared with 272 controls. *Psychosomatic Medicine* 59(1):32-41.

Malviya VK, Liu PY, Goldberg DA, Hantel A, O'Toole RV, Roach RW, Conrad ME, Alberts DS. (1996). A phase II trial of piroxantrone in endometrial cancer: Southwest Oncology Group study 8918. *Anticancer Drugs* 7(5):527-530.

Manandhar NP. (1998). Naïve phytotherapy among the Raute tribes of Dadeldhura district, Nepal. *Journal of Entopharmacology* 60(3):199-206.

Mandanas R, Einhorn LH, Wheeler B, Ansari R, Lutz T, Miller ME. (1993). Carboplatin (CBDCA) plus alpha interferon in metastatic non-small cell lung cancer: A Hoosier Oncology Group phase II trial. *American Journal of Clinical Oncology* 16(6):519-521.

Mani S, Poo WJ. (1996). Single institution experience with recombinant gamma-interferon in the treatment of patients with metastatic renal cell carcinoma. *American Journal of Clinical Oncology* 19(2):149-153.

Mani S, Schiano T, Garcia JC, Ansari RH, Samuels B, Sciortino DF, Tembe S, Shulman KL, Baker A, Benner SE, et al. (1998-1999). Phase II trial of uracil/tegafur (UFT) plus leucovorin in patients with advanced hepatocellular carcinoma. *Investigative New Drugs* 16(3):279-283.

Mani S, Sciortino D, Samuels B, Arrietta R, Schilsky RL, Vokes EE, Benner S. (1999). Phase II trial of uracil/tegafur (UFT) plus leucovorin in patients with advanced biliary carcinoma. *Investigative New Drugs* 17(1):97-101.

Mani S, Todd M, Poo WJ. (1996). Recombinant beta-interferon in the treatment of patients with metastatic renal cell carcinoma. *American Journal of Clinical Oncology* 19(2):187-189.

Mani S, Vogelzang NJ, Bertucci D, Stadler WM, Schilsky RL, Ratain MJ. (2001). Phase I study to evaluate multiple regimens of intravenous 5-fluorouracil administered in combination with weekly gemcitabine in patients with advanced solid tumors: A potential broadly active regimen for advanced solid tumor malignancies. *Cancer* 92(6):1567-1576.

Mannaerts GH, Rutten HJ, Martijn H, Hanssens PE, Wiggers T. (2002). Effects on functional outcome after IORT-containing multimodality treatment for locally advanced primary and locally recurrent rectal cancer. *International Journal of Radiation Oncology, Biology and Physics* 54(4):1082-1088.

Mannerkorpi K, Kroksmark T, Ekdahl C. (1999). How patients with fibromyalgia experience their symptoms in everyday life. *Physiotherapy Research International* 4(2):110-122.

Mannerkorpi K, Nyberg B, Ahlmen M, Ekdahl C. (2000). Pool exercise combined with an education program for patients with fibromyalgia syndrome: A prospective, randomized study. *Journal of Rheumatology* 27(10):2473-2481.

Mansur-Garza EM, Ishikawa T. (1994). "GS X pump" mediates ATP-dependent export of methotrexate. *Proceedings of the Annual Meeting of the American Association of Cancer Research* 35:A2240.

Mantovani G, Maccio A, Lai P, Massa E, Ghiani M, Santona MC. (1998). Cytokine involvement in cancer anorexia/cachexia: Role of megestrol acetate and medroxyprogesterone acetate on cytokien downregulation and improvement of clinical symptoms. *Critical Reviews in Oncogenesis* 9(2):99-106.

Manu P. (2000). *The Pharmacotherapy of Common Functional Syndromes: Evidence-Based Guidelines for Primary Care Practice.* Binghamton, NY: The Haworth Press.

Manuck SB, Cohen S, Rabin BS, Muldoon MF, Bachen EA. (1991). Individual differences in cellular immune response to stress. *Psychological Science* 2:111-115.

Manzullo EF, Escalante CP. (2002). Research into fatigue. *Hematology Oncology Clinics of North America* 16(3):619-628.

Maral J, Steinberg M, Weil M, Chleq C, Khayat D, Banzet P, Jacquillat C. (1987). [Human recombinant leukocyte interferon alpha-2-A in 22 cases of metastatic malignant melanoma]. *Presse Medicale* 16(21):1031-1034.

Marcel B, Komaroff AL, Fagioli LR, Kornish RJ II, Albert MS. (1996). Cognitive deficits in patients with chronic fatigue syndrome. *Biological Psychiatry* 40(6):535-541.

Marchant A, Goethebuer T, Ota MO, Wolfe I, Ceesay SJ, De Groote D, Corrah T, Bennett S, Wheeler J, Huygen K, et al. (1999). Newborns develop a Th1-type immune response to *Mycobacterium bovis* bacillus Calmette-Guérin vaccination. *Journal of Immunology* 163(4):2249-2255.

Marcovitch H. (1997). Managing chronic fatigue syndrome in children. *British Medical Journal* 314(7095):1635-1636.

Marcusson JA, Lindh G, Evengard B. (1999). Chronic fatigue syndrome and nickel allergy. *Contact Dermatitis* 40(5):269-272.

Margolin KA, Van Besien K, Wright C, Niland J, Champlin R, Fung HC, Kashyap A, Molina A, Nademanee AP, O'Donnell MR, et al. (1999). Interleukin-2-activated autologous bone marrow and peripheral blood stem cells in the treatment of acute leukemia and lymphoma. *Biology of Blood Marrow Transplantation* 5(1):36-45.

Mark L, Delmore F, Creech JL Jr, Ogden LL II, Fadell EH, Songster CL, Clanton J, Johnson MN, Christopherson WM. (1976). Clinical and morphologic features of hepatic angiosarcoma in vinyl chloride workers. *Cancer* 37(1):149-163.

Markowitz SB, Nunez CM, Klitzman S, Munshi AA, Kim WS, Eisinger J, Landrigan PJ. (1994). Lead poisoning due to hai ge fen: The porphyrin content of individual erythrocytes. *JAMA* 271(12):932-934.

Marks SM, McCaffrey R, Rosenthal DS, Moloney WC. (1978). Blastic transformation in chronic myelogenous leukemia: Experience with 50 patients. *Medical Pediatric Oncology* 4(2):159-167.

Marlowe SM. (1998). Calming the fire of fibromyalgia. *Advances in Nurse Practice* 6(1):51-53.

Marmion BP, Shannon M, Maddock I, Storm P, Penttila I. (1996). Protracted debility and fatigue after acute Q fever. *Lancet* 347(9006):977-978.

Marschalko M, Kovacs J, Somlai B, Berecz M, Hidvegi B, Harsing J, Desaknai M, Horvath A. (2001). [Interferon-alpha and PUVA therapy for mycosis fungoides]. *Orv Hetil* 142(37):2021-2023.

Marschner NW, Adler M, Nagel GA, Christmann D, Fenzl E, Upadhyaya B. (1991). Double-blind randomised trial of the antiemetic efficacy and safety of ondansetron and metoclopramide in advanced breast cancer patients treated with epirubicin and cyclophosphamide. *European Journal of Cancer* 27(9):1137-1140.

Marsh S, Kaplan M, Asano Y, Hoekzema D, Komaroff AL, Whitman JE Jr, Ablashi DV. (1996). Development and application of HHV-6 antigen capture assay for the detection of HHV-6 infections. *Journal of Virological Methods* 61(1-2):103-112.

Marshall JL, Bangalore N, El-Ashry D, Fuxman Y, Johnson M, Norris B, Oberst M, Ness E, Wojtowicz-Praga S, Bhargava P, et al. (2002). Phase I study of prolonged infusion bryostatin-1 in patients with advanced malignancies. *Cancer Biology and Therapy* 1(4):409-416.

Marshall JL, Richmond E, DeLap RJ. (1996). Biochemical modulation in the treatment of advanced cancer: A study of combined leucovorin, fluorouracil, and iododeoxyuridine. *Clinical Cancer Research* 2(9):1475-1480.

Marshall PS, Forstot M, Callies A, Peterson PK, Schenck CH. (1997). Cognitive slowing and working memory difficulties in chronic fatigue syndrome. *Psychosomatic Medicine* 59(1):58-66.

Marshall PS, Watson D, Steinberg P, Cornblatt B, Peterson PK, Callies A, Schenck CH. (1996). An assessment of cognitive function and mood in chronic fatigue syndrome. *Biological Psychiatry* 39(3):199-206.

Marth C, Mull R, Gastl G, Herold M, Steiner E, Daxenbichler G, Hetzel H, Flener R, Huber C, Dapunt O. (1989). [The intraperitoneal installation of gamma interferon for the treatment of refractory ovarian carcinoma]. *Geburtshilfe Frauenheilkunde* 49(11):987-991.

Marti B. (1992). Körperliche Bewegung und Krebs: Eine epidemiologische Kurzreview der Effekte von Physischer Aktivität auf das Karzinomrisiko. [Exercise and cancer: An epidemiological short review of the effects of physical activity on carcinoma risk]. *Schweizer Medizinische Wochenschrift* 122:1048-1056.

Marti B, Minder CE. (1989). Physische Berufsaktivität und Kolonkarzinommortalität bei Schweizer Männern, 1979-1982. [Physical occupational activity and colonic carcinoma mortality in Swiss men, 1979-1982]. *Soziale Preventivmedizin* 34:30-37.

Martin E, Muler JV, Dionel C. (1988). Disappearance of CD4 lymphocyte circadian cycles in HIV-infected patients: Early event during asymptomatic infection. *AIDS* 2:133-134.

Martin L. (1999). Silicone breast implants: The saga continues. *Journal of Rheumatology* 26(5):1020-1021.

Martin L, Nutting A, MacIntosh BR, Edworthy SM, Butterwick D, Cook J. (1996). An exercise program in the treatment of fibromyalgia. *Journal of Rheumatology* 23(6):1050-1053.

Martin WJ. (1996a). Genetic instability and fragmentation of a stealth viral genome. *Pathobiology* 64(1):9-17.

Martin WJ. (1996b). Severe stealth virus encephalopathy following chronic-fatigue syndrome-like illness: Clinical and histopathological features. *Pathobiology* 64(1):1-8.

Martin WJ. (1997). Detection of RNA sequences in cultures of a stealth virus isolated from the cerebrospinal fluid of a health care worker with chronic fatigue syndrome: Case report. *Pathobiology* 65(1):57-60.

Martin WJ. (1998). Cellular sequences in stealth viruses. *Pathobiology* 66(2):53-58.

Martinez FD. (1994). Role of viral infections in the inception of asthma and allergies during childhood: Could they be protective? *Thorax* 49:1189-1191.

Martinez-Lavin M, Hermosillo AG. (2000). Autonomic nervous system dysfunction may explain the multisystem features of fibromyalgia. *Seminars in Arthitis and Rheumatism* 29(4):197-199.

Martinez-Lavin M, Hermosillo AG, Mendoza C, Ortiz R, Cajigas JC, Pineda C, Nava A, Vallejo M. (1997). Orthostatic sympathetic derangement in subjects with fibromyalgia. *Journal of Rheumatology* 24(4):714-718.

Martinez-Lavin M, Hermosillo AG, Rosas M, Soto ME. (1998). Circadian studies of autonomic nervous balance in patients with fibromyalgia: A heart rate variability analysis. *Arthritis and Rheumatism* 41(11):1966-1971.

Marwick C. (2000). International plan focuses on eradication of polio and containment of the virus. *JAMA* 283(12):1553-1554.

Marx GM, Pavlakis N, McCowatt S, Boyle FM, Levi JA, Bell DR, Cook R, Biggs M, Little N, Wheeler HR. (2001). Phase II study of thalidomide in the treatment of recurrent glioblastoma multiforme. *Journal of Neurooncology* 54(1):31-38.

Masi AT. (1998). Concepts of illness in populations as applied to fibromyalgia syndromes: A biopsychosocial perspective. *Zeitschrift Rheumatologie* 57(Suppl. 2): 31-35.

Massey RU. (1996). Neurasthenia, psychoasthenia, CFS, and related matters. *Connecticut Medicine* 60(10):627-628.

Mast ME. (1998). Correlates of fatigue in survivors of breast cancer. *Cancer Nursing* 21(2):136-142.

Masuda A, Nozoe SI, Matsuyama T, Tanaka H. (1994). Psychobehavioral and immunological characteristics of adult people with chronic fatigue and patients with chronic fatigue syndrome. *Psychosomatic Medicine* 56(6):516-518.

Masuda N, Matsui K, Yamamoto N, Nogami T, Nakagawa K, Negoro S, Takeda K, Takifuji N, Yamada M, Kudoh S, et al. (2000). Phase I trial of oral 2'-deoxy-2'-methylidenecytidine: On a daily x 14-day schedule. *Clinical Cancer Research* 6(6):2288-2294.

Masuda N, Yayoi E, Furukawa J, Maruhashi S, Tokunaga M, Takiguchi S, Matsui S, Yano H, Tateishi H, Kinuta M, et al. (1998). [Analysis of 18 breast cancer patients with hypercalcemia]. *Gan To Kagaku Ryoho* 25(6):845-851.

Masutani K, Fujimaru M, Tsubota Y, Matsui N, Okamura T. (1997). [Double negative adult T-cell leukemia with hemophagocytic syndrome]. *Rinsho Ketsueki* 38(11):1199-1205.

Mathiak G, Meyer-Pannwitt U, Mathiak M, Schroder S, Henne-Bruns D, Froschle G. (1996). [Inflammatory pseudotumor of the liver—rare differential diagnosis of undetermined hepatic space-occupying lesion: Case report and review of the literature]. *Langenbecks Arch Chir* 381(6):309-317.

Matsuda A, Jinnai I, Mizuno H, Sakata T, Kusumoto S, Kayano H, Takeuchi H, Bessho M, Saito M, Katayama I, et al. (1992). [Hairy cell leukemia successfully treated with deoxycoformycin]. *Rinsho Ketsueki* 33(11):1685-1690.

Matsumoto S, Hayase M, Imamura H, Oda Y, Kikuchi H, Katayama M, Ishihara T. (2001). [A case of intrasellar meningioma mimicking pituitary adenoma]. *No Shinkei Geka* 29(6):551-557.

Matsumoto Y. (1999). [Fibromyalgia syndrome]. *Nippon Rinsho* 57(2):364-369.

Matsuoka H, Seo Y, Wakasugi H, Saito T, Tomoda H. (1997). Lentinan potentiates immunity and prolongs the survival time of some patients. *Anticancer Research* 17:2751-2755.

Matsuoka N, Yamamoto T, Haratake J, Hashimoto H, Unoki H. (1992). [Sarcomatoid liver carcinoma diagnosed clinically as hemangioma]. *Journal of Occupational and Environmental Health* 14(4):297-303.

Matsuyama H, Yamamoto M, Yoshihiro S, Ohmoto Y, Naito K. (1997). Efficacy of continuous subcutaneous infusion therapy using interferon alpha and the possible prognostic indicator of TNF-alpha in renal cell carcinoma. *International Journal of Urology* 4(5):447-450.

Mattei A, Bizollon T, Charles JD, Debat P, Fontanges T, Chevallier M, Trepo C. (1992). Liver damage induced by the ingestion of a product of phytotherapy containing wild germander: Four cases. *Gastroenterologie Clinique et Biologique* 16(10):798-800.

Matthys P, Billiau A. (1997). Cytokines and cachexia. *Nutrition* 13:763-770.

Mattioli R, Silva RR, Battelli N, Manocchi P, Pilone A, Rossini S, Delprete S, Mazzanti P, Bascioni R, Battelli T. (1993). Mitomycin C, 5-fluorouracil and folinic acid in combination with alpha 2b interferon for advanced colorectal cancer. *Tumori* 79(6):393-396.

Mattson K, Holsti LR, Niiranen A, Kivisaari L, Iivanainen M, Sovijarvi A, Cantell K. (1985). Human leukocyte interferon as part of a combined treatment for previously untreated small cell lung cancer. *Journal of Biological Response Modifiers* 4(1):8-17.

Mauff G, Gon M. (1991). CFS in Incline Village. *Southern Medical Association Journal* 3(March):15-20.

Maurizio SJ, Rogers JL. (1997). Recognizing and treating fibromyalgia. *Nurse Practice* 22(12):18-26, 28, 31.

Mavroudis D, Papadakis E, Veslemes M, Tsiafaki X, Stavrakakis J, Kouroussis C, Kakolyris S, Bania E, Jordanoglou J, Agelidou M, et al. (2001). A multicenter randomized clinical trial comparing paclitaxel-cisplatin-etoposide versus cisplatin-etoposide as first-line treatment in patients with small-cell lung cancer. *Annals of Oncology* 12(4):463-470.

Mawle AC, Nisembaum R, Dobbins JG, Gary HE Jr, Stewart JA, Reyes M, Steele L, Schmid DS, Reeves WC. (1997). Immune responses associated with chronic fatigue syndrome: A case-control study. *Journal of Infectious Diseases* 175(1):136-141.

Mazumder A, Rosenberg SA. (1984). Successive immunotherapy of natural killer-resistant established pulmonary melanoma metastases by the intravenous adoptive transfer of syngeneic lymphocytes activated in vitro by interleukin 2. *Journal of Experimental Medicine* 159:495-507.

McAllister CG, Rapaport MH, Pickar D, Podruchny TA, Christison G, Alphs LD, Paul SM. (1989). Increased numbers of CD5+ B lymphocytes in schizophrenic patients. *Archives of General Psychiatry* 46:890-894.

McClenathan JH. (1989). Metastatic melanoma involving the colon: Report of a case. *Diseases of Colon and Rectum* 32(1):70-72.

McCluskey DR. (1998). Chronic fatigue syndrome: Its cause and a strategy for management. *Comprehensive Therapy* 24(8):357-363.

McCully KK, Natelson BH, Iotti S, Sisto S, Leigh JS Jr. (1996). Reduced oxidative muscle metabolism in chronic fatigue syndrome. *Muscle and Nerve* 19(5):621-625.

McCully KK, Sisto SA, Natelson BH. (1996). Use of exercise for treatment of chronic fatigue syndrome. *American Journal of Sports Medicine* 21(1):35-48.

McCune JM, Namikawa R, Shih C-C, Rabin L, Kaneshima H. (1990). Suppression of HIV infection in AZT-treated SCID-hu mice. *Science* 247(4942):564-566.

McDonald AC, Vasey PA, Adams L, Walling J, Woodworth JR, Abrahams T, McCarthy S, Bailey NP, Siddiqui N, Lind MJ, et al. (1998). A phase I and pharmacokinetic study of LY231514, the multitargeted antifolate. *Clinical Cancer Research* 4(3):605-610.

McGregor NR, Dunstan RH, Zerbes M, Butt HL, Roberts TK, Klineberg IJ. (1996a). Preliminary determination of a molecular basis of chronic fatigue syndrome. *Biochemistry and Molecular Medicine* 57(2):73-80.

McGregor NR, Dunstan RH, Zerbes M, Butt HL, Roberts TK, Klineberg IJ. (1996b). Preliminary determination of the association between symptom expression and urinary metabolites in subjects with chronic fatigue syndrome. *Biochemistry and Molecular Medicine* 58(1):85-92.

McGuire WP, Blessing JA, Bookman MA, Lentz SS, Dunton CJ. (2000). Topotecan has substantial antitumor activity as first-line salvage therapy in platinum-sensitive epithelial ovarian carcinoma: A Gynecologic Oncology Group study. *Journal of Clinical Oncology* 18(5):1062-1067.

McIntyre M. (1999a). Alternative licensing for herbal medicine-like products in the European Union. European Herbal Practitioners Association. *Journal of Alternative and Complementary Medicine* 5(2):110-113.

McIntyre M. (1999b). Protecting the availability of herbal medicines. *Journal of Alternative and Complementary Medicine* 5(2):109-110.

McKenzie R, O'Fallon A, Dale J, Demitrack M, Sharma G, Deloria M, Garcia-Borreguero D, Blackwelder W, Straus SE. (1998). Low dose hydrocortisone for treatment of chronic fatigue syndrome: A randomized controlled trial. *JAMA* 280(12):1061-1066.

McLachlan SA, Devins GM, Goodwin PJ. (1999). Factor analysis of the psychosocial items of the EORTC QLQ-C30 in metastatic breast cancer patients participating in a psychosocial intervention study. *Quality of Life Research* 8(4):311-317.

McLaughlin CL, Rogan GJ, Ton J. (1992). Food intake and body temperature responses of rat to recombinant interleukin 1 beta and a tripeptide interleukin 1 beta antagonist. *Physiology and Behavior* 52:1155-1160.

McLaughlin P, Cabanillas F, Hagemeister FB, Swan F Jr, Romaguera JE, Taylor S, Rodriguez MA, Velasquez WS, Redman JR, Gutterman JU. (1993). CHOP-Bleo plus interferon for stage IV low-grade lymphoma. *Annals of Oncology* 4(3):205-211.

McLean AA. (1979). *Work Stress.* Reading, MA: Addison-Wesley.

McMillan SC. (1996). Pain and pain relief experienced by hospice patients with cancer. *Cancer Nursing* 19(4):298-307.

McNair D, Lorr D, Droppleman L. (1992). *Edits Manual for the Profile of Mood States.* San Diego, CA: Educational and Industrial Testing Services.

McNamara MJ, Alexander HR, Norton JA. (1992). Cytokines and their role in the pathophysiology of cancer cachexia. *Journal of Parenteral and Enteral Nutrition* 16(Suppl 6):50S-55S.

McNeil C. (2001). Cancer fatigue: One drug fails but more are in the pipeline. *Journal of the National Cancer Institute* 93(12):892-893.

McQuellon RP, Craven B, Russell GB, Hoffman S, Cruz JM, Perry JJ, Hurd DD. (1996). Quality of life in breast cancer patients before and after autologous bone marrow transplantation. *Bone Marrow Transplantation* 18(3):579-584.

McQuellon RP, Russell GB, Rambo TD, Craven BL, Radford J, Perry JJ, Cruz J, Hurd DD. (1998). Quality of life and psychological distress of bone marrow transplant recipients: The "time trajectory" to recovery over the first year. *Bone Marrow Transplantation* 21(5):477-486.

McRae S. (1996). Elevated serum digoxin levels in a patient taking digoxin and Siberian ginseng. *Canadian Medical Association Journal* 155(3):293-295, comment 115(9):1237.

Meadowcroft AM, Gilbert CJ, Maravich-May D, Hayward SL. (1998). Cost of managing anemia with and without prophylactic epoetin alfa therapy in breast cancer patients receiving combination chemotherapy. *American Journal of Health Systems and Pharmacy* 55(18):1898-1902.

Meadows LM, Walther P, Ozer H. (1991). Alpha-interferon and 5-fluorouracil: Possible mechanisms of antitumor action. *Seminars in Oncology* 18(5 Suppl 7): 71-76.

Meden H, Beneke A, Hesse T, Novophashenny I, Wischnewsky M. (2001). Weekly intravenous recombinant humanized anti-P185HER2 monoclonal antibody (herceptin) plus docetaxel in patients with metastatic breast cancer: A pilot study. *Anticancer Research* 21(2B):1301-1305.

MedLetter Associates (1998). Unraveling a mysterious cause of pain. Johns Hopkins Medical Letters. *Health After 50* 10(4):3.

Meek PM, Nail LM, Barsevick A, Schwartz AL, Stephen S, Whitmer K, Beck SL, Jones LS, Walker BL. (2000). Psychometric testing of fatigue instruments for use with cancer patients. *Nursing Research* 49(4):181-190.

Mehregan DA, Su WP, Kurtin PJ. (1994). Subcutaneous T-cell lymphoma: A clinical, histopathologic, and immunohistochemical study of six cases. *Journal of Cutaneous Pathology* 21(2):110-117.

Meisler JG. (1999). Chronic pain conditions in women. *Journal of Women's Health* 8(3):313-320.

Meiworm L, Jakob E, Walker UA, Peter HH, Keul J. (2000). Patients with fibromyalgia benefit from aerobic endurance exercise. *Clinical Rheumatology* 19(4): 253-257.

Melchart DM, Linde K, Worku F, Sarkady L, Holzmann M, Jurcic K, Wagner H. (1995). Results of five randomized studies on the immunomodulatory activity of preparations of echinacea. *Journal of Alternative and Complementary Medicine* 1(27):145-160.

Melchart DM, Wahlther E, Linde K, Brandmaaier R, Lersch C. (1998). Echinacea root extracts for the prevention of upper respiratory tract infections: A double-blind, placebo-controlled, randomized trial. *Archives of Family Medicine* 7(6): 541-545.

Melichar B, Malir F, Jandik P, Malirova E, Vavrova J, Mergancova J, Voboril Z. (1995). Increased urinary zinc excretion in cancer patients is linked to immune activation and renal tubular cell dysfunction. *Biometals* 8(3):205-208.

Mellergard M. (1997). Only extremely tired? *Ugeskrift for Laeger* 159(31):4769.

Mendell MJ, Fisk WJ, Deddens JA, Seavey WG, Smith AH, Smith DF, Hodgson AT, Daisey JM, Goldman LR. (1996). Elevated symptoms prevalence associated with ventilation type in office buildings. *Epidemiology* 7(6):583-589.

Mendelson WB. (1997). Efficacy of melatonin as a hypnotic agent. *Journal of Biological Rhythms* 12:651-656.

Mendoza TR, Wang XS, Cleeland CS, Morrissey M, Johnson BA, Wendt JK, Huber SL. (1999). The rapid assessment of fatigue severity in cancer patients: Use of the Brief Fatigue Inventory. *Cancer* 85(5):1186-1196.

Mendoza Montero J. (1990). [Epstein-Barr virus]. *Enfermedades Infecciosas y Microbiologia Clinica* 8(7):397-401.

Mengshoel AM. (1996). [Effect of physical exercise in fibromyalgia] Effekt av fysisk trening ved fibromyalgi. *Tidsskr Nor Largeforen* 116(6):746-748.

Mengshoel AM. (1997). [Physical therapy and fibromyalgia] Fysioterapi og fibromyalgi. *Tiddskr Nor Laegeforen* 117(30):4484-4485.

Mengshoel AM, Vollestad NK, Forre O. (1995). Pain and fatigue induced by exercise in fibromyalgia patients and sedentary healthy subjects. *Clinical and Experimental Rheumatology* 13(4):477-482.

Merchant RE, McVicar DW, Merchant LH, Young HF. (1992). Treatment of recurrent malignant glioma by repeated intracerebral injections of human recombinant interleukin-2 alone or in combination with systemic interferon-alpha: Results of a phase I clinical trial. *Journal of Neurooncology* 12(1):75-83.

Merchant TE, Kiehna EN, Miles MA, Zhu J, Xiong X, Mulhern RK. (2002). Acute effects of irradiation on cognition: Changes in attention on a computerized continuous performance test during radiotherapy in pediatric patients with localized primary brain tumors. *International Journal of Radiation Oncology, Biology and Physics* 53(5):1271-1278.

Merimsky O, Chaitchik S. (1992). Neurotoxicity of interferon-alpha. *Anticancer Drugs* 3(6):567-570.

Meropol NJ, Barresi GM, Fehniger TA, Hitt J, Franklin M, Caligiuri MA. (1998). Evaluation of natural killer cell expansion and activation in vivo with daily subcutaneous low-dose interleukin-2 plus periodic intermediate-dose pulsing. *Cancer Immunology and Immunotherapy* 46(6):318-326.

Meropol NJ, Rustum YM, Petrelli NJ, Rodriguez-Bigas M, Frank C, Ho DH, Kurowski M, Creaven PJ. (1996). A phase I and pharmacokinetic study of oral uracil, ftorafur, and leucovorin in patients with advanced cancer. *Cancer Chemotherapy Pharmacology* 37(6):581-586.

Mesch U, Lowenthal RM, Coleman D. (1996). Lead poisoning masquerading as chronic fatigue syndrome. *Lancet* 347(9009):1193.

Mettlin C. (1988). Descriptive and analytic epidemiology: Bridges to cancer control. *Cancer* 62:1680-1687.

Metz L. (1998). Multiple sclerosis: Symptomatic therapies. *Seminars in Neurology* 18(3):389-395.

Metz-Kurschel U, Wehr M. (1989). [Atrial myxoma and signs of autoimmune disease]. *Deutsche Medizinische Wochenschrift* 114(5):181-183.

Meyer BB, Lemley KJ. (2000). Utilizing exercise to affect the symptomatology of fibromyalgia: A pilot study. *Medical Science, Sports, and Exercise* 32(10):1691-1697.

Meyer R, Haggarty R. (1962). Streptococcal infections in families. *Pediatrics* 10: 539-549.

Meyer RM, Gyger M, Langley R, Lesperance B, Caplan SN. (1998). A phase I trial of standard and cyclophosphamide dose-escalated CHOP with granulocyte colony stimulating factor in elderly patients with non-Hodgkin's lymphoma. *Leukemia and Lymphoma* 30(5-6):591-600.

Meyer-Lindenberg A, Gallhofer B. (1998). Somatized depression as a subgroup of fibromyalgia syndrome. *Zeitschrift Rheumatologie* 57(Suppl. 2):92-93.

Meyerowitz BE, Sparks FC, Spears IK. (1979). Adjuvant chemotherapy for breast carcinoma: Psychosocial implications. *Cancer* 43(5):1613-1618.

Meyers CA. (2000). Neurocognitive dysfunction in cancer patients. *Oncology* 14(1):75-79; discussion 79, 81-82, 85.

Meyers FJ, Lew D, Lara PN Jr, Williamson S, Marshall E, Balcerzak SP, Rivkin SE, Samlowski W, Crawford ED. (1998-1999). Phase II trial of edatrexate in relapsed or refractory germ cell tumors: A Southwest Oncology Group study (SWOG 9124). *Investigative New Drugs* 16(4):347-351.

Miaskowski C, Lee KA. (1999). Pain, fatigue, and sleep disturbances in oncology outpatients receiving radiation therapy for bone metastasis: A pilot study. *Journal of Pain Symptomatology and Management* 17(5):320-332.

Miccinesi G, Paci E, Toscani F, Tamburini M, Brunelli C, Costantini M, Peruselli C, Di Giulio P, Gallucci M, Addington-Hall J, et al. (1999). [Quality of life at the end of life. Analysis of the quality of life of oncologic patients treated with palliative care. Results of a multicenter observational study (staging)]. *Epidemiology Previews* 23(4):333-345.

Michael A. (1998). Treating chronic fatigue with exercise: Exercise improved mood and sleep. *British Medical Journal* 317(7158):600.

Michaelson R, Kemeny N, Young C. (1982). Phase II evaluation of 4'-epi-doxorubicin in patients with advanced colorectal carcinoma. *Cancer Treatment Reports* 66(9):1757-1758.

Michiels V, Cluydts R, Fischler B. (1998). Attention and verbal learning in patients with chronic fatigue syndrome. *Journal of International Neuropsychology Society* 4(5):456-466.

Michiels V, Cluydts R, Fischler B, Hoffmann G, Le Bon O, De Meirleir K. (1996). Cognitive functioning in patients with chronic fatigue syndrome. *Journal of Clinical and Experimental Neuropsychology* 18(5):666-677.

Micieta I, Vagac M, Badalik L, Cechvalova A. (1972). [Diagnosis of bronchogenic carcinoma]. *Bratisl Lek Listy* 58(3):353-359.

Mier JW, Aronson FR, Numerof RP, Vachino G, Atkins MB. (1988). Toxicity of immunotherapy with interleukin-2 and lymphokine-activated killer cells. *Pathology and Immunopathology Research* 7(6):459-476.

Mihm S, Ennen J, Pessara U, Kurth R, Drogue W. (1991). Inhibition of HIV-1 replication and NF-kB activity by cysteine and cysteine derivatives. *AIDS* 5:497-503.

Mikkelsson M. (1999). One year outcome of preadolescents with fibromyalgia. *Journal of Rheumatology* 26(3):674-682.

Mikkelsson M, Salminen JJ, Kautiainen H. (1997). Non-specific musculoskeletal pain in preadolescents: Prevalence and 1-year persistence. *Pain* 73(1):29-35.

Mikkelsson M, Sourander A, Piha J, Salminen JJ. (1997). Psychiatric symptoms in preadolescents with musculoskeletal pain and fibromyalgia. *Pediatrics* 100 (2 Pt 1):220-227.

Miles A. (1998). Radio and the commodification of natural medicine in Ecuador. *Social Science Medicine* 47(12):2127-2137.

Milkovich G, Moleski RJ, Reitan JF, Dunning DM, Gibson GA, Paivanas TA, Wyant S, Jacobs RJ. (2000). Comparative safety of filgrastim versus sargramostim in patients receiving myelosuppressive chemotherapy. *Pharmacotherapy* 20(12):1432-1440.

Millea PJ, Holloway RL. (2000). Treating fibromyalgia. *American Family Physician* 62(7):1575-1582.

Miller JI, Mankin HT, Broadbent JC, Giuliani ER, Daniwlson GK. (1972). Primary cardiac tumors: Surgical considerations and results of operation. *Circulation* 45(Suppl 1):I134-I138.

Miller LG. (1998). Herbal medicinals: Selected clinical considerations focusing on known or potential drug-herb interactions. *Archives of Internal Medicine* 158(20): 2200-2211.

Miller NA, Carmichael HA, Hall FC, Calder BD. (1991). Antibody to coxsackie B virus in diagnosing postviral fatigue syndrome. *British Medical Journal* 302: 140-143.

Miller TA, Allen GM, Gandevia SC. (1996). Muscle force, perceived effort, and voluntary activation of the elbow flexors assessed with sensitive twitch interpolation in fibromyalgia. *Journal of Rheumatology* 23(9):1621-1627.

Miller WH Jr, Reyno LM, Loewen GR, Huan S, Winquist E, Moore M, Cato A III, Jaunakais D, Truglia JA, Matthews S, et al. (2000). A phase I-II study of 9-cis retinoic acid and interferon-alpha2b in patients with advanced renal-cell carcinoma: An NCIC Clinical Trials Group study. *Annals of Oncology* 11(11):1387-1389.

Millner L, Widerman E. (1994). Women's health issues: A review of the current literature in the social work journals, 1985-1992. *Social Work and Health Care* 19(3-4):145-172.

Mimori K, Kawauchi K, Watanabe H, Sugiyama H. (1989). [Complex karyotypic abnormality in an aged patient with acute myeloid leukemia (M 2)]. *Rinsho Ketsueki* 30(6):868-873.

Mings D. (1998a). Canadian Association of Nurses in Oncology position paper on cancer-related fatigue. *Canadian Oncology Nursing Journal* 8(S1):S4.

Mings D. (1998b). Correlates of fatigue. *Canadian Oncology Nursing Journal* 8(S1):S6.

Mings D. (1998c). Patient education resources: An annotated bibliography of fatigue resources for patients and their families. *Canadian Oncology Nursing Journal* 8(S1):S16.

Mings D. (1998d). [A trainer's perspective on the cancer fatigue workshops.] *Canadian Oncology Nursing Journal* 8(S1):S7-S8.

Minowa M, Jiamo M. (1996). Descriptive epidemiology of chronic fatigue syndrome based on a nationwide survey in Japan. *American Journal of Epidemiology* 6(2):75-80.

Minsky BD, Cohen AM, Kemeny N, Enker WE, Kelsen DP, Reichman B, Saltz L, Sigurdson ER, Frankel J. (1992). Enhancement of radiation-induced downstaging of rectal cancer by fluorouracil and high-dose leucovorin chemotherapy. *Journal of Clinical Oncology* 10(1):79-84.

Miro O, Font C, Fernandez-Sola J, Casademont J, Pedrol E, Grau JM, Urbano-Marquez A. (1997). Chronic fatigue syndrome: Study of the clinical course of 28 cases. *Medicina Clínica* 108(15):561-565.

Mischis-Troussard C, Goudet P, Verges B, Cougard P, Tavernier C, Maillefert JF. (2000). Primary hyperparathyroidism with normal serum intact parathyroid hormone levels. *Quarterly Journal of Medicine* 93(6):365-367.

Mishkin S. (1999). The DINs and don'ts of herbal/natural preparations. *Canadian Journal of Gastroenterology* 13(4):335-337.

Misonou J, Kanda M, Miyake T, Kawamura T, Maekawa I, Hishiyama H, Atsuta T. (1990). An autopsy case of triple cancers including signet-ring cell carcinoma of the breast—Report of a rare case with reference to a review of the literature. *Japanese Journal of Surgery* 20(6):720-725.

Misonou J, Kanda M, Shishido T, Abe M, Miyake T, Kawamura T, Maekawa I, Itou N, Atsuta T, Kubota H, et al. (1990). An autopsy case of malignant fibrous histiocytoma of the mediastinum, presenting multiple metastases to the small intestine and to the brain—A rare case report with a review of the literature. *Gastroenterology Japan* 25(6):746-752.

Mitsudo K, Tohnai I, Hayashi Y, Ueda M, Yambe M, Hirose Y. (2000). A case of Burkitt's lymphoma that presented initially with resorption of alveolar bone. *Oral Diseases* 6(4):256-258.

Mitsuya H, Broder S. (1987). Strategies for antiviral therapy in AIDS. *Nature* 325:773-778.

Mitsuya H, Yarchoan R, Broder S. (1990). Molecular targets for AIDS therapy. *Science* 249:1533-1544.

Mitsuyama S, Ohno S, Koga T, Takayama T, Yamashita J, Ogawa M, Shirouzu K, Sugimachi K, Nomura Y, Ogawa N. (1999). [Study on CAF + medroxy-progesterone acetate (MPA) therapy for advanced or recurrent breast cancer—Comparison between MPA 600 mg and 1,200 mg. Kyushu CAFT Therapy Study Group (third study)]. *Gan To Kagaku Ryoho* 26(13):2029-2036.

Mittelman A, Chun HG, Puccio C, Coombe N, Lansen T, Ahmed T. (1999). Phase II clinical trial of didemnin B in patients with recurrent or refractory anaplastic astrocytoma or glioblastoma multiforme (NSC 325319). *Investigative New Drugs* 17(2):179-182.

Mittelman A, Huberman M, Puccio C, Fallon B, Tessitore J, Savona S, Eyre R, Gafney E, Wick M, Skelos A, et al. (1990). A phase I study of recombinant human interleukin-2 and alpha-interferon-2a in patients with renal cell cancer, colorectal cancer, and malignant melanoma. *Cancer* 66(4):664-669.

Mittelman A, Puccio C, Ahmed T, Zeffren J, Choudhury A, Arlin Z. (1991). A phase II trial of interleukin-2 by continuous infusion and interferon by intramuscular injection in patients with renal cell carcinoma. *Cancer* 68(8):1699-1702.

Mitterer M, Pescosta N, Fend F, Larcher C, Prang N, Schwarzmann F, Coser P, Huemer HP. (1995). Chronic active Epstein-Barr virus disease in a case of persistent polyclonal B-cell lymphocytosis. *British Journal of Haematology* 90(3): 526-531.

Miyagawa H, Kamioka N, Kohara H, Yuube R, Takahashi T, Nakatoh H, Kawada M, Utsunomiya T, Izumiyama F, Akimori T, et al. (1993). [A case of advanced hepatocellular carcinoma, in which the tumor almost disappeared by orally administered UFT]. *Gan To Kagaku Ryoho* 20(14):2211-2215.

Miyakoshi H, Aoki T, Mizukoshi M. (1984). Acting mechanisms of lentinan in humans: II. Enhancement of non-specific cell-mediated cytotoxicity as an interferon-induced response. *International Journal of Immunopharmacology* 6(4): 373-379.

Miyauchi M, Yamamoto N, Nakajima N, Suzuki M, Takahashi M, Ohno K, Ogawa K, Tsukamoto T, Yamamoto K, Oheda Y; Chiba Epirubicin Cooperative Study Group. (2001). [Usefulness of ambulatory adjuvant chemotherapy with low-dose epirubicin in patients with axially-node positive breast cancer: Chiba Epirubicin Cooperative Study Group]. *Gan To Kagaku Ryoho* 28(1):43-48.

Miyazaki E, Ando M, Ih K, Matsumoto T, Kaneda K, Tsuda T. (1998). Pulmonary edema associated with the Chinese medicine Sho-saiko-to. *Nihon Kokyuki Gakkai Zasshi* 36(9):776-780.

Mizel SB. (1989). The interleukins. *FASEB Journal* 3:2379-2388.

Mizusawa H, Okaneya T, Yoneyama T, Taguchi I. (1995). [Primary malignant lymphoma of the adrenal gland: A case report]. *Hinyokika Kiyo* 41(12):991-994.

Mochitomi Y, Inoue A, Kawabata H, Ishida S, Kanzaki T. (1998). Stevens-Johnson syndrome caused by a health drink (Eberu) containing ophiopogonis tuber. *Journal of Dermatology* 25(10):662-665.

Mock V. (1998). Breast cancer and fatigue: Issues for the workplace. *American Association of Home Nursing Journal* 46(9):425-431.

Mock V. (2001a). Evaluating a model of fatigue in children with cancer. *Journal of Pediatric Oncology Nursing* 18(2 Suppl 1):13-16.

Mock V. (2001b). Fatigue management: Evidence and guidelines for practice. *Cancer* 92(6 Suppl):1699-1707.

Mock V, Atkinson A, Barsevick A, Cella D, Cimprich B, Cleeland C, Donnelly J, Eisenberger MA, Escalante C, Hinds P, et al. (2000). NCCN practice guidelines for cancer-related fatigue. *Oncology* 14(11A):151-161.

Mock V, Burke MB, Sheehan P, Creaton EM, Winningham ML, McKenney-Tedder S, Schwager LP, Liebman M. (1994). A nursing rehabilitation program for women with breast cancer receiving adjuvant chemotherapy. *Oncology Nursing Forum* 21(5):899-907; discussion 908.

Mock V, Dow KH, Meares CJ, Grimm PM, Dienemann JA, Haisfield-Wolfe ME, Quitasol W, Mitchell S, Chakravarthy A, Gage I. (1997). Effects of exercise on fatigue, physical functioning, and emotional distress during radiation therapy for breast cancer. *Oncology Nursing Forum* 24(6):991-1000.

Mock V, Pickett M, Ropka ME, Muscari Lin E, Stewart KJ, Rhodes VA, McDaniel R, Grimm PM, Krumm S, McCorkle R. (2001). Fatigue and quality of life outcomes of exercise during cancer treatment. *Cancer Practice* 9(3):119-127.

Mock V, Ropka ME, Rhodes VA, Pickett M, Grimm PM, McDaniel R, Lin EM, Allocca P, Dienemann JA, Haisfield-Wolfe ME, et al. (1998). Establishing mechanisms to conduct multi-institutional research—Fatigue in patients with cancer: An exercise intervention. *Oncology Nursing Forum* 25(8):1391-1397.

Modlin RL, Nutman TB. (1993). Type 2 cytokines and negative immunoregulation in human infections. *Current Opinions in Immunology* 5:511-517.

Moertel CG, Rubin J, Kvols LK. (1989). Therapy of metastatic carcinoid tumor and the malignant carcinoid syndrome with recombinant leukocyte A interferon. *Journal of Clinical Oncology* 7(7):865-868.

Mohiuddin M, Chen E, Ahmad N. (1996). Combined liver radiation and chemotherapy for palliation of hepatic metastases from colorectal cancer. *Journal of Clinical Oncology* 14(3):722-728.

Moinpour CM. (1994). Measuring quality of life: An emerging science. *Seminars in Oncology* 21(5 Suppl 10):48-60.

Molassiotis A. (1999). A correlational evaluation of tiredness and lack of energy in survivors of haematological malignancies. *European Journal of Cancer Care* 8(1):19-25.

Molassiotis A, Morris PJ. (1999). Quality of life in patients with chronic myeloid leukemia after unrelated donor bone marrow transplantation. *Cancer Nursing* 22(5):340-349.

Molassiotis A, Yam BM, Yung H, Chan FY, Mok TS. (2002). Pretreatment factors predicting the development of postchemotherapy nausea and vomiting in Chinese breast cancer patients. *Support Care in Cancer* 10(2):139-145.

Moldawer LL, Andersson C, Galin J. (1988). Regulation of food intake and hepatic protein synthesis by recombinant-derived cytokines. *American Journal of Physiology* 254:6450-6456.

Moldawer LL, Copeland EM. (1997). Proinflammatory cytokines, nutritional support, and the cachixia syndrome: Interactions and therapeutic options. *Cancer* 79:1828-1839.

Moldawer LL, Gelin J, Schersten T. (1987). Circulating interleukin 1 and tumor necrosis factor during inflammation. *American Journal of Physiology* 253:R922-R928.

Moldawer LL, Rogy MA, Lowry SF. (1992). The role of cytokines in cancer cachexia. *Journal of Parenteral and Enteral Nutrition* 16:43S-49S.

Moldofsky H. (1989a). Nonrestorative sleep and symptoms after a febrile illness in patients with fibrositis and chronic fatigue syndrome. *Journal of Rheumatology* 16(19):150-153.

Moldofsky H. (1989b). Sleep and fibrositis syndrome. *Rheumatic Diseases Clinics of North America* 15:91-103.

Moldofsky H, Lue FA, Mously C, Roth-Schechter B, Reynolds WJ. (1996). The effect of zolpidem in patients with fibromyalgia: A dose ranging, double blind, placebo controlled, modified crossover study. *Journal of Rheumatology* 23(3):529-533.

Moldofsky H, Scarisbrick P. (1976). Induction of neurasthenic musculoskeletal pain syndrome by selective sleep stage deprivation. *Psychosomatic Medicine* 38:35-44.

Moldofsky H, Scarisbrick P, England R, Smythe H. (1975). Musculoskeletal symptoms and non-REM sleep distubance in patients with "fibrositis syndrome" and healthy subjects. *Psychosomatic Medicine* 37:341-351.

Molony RR, MacPeek DM, Schiffman PL, Frank M, Neubauer JA, Schwartzberg M, Seibold JR. (1986). Sleep, sleep apnea, and fibromyalgia syndrome. *Journal of Rheumatology* 13:797-800.

Monga U, Jaweed M, Kerrigan AJ, Lawhon L, Johnson J, Vallbona C, Monga TN. (1997). Neuromuscular fatigue in prostate cancer patients undergoing radiation therapy. *Archives of Physical Medicine Rehabilitation* 78(9):961-966.

Monga U, Kerrigan AJ, Thornby J, Monga TN. (1999). Prospective study of fatigue in localized prostate cancer patients undergoing radiotherapy. *Radiation Oncology Investigation* 7(3):178-185.

Monroe BA. (1998). Fibromyalgia—A hidden link? *Journal of the American College of Nutrition* 17(3):300.

Montgomery GK. (1983). Uncommon tiredness among college undergraduates. *Journal of Consulting and Clinical Psychology* 51:517-525.

Monti M, Castellani L, Berlusconi A, Cunietti E. (1996). Use of red blood cell transfusions in terminally ill cancer patients admitted to a palliative care unit. *Journal of Pain Symptomatology and Management* 12(1):18-22.

Monto AS, Fleming DM, Henry D, De Groot R, Makela M, Klein T, Elliott M, Keene ON, Man CY. (1999). Efficacy and safety of the neuraminidase inhibitor zanamivir in the treatment of influenza A and B virus infections. *Journal of Infectious Diseases* 180(2):256-261.

Montoya-Cabrera MA, Simental-Toba A, Sanchez-Rodriguez S, Escalante-Galindo P, Aguilar-Conteras A. (1998). Cardiorespiratory depression in 8 newborn infants whose mothers took "yucuyahui" (Zoapatle-*Montanoa tomentosa*) during labor. *Gaceta Médica de México* 134(5):611-615.

Moore DF Jr, Pazdur R, Sugarman S, Jones D III, Lippman SM, Bready B, Abbruzzese JL. (1995). Pilot phase II trial of 13-cis-retinoic acid and interferon-alpha combination therapy for advanced pancreatic adenocarcinoma. *American Journal of Clinical Oncology* 18(6):525-527.

Moore MJ, Erlichman C, Kaizer L, Fine S. (1993). A phase II study of 5-fluorouracil, leucovorin and interferon-alpha in advanced pancreatic cancer. *Anticancer Drugs* 4(5):555-557.

Moore MJ, Kaizer L, Erlichman C, Myers R, Feld R, Thiessen JJ, Fine S. (1995). A clinical and pharmacological study of 5-fluorouracil, leucovorin and interferon alfa in advanced colorectal cancer. *Cancer Chemotherapy Pharmacology* 37 (1-2):86-90.

Moore P. (1998). It's time to wake up to cancer fatigue. *Nursing Spectrum* 8(8):19.

Moore P, Dimsdale JE. (2002). Opioids, sleep, and cancer-related fatigue. *Medical Hypotheses* 58(1):77-82.

Moorkens G, Keenoy M, Vertommen B, Meludu JS, Noe M, De Leeuw I. (1997). Magnesium deficiency in a sample of the Belgian population presenting with chronic fatigue. *Magnesium Research* 4(2):329-337.

Morag A, Tobi M, Ravid Z, Ravel M, Schattner A. (1982). Increased (2'-5')-oligo-a synthetase activity in patients with prolonged illness associated with serological evidence of persistent Epstein-Barr virus infection. *Lancet* 1:744.

Morales A, Johnston B, Emerson L, Heaton JW. (1997). Intralesional administration of biological response modifiers in the treatment of localized cancer of the prostate: A feasibility study. *Urology* 50(4):495-502.

Morales AJ, Nolan JJ, Nelson JC, Yen SS. (1994). Effects of replacement dose of dehydroepiandrosterone in men and women of advancing age. *Journal of Clinical Endocrinology and Metabolism* 78(6):1360-1367.

Morand EF, Cooley H, Leech M, Littlejohn GO. (1996). Advances in the understanding of neuroendocrine function in rheumatic disease. *Australian and New Zealand Journal of Medicine* 26(4):543-551.

Morant R, Bernhard J, Maibach R, Borner M, Fey MF, Thurlimann B, Jacky E, Trinkler F, Bauer J, Zulian G, et al. (2000). Response and palliation in a phase II trial of gemcitabine in hormone-refractory metastatic prostatic carcinoma. Swiss Group for Clinical Cancer Research (SAKK). *Annals of Oncology* 11(2):183-188.

Morawetz RA, Doherty TM, Giese NA, Hartley JW, Müller W, Kühn R, Rajewski K, Coffman R, Morse III HC. (1994). Resistance to murine acquired immunodeficiency syndrome (MAIDS). *Science* 265:264-266.

Morehouse RL, Flanigan M, MacDonald DD, Braha D, Shapiro C. (1998). Depression and short REM latency in subjects with chronic fatigue syndrome. *Psychosomatic Medicine* 60(3):347-351.

Moreira AL, Sampaio EP, Zmuidzinas A, Frindt P, Smith KA, Kaplan G. (1993). Thalidomide exerts its inhibitory action on tumor necrosis factor alpha by enhancing mRNA degradation. *Journal of Experimental Medicine* 177(6):1675-1680.

Morgan DA, Ruscetti FW, Gallo RC. (1976). Selective in vitro growth of T lymphocytes from normal human bone marrows. *Science* 193:1007-1008.

Morimoto C, Letvin NL, Distaso JA, Aldrich WR, Schlossman SF. (1985). The isolation and characterization of the human suppressor inducer T cell subset. *Journal of Immunology* 134(3):1508-1512.

Morimoto K, Abe O, Kinoshita H. (1998). [Steady state and disappearance of the metabolites of miproxifene phosphate in the treatment of breast cancer]. *Gan To Kagaku Ryoho* 25(10):1565-1573.

Morishima Y, Satoh H, Ohtsu I, Matsumura T, Sumi M, Ninomiya H, Inoue M, Uchida Y, Ohtsuka M, Hasegawa S. (1996). [Invasive thymoma associated with pure red cell aplasia and lung cancer]. *Nihon Kyobu Shikkan Gakkai Zasshi* 34(2):236-240.

Morishita T, Yamazaki J, Ohsawa H, Uchi T, Kawamura Y, Okuzumi K, Nakano H, Wakakura M, Okamoto K, Koyama N, et al. (1988). Malignant schwannoma of the heart. *Clinical Cardiology* 11(2):126-130.

Mormont MC, Waterhouse J. (2002). Contribution of the rest-activity circadian rhythm to quality of life in cancer patients. *Chronobiology International* 19(1):313-323.

Mormont MC, Waterhouse J, Bleuzen P, Giacchetti S, Jami A, Bogdan A, Lellouch J, Misset JL, Touitou Y, Levi F. (2000). Marked 24-h rest/activity rhythms are associated with better quality of life, better response, and longer survival in patients with metastatic colorectal cancer and good performance status. *Clinical Cancer Research* 6(8):3038-3045.

Morris MJ, Tong WP, Cordon-Cardo C, Drobnjak M, Kelly WK, Slovin SF, Terry KL, Siedlecki K, Swanson P, Rafi M, et al. (2002). Phase I trial of BCL-2 antisense oligonucleotide (G3139) administered by continuous intravenous infusion in patients with advanced cancer. *Clinical Cancer Research* 8(3):679-683.

Morris P. (1986). Coping with cancer: In the shadow of the crab. *Nursing Times* 82(13):47.

Morrison LJ, Behan WH, Behan PO. (1991). Changes in natural killer cell phenotype in patients with post-viral fatigue syndrome. *Clinical and Experimental Immunology* 83:441-446.

Morriss RK, Wearden AJ, Battersby L. (1997). The relation of sleep difficulties to fatigue, mood and disability in chronic fatigue syndrome. *Journal of Psychosomatic Research* 42(6):597-602.

Morrow GR, Andrews PL, Hickok JT, Roscoe JA, Matteson S. (2002). Fatigue associated with cancer and its treatment. *Support Care and Cancer* 10(5):389-398.

Morrow GR, Hickok JT, Andrews, PL, Stern RM. (2002). Reduction in serum cortisol after platinum based chemotherapy for cancer: A role for the HPA axis in treatment-related nausea? *Psychophysiology* 39(4):491-495.

Morte S, Castilla A, Civeira MP, Serrano M, Prieto J. (1988). Gamma-interferon and chronic fatigue syndrome. *Lancet* 2(8611):623-624.

Morte S, Castilla A, Civeira M-P, Serrano M, Prieto J. (1989). Production of interleukin-1 by peripheral blood mononuclear cells in patients with chronic fatigue syndrome. *Journal of Infectious Diseases* 159:362.

Mortimer JE, Schulman S, MacDonald JS, Kopecky K, Goodman G. (1990). High-dose cisplatin in disseminated melanoma: A comparison of two schedules. *Cancer Chemotherapy Pharmacology* 25(5):373-376.

Mosier DE, Gulizia RJ, Baird SM, Wilson DB, Spector DH, Spector SA. (1991). Human immunodeficiency virus infection of human PBL-SCID mice. *Science* 251(4995):791-794.

Moss RB, Mercandetti A, Vojdani A. (1999). TNF-alpha and chronic fatigue syndrome. *Journal of Clinical Immunology* 19(5):314-316.

Moss TM. (1998). Herbal medicine in the emergency department: A primer for toxicities and treatment. *Journal of Emergency Nursing* 24(6):509-513.

Moss-Morris R, Petrie KJ, Large RG, Kydd RR. (1996). Neuropsychological deficits in chronic fatigue syndrome: Artifact or reality? *Journal of Neurology, Neurosurgery and Psychiatry* 60(5):474-477.

Motohashi Y, Iizuka Y, Takeuchi K, Suzuki S, Ichii S, Takeuchi J, Kawamura M, Ohyashiki J, Toyama K, Ohshima T, et al. (1990). [Acute myeloblastic leukemia associated with 46, XY, del(5)(q22)]. *Rinsho Ketsueki* 31(7):979-983.

Motzer RJ, Rakhit A, Ginsberg M, Rittweger K, Vuky J, Yu R, Fettner S, Hooftman L. (2001). Phase I trial of 40-kd branched pegylated interferon alfa-2a for patients with advanced renal cell carcinoma. *Journal of Clinical Oncology* 19(5): 1312-1319.

Moyad MA. (1999a). Alternative therapies for advanced prostate cancer: What should I tell my patients? *Urology Clinics of North America* 26(2):413-417.

Moyad MA. (1999b). Nontraditional treatments for localized prostate cancer: Ten rules to know before talking to my patients. *Seminars in Urology and Oncology* 17(2):64-69.

Mraz L, Rusavy Z, Zdenek P, Heidenreichova M, Kozeluhova J, Steinigerova J, Tesinsky P. (1995). [A vasoactive-intestinal-polypeptide producing tumor (VIPoma) as an uncommon cause of life-threatening hypokalemia]. *Vnitr Lek* 41(8):535-537.

Mross K, Hauns B, Haring B, Bauknecht T, Meerpohl HG, Unger C, Maier-Lenz H. (1998). Clinical phase I study with one-hour paclitaxel infusion. *Annals of Oncology* 9(5):569-572.

Mu HH, Sewell WA. (1993). Enhancement of interleukin-4 production by pertussis toxin. *Infection and Immunity* 61(7):3190-3198.

Muggia FM, Brown TD, Goodman PJ, Macdonald JS, Hersh EM, Fleming TR, Leichman L. (1992). High incidence of coagualopathy in phase II studies of recombinant tumor necrosis factor in advanced pancreatic and gastric cancers. *Anticancer Drugs* 3(3):211-217.

Mukherjee M, Sahasrabuddhe MB. (1982). Effect of operation on peripheral lymphocyte counts and production of adenosine triphosphate (ATP) in cancer patients. *Journal of Surgical Oncology* 20:1-8.

Mulé JJ, Shu S, Rosenberg SA. (1984). The anti-tumor efficacy of lymphokine-activated killer cells and recombinant interleukin2 in vivo. *Journal of Immunology* 135:646-652.

Mulé JJ, Shu S, Schwarz SL, Rosenberg SA. (1984). Adoptive immunotherapy of established pulmonary metastases with LAK cells and recombinant interleukin-2. *Science* 225:1487-1489.

Muller R, Paneff J, Kollner V, Koch R. (2001). Quality of life of patients with laryngeal carcinoma: A post-treatment study. *European Archives of Otorhinolaryngology* 258(6):276-280.

Muller SO, Eckert I, Lutz WK, Stopper H. (1996). Genotoxicity of the laxative drug components emodin, aloe-emodin and danthron in mammalian cells: Topoisomerase II mediated? *Mutation Research* 371(3-4):165-173.

Muller W, Pongratz D, Barlin E, Eich W, Farber L, Haus U, Lautenschlager J, Mense S, Neeck G, Offenbacher M, et al. (2000). The challenge of fibromyalgia: New approaches. *Scandinavian Journal of Rheumatology* 113:86.

Muller WE, Ushijima H, Schroder HC. (1994). Mechanism of the antiretroviral effect of dsRNA. *Progress in Molecular and Subcellular Biology* 14:66-88.

Mullins RJ. (1998). Echinacea-associated anaphylaxis. *Medical Journal of Australia* 168(4):170-171.

Mulube M. (1996). Myths dispelled about chronic fatigue syndrome. *British Medical Journal* 313(7061):839.

Mura P, Piriou A, Tallineau C, Reiss D. (1986). La neopterine urinaire: Interet dans l'exploration de certains neoplasies. *Annales de Biologie et Clinique* 44:505-510.

Murad AM, Guimaraes RC, Aragao BC, Scalabrini-Neto AO, Rodrigues VH, Garcia R. (2001). Phase II trial of the use of paclitaxel and gemcitabine as a salvage treatment in metastatic breast cancer. *American Journal of Clinical Oncology* 24(3):264-268.

Muraoka A, Asami M, Ueno H, Yoneda R, Ogura M, Oribe T, Suzuki K, Maeda M, Chinzei T, Yamashiro K, et al. (1990). [B-chronic lymphocytic leukemia/prolymphocytic leukemia (CLL/PL)—A case report]. *Rinsho Ketsueki* 31(11): 1840-1844.

Murphy BJ. (1999). Test your knowledge: Fatigue assessment. *Clinical Journal of Oncology Nursing* 3(2):85-86.

Murren JR, Anderson S, Fedele J, Pizzorno G, Belliveau D, Zelterman D, Burtness BA, Tocino I, Flynn SD, Beidler D, et al. (1997). Dose-escalation and pharmacodynamic study of topotecan in combination with cyclophosphamide in patients with refractory cancer. *Journal of Clinical Oncology* 15(1):148-157.

Murren JR, Peccerillo K, DiStasio SA, Li X, Leffert JJ, Pizzorno G, Burtness BA, McKeon A, Cheng Y. (2000). Dose escalation and pharmacokinetic study of irinotecan in combination with paclitaxel in patients with advanced cancer. *Cancer Chemotherapy and Pharmacology* 46(1):43-50.

Murren JR, Pizzorno G, DiStasio SA, McKeon A, Peccerillo K, Gollerkari A, McMurray W, Burtness BA, Rutherford T, Li X, et al. (2002). Phase I study of perillyl alcohol in patients with refractory malignancies. *Cancer Biology and Therapy* 1(2):130-135.

Murthy MS, Meckstroth CV, Merkle BH, Huston JT, Cattaneo SM. (1976). Primary intimal sarcoma of pulmonary valve and trunk with osteogenic sarcomatous elements: Report of a case considered to be pulmonary embolus. *Archives of Pathology and Laboratory Medicine* 100(12):649-651.

Muscato JJ, Cirrincione C, Clamon G, Perry MC, Omura G, Berkowitz I, Reid T, Herndon JE II, Green MR. (1995). Etoposide (VP-16) and cisplatin at maximum tolerated dose in non-small cell lung carcinoma: A Cancer and Leukemia Group B study. *Lung Cancer* 13(3):285-294.

Muscio B. (1921). Is a fatigue test possible? *British Journal of Psychology* 12:31-46.

Muss HB, Capizzi RL, Atkins JN, Powell BL, Cooper MR, Ferree D, McMahan RA, Jobson V, Craig J, Homesley HD, et al. (1985). Phase I trials of high-dose cytosine arabinoside (HDara-C) and HDara-C plus cisplatin in patients with advanced malignancies. *Seminars in Oncology* 12(2 Suppl 3):166-170.

Muss HB, Spell N, Scudiery D, Capizzi RL, Cooper MR, Cruz J, Jackson DV, Richards F II, Spurr CL, White DR, et al. (1990). A phase II trial of PEG-L-asparaginase in the treatment of non-Hodgkins lymphoma. *Investigative New Drugs* 8(1):125-130.

Mystakidou K, Tsilika E, Kalaidopoulou O, Chondros K, Georgaki S, Papadimitriou L. (2002). Comparison of octreotide administration vs. conservative treatment in the management of inoperable bowel obstruction in patients with far advanced cancer: A randomized, double-blind, controlled clinical trial. *Anti-cancer Research* 22(2B):1187-1192.

Naftzger C, Takechi Y, Kohda H, Hara I, Vijayasaradhi S, Houghton AN. (1996). Immune response to a differentiation antigen induced by altered antigen: A study of tumor rejection and autoimmunity. *Proceedings of the National Academy of Sciences of the United States of America* 93:14809-14814.

Nagai T, Koyama R, Sasagawa Y, Matsumoto S, Kohgo Y, Niitsu Y, Konn S. (1993). [Follicular lymphoma associated with t(14;18)(q32;q21) chromosome translocation and bcl-2 gene rearrangement: Report of a case]. *Rinsho Ketsueki* 34(2):137-142.

Nagel GA, Wander HE, Blossey HC. (1982). Phase II study of aminoglutethimide and medroxyprogesterone acetate in the treatment of patients with advanced breast cancer. *Cancer Research* 42(8 Suppl):3442s-3444s.

Nagler A, Ackerstein A, Barak V, Slavin S. (1994). Treatment of chronic myelogenous leukemia with recombinant human interleukin-2 and interferon-alpha 2a. *Journal of Hematotherapy* 3(1):75-82.

Naglieri E, Procacci A, Galetta D, Abbate I, Della Erba L, Colucci G. (1999). Cisplatin, interleukin-2, interferon-alpha and tamoxifen in metastatic melanoma: A phase II study. *Journal of Chemotherapy* 11(2):150-155.

Nail LM. (2001). Long-term persistence of symptoms. *Seminars in Oncology Nursing* 17(4):249-254.

Nail LM. (2002). Fatigue in patients with cancer. *Oncology Nursing Forum* 29(3): 537.

Nail LM, Barsevick AM, Meek PM, Beck SL, Jones LS, Walker BL, Whitmer KR, Schwartz AL, Stephen S, King ME. (1998). Planning and conducting a multi-institutional project on fatigue. *Oncology Nursing Forum* 25(8):1398-1403.

Nail LM, Jones LS, Greene D, Schipper DL, Jensen R. (1991). Use and perceived efficacy of self-care activities in patients receiving chemotherapy. *Oncology Nursing Forum* 18(5):883-887.

Nail LM, King KB. (1987). Symptom distress: Fatigue. *Seminars in Oncology Nursing* 3(4):257-262.

Nail LM, Winningham ML. (1995). Fatigue and weakness in cancer patients: The symptoms experience. *Seminars in Oncology Nursing* 11(4):272-278.

Naito S, Yasumasu T, Kumazawa J, Hiratsuka Y, Sakamoto K, Iguchi A, Masaki Z, Hasui Y, Osada Y, Kurozumi T, et al. (1995). [Treatment of advanced renal cell carcinoma with a combination of interferon alpha and gamma]. *Nippon Hinyokika Gakkai Zasshi* 86(8):1346-1352.

Nakagomi H, Pisa P, Pisa EK, Yamamoto Y, Halapi E, Backlin K, Juhlin C, Kiessling R. (1995). Lack of interleukin-2 (IL-2) expression and selective expression of IL-10 mRNA in human renal cell carcinoma. *International Journal of Cancer* 63:366-371.

Nakajima T, Noguchi T, Kumahara Y, Sugihara A, Yamazaki T, Iwasaki T, Hamano T, Kakishita E. (1995). [Neuron specific enolase-producing IgD multiple myeloma with high serum amylase activity]. *Rinsho Ketsueki* 36(4):359-364.

Nakashima H, Nagafuchi K, Satoh H, Takeda K, Yamasaki T, Yonemasu H, Kishikawa H. (2000). Hepatoid adenocarcinoma of the gallbladder. *Journal of Hepatobiliary and Pancreatic Surgery* 7(2):226-230.

Nakaya T, Kuratsune H, Kitani T, Ikuta K. (1997). Demonstration of Borna disease virus in patients with chronic fatigue syndrome. *Nippon Rinsho—Japanese Journal of Clinical Medicine* 55(11):3064-3071.

Nakaya T, Takahashi H, Nakamura Y, Asahi S, Tobiume M, Kuratsune H, Kitani T, Yamanishi K, Ikuta K. (1996). Demonstration of Borna disease virus RNA in peripheral blood mononuclear cells derived from Japanese patients with chronic fatigue syndrome. *FEBS Letters* 378(2):145-149.

Nanjo H, Murakami M, Ebina T, Hoshi N, Sasaki T, Zhuang YJ, Kobayashi M, Kawamura K, Masuda H. (1996). Aortic intimal sarcoma with acute myocardial infarction. *Pathology International* 46(9):673-681.

Nasralla M, Haier J, Nicolson GL. (1999). Multiple mycoplasmal infections detected in blood of patients with chronic fatigue syndrome and/or fibromyalgia syndrome. *European Journal of Clinical Microbiology and Infectious Diseases* 18(12):859-865.

Natelson BH, Cheu J, Hill N, Bergen M, Korn L, Denny T, Dahl K (1998). Single-blind, placebo phase-in-trial of two escalating doses of selegiline in the chronic fatigue syndrome. *Neuropsychobiology* 37(3):150-154.

Natelson BH, Cheu J, Pareja J, Ellis SP, Policastro T, Findley TW. (1996). Randomized, double blind, controlled placebo-phase in trial of low dose phenelzine in the chronic fatigue syndrome. *Psychopharmacology* 124(3):226-230.

Natelson BH, LaManca JJ, Denny TN, Vladutiu A, Oleske J, Hill N, Bergen MT, Korn L, Hay J. (1998). Immunologic parameters in chronic fatigue syndrome, major depression, and multiple sclerosis. *American Journal of Medicine* 105(3A): 43S-49S.

National Institutes of Health (NIH) Consensus Conference. (1998). Acupuncture. *JAMA* 280(17):1518-1524.

National Institutes of Health Consensus Development Panel. (1997). Acupuncture. NIH Consensus Statement 107, November 3-5.

National Institutes of Health Consensus Development Panel. (2001). National Institutes of Health Consensus Development Conference statement: Adjuvant therapy for breast cancer, November 1-3, 2000. *Journal of the National Cancer Institutes Monographs* (30):5-15.

Natori H, Nakamura E, Tanaka K, Naito K, Egami K, Honda J, Osabe S, Imamura Y, Natori K, Yasuda K, et al. (1990). [Acute myelomonocytic leukemia with mastocytosis in bone marrow]. *Rinsho Ketsueki* 31(2):239-244.

Naughton M, Homsi J. (2002). Symptom assessment in cancer patients. *Current Oncology Reports* 4(3):256-263.

Neben K, Moehler T, Egerer G, Kraemer A, Hillengass J, Benner A, Ho AD, Goldschmidt H. (2001). High plasma basic fibroblast growth factor concentration is associated with response to thalidomide in progressive multiple myeloma. *Clinical Cancer Research* 7(9):2675-2681.

Neeck G. (1998). From the fibromyalgia challenge toward a new bio-psycho-social model of rheumatic diseases. *Zeitschrift Rheumatologie* 57(Suppl. 2):A13-A16.

Neeck G. (2000). Neuroendocrine and hormonal perturbations and relations to the serotonergic system in fibromyalgia patients. *Scandinavian Journal of Rheumatology* 113:8-12.

Neeck G, Riedel W. (1999). Hormonal perturbations in fibromyalgia syndrome. *Annals of the New York Academy of Sciences* 876:325-338.

Neeck G, Riedel W, Vaitl D, eds. (1997). Fibromyalgia syndrome: An interdisciplinary challenge of basic and clinical science. International conference, Bad Nauheim, Germany, October 23-25. *Zeitschrift für Rheumatologie* 57(Suppl. 2).

Needleman SW, Burns CP, Dick FR, Armitage JO. (1981). Hypoplastic acute leukemia. *Cancer* 48(6):1410-1414.

Neefe JR, Legha SS, Markowitz A, Salmon S, Meyskens F, Groopman J, Campion M, Evans L. (1990). Phase II study of recombinant alpha-interferon in malignant melanoma. *American Journal of Clinical Oncology* 13(6):472-476.

Neerinckx E, Van Houdenhove B, Lysens R, Vertommen H, Onghena P. (2000). Attributions in chronic fatigue syndrome and fibromyalgia syndrome in tertiary care. *Journal of Rheumatology* 27(4):1051-1055.

Neidhart JA, Gagen MM, Young D, Tuttle R, Melink TJ, Ziccarelli A, Kisner D. (1984). Interferon-alpha therapy of renal cancer. *Cancer Research* 44(9):4140-4143.

Neidhart JA, Gochnour D, Roach R, Hoth D, Young D. (1986). A comparison of mitoxantrone and doxorubicin in breast cancer. *Journal of Clinical Oncology* 4(5):672-677.

Neidhart JA, Gochnour D, Roach RW, Young D, Steinberg JA. (1984). A comparative trial of mitoxantrone and doxorubicin in patients with minimally pretreated breast cancer. *Seminars in Oncology* 11(3 Suppl 1):11-14.

Neidhart JA, Kohler W, Stidley C, Mangalik A, Plauche A, Anderson T, Quenzer RW, Rinehart JJ. (1990). Phase I study of repeated cycles of high-dose cyclophosphamide, etoposide, and cisplatin administered without bone marrow transplantation. *Journal of Clinical Oncology* 8(10):1728-1738.

Neilley LK, Goodin DS, Goodkin DE, Hauser SL. (1996). Side effect profile of interferon-beta-1b in MS: Results of an open label trial. *Neurology* 46(2):552-554.

Nelson K, Walsh D. (1991). Management of the anorexia/cachexia syndrome. *Cancer Bulletin* 43:403-406.

Nemoto K, Yamada S, Takai Y, Ogawa Y, Kakuto Y, Ariga H. (1997). [Radiation therapy for low-grade astrocytomas: Survival and QOL]. *Nippon Igaku Hoshasen Gakkai Zasshi* 57(6):336-340.

Nerenz DR, Love RR, Leventhal H, Easterling DV. (1986). Psychosocial consequences of cancer chemotherapy for elderly patients. *Health Services Research* 20(6 Pt 2):961-976.

Neri B, Doni L, Gemelli MT, Fulignati C, Turrini M, Di Cello V, Dominici A, Maleci M, Mottola A, Ponchietti R, et al. (2002). Phase II trial of weekly intravenous gemcitabine administration with interferon and interleukin-2 immunotherapy for metastatic renal cell cancer. *Journal of Urology* 168(3):956-958.

Neri G, Bianchedi M, Croce A, Moretti A. (1996). "Prolonged" decay test and auditory brainstem responses in the clinical diagnosis of the chronic fatigue syndrome. *Acta Otorhinolaryngologica Italica* 16(4):317-323.

Netea MG, Blok WL, Kullberg BJ, Bemelmans M, Vogels MT, Buurman WA, Van der Meer JW. (1995). Pharmacologic inhibitors of tumor necrosis factor production exert differential effects in lethal endotoxemia and in infection with live microorganisms in mice. *Journal of Infectious Diseases* 171(2):393-399.

Netter P, Hennig J. (1998). The fibromyalgia syndrome as a manifestation of neuroticism? *Zeitschrift Rheumatologie* 57(Suppl 2):105-108.

Neuhaus W, Ghaemi Y, Schmidt T, Lehmann E. (2000). [Treatment of perioperative anxiety in suspected breast carcinoma with a phytogenic tranquilizer]. *Zentralblatt Gynakologie* 122(11):561-565.

Neumann L, Buskila D. (1997). Quality of life and physical functioning of relatives of fibromyalgia patients. *Seminars in Arthritis and Rheumatism* 26(6):834-839.

Neumann L, Buskila D. (1998). Ethnocultural and educational differences in Israeli women correlate with pain perception in fibromyalgia. *Journal of Rheumatology* 25(7):1369-1373.

Newell S, Sanson-Fisher RW, Girgis A, Ackland S. (1999). The physical and psychosocial experiences of patients attending an outpatient medical oncology department: A cross-sectional study. *European Journal of Cancer Care* 8(2):73-82.

Newell S, Sanson-Fisher RW, Girgis A, Bonaventura A. (1998). How well do medical oncologists' perceptions reflect their patients' reported physicial and psychosocial problems? Data from a survey of five oncologists. *Cancer* 83(8):1640-1651.

Newman GE, Ravin CE. (1980). Weight loss, fatigue, and mediastinal and hilar adenopathy in a 67-year-old man. *Investigative Radiology* 15(3):174-177.

Newsholme EA, Blomstrand E. (1996). The plasma level of some amino acids and mental fatigue. *Experientia* 52(5):413-415.

Newton KA, Mackenzie DH, Spittle MF, Mikolajczuk A. (1973). Hodgkin's disease: A clinico-pathological study of 250 cases with a 5-year follow-up. *British Journal of Cancer* 27(1):80-91.

Ng YY, Yu S, Chen TW, Wu SC, Yang AH, Yang WC. (1998). Interstitial renal fibrosis in a young woman: Association with a Chinese preparation given for irregular menses. *Nephrology, Dialysis and Transplantation* 13(8):2115-2117.

Nicaise C, Rozencweig M, Crespeigne N, Dodion P, Gerard B, Lambert M, Decoster G, Kenis Y. (1986). Phase I study of triglycidylurazol given on a 5-day i.v. schedule. *Cancer Treatment Reports* 70(5):599-603.

Nicaise C, Rozencweig M, de Marneffe M, Crespeigne N, Dodion P, Piccart M, Sculier JP, Lenaz L, Kenis Y. (1983). Clinical phase I trial of marcellomycin with a single-dose schedule. *European Journal of Cancer and Clinical Oncology* 19(4):449-454.

Nicassio PM, Radojevic V, Weisman MH, Schuman C, Kim J, Schoenfeld-Smith K, Krall T. (1997). A comparison of behavioral and educational interventions for fibromyalgia. *Journal of Rheumatology* 24(10):2000-2007.

Nicolson GL, Bruton DM Jr, Nicolson NL. (1996). Chronic fatigue illness and Operation Desert Storm. *Journal of Occupational and Environmental Medicine* 38(1):14-16.

Nicolson GL, Nasralla M, Franco AR, De Meileir K, Nicolson NL, Ngwenya R, Haier J. (2000). Role of mycoplasmal infections in fatigue illnesses: Chronic fatigue and fibromyalgia syndromes, Gulf War illness, and rheumatoid arthritis. *Journal of Chronic Fatigue Syndrome* 6(3/4):23-39.

Nicolson GL, Nasralla M, Haier J. (1998). Diagnosis and treatment of mycoplasmal infections in fibromyalgia and chronic fatigue syndromes: Relationship to Gulf War illness. *Biomedical Therapy* 16:266-271.

Niederle N, Doberauer C, Kloke O, Hoffken K, Schmidt CG. (1987). [Effectiveness of gamma interferon and alpha interferon in hairy cell leukemia]. *Klinische Wochenschrift* 65(14):706-712.

Niederle N, Kurschel E, Schmidt CG. (1984). [Biological effect of recombined leukocyte alpha-2-interferon in metastasizing colorectal cancers]. *Deutsche Medizinsche Wochenschrift* 109(20):779-782.

Nielens H, Boisset V, Masquelier E. (2000). Fitness and perceived exertion in patients with fibromyalgia syndrome. *Clinical Journal of Pain* 16(3):209-213.

Niezgoda HE, Pater JL. (1993). A validation study of the domains of the core EORTC quality of life questionnaire. *Quality of Life Research* 2(5):319-325.

Niimoto M, Yoshinaka K, Hattori T, Kobayashi S, Hada Y, Hosoma S, Hatayama T, Ogawa Y, Iwamori S, Nagata N, et al. (1986). [Phase II study of THP patients with gastrointestinal cancer]. *Gan To Kagaku Ryoho* 13(2):362-367.

Niimoto M, Yoshinaka K, Hattori T, Kobayashi S, Hosoma S, Ogawa Y, Iwamori S, Nagata N, Yamagata S, Nishimawari K. (1985). [Phase II study on MCNU in patients with advanced or recurrent gastrointestinal cancer]. *Gan To Kagaku Ryoho* 12(9):1813-1819.

Niiranen A, Holsti LR, Cantell K, Mattson K. (1990). Natural interferon-alpha alone and in combination with conventional therapies in non-small cell lung cancer: A pilot study. *Acta Oncologica* 29(7):927-930.

Niitani H, Furuse K, Fukuoka M, Hasegawa K, Taguchi T. (1994). [Phase I clinical study on new vinca alkaloid derivative, KW-2307 (vinorelbine). KW-2307 Study Group]. *Gan To Kagaku Ryoho* 21(2):177-187.

Niloff JM, Knapp RC, Jones G, Schaetzl EM, Bast RC Jr. (1985). Recombinant leukocyte alpha interferon in advanced ovarian carcinoma. *Cancer Treatment Reports* 69(7-8):895-896.

Nilsson L, Kjellman NI, Storsaeter J, Gustafsson L, Olin P. (1996). Lack of association between pertussis vaccine and symptoms of asthma and allergy. *JAMA* 275(10):760.

Nisenbaum R, Reyes M, Mawle AC, Reeves WC. (1998). Factor analysis of unexplained severe fatigue and interrelated symptoms: Overlap with criteria for chronic fatigue syndrome. *American Journal of Epidemiology* 148(1):72-77.

Nishida Y, Deguchi T, Hayashi S, Kuriyama M, Ban Y, Kawada Y. (1992). [A case of Cushing's syndrome due to adrenal black adenoma]. *Hinyokika Kiyo* 38(1): 47-50.

Nishikai M. (1999). [Fibromyalgia]. *Nippon Naika Gakkai Zasshi* 88(10):1937-1942.

Nishikai M, Akiya K, Tojo T, Onoda N, Tani M, Shimizu K. (1996). "Seronegative" Sjögren's syndrome manifested as a subset of chronic fatigue syndrome. *British Journal of Rheumatology* 35(5):471-474.

Nishimura K, Nozawa M, Hara T, Sonoda T, Oka T. (1994). [A case of primary hyperparathyroidism associated with marked hypercalcemic crisis]. *Hinyokika Kiyo* 40(8):729-734.

Nishiyama K, Takahashi H, Okamoto M, Yao K, Inagi K, Nakayama M, Makoshi T. (1996). Combined chemotherapy and radiation therapy in head and neck cancer. *Acta Otolaryngologica Supplement* 524:79-82.

Nishiyama N, Kinoshita H, Kobayashi Y, Iwasa R, Katoh T, Inoue K, Inoue T. (1996). [Malignant lymphoma of the chest wall in a patient with chronic empyema]. *Nihon Kyobu Shikkan Gakkai Zasshi* 34(5):579-585.

Nixon PG. (1996a). Brainstem hypoperfusion in CFS. *Quarterly Journal of Medicine* 89(2):163-164.

Nixon PG. (1996b). Brainstem hypoperfusion in CFS. *Quarterly Journal of Medicine* 89(3):237.

Noble RL. (1984). Androgen use by athletes: A possible cancer risk. *Canadian Medical Association Journal* 130:549-550.

Noda K, Tanaka K, Ozaki M, Hirabayasi K, Hasegawa K, Nishiya I, Yakushiji M, Izumi R, Tomoda Y, Ogita Y, et al. (1998). [Early phase II trial of oral etoposide administered for 21 consecutive days in patients with cervical or ovarian cancer. ETP 21 Study Group—Cervical-Ovarian Cancer Group]. *Gan To Kagaku Ryoho* 25(13):2061-2068.

Noda K, Terajima Y, Ogita Y, Kono I, Hirabayashi K, Yakushiji M, Taguchi T. (1994). [Phase II clinical study of RP56976 (docetaxel) in patients with carcinoma ovarii or carcinoma colli uteri]. *Gan To Kagaku Ryoho* 21(14):2471-2477.

Noguchi Y, Yoshikawa T, Matsumoto A, Svaninger G, Gelin J. (1996). Are cytokines possible mediators of cancer cachexia? *Surgery Today* 26(7):467-475.

Nogue M, Saigi E, Segui MA. (1995). Clinical experience with tegafur and low dose oral leucovorin: A dose-finding study. *Oncology* 52(2):167-169.

Nole F, Munzone E, Mandala M, Catania C, Orlando L, Zampino MG, Minchella I, Colleoni M, Peruzzotti G, Marrocco E, et al. (2001). Vinorelbine, cisplatin and continuous infusion of 5-fluorouracil (ViFuP) in metastatic breast cancer patients: A phase II study. *Annals of Oncology* 12(1):95-100.

Nollet F, Ivanyi B, De Visser M, De Jong BA. (1996). Post-polio syndrome; the limit of neuromuscular adaptation? *Nederlands Tijdschrift voor Geneeskunde* 140(22):1169-1173.

Nomura Y, Abe O, Izuo M, Inoue K, Enomoto K, Kubo K, Koyama H, Sakai K, Terasawa T, Tominaga T. (1988). [Clinical evaluation of adriamycin in advanced and recurrent breast cancer (No. 4)—Joint study by 30 institutes on the duration of remission using various maintenance therapies in patients treated with CAF. Clinical Study Group of Adriamycin for Breast Cancer in Japan]. *Gan To Kagaku Ryoho* 15(6):1863-1871.

Nomura Y, Tominaga T, Abe O, Izuo M, Ogawa N. (1993). [Clinical evaluation of NK 622 (toremifene citrate) in advanced or recurrent breast cancer—A comparative study by a double blind method with tamoxifen]. *Gan To Kagaku Ryoho* 20(2):247-258.

Nortier J, Depierreux M, Vanherweghem JL. (1999). Herbal remedies and nephrotoxicity. *Revue Medicale de Bruxelles* 20(1):9-14.

Norton SA. (1998). Herbal medicines in Hawaii from tradition to convention. *Hawaii Medical Journal* 57(1):382-386.

Norum J, Wist EA. (1996). Quality of life in survivors of Hodgkin's disease. *Quality of Life Research* 5(3):367-374.

Notermans NC, Lokhorst HM, Wielaard R, Biesma DH, Rinkel GJ. (1998). [Clinical judgment and decision making in medical practice: A retiree with fatigue and foot drop]. *Nederlander Tijdschrift Geneeskunde* 142(4):174-179.

Notsu K, Oka N, Sohmiya M, Sato T, Ando S, Moritake K, Inada K, Osamura Y, Kato Y. (1994). Isolated adrenocorticotrophin deficiency associated with antipituitary antibodies, pituitary cyst, sphenoidal cyst and pineal tumor. *Endocrinology Journal* 41(6):631-637.

Novick SC, Warrell RP Jr. (2000). Arsenicals in hematologic cancers. *Seminars in Oncology* 27(5):495-501.

Nowak D, Zlatic T. (1999). Herbal products and the Internet: A marriage of convenience. *Journal of the American Pharmaceutical Association* 39(2):241-242.

Nozawa I, Imamura S, Fujimori I, Hashimoto K, Nakayama H, Hisamatsu K, Murakami Y. (1997). The relationship between psychosomatic factors and orthostatic dysregulation in young men. *Clinical Otolaryngology and Allied Sciences* 22(2):135-138.

Nukariya N, Kobayashi K, Ishihara Y, Yoneda S, Matsuda T, Yakushiji M, Yamakido M, Fukuoka M, Niitani H, Furue H. (1996). [Effects of an anti-emetic tropisetron capsule on QOL of patients with delayed nausea and vomiting induced by cancer chemotherapy. Group for Investigation of QOL Questionnaire for Anti-Emetics used in Cancer Chemotherapy. Joint Research Group for Tropisetron Double-Blind Comparative Study]. *Gan To Kagaku Ryoho* 23(6): 757-771.

Nwosu MO. (1998). Aspects of ethnobotanical medicine in southeast Nigeria. *Journal of Alternative and Complementary Medicine* 4(3):305-310.

Nygard R, Norum J, Due J. (2001). Goserelin (Zoladex) or orchiectomy in metastatic prostate cancer? A quality of life and cost-effectiveness analysis. *Anticancer Research* 21(1B):781-788.

Nyren O, Yin L, Josefsson S, McLaughlin JK, Blot WJ, Engqvist M, Hakelius L, Boice JD Jr, Adami HO. (1998). Risk of connective tissue disease and related disorders among women with breast implants: A nation-wide retrospective cohort study in Sweden. *British Medical Journal* 316(7129):417-422.

Obbens EA, Feun LG, Leavens ME, Savaraj N, Stewart DJ, Gutterman JU. (1985). Phase I clinical trial of intralesional or intraventricular leukocyte interferon for intracranial malignancies. *Journal of Neurooncology* 3(1):61-67.

Oberg K. (1992). Interferons in the management of neuroendocrine tumors and their possible mechanism of action. *Yale Journal of Biological Medicine* 65(5):519-529; discussion 531-536.

Oberg K. (1994). Endocrine tumors of the gastrointestinal tract: Systemic treatment. *Anticancer Drugs* 5(5):503-519.

Oberg K. (1996). Interferon-alpha versus somatostatin or the combination of both in gastro-enteropancreatic tumours. *Digestion* 57(Suppl 1):81-83.

Oberg K, Eriksson B. (1991a). The role of interferons in the management of carcinoid tumors. *Acta Oncologica* 30(4):519-522.

Oberg K, Eriksson B. (1991b). The role of interferons in the management of carcinoid tumours. *British Journal of Haematology* 79(Suppl 1):74-77.

Oberst MT, Hughes SH, Chang AS, McCubbin MA. (1991). Self-care burden, stress appraisal, and mood among persons receiving radiotherapy. *Cancer Nursing* 14(2):71-78.

O'Brien S, Talpaz M, Cortes J, Shan J, Giles FJ, Faderl S, Thomas D, Garcia-Manero G, Mallard S, Beth M, et al. (2002). Simultaneous homoharringtonine and interferon-alpha in the treatment of patients with chronic-phase chronic myelogenous leukemia. *Cancer* 94(7):2024-2032.

Obrist R, Paravicini U, Hartmann D, Nagel GA, Obrecht JP. (1979). Vindesine: A clinical trial with special reference to neurological side effects. *Cancer Chemotherapy Pharmacology* 2(4):233-237.

Ockenga J, Pirlich M, Gastell S, Lochs H. (2002). [Tumour anorexia–tumour cachexia in case of gastrointestinal tumours: Standards and visions]. *Zeitshrift Gastroenterologie* 40(11):929-936.

Odent MR, Culpin EE, Kimmel T. (1994). Pertussis vaccination and asthma: Is there a link? *JAMA* 272(8):592-593.

Odunsi K, Terry G, Ho L, Bell J, Cuzick J, Gansean TS. (1996). Susceptibility to human papillomavirus-associated cervical intra-epithelial neoplasia is determined by specific HLA DR-DQ alleles. *International Journal of Cancer* 67:595-602.

O'Dwyer PJ, Donehower M, Sigman LM, Fortner CL, Aisner J, Van Echo DA. (1985). Phase I trial of N-methylformamide (NMF, NSC 3051). *Journal of Clinical Oncology* 3(6):853-857.

O'Dwyer PJ, Laub PB, DeMaria D, Qian M, Reilly D, Giantonio B, Johnston AL, Wu EY, Bauman L, Clendeninn NJ, et al. (1996). Phase I trial of the thymidylate synthase inhibitor AG331 as a 5-day continuous infusion. *Clinical Cancer Research* 2(10):1685-1692.

Oettgen HC, Martin TR, Wynshaw-Boris A, Deng C, Drazen JM, Leder P. (1994). Active anaphylaxis in IgE-deficient mice. *Nature* 370:367-370.

Oevermann K, Buer J, Hoffmann R, Franzke A, Schrader A, Patzelt T, Kirchner H, Atzpodien J. (2000). Capecitabine in the treatment of metastatic renal cell carcinoma. *British Journal of Cancer* 83(5):583-587.

Offenbächer M, Glatzeder K, Ackenheil M. (1998). Self-reported depression, familial history of depression and fibromyalgia (FM), and psychological distress in patients with FM. *Zeitschrift Rheumatologie* 57(Suppl 2):94-96.

Offenbächer M, Stucki G. (2000). Physical therapy in the treatment of fibromyalgia. *Scandinavian Journal of Rheumatology* 113:78-85.

Ogasawara H, Toda F, Kumoi T, Sawada Y, Mitsunobu M, Uematsu K. (1984). Malignant histiocytosis in the oropharynx. *Journal of Surgical Oncology* 26(4): 272-277.

Ogata M, Uno N, Ohtsuka E, Kikuchi H, Nasu M. (1996). [Acute lymphoblastic leukemia with marked morphologic abnormalities after chemotherapy for gastric cancer]. *Rinsho Ketsueki* 37(1):29-34.

Ogawa K, Shineha H, Abe R, Shichishima T, Kimura H, Yui T, Kawaguchi M, Matsuda S, Uchida T, Kariyone S. (1989). [Acute promyelocytic leukemia with a history of RAEB in transformation and the 15/17 translocation]. *Rinsho Ketsueki* 30(1):67-71.

Ogawa M, Nishiura T, Yoshimura M, Horikawa Y, Yoshida H, Okajima Y, Matsumura I, Ishikawa J, Nakao H, Tomiyama Y, et al. (1998). Decreased nitric oxide-mediated natural killer cell activation in chronic fatigue syndrome. *European Journal of Clinical Investigation* 28(11):937-943.

Ogawa M, Takaku F, Maekawa T, Ota K, Ichimaru M, Izuo M, Takakura K, Ikeda S, Koiso K, Machida T, et al. (1987). [Phase I study of a recombinant gamma interferon (S-6810)]. *Gan To Kagaku Ryoho* 14(2):446-452.

Ogawa Y, Chung YS, Nakata B, Muguruma K, Fujimoto Y, Yoshikawa K, Shiba M, Fukuda T, Sowa M. (1995). A case of primary Hodgkin's disease of the stomach. *Journal of Gastroenterology* 30(1):103-107.

Ogawa Y, Ohshima H, Kawashima E, Akita N, Tanazawa S, Tobise K, Onodera S, Aoki H, Kubota H, Murakami C. (1991). [A case of right atrial myxoma—The availability of transesophageal echocardiography in the detection of right atrial myxoma]. *Kokyu To Junkan* 39(3):283-286.

Oh WK, George DJ, Kaufman DS, Moss K, Smith MR, Richie JP, Kantoff PW. (2001). Neoadjuvant docetaxel followed by radical prostatectomy in patients with high-risk localized prostate cancer: A preliminary report. *Seminars in Oncology* 28(4 Suppl 15):40-44.

Oh WK, Manola J, George DJ, Fierman A, Fontaine-Rothe P, Morrissey S, Prisby J, Kaufman DS, Shapiro CL, Kantoff PW, et al. (2002). A phase II trial of interferon-alpha and toremifene in advanced renal cell cancer patients. *Cancer Investigation* 20(2):186-191.

O'Hanlon DM, Harkin M, Karat D, Sergeant T, Hayes N, Griffin SM. (1995). Quality-of-life assessment in patients undergoing treatment for oesophageal carcinoma. *British Journal of Surgery* 82(12):1682-1685.

Ohe Y, Kasai T, Heike Y, Saijo N. (1998). [Clinical trial of IL-12 for cancer patients]. *Gan To Kagaku Ryoho* 25(2):177-184.

Ohe Y, Niho S, Kakinuma R, Kubota K, Matsumoto T, Ohmatsu H, Goto K, Kunitoh H, Saijo N, Nishiwaki Y. (2001). Phase I studies of cisplatin and docetaxel administered by three consecutive weekly infusions for advanced non-small cell lung cancer in elderly and non-elderly patients. *Japanese Journal of Clinical Oncology* 31(3):100-106.

Ohnishi N, Yonekawa Y, Nakasako S, Nagasawa K, Yokoyama T, Yoshioka M, Kuroda K. (1999). Studies on interactions between traditional herbal and Western medicines: I. Effects of Sho-seiryu-to on the pharmacokinetics of carbamazepine in rats. *Biological Pharmacy Bulletin* 22(5):527-531.

Ohsaki Y, Morimoto H, Osanai S, Nishigaki Y, Akiba Y, Hasebe C, Hirata S, Aburano T, Miyokawa N, Kikuchi K. (2000). Extensively calcified hemangioma of the diaphragm with increased 99mTc-hydroxymethylene diphosphonate uptake. *Internal Medicine* 39(7):576-578.

Ohshima K, Kikuchi M, Yoshida T, Masuda Y, Kimura N. (1991). Lymph nodes in incipient adult T-cell leukemia-lymphoma with Hodgkin's disease-like histologic features. *Cancer* 67(6):1622-1628.

Ojeda HF, Mech K Jr, Hicken WJ. (1998). Localized malignant mesothelioma: A case report. *American Surgery* 64(9):881-885.

Ojo-Amaise EA, Conley EJ, Peters JB. (1994). Decreased natural killer cell activity is associated with severity of chronic fatigue immune deficiency syndrome. *Clinical Infectious Diseases* 18:S157-S159.

Oka M, Fukuda M, Kuba M, Ichiki M, Rikimaru T, Soda H, Tsurutani J, Nakamura Y, Kawabata S, Nakatomi K, et al. (2002). Phase I study of irinotecan and cisplatin with concurrent split-course radiotherapy in limited-disease small-cell lung cancer. *European Journal of Cancer* 38(15):1998.

Okada S, Sakata Y, Matsuno S, Kurihara M, Sasaki Y, Ohashi Y, Taguchi T. (1999). Phase II study of docetaxel in patients with metastatic pancreatic cancer: A Japanese cooperative study. Cooperative Group of Docetaxel for Pancreatic Cancer in Japan. *British Journal of Cancer* 80(3-4):438-443.

Okamoto T. (2002). NSAID zaltoprofen improves the decrease in body weight in rodent sickness behavior models: Proposed new applications of NSAIDs (review). *International Journal of Molecular Medicine* 9(4):369-372.

Okuno K, Ohnishi H, Koh K, Shindo H, Yoshioka H, Yasutomi M. (1992). Clinical trials of intrasplenic arterial infusion of interleukin-2 (IS-IL-2) to patients with advanced cancer. *Biotherapy* 4(4):257-265.

Okuyama T, Akechi T, Kugaya A, Okamura H, Imoto S, Nakano T, Mikami I, Hosaka T, Uchitomi Y. (2000). Factors correlated with fatigue in disease-free breast cancer patients: Application of the Cancer Fatigue Scale. *Support Care Cancer* 8(3):215-222.

Okuyama T, Akechi T, Kugaya A, Okamura H, Shima Y, Maruguchi M, Hosaka T, Uchitomi Y. (2000). Development and validation of the Cancer Fatigue Scale: A brief, three-dimensional, self-rating scale for assessment of fatigue in cancer patients. *Journal of Pain Symptomatology Management* 19(1):5-14.

Okuyama T, Tanaka K, Akechi T, Kugaya A, Okamura H, Nishiwaki Y, Hosaka T, Uchitomi Y. (2001). Fatigue in ambulatory patients with advanced lung cancer: Prevalence, correlated factors, and screening. *Journal of Pain Symptomatology and Management* 22(1):554-564.

Older SA, Battafarano DF, Danning CL, Ward JA, Grady EP, Derman S, Russell IJ. (1998). The effects of delta wave sleep interruption on pain thresholds and fibromyalgia-like symptoms in healthy subjects: Correlations with insulin-like growth factor I. *Journal of Rheumatology* 25(6):1180-1186.

Oldham RK, Blumenschein G, Schwartzberg L, Birch R, Arnold J. (1992). Combination biotherapy utilizing interleukin-2 and alpha interferon in patients with advanced cancer: A National Biotherapy Study Group trial. *Molecular Biotherapy* 4(1):4-9.

Olencki T, Peereboom D, Wood L, Budd GT, Novick A, Finke J, McLain D, Elson P, Bukowski RM. (2001). Phase I and II trials of subcutaneously administered rIL-2, interferon alfa-2a, and fluorouracil in patients with metastatic renal carcinoma. *Journal of Cancer Research and Clinical Oncology* 127(5):319-324.

Olesen BK, Ernst P, Nissen MH, Hansen HH. (1987). Recombinant interferon A (IFL-rA) therapy of small cell and squamous cell carcinoma of the lung: A phase II study. *European Journal of Cancer and Clinical Oncology* 23(7):987-989.

Olin R, Lidbeck J. (1996). [Fibromyalgia—The explanatory mechanisms should be searched centrally, not peripherally (letter)] Fibromyalgi—forklaringarna skall sokas centralt, inte perifert. *Lakartidningen* 93(22):2125-2126.

Olsen EA, Rosen ST, Vollmer RT, Variakojis D, Roenigk HH Jr, Diab N, Zeffren J. (1989). Interferon alfa-2a in the treatment of cutaneous T cell lymphoma. *Journal of the American Academy of Dermatology* 20(3):395-407.

Olson GB, Kanaan MN, Gersuk GM, Kelley LM, Jones JF. (1986). Correlation between allergy and persistent Epstein-Barr virus infections in chronic Epstein-Barr virus infected patients. *Journal of Allergy and Clinical Immunology* 78(2): 308-314.

Olson GB, Kanaan MN, Kelley LM, Jones JF. (1986). Specific allergen-induced Epstein-Barr nuclear antigen-positive B cells from patients with chronic active Epstein-Barr virus infections. *Journal of Allergy and Clinical Immunology* 78(2):315-320.

Olson K, Tom B, Hewitt J, Whittingham J, Buchanan L, Ganton G. (2002). Evolving routines: Preventing fatigue associated with lung and colorectal cancer. *Qualitative Health Research* 12(5):655-670.

Olson TA, Virmani R, Ansinelli RA, Lee DH, Mosijczuk AD, Marsella RC, Ruymann FB. (1982). Cardiomyopathy in a child with hypereosinophilic syndrome. *Pediatric Cardiology* 3(2):161-169.

Olver IN, Hercus T, Lopez A, Vadas M, Somogyi AA, Doyle I, Foster DJ, Keefe D, Taylor A, Brown M, et al. (2002). A phase I study of the GM-CSF antagonist E21R. *Cancer Chemotherapy and Pharmacology* 50(3):171-178.

O'Malley PG, Balden E, Tomkins G, Santoro J, Kroenke K, Jackson JL. (2000). Treatment of fibromyalgia with antidepressants: A meta-analysis. *Journal of General Internal Medicine* 15(9):659-666.

O'Malley PG, Jackson JL, Santoro J, Tomkins G, Balden E, Kroenke K. (1999). Antidepressant therapy for unexplained symptoms and symptom syndromes. *Journal of Family Practice* 48(12):980-990.

Ondrizek RR, Chan PJ, Patton WC, King A. (1999a). An alternative medicine study of herbal effects on the penetration of zona-free hamster oocytes and the integrity of sperm deoxyribonucleic acid. *Fertility and Sterility* 71(3):517-522.

Ondrizek RR, Chan PJ, Patton WC, King A. (1999b). Inhibition of human sperm motility by specific herbs used in alternative medicine. *Journal of Assisted Reproductive Genetics* 16(2):87-91.

Onishi Y, Yamaura T, Tauchi K, Sakamoto T, Tsukada K, Numone S, Komatsu Y, Saiki I. (1998). Expression of the anti-metastatic effect induced by Juzen-taihoto is based on the content of Shimotsu-to constituents. *Biological Pharmacy Bulletin* 21(7):761-765.

Onopa J. (1999). Complementary and alternative medicine (CAM): A review for the primary care physician. *Hawaii Medical Journal* 58(2):9-19.

Oostendorp RAJ, Schaaper WMMM, Post J, Von Blomberg BM, Meloen RH, Scheper RJ. (1992). Suppression of lymphocyte proliferation by a retroviral p15E-derived hexapeptide. *European Journal of Immunology* 22:1505-1511.

Ophüls W. (1921). Arteriosclerosis and cardiovascular disease: Their relation to infectious diseases. *JAMA* 76:700-701.

Opp MR, Hughes TK Jr, Rady P, Smith EM. (1996). Mechanisms of HIV-induced alterations in sleep: The role of cytokines in the CNS. *SRS Bulletin* 2:31-37.

Opp MR, Toth LA. (1998). Somnogenic and pyrogenic effects of interleukin-1beta and lipopolysaccharide in intact and vagotomized rats. *Life Scientist* 62:923-936.

O'Quinn K. (2001). Pathologic quiz case: A 43-year-old man with fatigue and night sweats. *Archives of Pathology and Laboratory Medicine* 125(6):838-840.

O'Reilly EM, Stuart KE, Sanz-Altamira PM, Schwartz GK, Steger CM, Raeburn L, Kemeny NE, Kelsen DP, Saltz LB. (2001). A phase II study of irinotecan in patients with advanced hepatocellular carcinoma. *Cancer* 91(1):101-105.

O'Reilly SE, Gelmon KA. (1995). Biweekly paclitaxel and cisplatin: A phase I/II study in the first-line treatment of metastatic breast cancer. *Seminars in Oncology* 22(3 Suppl 6):109-111.

Orii K, Kobayashi H, Ueno M, Ishida F, Saito H, Hata S, Aoki K, Narita A, Shimodaira S, Kitano K, Uchimaru K, Motokura T. (1997). [Mantle cell lymphoma with multiple extranodal involvement]. *Rinsho Ketsueki* 38(6):520-525.

Ormrod D, Spencer CM. (1999). Topotecan: A review of its efficacy in small cell lung cancer. *Drugs* 58(3):533-551.

Osborne CK, Sunderland MC, Neidhart JA, Ravdin PM, Abeloff MD. (1994). Failure of GM-CSF to permit dose-escalation in an every other week dose-intensive regimen for advanced breast cancer. *Annals of Oncology* 5(1):43-47.

Osoba D. (2000). Health-related quality-of-life assessment in clinical trials of supportive care in oncology. *Support Care in Cancer* 8(2):84-88.

Osoba D, Aaronson NK, Muller M, Sneeuw K, Hsu MA, Yung WK, Brada M, Newlands E. (1997). Effect of neurological dysfunction on health-related quality of life in patients with high-grade glioma. *Journal of Neurooncology* 34(3):263-278.

Osoba D, Brada M, Prados MD, Yung WK. (2000). Effect of disease burden on health-related quality of life in patients with malignant gliomas. *Neuro-oncology* 2(4):221-228.

Osoba D, Burchmore M. (1999). Health-related quality of life in women with metastatic breast cancer treated with trastuzumab (Herceptin). *Seminars in Oncology* 26(4 Suppl 12):84-88.

Osoba D, Murray N, Gelmon K, Karsai H, Knowling M, Shah A, McLaughlin M, Fetherstonhaugh E, Page R, Bowman CA. (1994). Quality of life, appetite, and weight change in patients receiving dose-intensive chemotherapy. *Oncology* 8(4):61-65; discussion 65-66, 69.

Osoba D, Northfelt DW, Budd DW, Himmelberger D. (2001). Effect of treatment on health-related quality of life in acquired immunodeficiency syndrome (AIDS)-

related Kaposi's sarcoma: A randomized trial of pegylated-liposomal doxorubicin versus doxorubicin, bleomycin, and vincristine. *Cancer Investigation* 19(6): 573-580.

Osoba D, Rusthoven JJ, Turnbull KA, Evans WK, Shepherd FA. (1985). Combination chemotherapy with bleomycin, etoposide, and cisplatin in metastatic non-small-cell lung cancer. *Journal of Clinical Oncology* 3(11):1478-1485.

Osoba D, Slamon DJ, Burchmore M, Murphy M. (2002). Effects on quality of life of combined trastuzumab and chemotherapy in women with metastatic breast cancer. *Journal of Clinical Oncology* 20(14):3106-3113.

Osoba D, Zee B, Pater J, Warr D, Kaizer L, Latreille J. (1994). Psychometric properties and responsiveness of the EORTC quality of Life Questionnaire (QLQ-C30) in patients with breast, ovarian and lung cancer. *Quality of Life Research* 3(5):353-364.

Osoba D, Zee B, Pater J, Warr D, Latreille J, Kaizer L. (1997). Determinants of postchemotherapy nausea and vomiting in patients with cancer: Quality of Life and Symptom Control Committees of the National Cancer Institute of Canada Clinical Trials Group. *Journal of Clinical Oncology* 15(1):116-123.

Osoba D, Zee B, Warr D, Kaizer L, Latreille J, Pater J. (1996). Quality of life studies in chemotherapy-induced emesis. *Oncology* 53(Suppl 1):92-95.

Osoba D, Zee B, Warr D, Latreille J, Kaizer L, Pater J. (1997). Effect of post-chemotherapy nausea and vomiting on health-related quality of life: The Quality of Life and Symptom Control Committees of the National Cancer Institute of Canada Clinical Trials Group. *Support Care in Cancer* 5(4):307-313.

Osse BH, Vernooij-Dassen MJ, Schade E, De Vree B, Van den Muijsenbergh ME, Grol RP. (2002). Problems to discuss with cancer patients in palliative care: A comprehensive approach. *Patient Education and Counseling* 47(3):195-204.

Ostensen M, Rugelsjoen A, Wigers SH. (1997). The effect of reproductive events and alterations of sex hormone levels on the symptoms of fibromyalgia. *Scandinavian Journal of Rheumatology* 26(5):355-360.

Ostensen M, Schei B. (1997). Sociodemographic characteristics and gynecological disease in 40-42 year old women reporting musculoskeletal disease. *Scandinavian Journal of Rheumatology* 26(6):426-434.

Oster W, Herman F, Gamm H. (1990). Erythropoietin for the treatment of anemia of malignancy associated with neoplastic bone marrow infiltration. *Journal of Clinical Oncology* 8:956-962.

Osterbor A. (2000). The role of recombinant human erythropoietin in the management of anaemic cancer patients: Focus on haematological malignancies. *Medical Oncology* 17(Suppl 1):S17-S22.

Osterholm MT. (2000). Emerging infections—Another warning. *The New England Journal of Medicine* 342(17):1280-1281.

Osterlund P, Elomaa I, Virkkunen P, Joensuu H. (2001). A phase I study of raltitrexed (Tomudex) combined with carmofur in metastatic colorectal cancer. *Oncology* 61(2):113-119.

Osterlund P, Orpana A, Elomaa I, Repo H, Joensuu H. (2002). Raltitrexed treatment promotes systemic inflammatory reaction in patients with colorectal carcinoma. *British Journal of Cancer* 87(6):591-599.

Osterwalder P, Koch J, Iten M, Vetter W. (1998). [Fatigue, general weakness, subcutaneous nodules]. *Schweizerische Rundschau fur Medizin Praxis* 87(4): 116-121.

Ostrow S, Van Echo D, Whitacre M, Aisner J, Simon R, Wiernik PH. (1981). Physiologic response and toxicity in patients undergoing whole-body hyperthermia for the treatment of cancer. *Cancer Treatment Reports* 65(3-4):323-325.

Otani M, Shimizu T, Serizawa H, Ebihara Y, Nagashima Y. (2001). Low-grade renal cell carcinoma arising from the lower nephron: A case report with immunohistochemical, histochemical and ultrastructural studies. *Pathology International* 51(12):954-960.

Otsuji Y, Arima N, Fujiwara H, Saito K, Kisanuki A, Tanaka H. (1994). Reversible complete atrioventricular block due to malignant lymphoma. *European Heart Journal* 15(3):407-408.

Otsuka F, Ogura T, Hayakawa N, Hashimoto M, Makino H, Ota Z, Kageyama J. (1996). A case of Schmidt syndrome accompanied by a pituitary adenoma. *Endocrinology Journal* 43(5):495-502.

Oura S, Sakurai T, Yoshimura G, Tamaki T, Umemura T, Kokawa Y. (1999). [A study of the safety of rapid infusion of alendronate]. *Gan To Kagaku Ryoho* 26(3):345-351.

Oyama H, Kaneda M, Katsumata N, Akechi T, Ohsuga M. (2000). Using the bedside wellness system during chemotherapy decreases fatigue and emesis in cancer patients. *Journal of Medical Systems* 24(3):173-182.

Oye I, Morland LM, Gustafsson H. (1996). [Fibromyalgia and central sensitization] Fibromyalgi og sentral sensitivisering. *Lakartidningen* 93(21):2040.

Ozata M, Odabasi Z, Musabak U, Corakci A, Gundogan MA. (1997). A case of Addison's disease associated with the Lambert-Eaton myasthenic syndrome. *Journal of Endocrinological Investigation* 20(6):338-341.

Ozawa A, Iwasaki T, Miyake F, Murayama M, Miyamoto S, Aida Y, Takakuwa T, Tadokoro M, Ohkawa S. (1997). A case of primary malignant fibrous histiocytoma of the heart with a left-to-right atrial shunt. *Japanese Circulation Journal* 61(11):943-946.

Ozer H, Gavigan M, O'Malley J, Thompson D, Dadey B, Nussbaum-Blumenson A, Snider C, Rudnick S, Ferraresi R, Norred S, et al. (1983). Immunomodulation by recombinant interferon-alpha 2 in a phase I trial in patients with lymphoproliferative malignancies. *Journal of Biological Response Modifiers* 2(6):499-515.

Paal E, Thompson LD, Frommelt RA, Przygodzki RM, Heffess CS. (2001). A clinicopathologic and immunohistochemical study of 35 anaplastic carcinomas of the pancreas with a review of the literature. *Annals of Diagnostic Pathology* 5(3):129-140.

Paciucci PA, Holland JF, Glidewell O, Odchimar R. (1989). Recombinant interleukin-2 by continuous infusion and adoptive transfer of recombinant interleukin-2-activated cells in patients with advanced cancer. *Journal of Clinical Oncology* 7(7):869-878.

Paciucci PA, Raptis G, Bleiweiss I, Weltz C, Lehrer D, Gurry R. (2002). Neo-adjuvant therapy with dose-dense docetaxel plus short-term filgrastim rescue for locally advanced breast cancer. *Anticancer Drugs* 13(8):791-795.

Padgett DA, Sheridan JF, Loria RM. (1995). Steroid hormone regulation of a polyclonal Th2 immune response. *Annals of the New York Academy of Sciences* 774:323-325.

Padilla GV. (1990). Gastrointestinal side effects and quality of life in patients receiving radiation therapy. *Nutrition* 6(5):367-370.

Padilla GV. (1992). Validity of health-related quality of life subscales. *Progress in Cardiovascular Nursing* 7(1):13-20.

Padmanabhan N, Balkwill FR, Bodmer JG, Rubens RD. (1985). Recombinant DNA human interferon alpha 2 in advanced breast cancer: A phase 2 trial. *British Journal of Cancer* 51(1):55-60.

Paelinck BP, Vermeersch PH, Convens CG, Van Cauwelaert PA, Van Den Branden FL. (1995). [Cardiac myxoma in 13 patients]. *Nederlander Tijdschrift Geneeskunde* 139(38):1931-1935.

Paffenbarger RS, Lee I-M, Wing AL. (1992). The influence of physical activity on the incidence of site-specific cancers in college alumni. *Advances in Experimental Medicine and Biology* 322:7-15.

Paganelli R, Scala E, Ansotegui IJ, Ausiello CM, Halapi E, Fanales-Belasio E, D'Offizi G, Mezzaroma I, Pandolfi F, Fiorilli M, et al. (1995). CD8+ T lymphocytes provide helper activity for IgE synthesis in human immunodeficiency virus-infected patients with hyper-IgE. *Journal of Experimental Medicine* 181: 423-428.

Paintal AS. (1973). Vadal sensory receptors and their reflex effects. *Physiology Reviews* 53:159-227.

Paintal AS. (1995). Sensations from J receptors. *News in Physiological Science* 10:238-243.

Paintal AS, Damodaran VN, Guz A. (1973). Mechanism of excitation of type J receptors. *Acta Neurobiologica Experimenta* 33:15-19.

Paiva T, Batista A, Martins P, Martins A. (1995). The relationship between headaches and sleep disturbances. *Headache* 35(10):590-596.

Pajkos G, Bodoky G, Padi E, Izso J, Szanto J. (1998). [Low-dose leucovorin and interferon-alpha as modulators of 5-fluorouracil for adjuvant chemotherapy of colorectal cancer]. *Orv Hetil* 139(26):1571-1575.

Palani V, Senthilkumaran RK, Govindasamy S. (1999). Biochemical evaluation of antitumor effect of Muthu Marunthu (a herbal formulation) on experimental fibrosarcoma in rats. *Journal of Ethnopharmacology* 65(3):257-265.

Palmer FJ. (1983). The clinical manifestations of primary hyperparathyroidism. *Comprehensive Therapy* 9(2):56-64.

Palmeri S, Gebbia V, Rausa L. (1990). 5-Fluorouracil and recombinant alpha interferon-2a in the treatment of advanced colorectal carcinoma: A dose optimization study. *Journal of Chemotherapy* 2(5):327-330.

Paltiel O, Avitzour M, Peretz T, Cherny N, Kaduri L, Pfeffer RM, Wagner N, Soskolne V. (2001). Determinants of the use of complementary therapies by patients with cancer. *Journal of Clinical Oncology* 19(9):2439-2448.

Paoletti C, Le Pecq JB, Dat-Xuong N, Juret P, Garnier H, Amiel JL, Rouesse J. (1980). Antitumor activity, pharmacology, and toxicity of ellipticines, ellipticinium, and 9-hydroxy derivatives: Preliminary clinical trials of 2-methyl-9-hydroxy ellipticinium (NSC 264-137). *Recent Results in Cancer Research* 74: 107-123.

Papakostas P, Kouroussis C, Androulakis N, Samelis G, Aravantinos G, Kalbakis K, Sarra E, Souglakos J, Kakolyris S, Georgoulias V. (2001). First-line chemotherapy with docetaxel for unresectable or metastatic carcinoma of the biliary tract: A multicentre phase II study. *European Journal of Cancer* 37(15):1833-1838.

Parcell S. (2002). Sulfur in human nutrition and applications in medicine. *Alternative Medicine Reviews* 7(1):22-44.

Paredes Espinoza M, Lippman SM, Kavanagh JJ, Delgadillo Madrueno F, Paredes Casillas P, Banuelos Acosta O, Alvarez Marquez V, Buenrostro Ahued MA, de Alba Ayala I, Arias Castro G. (1994). [Treatment of 32 cervico-uterine cancer patients with 13-cis-retinoic acid and interferon alpha]. *Revista de Investigacion Clinica* 46(2):105-111.

Paridaens R, Uges DR, Barbet N, Choi L, Seeghers M, van der Graaf WT, Groen HJ, Dumez H, Buuren IV, Muskiet F, et al. (2000). A phase I study of a new polyamine biosynthesis inhibitor, SAM486A, in cancer patients with solid tumours. *British Journal of Cancer* 83(5):594-601.

Parish JG. (1978). Early outbreaks of "epidemic neuromyasthenia." *Postgraduate Medical Journal* 54:711-717.

Park IS, Lee YS, Kim JC, Hwang SG. (1995). Serum neopterin levels in ovarian tumors. *International Journal of Gynaecology and Obstetrics* 51(3):229-234.

Park JH, Phothimat P, Oates CT, Hernanz-Schulman M, Olsen NJ. (1998). Use of P-31 magnetic resonance spectroscopy to detect metabolic abnormalities in muscles of patients with fibromyalgia. *Arthritis and Rheumatism* 41(3):406-413.

Parra HS, Tixi L, Latteri F, Bretti S, Alloisio M, Gravina A, Lionetto R, Bruzzi P, Dani C, Rosso R, et al. (2001). Combined regimen of cisplatin, doxorubicin, and alpha-2b interferon in the treatment of advanced malignant pleural mesothelioma: A phase II multicenter trial of the Italian Group on Rare Tumors (GITR) and the Italian Lung Cancer Task Force (FONICAP). *Cancer* 92(3):650-656.

Parsaie FA, Golchin M, Asvadi I. (2000). A comparison of nurse and patient perceptions of chemotherapy treatment stressors. *Cancer Nursing* 23(5):371-374.

Parth P, Dunlap WP, Kennedy RS, Ordy JM, Lane NE. (1989). Motor and cognitive testing of bone marrow transplant patients after chemoradiotherapy. *Perception and Motor Skills* 68(3 Pt 2):1227-1241.

Parziale JR, Chen JJ. (1996). Fibromyalgia. *Medical Health Rhode Island* 79(5): 188-192.

Pasero CL. (1998). Understanding fibromyalgia syndrome. *American Journal of Nursing* 98(10):17-18.

Passik SD, Kirsh KL, Rosenfeld B, McDonald MV, Theobald DE. (2001). The changeable nature of patients' fears regarding chemotherapy: Implications for palliative care. *Journal of Pain Symptomatology and Management* 21(2):113-120.

Passik SD, Kirsh KL, Theobald D, Donaghy K, Holtsclaw E, Edgerton S, Dugan W. (2002). Use of a depression screening tool and a fluoxetine-based algorithm to improve the recognition and treatment of depression in cancer patients: A demonstration project. *Journal of Pain Symptomatology and Management* 24(3): 318-327.

Passik SD, Roth AJ. (1999). Anxiety symptoms and panic attacks preceding pancreatic cancer diagnosis. *Psychooncology* 8(3):268-272.

Pastoris O, Aquilani R, Foppa P, Bovio G, Segagni S, Baiardi P, Catapano M, Maccario M, Salvadeo A, Dossena M. (1997). Altered muscle energy metabolism in post-absoptive patients with chronic renal failure. *Scandinavian Journal of Urology and Nephrology* 31:281-287.

Patarca R. (2000). *Concise Encyclopedia of Chronic Fatigue Syndrome.* Binghamton, NY: The Haworth Medical Press.

Patarca R, Dorta B, Ramirez JL. (1982). Creation of a database for sequences of ribosomal nucleic acids and detection of conserved restriction endonucleases sites through computerized processing. *Nucleic Acids Research* 10(1):175-182.

Patarca R, Fletcher MA. (1997). Interleukin-1: Basic science and clinical applications. *Critical Reviews in Oncogenesis* 8(2-3):143-188.

Patarca R, Fletcher MA. (1998). Interleukin-6 and disease: Two case reports that point to the usefulness of measuring cytokine levels in clinical settings. *Journal of Chronic Fatigue Syndrome* 4(1):53-69.

Patarca R, Fletcher MA, Podack ER. (1995). Cytolytic cell functions. In *Manual of Clinical Laboratory Immunology,* Rose NR, De Macario EC, Folds JD, Lane HC, Nakamura RM, eds. Washington DC: American Society for Microbiology, pp. 296-303.

Patarca R, Haseltine WA. (1984). Similarities among retrovirus proteins. *Nature* 312:496.

Patarca R, Haseltine WA. (1985). A major retroviral core protein related to EPA and TIMP. *Nature* 318:390.

Patarca R, Haseltine WA. (1986). Variation among the human T-lymphotropic virus type III (HTLV-III/LAV) strains. *Journal of Theoretical Biology* 125:213-217.

Patarca R, Haseltine WA. (1987). Letter to the editor. *AIDS Research and Human Retroviruses* 3:1-2.

Patarca R, Haseltine WA, Webster T, Smith TF. (1987). Of how great significance. *Nature* 326:749.

Patarca R, Heath C, Goldenberg GJ, Rosen CA, Sodroski JG, Haseltine WA, Hansen UM. (1987). In vitro transcription directed by the HIV LTR. *AIDS Research and Human Retroviruses* 3:41-56.

Patarca R, Klimas NG, Lutgendorf S, Antoni M, Fletcher MA. (1994). Dysregulated expression of tumor necrosis factor in chronic fatigue syndrome: Interrelations with cellular sources and patterns of soluble immune mediator expression. *Clinical Infectious Diseases* 18(Suppl 1):S147-S153.

Patarca R, Klimas NG, Sandler D, Garcia MN, Fletcher MA. (1995). Interindividual immune status variation patterns in patients with chronic fatigue syndrome: Association with gender and the tumor necrosis factor system. *Journal of Chronic Fatigue Syndrome* 2(1):13-40.

Patarca R, Klimas NG, Walling J, Mayer V, Baum M, Yue X-S, Garcia MN, Pons H, Sandler D, Friedlander A, et al. (1994). CD8 T-cell immunotherapy in AIDS: Rationale and lessons learned at the cellular and molecular biology levels. *Clinical Immunology Newsletter* 14:105-111.

Patarca R, Klimas NG, Walling J, Sandler D, Friedlander A, Jin X-Q, Garcia MN, Fletcher MA. (1995). Adoptive CD8+ T-cell immunotherapy of AIDS patients with Kaposi's sarcoma. *Critical Reviews in Oncogenesis* 6(3-6):179-234.

Patarca R, Lutgendorf S, Antoni M, Klimas NG, Fletcher MA. (1994). Dysregulated expression of tumor necrosis factor in the chronic fatigue immune dysfunction syndrome: Interrelations with cellular sources and patterns of soluble immune mediator expression. *Clinical Infectious Diseases* 18:S147-S153.

Patarca R, Perez G, Gonzalez A, Garcia-Morales RO, Gamble R, Klimas N, Fletcher MA. (1992). Comprehensive evaluation of acute immunological changes induced by cuprophane and polysulfone membranes in a patient on chronic hemodialysis. *American Journal of Nephrology* 12:274-278.

Patarca R, Sandler D, Walling J, Klimas NG, Fletcher MA. (1995). Assessment of immune mediator expression levels in biological fluids and cells: A critical appraisal. *Critical Reviews in Oncogenesis* 6(2):117-149.

Patarca-Montero R, Klimas NG, Fletcher MA. (2000). Immunotherapy of chronic fatigue syndrome: Therapeutic interventions aimed at modulating the Th1/Th2 cytokine expression balance. *Journal of Chronic Fatigue Syndrome* 8(1):3-37.

Patenaude H, Gelinas C, Vandal S, Fillion L. (2002). [Elaboration of a conceptual frame to explain fatigue secondary to a health difficulty and implications for nursing practice]. *Rech Soins Infirmieres* 70:66-81.

Pater JL, Zee B, Palmer M, Johnston D, Osoba D. (1997). Fatigue in patients with cancer: Results with National Cancer Institute of Canada Clinical Trials Group studies employing the EORTC QLQ-C30. *Supportive Care in Cancer* 5(5):410-413.

Paterson DL, Georghiou PR, Allworth AM, Kemp RJ. (1995). Thalidomide as treatment of refractory aphthous ulceration related to human immunodeficiency virus infection. *Clinical Infectious Diseases* 20(2):250-254.

Patnaik A, Rowinsky EK, Villalona MA, Hammond LA, Britten CD, Siu LL, Goetz A, Felton SA, Burton S, Valone FH, et al. (2002). A phase I study of pivaloyloxymethyl butyrate, a prodrug of the differentiating agent butyric acid, in patients with advanced solid malignancies. *Clinical Cancer Research* 8(7):2142-2148.

Patt YZ, Hassan MM, Lozano RD, Waugh KA, Hoque AM, Frome AI, Lahoti S, Ellis L, Vauthey JN, Curley SA, Schnirer II, Raijman I. (2001). Phase II trial of cisplatin, interferon alpha-2b, doxorubicin, and 5-fluorouracil for biliary tract cancer. *Clinical Cancer Research* 7(11):3375-3380.

Patt YZ, Jones DV Jr, Hoque A, Lozano R, Markowitz A, Raijman I, Lynch P, Charnsangavej C. (1996). Phase II trial of intravenous flourouracil and subcutaneous interferon alfa-2b for biliary tract cancer. *Journal of Clinical Oncology* 14(8):2311-2315.

Paul WE, Ohara J. (1987). B-cell stimulatory factor-1/interleukin-4. *Annual Reviews of Immunology* 5:429-459.

Paul WE, Seder RA. (1994). Lymphocyte responses and cytokines. *Cell* 76:241-251.

Pawelec G, Zeuthen J, Kiessling R. (1997). Escape from host-antitumor immunity. *Critical Reviews in Oncogenesis* 8(2-3):111-141.

Payne JK. (2002). The trajectory of fatigue in adult patients with breast and ovarian cancer receiving chemotherapy. *Oncology Nursing Forum* 29(9):1334-1340.

Paz-Ares L, Kunka R, DeMaria D, Cassidy J, Alden M, Beranek P, Kaye S, Littlefield D, Reilly D, Depee S, et al. (1998). A phase I clinical and pharmacokinetic study of the new topoisomerase inhibitor GI147211 given as a 72-h continuous infusion. *British Journal of Cancer* 78(10):1329-1336.

Pazdur R. (1997). Phase II study of UFT plus leucovorin in colorectal cancer. *Oncology* 54(Suppl 1):19-23.

Pazdur R, Ajani JA, Abbruzzese JL, Belt RJ, Dakhil SR, Dubovsky D, Graham S, Pilat S, Winn R, Levin B. (1992). Phase II evaluation of fluorouracil and recombinant alpha-2a-interferon in previously untreated patients with pancreatic adenocarcinoma. *Cancer* 70(8):2073-2076.

Pazdur R, Ajani JA, Patt YZ, Gomez J, Bready B, Levin B. (1993). Phase II evaluation of recombinant alpha-2a-interferon and continuous infusion fluorouracil in previously untreated metastatic colorectal adenocarcinoma. *Cancer* 71(4):1214-1218.

Pazdur R, Ajani JA, Winn R, Bearden J, Belt RJ, Pilat S, Hallinan R, Levin B. (1992). A phase II trial of 5-fluorouracil and recombinant alpha-2a-interferon in previously untreated metastatic gastric carcinoma. *Cancer* 69(4):878-882.

Pazdur R, Bready B, Ajani JA, Abbruzzese JL, Markowitz A, Sugarman S, Jones D, Levin B. (1995). Phase II trial of isotretinoin and recombinant interferon alfa-2a in metastatic colorectal carcinoma. *American Journal of Clinical Oncology* 18(5):436-438.

Pazdur R, Bready B, Scalzo AJ, Brandof JE, Close DR, Kolbye S, Winn RJ. (1994). Phase II trial of piroxantrone in metastatic gastric adenocarcinoma. *Investigative New Drugs* 12(3):263-265.

Pazdur R, Diaz-Canton E, Ballard WP, Bradof JE, Graham S, Arbuck SG, Abbruzzese JL, Winn R. (1997). Phase II trial of 9-aminocamptothecin administered as a 72-hour continuous infusion in metastatic colorectal carcinoma. *Journal of Clinical Oncology* 15(8):2905-2909.

Pazdur R, Lassere Y, Diaz-Canton E, Bready B, Ho DH. (1997). Phase I trial of uracil-tegafur (UFT) plus oral leucovorin: 14-day schedule. *Investigative New Drugs* 15(2):123-128.

Pazdur R, Lassere Y, Rhodes V, Ajani JA, Sugarman SM, Patt YZ, Jones DV Jr, Markowitz AB, Abbruzzese JL, Bready B, et al. (1994). Phase II trial of uracil and tegafur plus oral leucovorin: An effective oral regimen in the treatment of metastatic colorectal carcinoma. *Journal of Clinical Oncology* 12(11):2296-2300.

Pazdur R, Moore DF, Bready B, Giannone L, Maldonado A, Lin YG, Fueger RH, Winn RJ, Levin B. (1994). Phase II trial of edatrexate in patients with advanced hepatocellular carcinoma. *Annals of Oncology* 5(7):646-648.

Pazdur R, Royce ME, Rodriguez GI, Rinaldi DA, Patt YZ, Hoff PM, Burris HA. (1999). Phase II trial of docetaxel for cholangiocarcinoma. *American Journal of Clinical Oncology* 22(1):78-81.

Peakman M, Deale A, Field R, Mahalingam M, Wessely S. (1997). Clinical improvement in chronic fatigue syndrome is not associated with lymphocyte subsets of function or activation. *Clinical Immunology and Immunopathology* 82(1): 83-91.

Pearce S, Richardson A. (1994). Fatigue and cancer: A phenomenological study. *Journal of Clinical Nursing* 3(6):381-382.

Pearce S, Richardson A. (1996). Fatigue in cancer: A phenomenological perspective. *European Journal of Cancer Care* 5(2):111-115.

Pearn JH. (1996). Chronic ciguatera: One organic cause of the chronic fatigue syndrome. *Journal of Chronic Fatigue Syndrome* 2(2/3):29-34.

Pearn JH. (1997). Chronic ciguatera poisoning as a differential diagnosis. *Medical Journal of Australia* 166(6):309-310.

Pectasides D, Dimopoulos MA, Aravantinos G, Kalophonos HP, Papacostas P, Briasoulis E, Cogas E, Papadimitriou C, Skarlos D, Kosmidis P, Fountzilas G. (2001). First line combination chemotherapy with docetaxel and vinorelbine in advanced breast cancer: A phase II study. *Anticancer Research* 21(5):3575-3580.

Pectasides D, Kalofonos HP, Samantas E, Nicolaides C, Papacostas P, Onyenadum A, Visvikis A, Skarlos D, et al. (2001). An out-patient second-line chemotherapy with gemcitabine and vinorelbine in patients with non-small cell lung cancer previously treated with cisplatin-based chemotherapy: A phase II study of the Hellenic Co-operative Oncology Group. *Anticancer Research* 21(4B):3005-3010.

Pectasides D, Visvikis A, Kouloubinis A, Glotsos J, Bountouroglou N, Karvounis N, Ziras N, Athanassiou A. (2002). Weekly chemotherapy with carboplatin, docetaxel and irinotecan in advanced non-small-cell-lung cancer: A phase II study. *European Journal of Cancer* 38(9):1194-1200.

Pedersen-Bjergaard J, Worm AM, Hainau B. (1977). Blastic transformation of chronic myelocytic leukaemia: Clinical manifestations, prognostic factors and results of therapy. *Scandinavian Journal of Haematology* 18(4):292-300.

Pelcovitz D, Septimus A, Friedman SB, Krilov LR, Mandel F, Kaplan S. (1995). Psychosocial correlates of chronic fatigue syndrome in adolescent girls. *Journal of Developmental and Behavioral Pediatrics* 16(5):333-338.

Pellegrini P, Berghella AM, Del Beato T, Adorno D, Casciani CU. (1996). Immunological directives for biotherapy improvement in the treatment of colorectal cancer. *Cancer Biotherapy and Radiopharmacology* 11(2):113-118.

Pellegrini P, Berghella AM, Del Beato T, Cicia S, Adorno D, Casciani CU. (1996). Disregulation in TH1 and TH2 subsets of CD4+ T cells in peripheral blood of colorectal cancer patients and involvement in cancer establishment and progression. *Cancer Immunology and Immunotherapy* 42(1):1-8.

Pellegrini P, Berghella AM, Di Loreto S, Del Beato T, Di Marco F, Adorno D, Casciani CU. (1996). Cytokine contribution to the repair processes and homeostasis recovery following anoxic insult: A possible IFN-gamma-regulating role in IL-1beta neurotoxic action in physiological or damaged CNS. *Neuroimmunomodulation* 3(4):213-218.

Pelletier G, Verhoef MJ, Khatri N, Hagen N. (2002). Quality of life in brain tumor patients: The relative contributions of depression, fatigue, emotional distress, and existential issues. *Journal of Neurooncology* 57(1):41-49.

Pelley RP, Strickland FM. (2000). Plants, polysaccharides, and the treatment and prevention of neoplasia. *Critical Reviews in Oncogenesis* 13(3-4):189-225.

Peloso PM. (1998). The fibromyalgia problem. *Journal of Rheumatology* 25(5): 1024-1025, discussion 1028-1030.

Peng CY, Manz BD, Keck J. (2001). Modeling categorical variables by logistic regression. *American Journal of Health Behavior* 25(3):278-284.

Penttila IA, Harris RJ, Storm P, Haynes D, Worswick DA, Marmion BP. (1998). Cytokine dysregulation in the post-Q-fever fatigue syndrome. *Quarterly Journal of Medicine* 91(8):549-560.

Pepping J. (1999). Echinacea. *American Journal of Health System Pharmacy* 56(2):121-122.

Perel'man LB, Almazova EG, Kasatkina LF, Kolomenskaia EA, Nozdracheva LV. (1979). [Clinical and electromyographic characteristics of syndromes of pathologic muscular fatigue of the myasthenic type]. *Zh Nevropatol Psikhiatr Im S S Korsakova* 79(11):1503-1510.

Perel'man LB, Almazova EG, Kasatkina LF, Kolomenskaya EA, Nozdracheva LV, Gekht BM. (1984). Clinical and electromyographic characteristics of pathological muscular-fatigue syndromes of the myasthenia type. *Neurosciences and Behavioral Physiology* 14(4):261-267.

Perez JE, Lacava JA, Dominguez ME, Rodriguez R, Barbieri MR, Romero Acuna LA, Romero Acuna JM, Langhi MJ, Amato S, Marrone N, et al. (1998). Biomodulation with sequential intravenous IFN-alpha2b and 5-fluorouracil as second-line treatment in patients with advanced colorectal cancer. *Journal of Interferon and Cytokine Research* 18(8):565-569.

Perez-Soler R, Fossella FV, Glisson BS, Lee JS, Murphy WK, Shin DM, Kemp BL, Lee JJ, Kane J, Robinson RA, et al. (1996). Phase II study of topotecan in patients with advanced non-small-cell lung cancer previously untreated with chemotherapy. *Journal of Clinical Oncology* 14(2):503-513.

Perl A, Gorevic PD, Condemi JJ, Papsidero L, Poiesz BJ, Abraham GN. (1991). Antibodies to retroviral proteins and reverse transcriptase activity in patients with essential cryoglobulinemia. *Arthritis and Rheumatism* 34(10):313-318.

Perlis ML, Giles DE, Bootzin RR, Dikman ZV, Fleming GV, Drummond SP, Rose MW. (1997). Alpha sleep and information processing, perception of sleep, pain, and arousability in fibromyalgia. *International Journal of Neurosciences* 89 (3-4):265-280.

Peroutka SJ. (1998). Chronic fatigue disorders: An inappropriate response to arginine vasopressin? *Medical Hypotheses* 50(6):521-523.

Pershagen G. (2000). Can immunization affect the development of allergy? *Pediatric Allergy and Immunology* 11(Suppl 13):26-28.

Persson CR, Johansson BB, Sjoden PO, Glimelius BL. (2002). A randomized study of nutritional support in patients with colorectal and gastric cancer. *Nutrition and Cancer* 42(1):48-58.

Persson L, Hallberg IR. (1995). Acute leukaemia and malignant lymphoma patients' experiences of disease, treatment and nursing care during the active treatment phase: An explorative study. *European Journal of Cancer Care* 4(3): 133-142.

Persson L, Hallberg IR, Ohlsson O. (1997). Survivors of acute leukaemia and highly malignant lymphoma—Retrospective views of daily life problems during treatment and when in remission. *Journal of Advanced Nursing* 25(1):68-78.

Peters MN, Hall RJ, Cooley DA, Leachman RD, Garcia E. (1974). The clinical syndrome of atrial myxoma. *JAMA* 230(5):695-701.

Peters W, Smith D, Fornasier V, Lugowski S, Ibanez D. (1997). An outcome analysis of 100 women after explantation of silicone gel breast implants. *Annals of Plastic Surgery* 39(1):9-19.

Petit T, Aylesworth C, Burris H, Ravdin P, Rodriguez G, Smith L, Peacock N, Smetzer L, Bellet R, Von Hoff DD, et al. (1999). A phase I study of docetaxel and 5-fluorouracil in patients with advanced solid malignancies. *Annals of Oncology* 10(2):223-229.

Petri G. (1999). Possibilities of advanced education in phytotherapy. *Orv Hetil* 140(18):1030-1031.

Petrie K, Moss-Morris R, Weinman J. (1995). The impact of catastrophic beliefs on functioning in chronic fatigue syndrome. *Journal of Psychosomatic Research* 39(1):31-37.

Petz T, Diete S, Gademann G, Wallesch CW. (2001). [Coping in patients with malignant glioma in the course of radiation therapy]. *Psychotherapy and Psychosomatic Medicine and Psychology* 51(7):281-287.

Petzke F, Radbruch L, Sabatowski R, Karthaus M, Mertens A. (2001). Slow-release tramadol for treatment of chronic malignant pain—An open multicenter trial. *Support Care in Cancer* 9(1):48-54.

Phillips GD, Cousins MJ. (1986). Neurological mechanisms of pain and the relationship of pain, anxiety, and sleep. In *Acute Pain Management,* Cousins MJ, Phillips GD, eds. New York: Churchill Livingstone, pp. 21-48.

Pickar JG. (1998). The thromboxane A2 mimetic U-46619 inhibits somatomotor activity via a vagal reflex from the lung. *American Journal of Physiology* 275: R706-R712.

Pickar JG, Hill JM, Kaufman MP. (1993). Stimulation of vagal afferents inhibits locomotion in mesencephalic cats. *Journal of Applied Physiology* 74:103-110.

Pickard-Holley S. (1991). Fatigue in cancer patients: A descriptive study. *Cancer Nursing* 14(1):13-19.

Pickett M, Mock V, Ropka ME, Cameron L, Coleman M, Podewils L. (2002). Adherence to moderate-intensity exercise during breast cancer therapy. *Cancer Practice* 10(6):284-292.

Picus J, Schultz M. (1999). Docetaxel (Taxotere) as monotherapy in the treatment of hormone-refractory prostate cancer: Preliminary results. *Seminars in Oncology* 26(5 Suppl 17):14-18.

Pilcher JJ, Huffcutt AI. (1996). Effects of sleep deprivation on performance: A meta-analysis. *Sleep* 19(4):318-326.

Pillemer SR, Bradley LA, Crofford LJ, Moldofsky H, Chrousos GP. (1997). The neuroscience and endocrinology of fibromyalgia. *Arthritis and Rheumatism* 40(11):1928-1939.

Pilowski I, Crettenden I, Townly M. (1985). Sleep disturbance in pain clinic patients. *Pain* 23:27-33.

Pinto BM, Maruyama NC. (1999). Exercise in the rehabilitation of breast cancer survivors. *Psychooncology* 8(3):191-206.

Pipas JM, Mitchell SE, Barth RJ Jr, Vera-Gimon R, Rathmann J, Meyer LP, Wagman RS, Lewis LD, McDonnell C, Colacchio TA, et al. (2001). Phase I study of twice-weekly gemcitabine and concomitant external-beam radiotherapy in patients with adenocarcinoma of the pancreas. *International Journal of Radiation Oncology, Biology and Physics* 50(5):1317-1322.

Piper BF. (1990). Piper Fatigue Scale available for clinical testing. *Oncology Nursing Forum* 17(5):661-662.

Piper BF. (1993). Fatigue and cancer: Inevitable companions? *Support Care in Cancer* 1(6):285-286.

Piper BF, Dibble SL, Dodd MJ, Weiss MC, Slaughter RE, Paul SM. (1998). The revised Piper Fatigue Scale: Psychometric evaluation in women with breast cancer. *Oncology Nursing Forum* 25(4):677-684.

Piper BF, Lindsey AM, Dodd MJ. (1987). Fatigue mechanisms in cancer patients: Developing nursing theory. *Oncology Nursing Forum* 14(6):17-23.

Piper BF, Lindsey A, Dodd M, Ferketich S, Paul S. (1989). The development of an instrument to measure the subjective dimension of fatigue. In *Key Aspects of Comfort: Management of Pain, Fatigue, and Nausea,* Funk S, Tornquist M, Champagne M, Copp L, Wiese R, eds. New York: Springer, pp. 199-207.

Piper BF, Rieger PT, Brophy L, Haeuber D, Hood LE, Lyver A, Sharp E. (1989). Recent advances in the management of biotherapy-related side effects: Fatigue. *Oncology Nursing Forum* 16(6 Suppl):27-34.

Piper DW. (1995). A comparative overview of the adverse effects of antiulcer drugs. *Drug Safety* 12(2):120-138.

Pisa P, Cannon MJ, Pisa EK, Cooper NR, Fox RI. (1992). Epstein-Barr virus induced lymphoproliferative tumors in severe combined immunodeficient mice are oligoclonal. *Blood* 79(1):173-179.

Pisa P, Halapi E, Pisa EK, Gerdin E, Hising C, Bucht A, Gerdin B, Kiessling R. (1992). Selective expression of interleukin-10, interferon-gamma, and granulocyte macrophage colony-stimulating factor in ovarian cancer biopsies. *Proceedings of the National Academy of Sciences of the United States of America* 89:7708-7712.

Pisters KM, Tyson LB, Tong W, Fleisher M, Miller VA, Grant SC, Pfister DG, Rigas JR, Densmore CL, Krol G, et al. (1996). High-dose edatrexate with oral leucovorin rescue: A phase I and clinical pharmacological study in adults with advanced cancer. *Clinical Cancer Research* 2(11):1819-1824.

Pizzocaro G, Piva L, Faustini M, Nicolai N, Salvioni R, Pisani E, Maggioni A, Mandressi A, Dormia E, Minervini S, et al. (1993). [Adjuvant interferon alpha in renal carcinoma with a high risk of recurrence: Multicenter pilot study]. *Archives of Italian Urology and Andrology* 65(2):173-176.

Pizzorno G, Yee L, Burtness BA, Marsh JC, Darnowski JW, Chu MY, Chu SH, Chu E, Leffert JJ, Handschumacher RE, et al. (1998). Phase I clinical and pharmacological studies of benzylacyclouridine, a uridine phosphorylase inhibitor. *Clinical Cancer Research* 4(5):1165-1175.

Platanias LC, Vogelzang NJ. (1990). Interleukin-1: Biology, pathophysiology, and clinical prospects. *American Journal of Medicine* 89(5):621-629.

Player MR, Torrence PF. (1998). The 2-5A system: Modulation of viral and cellular processes through acceleration of RNA degradation. *Pharmacological Therapy* 78:55-113.

Plioplys AV. (1997a). Antimuscle and anti-CNS circulating antibodies in chronic fatigue syndrome. *Neurology* 48(6):1717-1719.

Plioplys AV. (1997b). Chronic fatigue syndrome should not be diagnosed in children. *Pediatrics* 100(2 Pt 1):270-271.

Plioplys AV, Plioplys S. (1997). Amantadine and L-carnitine treatment for chronic fatigue syndrome. *Neuropsychobiology* 35(1):16-23.

Plioplys AV, Plioplys S, Davis JS IV. (1997). Meeeting the frustrations of chronic fatigue syndrome. *Hospital Practice* 32(6):147-150, 153-156, 160-161.

Plotnikoff GA, George H. (1999). Herbalism in Minnesota: What should physicians know? *Minnesota Medicine* 82(5):12-26.

Plummer R, Ghielmini M, Calvert P, Voi M, Renard J, Gallant G, Gupta E, Calvert H, Sessa C. (2002). Phase I and pharmacokinetic study of the new taxane analog BMS-184476 given weekly in patients with advanced malignancies. *Clinical Cancer Research* 8(9):2788-2797.

Pocinki AG. (1997). Fireworks over fibromyalgia, CFS, and IBS. *Postgraduate Medicine* 102(6):43.

Poggi MM, Kroog GS, Russo A, Muir C, Cook J, Smith J, Mitchell JB, Herscher LL. (2002). Phase I study of weekly gemcitabine as a radiation sensitizer for unresectable pancreatic cancer. *International Journal of Radiation Oncology, Biology and Physics* 54(3):670-676.

Pongratz DE, Sievers M. (2000). Fibromyalgia—symptom or diagnosis: A definition of the position. *Scandinavian Journal of Rheumatology* 113:3-7.

Popa IE, Stewart K, Smith FP, Rizvi NA. (2002). A phase II trial of gemcitabine and docetaxel in patients with chemotherapy-naive, advanced nonsmall cell lung carcinoma. *Cancer* 95(8):1714-1719.

Porock D, Kristjanson LJ, Tinnelly K, Duke T, Blight J. (2000). An exercise intervention for advanced cancer patients experiencing fatigue: A pilot study. *Journal of Palliative Care* 16(3):30-36.

Portenoy RK. (2000). Cancer-related fatigue: An immense problem. *Oncologist* 5(5):350-352.

Portenoy RK, Itri LM. (1999). Cancer-related fatigue: Guidelines for evaluation and management. *Oncologist* 4(1):1-10.

Portenoy RK, Kornblith AB, Wong G, Vlamis V, Lepore JM, Loseth DB, Hakes T, Foley KM, Hoskins WJ. (1994). Pain in ovarian cancer patients: Prevalence, characteristics, and associated symptoms. *Cancer* 74(3):907-915.

Poser CM. (1996). Fatigue in MS. *Neurology* 47(5):1351.

Posner M, Martin A, Slapak CA, Clark JW, Cummings FJ, Robert NJ, Sikov W, Akerley W. (1992). A phase II trial of continuous infusion cisplatin and 5-fluorouracil with oral calcium leucovorin in colorectal carcinoma. *American Journal of Clinical Oncology* 15(3):239-241.

Posner M, Slapak CA, Browne MJ, Clark JW, Curt G, Weitberg A, Calabresi P, Cummings FJ, Wiemann M, Urba S, et al. (1990). A phase I-II trial of continuous-infusion cisplatin, continuous-infusion 5-fluorouracil, and VP-16 in colorectal carcinoma. *American Journal of Clinical Oncology* 13(5):455-458.

Poteliakhoff A. (1998). Fatigue syndromes and the aetiology of autoimmune diseases. *Journal of Chronic Fatigue Syndrome* 4(4):31-50.

Potempa KM. (1993). Chronic fatigue. *Annual Reviews of Nursing Research* 11: 57-76.

Potter JD. (1995). Risk factors for colon neoplasia—Epidemiology and biology. *European Journal of Cancer* 31A:1033-1038.

Potter JD, Slattery ML, Bostick RM, Gapstur SM. (1993). Colon cancer: A review of the epidemiology. *Epidemiological Reviews* 15:499-545.

Potter PJ. (1997). Musculoskeletal complaints and fibromyalgia in patients attending a respiratory sleep disorders clinic. *Journal of Rheumatology* 24(8):1657-1658.

Potter PJ. (1998). The fatigue of cancer. *Canadian Medical Association Journal* 159(8):921.

Poulson J. (1998). Dead tired. *Canadian Medical Association Journal* 158(13): 1748-1750.

Poulson MJ. (2001). Not just tired. *Journal of Clinical Oncology* 19(21):4180-4181.

Pourel N, Peiffert D, Lartigau E, Desandes E, Luporsi E, Conroy T. (2002). Quality of life in long-term survivors of oropharynx carcinoma. *International Journal of Radiation Oncology, Biology and Physics* 54(3):742-751.

Povoa P, Ducla-Soares J, Fernandes A, Palma-Carlos AG. (1991). A case of systemic mastocytosis; therapeutic efficacy of ketotifen. *Journal of Internal Medicine* 229(5):475-477.

Press J, Phillip M, Neumann L, Barak R, Segev Y, Abu-Shakra M, Buskila D. (1998). Normal melatonin levels in patients with fibromyalgia syndrome. *Journal of Rheumatology* 25(3):551-555.

Prian GW, Scott M, Robinson W. (1978). Surgical leukemia. *Surgical Gynecology and Obstetrics* 147(3):397-400.

Prieto J, Subira ML, Castilla A, Castilla A, Serrano M (1989). Naloxone-reversible monocyte dysfunction in patients with chronic fatigue syndrome. *Scandinavian Journal of Immunology* 30(1):13-20.

Prince HE, Kleinman S, Czaplicki C, John J, Williams AEW. (1990). Interrelationships between serologic markers of immune activation and T lymphocyte subsets in HIV infection. *Journal of Acquired Immune Deficiency Syndromes* 3:525-530.

Pringle W, Swan E. (2001). Continuing care after discharge from hospital for stoma patients. *British Journal of Nursing* 10(19):1275-1288.

Proceedings of the International Fibromyalgia Conference. (1998). Bad Nauheim, Germany, October 1997. *Zeitschrift Rheumatologie* 57(Suppl 2):V-X, 1-108.

Prophet S. (1999). Alternative medicine: Growing trend for the new millenium, part II. *Journal AHIMA* 70(5):65-70.

Propper DJ, Macaulay V, O'Byrne KJ, Braybrooke JP, Wilner SM, Ganesan TS, Talbot DC, Harris AL. (1998). A phase II study of bryostatin 1 in metastatic malignant melanoma. *British Journal of Cancer* 78(10):1337-1341.

Propper DJ, McDonald AC, Man A, Thavasu P, Balkwill F, Braybrooke JP, Caponigro F, Graf P, Dutreix C, Blackie R, et al. (2001). Phase I and pharmacokinetic study of PKC412, an inhibitor of protein kinase C. *Journal of Clinical Oncology* 19(5):1485-1492.

Pruessner JC, Hellhammer DH, Kirschbaum C. (1999). Burnout, perceived stress, and cortisol responses to awakening. *Psychosomatic Medicine* 61(2):197-204.

Puccio M, Nathanson L. (1997). The cancer cachexia syndrome. *Seminars in Oncology* 24(3):277-287.

Pui CH. (1989). Serum interleukin-2 receptor: Clinical and biological implications. *Leukemia* 3(5):323-327.

Punt CJ, Kingma BJ. (1994). Severe asthenia and fatigue caused by recombinant human granulocyte colony-stimulating factor (rh G-CSF). *Annals of Oncology* 5(5):473.

Punt CJ, van Herpen CM, Jansen RL, Vreugdenhil G, Muller EW, de Mulder PH. (1997). Chemoimmunotherapy with bleomycin, vincristine, lomustine, dacarbazine (BOLD) plus interferon alpha for metastatic melanoma: A multicentre phase II study. *British Journal of Cancer* 76(2):266-269.

Punt CJ, van Maanen L, Bol CJ, Seifert WF, Wagener DJ. (2001). Phase I and pharmacokinetic study of the orally administered farnesyl transferase inhibitor R115777 in patients with advanced solid tumors. *Anticancer Drugs* 12(3):193-197.

Pyrhonen S, Hahka-Kemppinen M, Muhonen T. (1992). A promising interferon plus four-drug chemotherapy regimen for metastatic melanoma. *Journal of Clinical Oncology* 10(12):1919-1926.

Qin Z, Noffz G, Mohaupt M, Blankenstein T. (1997). Interleukin-10 prevents dendritic cell accumulation and vaccination with granulocyte-macrophage colony-stimulating factor gene-modified tumor cells. *Journal of Immunology* 159:770-776.

Quan WD Jr, Casal R, Rosenfeld M, Walker PR. (1996). Alpha interferon-2b, leucovorin, and 5-fluorouracil (ALF) in non-small cell lung cancer. *Cancer Biotherapy and Radiopharmacology* 11(4):229-234.

Quan WD Jr, Dean GE, Lieskovsky G, Mitchell MS, Kempf RA. (1994). Phase II study of low dose cyclophosphamide and intravenous interleukin-2 in metastatic renal cancer. *Investigative New Drugs* 12(1):35-39.

Quan WD Jr, Madajewicz S, Smith MR, Skeel RT. (1994). Alpha interferon, leucovorin, and 5-fluorouracil (ALF) in advanced cancer: Results of a dose-finding study and evidence of activity in non-small cell lung cancer. *Cancer Investigation* 12(4):367-374.

Quan WD Jr, Mitchell MS. (1993). Phase II trial of carbetimer in metastatic melanoma. *Investigative New Drugs* 11(2-3):231-233.

Quesada JR, Alexanian R, Hawkins M, Barlogie B, Borden E, Itri L, Gutterman JU. (1986). Treatment of multiple myeloma with recombinant alpha-interferon. *Blood* 67(2):275-278.

Quesada JR, Alexanian R, Kurzrock R, Barlogie B, Saks S, Gutterman JU. (1988). Recombinant interferon gamma in hairy cell leukemia, multiple myeloma, and Waldenstrom's macroglobulinemia. *American Journal of Hematology* 29(1): 1-4.

Quesada JR, Gutterman JU, Hersh EM. (1982). Clinical and immunological study of beta interferon by intramuscular route in patients with metastatic breast cancer. *Journal of Interferon Research* 2(4):593-599.

Quesada JR, Hawkins M, Horning S, Alexanian R, Borden E, Merigan T, Adams F, Gutterman JU. (1984). Collaborative phase I-II study of recombinant DNA-produced leukocyte interferon (clone A) in metastatic breast cancer, malignant lymphoma, and multiple myeloma. *American Journal of Medicine* 77(3):427-432.

Quesada JR, Hersh EM, Manning J, Reuben J, Keating M, Schnipper E, Itri L, Gutterman JU. (1986). Treatment of hairy cell leukemia with recombinant alpha-interferon. *Blood* 68(2):493-497.

Quesada JR, Kurzrock R, Sherwin SA, Gutterman JU. (1987). Phase II studies of recombinant human interferon gamma in metastatic renal cell carcinoma. *Journal of Biological Response Modifiers* 6(1):20-27.

Quesada JR, Swanson DA, Gutterman JU. (1985). Phase II study of interferon alpha in metastatic renal-cell carcinoma: A progress report. *Journal of Clinical Oncology* 3(8):1086-1092.

Quesada JR, Talpaz M, Rios A, Kurzrock R, Gutterman JU. (1986). Clinical toxicity of interferons in cancer patients: A review. *Journal of Clinical Oncology* 4(2):234-243.

Quintner JL, Cohen ML. (1997). Fibromyalgia syndrome. *Medical Journal of Australia* 166(3):168.

Quintner JL, Cohen ML. (1999). Fibromyalgia falls foul of a fallacy. *Lancet* 353(9158):1092-1094.

Raats JI, Falkson G, Falkson HC. (1992). A study of fadrozole, a new aromatase inhibitor, in postmenopausal women with advanced metastatic breast cancer. *Journal of Clinical Oncology* 10(1):111-116.

Raber MN. (2001). A patient's perspective on cancer-related fatigue. *Cancer* 92 (6 Suppl):1662-1663.

Rabinowe SL, Jackson RA, Dluhy RG, Williams GH. (1984). Ia-positive T lymphocytes in recently diagnosed idiopathic Addison's disease. *American Journal of Medicine* 77:597-601.

Rabinowich H, Suminami Y, Reichert TE, Crowley-Nowick P, Bell M, Edwards R, Whiteside TL. (1996). Expression of cytokine genes or proteins and signaling molecules in lymphocytes associated with human ovarian carcinoma. *International Journal of Cancer* 68:276-284.

Racciatti D, Vecchiet J, Ceccomancini A, Ricci F, Pizzigallo E. (2001). Chronic fatigue syndrome following a toxic exposure. *Science and Total Environment* 270(1-3):27-31.

Raizner AE, Heck KA. (1995). 37-year-old woman with progressive fatigue, syncope, and chest pain. *Circulation* 91(1):231-235.

Rajkumar SV. (2000). Thalidomide in multiple myeloma. *Oncology* 14(12 Suppl 13):11-16.

Rajkumar SV. (2001a). Current status of thalidomide in the treatment of cancer. *Oncology* 15(7):867-874; discussion 877-879.

Rajkumar SV. (2001b). Thalidomide in the treatment of multiple myeloma. *Expert Reviews on Anticancer Therapy* 1(1):20-28.

Rajkumar SV, Witzig TE. (2000). A review of angiogenesis and antiangiogenic therapy with thalidomide in multiple myeloma. *Cancer Treatment Reviews* 26(5):351-362.

Ralston SH, Gallacher SJ, Patel U, Campbell J, Boyle IT. (1990). Cancer-associated hypercalcemia: Morbidity and mortality—Clinical experience in 126 treated patients. *Annals of Internal Medicine* 112(7):499-504.

Ramalingam S, Belani CP. (2002). Meaningful survival in lung cancer patients. *Seminars in Oncology* 29(1 Suppl 4):125-131.

Ramiya VK, Shang XZ, Pharis PG, Wasserfall CH, Stabler TV, Muir AB, Schatz DA, Maclaren NK. (1996). Antigen based therapies to prevent diabetes in NOD mice. *Journal of Autoimmunity* 9:349-356.

Ramot Y, Rapoport MJ, Hagag P, Wysenbeek AJ. (1996). A study of the clinical differences between women and men with hyperprolactinemia. *Gynecological Endocrinology* 10(6):397-400.

Ramsay C, Moreland J, Ho M, Joyce S, Walker S, Pullar T. (2000). An observer-blinded comparison of supervised and unsupervised aerobic exercise regimens in fibromyalgia. *Rheumatology* (Oxford) 39(5):501-505.

Rankin DB. (1999). The fibromyalgia syndrome: A consensus report. *New Zealand Medical Journal* 112(1080):18-19.

Raphael KG, Marbach JJ. (2000). Comorbid fibromyalgia accounts for reduced fecundity in women with myofascial face pain. *Clinical Journal of Pain* 16(1):29-36.

Rapoport BL, Falkson G, Raats JI, de Wet M, Lotz BP, Potgieter HC. (1993). Suramin in combination with mitomycin C in hormone-resistant prostate cancer: A phase II clinical study. *Annals of Oncology* 4(7):567-573.

Rasmussen AK, Nielsen AH, Andersen V, Barlington T, Bendtzen K, Hansen MB, Nielsen L, Pederson BK, Wiik A. (1994). Chronic fatigue syndrome—A controlled cross sectional study. *The Journal of Rheumatology* 21(8):1527-1531.

Raspe H. (1996). [Fibromyalgia—An artifact?] Fibromyalgie—ein artefakt? *Zeitschrift Rheumatologie* 55(1):1-3.

Raspe H, Croft P. (1995). Fibromyalgia. *Baillieres Clinical Rheumatology* 9(3): 599-614.

Ratain MJ, Priest ER, Janisch L, Vogelzang NJ. (1993). A phase I study of subcutaneous recombinant interleukin-2 and interferon alfa-2a. *Cancer* 71(7):2371-2376.

Ratain MJ, Skoog LA, O'Brien SM, Cooper N, Schilsky RL, Vogelzang NJ, Gerber M, Narang PK, Nicol SJ. (1997). Phase I study of 3'-deamino-3'-(2-methoxy-4-morpholinyl)doxorubicin (FCE 23762, PNU 152243) administered on a daily x3 schedule. *Annals of Oncology* 8(8):807-809.

Ratanatharathorn V, Jirajarus M, Sirachainan E, Sirilerttrakul S, Euaree A, Supatchaipisit P. (1998). Paclitaxel and carboplatin in combination in the treatment of advanced non-small-cell lung cancer (NSCLC): A preliminary study. *Journal of the Medical Association of Thailand* 81(10):763-771.

Ratner L, Haseltine WA, Patarca R, Livak K, Starcich B, Josephs SF, Doran ER, Rafalski JA, Whitehorn EA, Baumeister K, et al. (1985). Complete nucleotide sequence of the AIDS virus, HTLV-III. *Nature* 313:277-284.

Rau CL, Russell IJ. (2000). Is fibromyalgia a distinct clinical syndrome? *Current Reviews in Pain* 4(4):287-294.

Rauthe G, Sistermanns J. (1997). Recombinant tumour necrosis factor in the local therapy of malignant pleural effusion. *European Journal of Cancer* 33(2):226-231.

Rauthe G, Sistermanns J. (1998). Pleurodesis with recombinant tumour necrosis factor in gynaecological neoplasms. *European Journal of Gynaecological Oncology* 19(2):108-112.

Ravaud A, Negrier S, Cany L, Merrouche Y, Le Guillou M, Blay JY, Clavel M, Gaston R, Oskam R, Philip T. (1994). Subcutaneous low-dose recombinant interleukin 2 and alpha-interferon in patients with metastatic renal cell carcinoma. *British Journal of Cancer* 69(6):1111-1114.

Ravdin LD, Hilton E, Primeau M, Clements C, Barr WB. (1996). Memory functioning in Lyme borreliosis. *Journal of Clinical Psychiatry* 57(7):282-286.

Ravdin PM, Havlin KA, Marshall MV, Brown TD, Koeller JM, Kuhn JG, Rodriguez G, Von Hoff DD. (1991). A phase I clinical and pharmacokinetic trial of hepsulfam. *Cancer Research* 51(23 Pt 1):6268-6272.

Rawls WH, Lamm DL, Lowe BA, Crawford ED, Sarosdy MF, Montie JE, Grossman HB, Scardino PT. (1990). Fatal sepsis following intravesical BCG administration for bladder cancer: A Southwest Oncology Group study. *Journal of Urology* 144:1328-1330.

Rawsthorne P, Shanahan F, Cronin NC, Anton PA, Lofberg R, Bohman L, Bernstein CN. (1999). An international survey of the use and attitudes regarding alternative medicine by patients with inflammatory bowel disease. *American Journal of Gastroenterology* 94(5):1298-1303.

Ray C, Jefferies S, Weir WRC. (1995). Coping with chronic fatigue syndrome: Illness responses and their relationships with fatigue, functional impairment and emotional status. *Psychological Medicine* 25:937-945.

Ray C, Jefferies S, Weir W. (1997). Coping and other predictors of outcome in chronic fatigue syndrome: A 1 year follow up. *Journal of Psychosomatic Research* 43(4):405-415.

Ray C, Weir WRC, Phillips S, Cullen S. (1992). Development of a measure of symptoms in chronic fatigue syndrome: The Profile of Fatigue-Related Symptoms (PFRS). *Psychology and Health* 7:27-43.

Raymond E, Ten Bokkel Huinink WW, Taieb J, Beijnen JH, Faivre S, Wanders J, Ravic M, Fumoleau P, Armand JP, Schellens JH. (2002). Phase I and pharmacokinetic study of E7070, a novel chloroindolyl sulfonamide cell-cycle inhibitor, administered as a one-hour infusion every three weeks in patients with advanced cancer. *Journal of Clinical Oncology* 20(16):3508-3521.

Raymond MC, Brown JB. (2000). Experience of fibromyalgia: Qualitative study. *Canadian Family Physician* 46:1100-1106.

Raziuddin S, Elawad ME. (1990). Immunoregulatory CD4+CD45R+ suppressor/ inducer T lymphocyte subsets and impaired cell-mediated immunity in patients with Down's syndrome. *Clinical and Experimental Immunology* 79:67-71.

Rea TD, Russo JE, Katon W, Ashley RL, Buchwald DS. (2001). Prospective study of the natural history of infectious mononucleosis caused by Epstein-Barr virus. *Journal of the American Board Family Practice* 14(4):234-242.

Ream E, Richardson A. (1996). Fatigue: A concept analysis. *International Journal of Nursing Studies* 33(5):519-529.

Ream E, Richardson A. (1997). Fatigue in patients with cancer and chronic obstructive airways disease: A phenomenological enquiry. *International Journal of Nursing Studies* 34(1):44-53.

Ream E, Richardson A. (1999). From theory to practice: Designing interventions to reduce fatigue in patients with cancer. *Oncology Nursing Forum* 26(8):1295-1303; quiz 1304-1305.

Ream E, Richardson A, Alexander-Dann C. (2002). Facilitating patients' coping with fatigue during chemotherapy-pilot outcomes. *Cancer Nursing* 25(4):300-308.

Recchia F, De Filippis S, Rosselli M, Saggio G, Cesta A, Fumagalli L, Rea S. (2001). Phase 1B study of subcutaneously administered interleukin 2 in combination with 13-cis retinoic acid as maintenance therapy in advanced cancer. *Clinical Cancer Research* 7(5):1251-1257.

Rector JT, Gray CL, Sharpe RW, Hall FW, Thomas W, Jones W. (1993). Acute lymphoid leukemia associated with Maffucci's syndrome. *American Journal of Pediatric Hematology and Oncology* 15(4):427-429.

Reddy SP, Harwood RM, Moore DF, Grimm EA, Murray JL, Vadhan-Raj S. (1997). Recombinant interleukin-2 in combination with recombinant interferon-gamma in patients with advanced malignancy: A phase 1 study. *Journal of Immunotherapy* 20(1):79-87.

Redeker NS, Lev EL, Ruggiero J. (2000). Insomnia, fatigue, anxiety, depression, and quality of life of cancer patients undergoing chemotherapy. *School Nursing Practice* 14(4):275-290; discussion 291-298.

Redmond K. (1996). Advances in supportive care. *European Journal of Cancer Care* 5(2 Suppl):1-7.

Redrizzani M, Benedetti B, Castelli C, Longo A, Ferrara GB, Herlyn M, Parmiani G, Fossati G. (1991). Human allogeneic melanoma-reactive T-helper lymphocyte clones: Functional analysis of lymphocyte-melanoma interactions. *International Journal of Cancer* 49:823-830.

Ree HJ, Crowley JP, Dinarello CA. (1987). Anti-interleukin-1 reactive cells in Hodgkin's disease. *Cancer* 59(10):1717-1720.

Reese DM, Corry M, Small EJ. (2000). Infusional floxuridine-based therapy for patients with metastatic renal cell carcinoma. *Cancer* 88(6):1310-1316.

Regland B, Andersson M, Abrahamsson L, Bagby J, Dyrehag LE, Gottfries CG. (1997). Increased concentrations of homocysteine in the cerebrospinal fluid in patients with fibromyalgia and chronic fatigue syndrome. *Scandinavian Journal of Rheumatology* 26(4):301-307.

Regland B, Zachrisson O, Stejskal V, Gottfries CG. (2000). Nickel allergy is found in a majority of women with chronic fatigue syndrome and muscle pain and may be triggered by cigarette smoke and dietary nickel intake. *Journal of Chronic Fatigue Syndrome* 8(1):57-65.

Reh M. (1998). Specialists help cancer survivors face unexpected challenges. *Journal of the National Cancer Institutes* 90(8):566-567.

Reid GJ, Lang BA, McGrath PJ. (1997). Primary juvenile fibromyalgia: Psychological adjustment, family functioning, coping, and functional disability. *Arthritis and Rheumatism* 40(4):752-760.

Reiffenberger DH, Amundson LH. (1996). Fibromyalgia syndrome: A review. *American Family Physician* 53(5):1698-1712.

Reilly PA, Littlejohn GO. (1993). Diurnal variation in symptoms and signs of the fibromyalgia syndrome (FS). *Journal of Musculoskeletal Pain* 1:237-243.

Reinherz EL, Schlossman SF. (1981). The characterization and function of human immunoregulatory T lymphocyte subsets. *Immunology Today* 2:6975-6979.

Reinhold-Keller E. (1997). [Diagnosis of fibromyalgia syndrome] Diagnose de fibromyalgiesyndroms. *Internist* (Berlin) 38(10):993-994.

Rekola KE, Levoska S, Takala J, Keinanen-Kiukaanniemi S. (1997). Patients with neck and shoulder complaints and multisite musculoskeletal symptoms—A prospective study. *Journal of Rheumatology* 24(12):2424-2428.

Rettig MB, Ma HJ, Vescio RA, Pold M, Schiller G, Belson D, Savage A, Nishikubo C, Wu C, Fraser I, et al. (1997). Kaposi-sarcoma associated herpesvirus infection of bone marrow dendritic cells from multiple myeloma patients. *Science* 276 (5320):1851-1854.

Rettmar K, Stierle U, Sheikhzadeh A, Diederich KW. (1993). Primary angiosarcoma of the heart: Report of a case and review of the literature. *Japanese Heart Journal* 34(5):667-683.

Rettori V, Gimeno MF, Karana A, Gonzalez MC, McCann SM. (1991). Interleukin-1a inhibits prostaglandin E_2 release to suppress pulsatile release of luteinizing hormone but not follicle-stimulating hormone. *Proceedings of the National Academy of Sciences of the United States of America* 88:2763-2767.

Reuille KM. (2002). Using self-regulation theory to develop an intervention for cancer-related fatigue. *Clinical Nurse Specialist* 16(6):312-319.

Reveille JD. (1997). Soft-tissue rheumatism: Diagnosis and treatment. *American Journal of Medicine* 102(1A):23S-29S.

Rexilius SJ, Mundt C, Erickson Megel M, Agrawal S. (2002). Therapeutic effects of massage therapy and handling touch on caregivers of patients undergoing autologous hematopoietic stem cell transplant. *Oncology Nursing Forum* 29(3): E35-E44.

Reyno LM, Egorin MJ, Eisenberger MA, Sinibaldi VJ, Zuhowski EG, Sridhara R. (1995). Development and validation of a pharmacokinetically based fixed dosing scheme for suramin. *Journal of Clinical Oncology* 13(9):2187-2195.

Reynolds WJ. (1996). Fibromyalgia 20 years later: What have we really accomplished? *Journal of Rheumatology* 23(1):192; discussion 193-194.

Rhodes VA, McDaniel RW, Homan SS, Johnson M, Madsen R. (2000). An instrument to measure symptom experience: Symptom occurrence and symptom distress. *Cancer Nursing* 23(1):49-54.

Rhodes VA, Watson PM, Hanson BM. (1988). Patients' descriptions of the influence of tiredness and weakness on self-care abilities. *Cancer Nursing* 11(3):186-194.

Rhoten D. (1982). Fatigue and the post-surgical patient. In *Concept Clarification and Nursing,* Norris DM, ed. Rockville, MD: Aspen Publishers, pp. 277-300.

Richardson A. (1995). Fatigue in cancer patients: A review of the literature. *European Journal of Cancer Care* 4(1):20-32.

Richardson A. (1998). Measuring fatigue in patients with cancer. *Support Care in Cancer* 6(2):94-100.

Richardson A, Ream E. (1996). The experience of fatigue and other symptoms in patients receiving chemotherapy. *European Journal of Cancer Care* 5(2 Suppl): 24-30.

Richardson A, Ream E. (1997). Self-care behaviours initiated by chemotherapy patients in response to fatigue. *International Journal of Nursing Studies* 34(1): 35-43.

Richardson A, Ream E, Wilson-Barnett J. (1998). Fatigue in patients receiving chemotherapy: Patterns of change. *Cancer Nursing* 21(1):17-30.

Richardson J, Campos Costa D. (1998). Relationship between SPECT scans and buspirone tests in patients with ME/CFS. *Journal of Chronic Fatigue Syndrome* 4(3):23-38.

Richner J, Joss RA, Goldhirsch A, Brunner KW. (1992). Phase II study of continuous subcutaneous interferon-alfa combined with cisplatin in advanced malignant melanoma. *European Journal of Cancer* 28A(6-7):1044-1047.

Richter G, Kruger-Krasagakes S, Hein G, Huls S, Schmitt E, Diamantstein T, Blankenstein T. (1993). Interleukin-10 transfected into Chinese hamster ovary cells prevents tumor growth and macrophage infiltration. *Cancer Research* 53(18):4134-4137.

Riddle JM. (1999). Historical data as an aid in pharmaceutical prospecting and drug safety determination. *Journal of Alternative and Complementary Medicine* 5(2): 195-201.

Ridgway K. (1999). Acupuncture as a treatment modality for back problems. *Veterinary Clinics of North America and Equine Practice* 15(1):211-221.

Riedel W, Layka H, Neeck G. (1998). Secretory pattern of GH, TSH, thyroid hormones, ACTH, cortisol, FSH, and LH in patients with fibromyalgia syndrome following systemic injection of the relevant hypothalamic-releasing hormones. *Zeitschrift Rheumatologie* 57(Suppl 2):81-87.

Rieger PT. (1988). Management of cancer-related fatigue. *Dimensions in Oncology Nursing* 2(3):5-8.

Rieger PT. (2001). Assessment and epidemiologic issues related to fatigue. *Cancer* 92(6 Suppl):1733-1736.

Riem L. (1999). [Etiology and therapy of chronic fatigue syndrome: Too tired for life. Press Conference: Fatigue—Paralyzing Symptom in Cancer Patients, Cologne, September 17, 1999]. *MMW Fortschrift Medizin* 141(45):16-18.

Riemsma RP, Rasker JJ, Taal E, Griep EN, Wouters JM, Wiegman O. (1998). Fatigue in rheumatoid arthritis: The role of self-efficacy and problematic social support. *British Journal of Rheumatology* 37(10):1042-1046.

Rifkin RM, Hersh EM, Salmon SE. (1988). A phase I study of therapy with recombinant granulocyte-macrophage colony-stimulating factor administered by IV bolus or continuous infusion. *Behring Institut Mittwochlich* 83:125-133.

Rimoldi D, Romero P, Carrel S. (1993). The human melanoma antigen-encoding gene MAGE-1 is expressed by other tumor cells of neuroextodermal origin such as glioblastomas and neuroblastoma. *International Journal of Cancer* 54:527-528.

Rinaldi DA, Burris HA, Dorr FA, Woodworth JR, Kuhn JG, Eckardt JR, Rodriguez G, Corso SW, Fields SM, Langley C, et al. (1995). Initial phase I evaluation of the novel thymidylate synthase inhibitor, LY231514, using the modified continual reassessment method for dose escalation. *Journal of Clinical Oncology* 13(11):2842-2850.

Rinaldi DA, Kuhn JG, Burris HA, Dorr FA, Rodriguez G, Eckhardt SG, Jones S, Woodworth JR, Baker S, Langley C, et al. (1999). A phase I evaluation of multitargeted antifolate (MTA, LY231514), administered every 21 days, utilizing the modified continual reassessment method for dose escalation. *Cancer Chemotherapy Pharmacology* 44(5):372-380.

Rinaldi DA, Lippman SM, Burris HA III, Chou C, Von Hoff DD, Hong WK. (1993). Phase II study of 13-cis-retinoic acid and interferon-alpha 2a in patients with advanced squamous cell lung cancer. *Anticancer Drugs* 4(1):33-36.

Rinaldi DA, Lormand NA, Brierre JE, Cole JL, Barnes BC, Mills G, Yadlapati S, Felicia Fontenot M, Buller EJ, Rainey JM. (2002). A phase II trial of topotecan and gemcitabine in patients with previously treated, advanced nonsmall cell lung carcinoma. *Cancer* 95(6):1274-1278.

Rinehart J, Hersh E, Issell B, Triozzi P, Buhles W, Neidhart J. (1997). Phase 1 trial of recombinant human interleukin-1 beta (rhIL-1 beta), carboplatin, and etoposide in patients with solid cancers: Southwest Oncology Group Study 8940. *Cancer Investigation* 15(5):403-410.

Rinehart J, Margolin KA, Triozzi P, Hersh E, Campion M, Resta D, Levitt D. (1995). Phase I trial of recombinant interleukin 3 before and after carboplatin/etoposide chemotherapy in patients with solid tumors: A Southwest Oncology Group study. *Clinical Cancer Research* 1(10):1139-1144.

Rini BI, Stadler WM, Spielberger RT, Ratain MJ, Vogelzang NJ. (1998). Granulo-cyte-macrophage-colony stimulating factor in metastatic renal cell carcinoma: A phase II trial. *Cancer* 82(7):1352-1358.

Rini BI, Vogelzang NJ, Dumas MC, Wade JL III, Taber DA, Stadler WM. (2000). Phase II trial of weekly intravenous gemcitabine with continuous infusion fluorouracil in patients with metastatic renal cell cancer. *Journal of Clinical Oncology* 18(12):2419-2426.

Rios A, Mansell PW, Newell GR, Reuben JM, Hersh EM, Gutterman JU. (1985). Treatment of acquired immunodeficiency syndrome-related Kaposi's sarcoma with lymphoblastoid interferon. *Journal of Clinical Oncology* 3(4):506-512.

Ripple GH, Gould MN, Stewart JA, Tutsch KD, Arzoomanian RZ, Alberti D, Feierabend C, Pomplun M, Wilding G, Bailey HH. (1998). Phase I clinical trial of perillyl alcohol administered daily. *Clinical Cancer Research* 4(5):1159-1164.

Rischin D, Boyer M, Smith J, Millward M, Michael M, Bishop J, Zalcberg J, Davison J, Emmett E, McClure B. (2000). A phase I trial of docetaxel and gemcitabine in patients with advanced cancer. *Annals of Oncology* 11(4):421-426.

Rivera E, Sutton L, Colwell B, Graham M, Frye D, Somerville M, Conklin HS, McGuirt C, Levin J, Hortobagyi GN. (2002). Multicenter phase II study of a 28-day regimen of orally administered eniluracil and fluorouracil in the treatment of patients with anthracycline- and taxane-resistant advanced breast cancer. *Journal of Clinical Oncology* 20(4):987-993.

Rivera E, Valero V, Esteva FJ, Syrewicz L, Cristofanilli M, Rahman Z, Booser DJ, Hortobagyi GN. (2002). Lack of activity of stealth liposomal doxorubicin in the treatment of patients with anthracycline-resistant breast cancer. *Cancer Chemotherapy and Pharmacology* 49(4):299-302.

Rivoire M. (1992). [Cancers of the colon and the rectum: News in 1992]. *Pathological Biology* 40(9 Pt 2):943-948.

Rizvi NA, Marshall JL, Ness E, Hawkins MJ, Kessler C, Jacobs H, Brenckman WD, Lee JS, Petros W, Hong WK, et al. (2002). Initial clinical trial of oral TAC-101, a novel retinoic acid receptor-alpha selective retinoid, in patients with advanced cancer. *Journal of Clinical Oncology* 20(16):3522-3532.

Robbins JM, Kirmayer LJ, Hemami S. (1997). Latent variable models of functional somatic distress. *Journal of Nervous and Mental Disorders* 185(10):606-615.

Roberts JD, Shibata S, Spicer DV, McLeod HL, Tombes MB, Kyle B, Carroll M, Sheedy B, Collier MA, Pithavala YK, et al. (2000). Phase I study of AG2034, a targeted GARFT inhibitor, administered once every 3 weeks. *Cancer Chemotherapy Pharmacology* 45(5):423-427.

Roberts TK, McGregor NR, Dunstan RH, Donohoe M, Murdoch RN, Hope D, Zhang S, Butt HL, Watkins JA, Taylor WG. (1998). Immunological and haematological parameters in patients with chronic fatigue syndrome. *Journal of Chronic Fatigue Syndrome* 4(4):51-66.

Robertson MJ, Pelloso D, Abonour R, Hromas RA, Nelson RP Jr, Wood L, Cornetta K. (2002). Interleukin 12 immunotherapy after autologous stem cell transplantation for hematological malignancies. *Clinical Cancer Research* 8(11):3383-3393.

Robertson TJ. (1999). Misunderstood illnesses: Fibromyalgia and chronic fatigue syndrome. *Alta RN* 55(3):6-7.

Robins HI, Chang SM, Prados MD, Yung WK, Hess K, Schiff D, Greenberg H, Fink K, Nicolas K, Kuhn JG, et al. (2002). A phase II trial of thymidine and carboplatin for recurrent malignant glioma: A North American Brain Tumor Consortium study. *Neuro-oncology* 4(2):109-114.

Robins HI, Jonsson GG, Jacobson EL, Schmitt CL, Cohen JD, Jacobson MK. (1991). Effect of hyperthermia in vitro and in vivo on adenine and pyridine nucleotide pools in human peripheral lymphocytes. *Cancer* 67:2096-2102.

Robins RK. (1986). Synthetic antiviral agents. *Chemical Engineering News* 27: 28-40.

Robinson KD, Posner JD. (1992). Patterns of self-care needs and interventions related to biologic response modifier therapy: Fatigue as a model. *Seminars in Oncology Nursing* 8(4 Suppl 1):17-22.

Roelcke U, Kappos L, Lechner-Scott J, Brunnschweiler H, Huber S, Ammann W, Plohmann A, Dellas S, Maguire RP, Missimer J, et al. (1997). Reduced glucose metabolism in the frontal cortex and basal ganglia of multiple sclerosis patients with fatigue: A 18F-fluorodeoxyglucose positron emission tomography study. *Neurology* 48(6):1566-1571.

Rogers BB. (1993). Taxol: A promising new drug of the '90s. *Oncology Nursing Forum* 20(10):1483-1489.

Roitt IM. (1994). The T-cell priming hurdle in autoimmune disease and tumor immunity. *The Immunologist* 2:41-46.

Roizenblatt S, Moldofsky H, Benedito-Silva AA, Tufik S. (2001). Alpha sleep characteristics in fibromyalgia. *Arthritis and Rheumatism* 44(1):222-230.

Roizenblatt S, Tufik S, Goldenberg J, Pinto LR, Feldman DP. (1997). Juvenile fibromyalgia: Clinical and polysomnographic aspects. *Journal of Rheumatology* 24:579-585.

Rokos H, Rokos K, Frisius H, Kirstaedter HJ. (1980). Altered urinary excretion of pteridines in neoplastic disease: Determination of biopterin, neopterin, xanthopterin and pterin. *Clinica Chimica Acta* 105:275-286.

Romagnani S. (1994). Lymphokine production by human T cells in disease states. *Annual Reviews of Immunology* 12:227-257.

Romain P, Schlossman S. (1984). Human T lymphocyte subsets: Functional heterogeneity and surface recognition structures. *Journal of Clinical Investigation* 74:1559-1565.

Romano TJ. (1996). Breast implants and connective-tissue disease. *JAMA* 276(2): 102, discussion 103.

Romano TJ. (1998). The fibromyalgia problem. *Journal of Rheumatology* 25(5): 1026-1027; discussion 1028-1030.

Romano TJ. (1999). Patients with fibromyalgia must be treated fairly. *Archives of Internal Medicine* 159(20):2481-2483.

Romanus V, Svensson A, Hallander HO. (1992). The impact of changing BCG coverage on tuberculosis incidence in Swedish-born children between 1969 and 1989. *Tuberculosis and Lung Diseases* 73:150-161.

Rook GA, Zumla A. (1997). Gulf War syndrome: Is it due to a systemic shift in cytokine balance towards a Th2 profile? *Lancet* 349(9068):1831-1833.

Roscoe JA, Morrow GR, Hickok JT, Bushunow P, Matteson S, Rakita D, Andrews PL. (2002). Temporal interrelationships among fatigue, circadian rhythm and depression in breast cancer patients undergoing chemotherapy treatment. *Support Care and Cancer* 10(4):329-336.

Rose L, Pugh LC, Lears K, Gordon DL. (1998). The fatigue experience: Persons with HIV infection. *Journal of Advanced Nursing* 28(2):295-304.

Rosen LS, Gordon D, Kaminski M, Howell A, Belch A, Mackey JA, Apffelstaedt J, Hussein M, Coleman RE, Reitsma DJ, et al. (2001). Zoledronic acid versus pamidronate in the treatment of skeletal metastases in patients with breast cancer or osteolytic lesions of multiple myeloma: A phase III, double-blind, comparative trial. *Cancer Journal* 7(5):377-387.

Rosen PJ, Mendoza EF, Landaw EM, Mondino B, Graves MC, McBride JH, Turcillo P, deKernion J, Belldegrun A. (1996). Suramin in hormone-refractory metastatic prostate cancer: A drug with limited efficacy. *Journal of Clinical Oncology* 14(5):1626-1636.

Rosenberg NL. (1996). The neuromythology of silicone breast implants. *Neurology* 46(2):308-314.

Rosenberg SA. (1984). Adoptive immunotherapy of cancer: Accomplishments and prospects. *Cancer Treatment Reports* 68:233-255.

Rosenberg SA. (1985). Lymphokine-activated killer cells: A new approach to immunotherapy of cancer. *Journal of the National Cancer Institute* 75:595-603.

Rosenberg SA, Terry W. (1977). Passive immunotherapy of cancer in animals and man. *Advances in Cancer Research* 25:328-388.

Rosenberg SA, White DE. (1996). Vitiligo in patients with melanoma: Normal tissue antigens can be targets for cancer immunotherapy. *Journal of Immunotherapy* 18:81-84.

Rosenbloom AJ, Pinsky MR, Bryant JL, Shin A, Than T, Whiteside T. (1995). Leukocyte activation in the peripheral blood of patients with cirrhosis of the liver and SIRS: Correlation with serum interleukin-6 levels and organ dysfunction. *JAMA* 274(1):58-65.

Rosenblum D, Saffir M. (1998). Therapeutic and symptomatic treatment of multiple sclerosis. *Physical Medicine and Rehabilitation Clinics of North America* 9(3):587-601.

Rosenfeld WD, Walco GA. (1997). One test too many: Toward an integrated approach to psychosomatic disorders. *Adolescent Medicine* 8(3):483-487.

Rosenstein M, Yron I, Kaufmann Y, Rosenberg SA. (1984). Lymphokine-activated killer cells: Lysis of fresh syngeneic natural killer resistant murine tumor cells by lymphocytes cultured in interleukin 2. *Cancer Research* 44:1946-1953.

Rosenthal MA, Oratz R. (1998). Phase II clinical trial of recombinant alpha 2b interferon and 13 cis retinoic acid in patients with metastatic melanoma. *American Journal of Clinical Oncology* 21(4):352-354.

Rosing H, Lustig V, van Warmerdam LJ, Huizing MT, Ten Bokkel Huinink WW, Schellens JH, Rodenhuis S, Bult A, Beijnen JH. (2000). Pharmacokinetics and metabolism of docetaxel administered as a 1-h intravenous infusion. *Cancer Chemotherapy Pharmacology* 45(3):213-218.

Ross DD, Alexander CS. (2001). Management of common symptoms in terminally ill patients: Part I. Fatigue, anorexia, cachexia, nausea and vomiting. *American Family Physician* 64(5):807-814.

Ross E. (1996). The history and treatment of chronic fatigue syndrome. *Nursing Times* 92(44):34-36.

Rosso R, Sertoli MR, Queirolo P, Sanguineti O, Barzacchi MC, Mariani GL, Miglio L, Venturini M, Toma S. (1992). An outpatient phase I study of a subcutaneous interleukin-2 and intramuscular alpha-2a-interferon combination in advanced malignancies. *Annals of Oncology* 3(7):559-563.

Rostoker G, Uzzan B, Baumelou E, Chapman A. (1986). [Familial IgG kappa myeloma in a mother and her daughter: Review of the literature]. *Nouvelle Revue Francaise de Hematologie* 28(1):27-32.

Roth AD, Maibach R, Martinelli G, Fazio N, Aapro MS, Pagani O, Morant R, Borner MM, Herrmann R, Honegger H, et al. (2000). Docetaxel (Taxotere)-cisplatin (TC): An effective drug combination in gastric carcinoma. Swiss Group for Clinical Cancer Research (SAKK), and the European Institute of Oncology (EIO). *Annals of Oncology* 11(3):301-306.

Roth AD, Morant R, Alberto P. (1999). High dose etretinate and interferon-alpha— A phase I study in squamous cell carcinomas and transitional cell carcinomas. *Acta Oncologica* 38(5):613-617.

Rothenberg ML, Liu PY, Wilczynski S, Hannigan EV, Weiner SA, Weiss GR, Hunter VJ, Chapman JA, Tiersten A, Kohler PC, et al. (2001). Phase II trial of oral altretamine for consolidation of clinical complete remission in women with stage III epithelial ovarian cancer: A Southwest Oncology Group trial (SWOG-9326). *Gynecological Oncology* 82(2):317-322.

Rougier P, Bugat R. (1996). CPT-11 in the treatment of colorectal cancer: Clinical efficacy and safety profile. *Seminars in Oncology* 23(1 Suppl 3):34-41.

Rougier P, Bugat R, Douillard JY, Culine S, Suc E, Brunet P, Becouarn Y, Ychou M, Marty M, Extra JM, et al. (1997). Phase II study of irinotecan in the treatment of advanced colorectal cancer in chemotherapy-naive patients and patients pretreated with fluorouracil-based chemotherapy. *Journal of Clinical Oncology* 15(1):251-260.

Rousseau P. (2001). The palliative use of high-dose corticosteroids in three terminally ill patients with pain. *American Journal of Hospital Palliative Care* 18(5):343-346.

Rowbottom DG, Keast D, Green S, Kakulas B, Morton AR. (1998). The case history of an elite ultra-endurance cyclist who developed chronic fatigue syndrome. *Medical Science in Sports and Exercise* 30(9):1345-1348.

Rowbottom DG, Keast D, Pervan Z, Goodman C, Bhagat C, Kakulas B, Morton A. (1998). The role of glutamine in the aetiology of the chronic fatigue syndrome: A prospective study. *Journal of Chronic Fatigue Syndrome* 4(2):3-22.

Rowe PC, Calkins H. (1998). Neurally mediated hypotension and chronic fatigue syndrome. *American Journal of Medicine* 105(3A):15S-21S.

Royal Colleges of Physicians, General Practitioners and Psychiatrists. (1996). *Report: Chronic Fatigue Syndrome*. London: Royal College of Physicians.

Royce ME, Hoff PM, Dumas P, Lassere Y, Lee JJ, Coyle J, Ducharme MP, De Jager R, Pazdur R. (2001). Phase I and pharmacokinetic study of exatecan mesylate (DX-8951f): A novel camptothecin analog. *Journal of Clinical Oncology* 19(5): 1493-1500.

Royce ME, McGarry W, Bready B, Dakhil SR, Belt RJ, Goodwin JW, Gray R, Hoff PM, Winn R, Pazdur R. (1999). Sequential biochemical modulation of fluorouracil with folinic acid, N-phosphonacetyl-L-aspartic acid, and interferon alfa-2a in advanced colorectal cancer. *Journal of Clinical Oncology* 17(10):3276-3282.

Rozencweig M, Nicaise C, Beer M, Crespeigne N, Van Rijmenant M, Lenaz L, Kenis Y. (1983). Phase I study of carboplatin given on a five-day intravenous schedule. *Journal of Clinical Oncology* 1(10):621-626.

Rozman C, Montserrat E, Vinolas N, Urbano-Ispizua A, Ribera JM, Gallart T, Compernolle C. (1988). Recombinant alpha 2-interferon in the treatment of B chronic lymphocytic leukemia in early stages. *Blood* 71(5):1295-1298.

Rubel DM, Freeman S, Southwell IA. (1998). Tea tree oil allergy: What is the offending agent? Report of three cases of tea tree oil allergy and review of the literature. *Australasian Journal of Dermatology* 39(4):244-247.

Rubenstein EB. (1998). Evaluating cost-effectiveness in outpatient management of medical complications in cancer patients. *Current Opinions in Oncology* 10(4): 297-301.

Rubin RT, Heist EK, McGeoy SS, Hanada K, Lesser IM. (1992). Neuroendocrine aspects of primary endogenous depression: XI. Serum melatonin measures in patients and matched control subjects. *Archives of General Psychiatry* 49:558-567.

Ruck B, Shih RD, Marcus SM. (1999). Hypertensive crisis from herbal treatment of impotence. *American Journal of Emergency Medicine* 17(3):317-318.

Rudin CM, Homlund J, Fleming GF, Mani S, Stadler WM, Schumm P, Monia BP, Johnston JF, Geary R, Yu RZ, et al. (2001). Phase I trial of ISIS 5132, an antisense oligonucleotide inhibitor of c-raf-1, administered by 24-hour weekly infusion to patients with advanced cancer. *Clinical Cancer Research* 7(5):1214-1220.

Ruiz Moral R, Munoz Alamo M, Perula de Torres L, Aguayo Galeote M. (1997). Biopsychosocial features of patients with widespread chronic musculoskeletal pain in family medicine clinics. *Family Practice* 14(3):242-248.

Rundles RW, Moore JO. (1978). Chronic lymphocytic leukemia. *Cancer* 42(2 Suppl):941-945.

Ruof J, Hulsemann JL, Stucki G. (1999). Evaluation of costs in rheumatic diseases: A literature review. *Current Opinions in Rheumatology* 11(2):104-109.

Russell IJ. (1998). Neurochemical pathogenesis of fibromyalgia. *Zeitschrift Rheumatologie* 57(Suppl 2):63-66.

Russell IJ. (1999). Is fibromyalgia a distinct clinical entity? The clinical investigator's evidence. *Baillieres Best Practice Research in Clinical Rheumatology* 13(3):445-454.

Russo D, Fanin R, Zuffa E, Gallizia C, Grazia Michieli M, Damiani D, Testoni N, Pecile V, Visani G, Colombini R, et al. (1989). Treatment of Ph+ chronic myeloid leukemia by gamma interferon. *Blut* 59(1):15-20.

Rusy LM, Harvey SA, Beste DJ. (1999). Pediatric fibromyalgia and dizziness: Evaluation of vestibular function. *Journal of Developmental Behavioral Pediatrics* 20(4):211-215.

Rutgeerts P, D'Haens G, Targan S, Vasiliauskas E, Hanauer SB, Present DH, Mayer L, Van Hogezand RA, Braakman T, De Woody SL, et al. (1999). Efficacy and safety of retreatment with anti-tumor necrosis factor antibody (Infliximab) to maintain remission in Crohn's disease. *Gastroenterology* 117(4):761-769.

Ryan CW, Vogelzang NJ, Dumas MC, Kuzel T, Stadler WM. (2000). Granulocyte-macrophage-colony stimulating factor in combination immunotherapy for patients with metastatic renal cell carcinoma: Results of two phase II clinical trials. *Cancer* 88(6):1317-1324.

Ryan CW, Vogelzang NJ, Stadler WM. (2002). A phase II trial of intravenous gemcitabine and 5-fluorouracil with subcutaneous interleukin-2 and interferon-alpha in patients with metastatic renal cell carcinoma. *Cancer* 94(10):2602-2609.

Ryan CW, Vokes EE, Vogelzang NJ, Janisch L, Kobayashi K, Ratain MJ. (2002). A phase I study of suramin with once- or twice-monthly dosing in patients with advanced cancer. *Cancer Chemotherapy Pharmacology* 50(1):1-5.

Ryan J, Straus DJ, Lange C, Filippa DA, Botet JF, Sanders LM, Shiu MH, Fortner JG. (1988). Primary lymphoma of the liver. *Cancer* 61(2):370-375.

Sabal, N. (1997). Fireworks over fibromyalgia, CFS, and IBS. *Postgraduate Medicine* 102(6):44.

Sabbatini P. (2000). Contribution of anemia to fatigue in the cancer patient. *Oncology* 14(11A):69-71.

Sabeh F, Wright T, Norton SJ. (1996). Isozymes of superoxide dismutase from *Aloë vera*. *Enzyme and Protein* 49(4):212-221.

Sabin TD, Dawson DM. (1993). History and epidemiology. In *Chronic Fatigue Syndrome,* Dawson DM, Sabin TD, eds. Boston: Little, Brown, pp. 1ff.

Sackheim HA, Weber SL. (1982). Functional brain asymmetry in regulation of emotion: Implications for bodily manifestations of stress. In *Handbook of Stress: Theoretical and Clinical Aspects,* Goldberger L, Breznits I, eds. New York: Free Press, pp. 1ff.

Sadigh MR. (2001). *Autogenic Training: A Mind-Body Approach for the Treatment of Fibromyalgia and Chronic Pain Syndrome.* Binghamton, NY: The Haworth Medical Press.

Sadler IJ, Jacobsen PB. (2001). Progress in understanding fatigue associated with breast cancer treatment. *Cancer Investigation* 19(7):723-731.

Sadler IJ, Jacobsen PB, Booth-Jones M, Belanger H, Weitzner MA, Fields KK. (2002). Preliminary evaluation of a clinical syndrome approach to assessing cancer-related fatigue. *Journal of Pain Symptomatology Management* 23(5): 406-416.

Sadler M. (1997). Graded exercise in chronic fatigue syndrome: Patients were a selected group. *British Medical Journal* 315(7113):947-948.

Saeki T, Jinushi K, Kim R, Toi M, Saeki K, Yoshinaka K, Yanagawa E, Niimoto M, Hattori T. (1989). [Combination chemotherapy of CPM-MTX-5-FU in nonresectable and recurrent cancer patients]. *Gan To Kagaku Ryoho* 16(4 Pt 1):827-831.

Saeki T, Saeki S, Yokoyama H, Fukuda T, Sato R, Morooka C, Inoue S, Uesaka Y. (1990). [A case of colony stimulating factor (CSF) producing gastric carcinoma]. *Gan No Rinsho* 36(14):2469-2474.

Safran S. (1998). Lack of control group deemed problematic in fibromyalgia pilot study. *Alternative Therapy Health Medicine* 4(5):114, 116.

Saggini R, Pizzigallo E, Vecchiet J, Macellari V, Giacomozzi C. (1998). Alteration of spatial-temporal parameters of gait in chronic fatigue syndrome. *Journal of Neurological Sciences* 154(1):18-25.

Sahlberg-Blom E, Ternestedt BM, Johansson JE. (2001). Is good "quality of life" possible at the end of life? An explorative study of the experiences of a group of cancer patients in two different care cultures. *Journal of Clinical Nursing* 10(4):550-562.

Said JW, Rettig MR, Heppner K, Vescio RA, Schiller G, Ma HJ, Belson D, Savage A, Shintaku IP, Koeffler HP, et al. (1997). Localization of Kaposi's sarcoma-associated herpesvirus in bone marrow biopsy samples from patients with multiple myeloma. *Blood* 90(11):4278-4282.

Saiki I. (2000). A Kampo medicine "Juzen-taiho-to"—Prevention of malignant progression and metastasis of tumor cells and the mechanism of action. *Biological Pharmacology Bulletin* 23(6):677-688.

Saita L, Polastri D, De Conno F. (1999). Visual disturbances in advanced cancer patients: Clinical observations. *Journal of Pain Symptomatology and Management* 17(3):224-226.

Saito K. (1995). Biochemical studies on AIDS dementia complex—Possible contribution of quinolinic acid during brain damage. *Rinsho Byori—Japanese Journal of Clinical Pathology* 43(9):891-901.

Sakai C, Minamihisamatsu M, Takagi T, Oguro M, Maruyama K, Tanaka K, Kamada N. (1990). [Prominent lymphadenopathy and double Ph1 chromosomes as initial and recurrent manifestations of chronic myelogenous leukemia in blast crisis: Report of a case and review of the literature]. *Rinsho Ketsueki* 31(9):1506-1511.

Sakai M, Sagara K, Tashiro A, Fujiyama S, Shiraoku H, Sato T, Nakamura T. (1984). [A case of advanced gastric cancer associated with smouldering adult T-cell leukemia (ATL)]. *Gan No Rinsho* 30(3):301-306.

Sakai Y, Yamada T, Nagahama K, Ichiyanagi N, Kamata S, Tanizawa A, Fukuda H, Watanabe T, Saitoh H. (2000). [A case of giant hemorrhagic adrenal pseudocyst with infection]. *Hinyokika Kiyo* 46(5):315-317.

Sakuda M, Hiura S, Usui M, Sugi M, Nukata J, Miyazaki T. (1980). Effect of a bleomycin derivative on oral carcinoma: A clinical and immunologic study of five cases. *International Journal of Oral Surgery* 9(2):103-112.

Sakuma F, Kuroda M, Takagi T, Terashima K, Ohishi A, Noguchi S, Mizuno A. (1999). [Evaluation of chemotherapy with docetaxel and cisplatin in advanced non-small cell lung cancer]. *Gan To Kagaku Ryoho* 26(7):927-932.

Salit IE. (1985). Sporadic postinfectious neuromyasthenia. *Canadian Medical Association Journal* 133:659-663.

Salit IE. (1996). The chronic fatigue syndrome: A position paper. *The Journal of Rheumatology* 23(3):540-544.

Salit IE. (1997). Precipitating factors for the chronic fatigue syndrome. *Journal of Psychiatric Research* 31(1):59-65.

Salminen E, Bergman M, Huhtala S, Ekholm E. (1999). Docetaxel: Standard recommended dose of 100 mg/m^2 is effective but not feasible for some metastatic breast cancer patients heavily pretreated with chemotherapy—A phase II single-center study. *Journal of Clinical Oncology* 17(4):1127.

Salminen E, Nikkanen V, Lindholm L. (1997). Palliative chemotherapy in non-Hodgkin's lymphoma. *Oncology* 54(2):108-111.

Saltz L, Kemeny N, Schwartz G, Kelsen D. (1994). A phase II trial of alpha-interferon and 5-fluorouracil in patients with advanced carcinoid and islet cell tumors. *Cancer* 74(3):958-961.

Saltz L, Sirott M, Young C, Tong W, Niedzwiecki D, Tzy-Jyun Y, Tao Y, Trochanowski B, Wright P, Barbosa K, et al. (1993). Phase I clinical and pharmacology study of topotecan given daily for 5 consecutive days to patients with advanced solid tumors, with attempt at dose intensification using recombinant granulocyte colony-stimulating factor. *Journal of the National Cancer Institutes* 85(18):1499-1507.

Saltzstein BJ, Wyshak G, Hubbuch JT, Perry JC. (1998). A naturalistic study of the chronic fatigue syndrome among women in primary care. *General Hospital Psychiatry* 20(5):307-316.

Salvatore M, Morozunov M, Schnemake M, Lipkin WI, the Bornavirus Study Group. (1998). Borna disease virus in brains of North American and European people with schizophrenia and bipolar disorders. *Lancet* 349:1813-1814.

Samaniego F, Markham PD, Gallo RC, Ensoli B. (1995). Inflammatory cytokines induce AIDS-Kaposi's sarcoma-derived spindle cells to produce and release basic fibroblast growth factor and enhance Kaposi's sarcoma-like lesion formation in nide mice. *Journal of Immunology* 154:3582-3592.

Samarel N, Leddy SK, Greco K, Cooley ME, Torres SC, Tulman L, Fawcett J. (1996). Development and testing of the symptom experience scale. *Journal of Pain Symptomatology and Management* 12(4):221-228.

Samborski W, Stratz T, Schochat T, Mennet P, Muller W. (1996). [Biochemical changes in fibromyalgia] Biochemicsche veranderungen bei der fibromyalgie. *Zeitschrift Rheumatologie* 55(3):168-173.

Samii A, Wassermann EM, Ikoma K, Mercuri B, George MS, O'Fallon A, Dale JK, Straus SE, Hallett M. (1996). Decreased postexercise facilitation of motor evoked potentials in patients with chronic fatigue syndrome or depression. *Neurology* 47(6):1410-1414.

Sampaio EP, Kaplan G, Miranda A, Neri JA, Miguel CP, Viana SM, Sarno EN. (1993). The influence of thalidomide on the clinical and immunologic manifestation of erythema nodosum leprosum. *Journal of Infectious Diseases* 168(2): 408-414.

Sampaio EP, Sarno EN, Galilly R, Cohn ZA, Kaplan G. (1991). Thalidomide selectively inhibits tumor necrosis alpha production by stimulated human monocytes. *Journal of Experimental Medicine* 173(3):699-703.

Sanchez-Ortiz RF, Broderick GA, Rovner ES, Wein AJ, Whittington R, Malkowicz SB. (2000). Erectile function and quality of life after interstitial radiation therapy for prostate cancer. *International Journal of Impotence Research* 12(Suppl 3): S18-S24.

Sanders L, Silverman M, Rossi R, Braasch J, Munson L. (1996). Gastric smooth muscle tumors: Diagnostic dilemmas and factors affecting outcome. *World Journal of Surgery* 20(8):992-995.

Sandler A, Blanke C, Monaco F, Carey MA, Ansari R, Fisher B, Spiridonidis CH, Einhorn L, Nichols C. (1998). CODE (cisplatin, vincristine, doxorubicin, etoposide) plus granulocyte colony-stimulating factor in advanced non-small-cell lung cancer: A Hoosier Oncology Group phase II trial. *American Journal of Clinical Oncology* 21(3):294-297.

Sandler RS. (1996). Epidemiology and risk factor for cancer. *Gastroenterology Clinics of North America* 25:717-735.

Sandman CA, Barron JL, Nackoul KA, Fidler PL, Goldstein J. (1992). Is there a chronic fatigue syndrome (CFS) dementia? In *The Clinical and Scientific Basis of Myalgic Encephalomyelitis/Chronic Fatigue Syndrome,* Hyde B, Levine P, Goldstein J, eds. Ottawa, Canada: Nightingale Research Foundation, pp. 467-479.

Sandor V, Bakke S, Robey RW, Kang MH, Blagosklonny MV, Bender J, Brooks R, Piekarz RL, Tucker E, Figg WD, et al. (2002). Phase I trial of the histone deacetylase inhibitor, depsipeptide (FR901228, NSC 630176), in patients with refractory neoplasms. *Clinical Cancer Research* 8(3):718-728.

Sane AC, Roggli VL. (1995). Curative resection of a well-differentiated papillary mesothelioma of the pericardium. *Archives of Pathology and Laboratory Medicine* 119(3):266-267.

Santiago-Palma J, Payne R. (2001). Palliative care and rehabilitation. *Cancer* 92 (4 Suppl):1049-1052.

Santra S, Ghosh SK. (1997). Interleukin-4 is effective in restoring cytotoxic T-cell activity that declines during in vivo progression of a murine B lymphoma. *Cancer Immunology and Immunotherapy* 44:291-300.

Sanyaolu AO, Fagbenro-Beyioku AF, Oyibo WA. (1997). Induced immunity to *Plasmodium yoelli nigeriensis* in albino mice by antigenic mice organs. *East African Medical Journal* 74(9):566-569.

Sapolsky R, Rivier C, Yamamoto G, Plotsky P, Vale W. (1987). Interleukin-1 stimulates the secretion of hypothalamic corticotropin-releasing factor. *Science* 238 (4826):522-524.

Sarhill N, Walsh D, Nelson KA, Homsi J, Le Grand S, Davis MP. (2001). Methylphenidate for fatigue in advanced cancer: A prospective open-label pilot study. *American Journal of Hospital Palliative Care* 18(3):187-192.

Sarna GP, Figlin RA. (1985). Phase II trial of alpha-lymphoblastoid interferon given weekly as treatment of advanced breast cancer. *Cancer Treatment Reports* 69(5):547-549.

Sarna GP, Figlin RA, Pertcheck M. (1987). Phase II study of betaseron (beta ser17-interferon) as treatment of advanced malignant melanoma. *Journal of Biological Response Modifiers* 6(4):375-378.

Sarna GP, Figlin RA, Pertcheck M, Altrock B, Kradjian SA. (1989). Systemic administration of recombinant methionyl human interleukin-2 (Ala 125) to cancer patients: Clinical results. *Journal of Biological Response Modifiers* 8(1):16-24.

Sarna L. (1993a). Correlates of symptom distress in women with lung cancer. *Cancer Practice* 1(1):21-28.

Sarna L. (1993b). Fluctuations in physical function: Adults with non-small cell lung cancer. *Journal of Advanced Nursing* 18(5):714-724.

Sarna L. (1993c). Women with lung cancer: Impact on quality of life. *Quality of Life Research* 2(1):13-22.

Sarna L. (1994). Functional status in women with lung cancer. *Cancer Nursing* 17(2):87-93.

Sarna L. (1998). Effectiveness of structured nursing assessment of symptom distress in advanced lung cancer. *Oncology Nursing Forum* 25(6):1041-1048.

Sarna L, Brecht ML. (1997). Dimensions of symptom distress in women with advanced lung cancer: A factor analysis. *Heart and Lung* 26(1):23-30.

Sarna L, Conde F. (2001). Physical activity and fatigue during radiation therapy: A pilot study using actigraph monitors. *Oncology Nursing Forum* 28(6):1043-1046.

Sarna L, Ganley BJ. (1995). A survey of lung cancer patient-education materials. *Oncology Nursing Forum* 22(10):1545-1550.

Sarosdy MF, Lamm DL. (1989). Long-term results of intravesical bacillus Calmette-Guérin for superficial bladder cancer. *Journal of Urology* 142:719.

Sastre-Garau X, Loste MN, Vicent-Salamon A, Favre M, Mouret E, Dela Rockefordiere A, Durande JC, Tartour E, Le Page V, Charron D. (1996). Decreased frequency of HLA-DRB1*13 alleles in Frenchwomen with HPV-positive carcinoma of the cervix. *International Journal of Cancer* 69:159-164.

Satake M. (1998). The utilization and safety of medicinal plants and crude drugs. *Kokuritsu Iyakuhin Shokuhin Eisei Kenkyusho Hokoku* 116:13-29.

Sato K, Miyasaka N, Yamaoka K, Okuda M, Yata J, Nishioka K. (1987). Quantitative defect of CD4+2H4+ cells in systemic lupus erythematosus and Sjögren's syndrome. *Arthritis and Rheumatism* 30(12):1407-1411.

Sato K, Tsuchiya S, Minato K, Takei Y, Watanabe S, Saitoh R, Mori M. (2001). A phase I study of weekly docetaxel and cisplatin in advanced non-small cell lung cancer. *Lung Cancer* 33(1):69-73.

Sato M, Kanai N, Kanai H, Sugase T, Hanada M, Hayakawa T, Saito Y, Oonishi T, Oda Y, Miyagawa J. (1995). [TSH-secreting fibrous pituitary adenoma showing calcification: A case report]. *No Shinkei Geka* 23(3):259-263.

Sauder C, Muller A, Cubitt B, Mayer J, Steimetz J, Trabert W, Ziegler B, Wanke K, Mueller-Lantzch N, De la Torre JC, et al. (1996). Detection of Borna disease virus (BDV) antibodies and BDV RNA in psychiatic patients: Evidence of high sequence conservation of human blood-derived RNA. *Journal of Virology* 70(1): 7713-7724.

Savage DG, Szydlo RM, Goldman JM. (1997). Clinical features at diagnosis in 430 patients with chronic myeloid leukaemia seen at a referral centre over a 16-year period. *British Journal of Haematology* 96(1):111-116.

Savarese DM, Halabi S, Hars V, Akerley WL, Taplin ME, Godley PA, Hussain A, Small EJ, Vogelzang NJ. (2001). Phase II study of docetaxel, estramustine, and low-dose hydrocortisone in men with hormone-refractory prostate cancer: A final report of CALGB 9780. Cancer and Leukemia Group B. *Journal of Clinical Oncology* 19(9):2509-2516.

Sawada Y, Yamamoto S, Ogawa T, Ohkawa T. (1986). [Malignant fibrous histiocytoma of the perirenal tissue: Report of a case—a statistical study of 58 cases of urological malignant fibrous histiocytoma in Japanese literature]. *Hinyokika Kiyo* 32(6):853-864.

Sawaki S. (1990). [A phase 2 study of recombinant interleukin 2 (S-6820) for head and neck cancer]. *Gan No Rinsho* 36(2):111-120.

Sawayama Y, Hayashi J, Yano Y, Takeya S, Tani Y, Pei Y, Kashiwagi S. (1996). [Efficiency of combination chemotherapy and interferon-alpha therapy in a patient with AIDS-related cutaneous and gastrointestinal Kaposi's sarcoma]. *Kansenshogaku Zasshi* 70(6):621-626.

Scagliotti GV, Novello S. (2001). Role of erythropoietin in the treatment of lung cancer associated anaemia. *Lung Cancer* 34(Suppl 4):S91-S94.

Scamps RA, O'Neill BJ, Purser BN. (1971). Histiocytic medullary reticulosis. *Medical Journal of Australia* 2(19):956-960.

Schaafsma J, Osoba D. (1994). The Karnofsky Performance Status Scale re-examined: A cross-validation with the EORTC-C30. *Quality of Life Research* 3(6): 413-424.

Schaefer K, Saupe J, Pauls A, von Herrath D. (1986). Hypercalcemia and elevated serum 1,25-dihydroxyvitamin D3 in a patient with Hodgkin's lymphoma. *Klinische Wochenschrift* 64(2):89-91.

Schaefer KM. (1995). Sleep disturbance and fatigue in women with fibromyalgia and chronic fatigue syndrome. *Journal of Obstetrics, Gynecology, and Neonatal Nursing* 24:229-233.

Schaefer KM. (1997). Health patterns of women with fibromyalgia. *Journal of Advanced Nursing* 26(3):565-571.

Schagen SB, Hamburger HL, Muller MJ, Boogerd W, van Dam FS. (2001). Neurophysiological evaluation of late effects of adjuvant high-dose chemotherapy on cognitive function. *Journal of Neurooncology* 51(2):159-165.

Schagen SB, van Dam FS, Muller MJ, Boogerd W, Lindeboom J, Bruning PF. (1999). Cognitive deficits after postoperative adjuvant chemotherapy for breast carcinoma. *Cancer* 85(3):640-650.

Schanberg LE, Keefe FJ, Lefebvre JC, Kredich DW, Gil KM. (1996). Pain coping strategies in children with juvenile primary fibromyalgia syndrome: Correlation with pain, physical function, and psychological distress. *Arthritis Care Research* 9(2):89-96.

Schanberg LE, Keefe FJ, Lefebvre JC, Kredich DW, Gil KM. (1998). Social context of pain in children with juvenile primary fibromyalgia syndrome: Parental pain history and family environment. *Clinical Journal of Pain* 14(2):107-115.

Schanke AK. (1997). Psychological distress, social support and coping behaviour among polio survivors: A 5-year perspective in 63 polio patients. *Disability and Rehabilitation* 19(3):108-116.

Schantz SP, Dimery I, Lippman SM, Clayman GL, Pellegrino C, Morice R. (1992). A phase II study of interleukin-2 and interferon-alpha in head and neck cancer. *Investigative New Drugs* 10(3):217-223.

Scharf MB, Hauck M, Stover R, McDonald M, Berkowitz D. (1998). Effect of gamma-hydroxybutyrate on pain, fatigue, and the alpha sleep anomaly in patients with fibromyalgia: Preliminary report. *Journal of Rheumatology* 25(10): 1986-1990.

Scherrer M, Tschumi HJ, Zeller C, Zimmermann C. (1980). [Subjective early symptoms of bronchial neoplasms: Retrospective computer analysis of case histories, written in free prose]. *Schweize Medizinische Wochenschrift* 110(19): 715-721.

Scheulen ME, Hilger RA, Oberhoff C, Casper J, Freund M, Josten KM, Bornhauser M, Ehninger G, Berdel WE, Baumgart J, et al. (2000). Clinical phase I dose escalation and pharmacokinetic study of high-dose chemotherapy with treosulfan and autologous peripheral blood stem cell transplantation in patients with advanced malignancies. *Clinical Cancer Research* 6(11):4209-4216.

Schikler KN. (2000). Is it juvenile rheumatoid arthritis or fibromyalgia? *Medicine Clinics of North America* 84(4):967-982.

Schiller JH, Storer B, Bittner G, Willson JK, Borden EC. (1988). Phase II trial of a combination of interferon-beta ser and interferon-gamma in patients with advanced malignant melanoma. *Journal of Interferon Research* 8(5):581-589.

Schiller JH, Storer B, Willson JK, Borden EC. (1987). Phase I trial of combinations of recombinant interferons beta(ser) and gamma in patients with advanced malignancy. *Cancer Treatment Reports* 71(10):945-952.

Schiller JH, Storer B, Witt PL, Alberti D, Tombes MB, Arzoomanian R, Proctor RA, McCarthy D, Brown RR, Voss SD, et al. (1991). Biological and clinical effects of intravenous tumor necrosis factor-alpha administered three times weekly. *Cancer Research* 51(6):1651-1658.

Schiller JH, Storer B, Witt PL, Nelson B, Brown RR, Horisberger M, Grossberg S, Borden EC. (1990). Biological and clinical effects of the combination of beta- and gamma-interferons administered as a 5-day continuous infusion. *Cancer Research* 50(15):4588-4594.

Schilsky RL, Dolan ME, Bertucci D, Ewesuedo RB, Vogelzang NJ, Mani S, Wilson LR, Ratain MJ. (2000). Phase I clinical and pharmacological study of O6-benzylguanine followed by carmustine in patients with advanced cancer. *Clinical Cancer Research* 6(8):3025-3031.

Schilsky RL, Hohneker J, Ratain MJ, Janisch L, Smetzer L, Lucas VS, Khor SP, Diasio R, Von Hoff DD, Burris HA III. (1998). Phase I clinical and pharmacologic study of eniluracil plus fluorouracil in patients with advanced cancer. *Journal of Clinical Oncology* 16(4):1450-1457.

Schilsky RL, Janisch L, Berezin F, Mick R, Vogelzang NJ, Ratain MJ. (1993). Phase I clinical and pharmacological study of iododeoxyuridine and bleomycin in patients with advanced cancer. *Cancer Research* 53(6):1293-1296.

Schleef J, Wagner A, Kleta R, Schaarschmidt K, Dockhorn-Dworniczak B, Willital G, Jurgens H. (1999). Small-cell carcinoma of the ovary of the hypercalcemic type in an 8-year-old girl. *Pediatric Surgery International* 15(5-6):431-434.

Schlenk EA, Erlen JA, Dunbar-Jacob J, McDowell J, Engebrg S, Sereika SM, Rohay JM, Bernier MJ. (1998). Health-related quality of life in chronic disorders: A comparison across studies using the MOS SF-36. *Quality of Life Research* 7(1):57-65.

Schloss M, Kronzon I, Gelber PM, Reed GE, Berger A. (1975). Cystic thymoma simulating contrictive pericarditis: The role of echocardiography in the differential diagnosis. *Journal of Thoracic and Cardiovascular Surgery* 70(1):143-146.

Schmaling KB, Jones JF. (1996). MMPI profiles of patients with chronic fatigue syndrome. *Journal of Psychosomatic Research* 40(1):67-74.

Schmid HP, Maibach R, Bernhard J, Hering F, Hanselmann S, Gusset H, Morant R, Pestalozzi D, Castiglione M. (1997). A phase II study of oral idarubicin as a treatment for metastatic hormone-refractory prostate carcinoma with special focus on prostate specific antigen doubling time. Swiss Group for Clinical Cancer Research, Berne, Switzerland. *Cancer* 79(9):1703-1739.

Schmidt KD. (2001). Cancer rehabilitation services in a tertiary care center. *Cancer* 92(4 Suppl):1053-1054.

Schneider RA. (1998a). Concurrent validity of the Beck Depression Inventory and the Multidimensional Fatigue Inventory-20 in assessing fatigue among cancer patients. *Psychology Reports* 82(3 Pt 1):883-886.

Schneider RA. (1998b). Reliability and validity of the Multidimensional Fatigue Inventory (MFI-20) and the Rhoten Fatigue Scale among rural cancer outpatients. *Cancer Fatigue* 21(5):370-373.

Schneider SM. (1999). I look funny and I feel bad: Measurement of symptom distress. *Journal of Child Family Nursing* 2(5):380-384.

Schneider T, Seydlitz F, Zimmermann U, Sontag B, Boesken WH. (2001). [Life threatening hypercalcemia in a young man with ALL]. *Deutsche Medizinische Wochenschrift* 126(1-2):7-11.

Schoffski P, Hagedorn T, Grunwald V, Paul H, Merkle K, Kowalski R, Ganser A. (2000). Repeated administration of short infusions of bendamustine: A phase I study in patients with advanced progressive solid tumours. *Journal of Cancer Research and Clinical Oncology* 126(1):41-47.

Schoffski P, Seeland G, Engel H, Grunwald V, Paul H, Merkle K, Kowalski R, Ganser A. (2000). Weekly administration of bendamustine: A phase I study in patients with advanced progressive solid tumours. *Annals of Oncology* 11(6): 729-734.

Schomburg A, Kirchner H, Fenner M, Menzel T, Poliwoda H, Atzpodien J. (1993). Lack of therapeutic efficacy of tamoxifen in advanced renal cell carcinoma. *European Journal of Cancer* 29A(5):737-740.

Schornagel JH, Verweij J, ten Bokkel Huinink WW, Klijn JG, de Mulder PH, Debruyne FM, van Deijk WA, Roozendaal K, Kok TC, Veenhof KH, et al. (1989). Phase II study of recombinant interferon alpha-2a and vinblastine in advanced renal cell carcinoma. *Journal of Urology* 142(2 Pt 1):253-256.

Schroeder D, Hill GL. (1993). Predicting postoperative fatigue: Importance of preoperative factors. *World Journal of Surgery* 17(2):226-231.

Schuchter LM, Wohlganger J, Fishman EK, MacDermott ML, McGuire WP. (1992). Sequential chemotherapy and immunotherapy for the treatment of metastatic melanoma. *Journal of Immunotherapy* 12(4):272-276.

Schuck JR, Chappel LT, Kindness G. (1997). Causal modeling and alternative medicine. *Alternative Therapy Health Medicine* 3(2):40-47.

Schuler M, Bruntsch U, Spath-Schwalbe E, Schrezenmeier H, Peschel C, Farber L, Burger KJ, Leissner J, Huber C, Aulitzky WE. (1998). Lack of efficacy of recombinant human interleukin-6 in patients with advanced renal cell cancer: Results of a phase II study. *European Journal of Cancer* 34(5):754-756.

Schult C. (1984). [Side effects of BCG immune therapy in 511 patients with malignant melanoma]. *Hautarzt* 35(2):78-83.

Schulte PA. (1991). Validation of biologic markers for use in research on chronic fatigue syndrome. *Reviews of Infectious Diseases* 13:S87-S89.

Schulz V, Hänsel R, Tyler VE. (1998). *Rational Phytotherapy: A Physician's Guide to Herbal Medicine,* Third Edition. Berlin: Springer.

Schumacher A, Kessler T, Buchner T, Wewers D, van de Loo J. (1998). Quality of life in adult patients with acute myeloid leukemia receiving intensive and prolonged chemotherapy—A longitudinal study. *Leukemia* 12(4):586-592.

Schumacher A, Wewers D, Heinecke A, Sauerland C, Koch OM, Van de Loo J, Buchner T, Berdel WE. (2002). Fatigue as an important aspect of quality of life in patients with acute myeloid leukemia. *Leukemia Research* 26(4):355-362.

Schutzer SE, Natelson BH. (1999). Absence of *Borrelia burgdorferi*-specific immune complexes in chronic fatigue syndrome. *Neurology* 53(6):1340-1341.

Schwartz AH. (2002). Validity of cancer-related fatigue instruments. *Pharmacotherapy* 22(11):1433-1441.

Schwartz AL. (1998a). Patterns of exercise and fatigue in physically active cancer survivors. *Oncology Nursing Forum* 25(3):485-491.

Schwartz AL. (1998b). The Schwartz Cancer Fatigue Scale: Testing reliability and validity. *Oncology Nursing Forum* 25(4):711-717.

Schwartz AL. (1999). Fatigue mediates the effects of exercise on quality of life. *Quality of Life Research* 8(6):529-538.

Schwartz AL. (2000a). Daily fatigue patterns and effect of exercise in women with breast cancer. *Cancer Practice* 8(1):16-24.

Schwartz AL. (2000b). Exercise and weight gain in breast cancer patients receiving chemotherapy. *Cancer Practice* 8(5):231-237.

Schwartz AL, Meek P. (1999). Additional construct validity of the Schwartz Cancer Fatigue Scale. *Journal of Nursing Measurements* 7(1):35-45.

Schwartz AL, Meek PM, Nail LM, Fargo J, Lundquist M, Donofrio M, Grainger M, Throckmorton T, Mateo M. (2002). Measurement of fatigue: Determining minimally important clinical differences. *Journal of Clinical Epidemiology* 55(3): 239-244.

Schwartz AL, Mori M, Gao R, Nail LM, King ME. (2001). Exercise reduces daily fatigue in women with breast cancer receiving chemotherapy. *Medical Science, Sports, and Exercise* 33(5):718-723.

Schwartz AL, Nail LM, Chen S, Meek P, Barsevick AM, King ME, Jones LS. (2000). Fatigue patterns observed in patients receiving chemotherapy and radiotherapy. *Cancer Investigation* 18(1):11-19.

Schwartz AL, Thompson JA, Masood N. (2002). Interferon-induced fatigue in patients with melanoma: A pilot study of exercise and methylphenidate. *Oncology Nursing Forum* 29(7):E85-E90.

Schwartz GK, Ilson D, Saltz L, O'Reilly E, Tong W, Maslak P, Werner J, Perkins P, Stoltz M, Kelsen D. (2001). Phase II study of the cyclin-dependent kinase inhibitor flavopiridol administered to patients with advanced gastric carcinoma. *Journal of Clinical Oncology* 19(7):1985-1992.

Schwartz JE, Jandorf L, Krupp LB. (1993). The measurement of fatigue: A new instrument. *Journal of Psychosomatic Research* 37:753-762.

Schwartz JE, Scuderi P, Wiggins C, Rudolph A, Hersh EM. (1989). A phase I trial of recombinant tumor necrosis factor (rTNF) administered by continuous intravenous infusion in patients with disseminated malignancy. *Biotherapy* 1(3):207-214.

Schweiger LM, Hsiang HY. (2002). Pathological case of the month: Acute symptomatic hypercalcemia associated with ovarian small cell carcinoma. *Archives of Pediatric and Adolescent Medicine* 156(1):83-84.

Schweitzer A, Wright S. (1937). The anti-strychinine action of acetylcholine, prostigmine and related substances, and of central vagus stimulation. *Journal of Physiology* 90:310-329.

Schwenk W, Bohm B, Muller JM. (1998). Postoperative pain and fatigue after laparoscopic or conventional colorectal resections: A prospective randomized trial. *Surgical Endoscopy* 12(9):1131-1136.

Scott HR, McMillan DC, Forrest LM, Brown DJ, McArdle CS, Milroy R. (2002). The systemic inflammatory response, weight loss, performance status and survival in patients with inoperable non-small cell lung cancer. *British Journal of Cancer* 87(3):264-267.

Scott LJ, Wiseman LR. (1999). Exemestane. *Drugs* 58(4):675-680; discussion 681-682.

Scott LV, Burnett F, Medbak S, Dinan TG. (1998). Naloxone-mediated activation of the hypothalamic-pituitary-adrenal axis in chronic fatigue syndrome. *Psychological Medicine* 28(2):285-293.

Scott LV, Dinan TG. (1998). Urinary cortisol excretion in chronic fatigue syndrome, major depression and in health volunteers. *Journal of Affective Disorders* 47(1-3):49-54.

Scott LV, Dinan TG. (1999). The neuroendocrinology of chronic fatigue syndrome. Focus on the hypothalamic-pituitary-adrenal axis. *Functional Neurology* 14(1): 3-11.

Scott LV, Medbak S, Dinan TG. (1998a). Blunted adrenocorticotropin and cortisol responses to corticotropin-releasing hormone stimulation in chronic fatigue syndrome. *Acta Psychiatrica Scandinavica* 97(6):450-457.

Scott LV, Medbak S, Dinan TG. (1998b). The low dose ACTH test in chronic fatigue syndrome and in health. *Clinical Endocrinology* 48(6):733-737.

Scott LV, Medbak S, Dinan TG. (1999). Desmospressin augments pituitary adrenal responsivity to corticotropin-releasing hormone in subjects with chronic fatigue syndrome and in healthy volunteers. *Biological Psychiatry* 45(11):1447-1454.

Scott LV, Salahuddin F, Cooney J, Svec F, Dinan TG. (1999). Differences in adrenal steroid profile in chronic fatigue syndrome, in depression and in health. *Journal of Affective Disorders* 54(1-2):129-137.

Scott LV, The J, Reznek R, Martin A, Sohaib A, Dinan TG. (1999). Small adrenal glands in chronic fatigue syndrome: A preliminary computer tomography study. *Psychoneuroendocrinology* 24(7):759-768.

Sebastian P, Varghese C, Sankaranarayanan R, Zaina CP, Nirmala G, Jeevy G, Nair MK. (1993). Evaluation of symptomatology in planning palliative care. *Palliative Medicine* 7(1):27-34.

See DM, Broumand N, Sahl L, Tilles TG. (1997). In vitro effects of echinacea and ginseng on natural killer and antibody-dependent cell cytotoxicity in healthy subjects and chronic fatigue syndrome or acquired immunodeficiency syndrome patients. *Immunopharmacology* 35(3):229-235.

See DM, Cimoch P, Chou S, Chang J, Tilles J. (1998). The in vitro immunomodulatory effects of glyconutrients on peripheral blood mononuclear cells of patients with chronic fatigue syndrome. *Integrative Physiological and Behavioral Science* 33(3):280-287.

See DM, Tilles JG. (1996). Alpha-interferon treatment of patients with chronic fatigue syndrome. *Immunological Investigations* 25(1-2):153-164.

Seelig M. (1998). Review and hypothesis: Might patients with the chronic fatigue syndrome have latent tetany of magnesium deficiency? *Journal of Chronic Fatigue Syndrome* 4(2):77-108.

Sehgal AR. (2003). Impact of quality improvement efforts on race and sex disparities in hemodialysis. *JAMA* 289(8):996-1000.

Sehgal VN, Luthra A, Bajaj P. (2002). Epidermodysplasia verruciformis: 14 members of a pedigree with an intriguing squamous cell carcinoma transformation. *International Journal of Dermatology* 41(8):500-503.

Selner JC. (1996). Chamber challenges: The necessity of objective observation. *Regulatory Toxicology and Pharmacology* 24(1 Pt 2):S87-S95.

Selye H. (1982). History and present status of the stress concept. In *Handbook of Stress: Theoretical and Clinical Aspects,* Goldberger L, Breznitz S, eds. New York: Free Press, pp. 7-17.

Semb KA, Aamdal S, Mette E, Ingvar C, Gullaksen N, Osmundsen K. (1998). Zilascorb(2H), a low-toxicity protein synthesis inhibitor that exhibits signs of anticancer activity in malignant melanoma. *Anticancer Drugs* 9(9):797-802.

Sen GC, Ransohoff RM. (1993). Interferon-induced antiviral actions and their regulation. *Advances in Virus Research* 42:57-102.

Sendrowski DP, Buker EA, Gee SS. (1997). An investigation of sympathetic hypersensitivity in chronic fatigue syndrome. *Optometry and Visual Sciences* 74(8): 660-663.

Seo P. (2002). Cases from the medical grand rounds of the Osler Medical Service at Johns Hopkins University. *American Journal of Medicine* 112(9):730-732.

Serenelli G, Petturiti G, Tognellini R, Frascarelli M, Sabbagh M, Viola-Magni MP. (1997). Apoptosis induced in glioma rat cells cultivated in the presence of a medicinal infusion of green tea. *European Journal of Histochemistry* 41(Suppl. 2): 85-86.

Sergi M, Rizzi M, Braghiroli A, Puttini PS, Greco M, Cazzola M, Andreoli A. (1999). Periodic breathing during sleep in patients affected by fibromyalgia syndrome. *European Respiration Journal* 14(1):203-208.

Sertoli MR, Bernengo MG, Ardizzoni A, Brunetti I, Falcone A, Vidili MG, Cusimano MP, Appino A, Doveil G, Fortini C, et al. (1989). Phase II trial of recombinant alpha-2b interferon in the treatment of metastatic skin melanoma. *Oncology* 46(2):96-98.

Sertoli MR, Brunetti I, Ardizzoni A, Falcone A, Guarneri D, Boccardo F, Martorana G, Curotto A, Sicignano A, Rosso R, et al. (1989). Recombinant alpha-2a interferon plus vinblastine in the treatment of metastatic renal cell carcinoma. *American Journal of Clinical Oncology* 12(1):43-45.

Servaes P, Prins J, Verhagen S, Bleijenberg G. (2002). Fatigue after breast cancer and in chronic fatigue syndrome: Similarities and differences. *Journal of Psychosomatic Research* 52(6):453-459.

Servaes P, van der Werf S, Prins J, Verhagen S, Bleijenberg G. (2001). Fatigue in disease-free cancer patients compared with fatigue in patients with chronic fatigue syndrome. *Support Care Cancer* 9(1):11-17.

Servaes P, Verhagen CA, Bleijenberg G. (2002a). Fatigue in cancer patients during and after treatment: Prevalence, correlates and interventions. *European Journal of Cancer* 38(1):27-43.

Servaes P, Verhagen CA, Bleijenberg G. (2002b). Relations between fatigue, neuropsychological functioning, and physical activity after treatment for breast carcinoma: Daily self-report and objective behavior. *Cancer* 95(9):2017-2026.

Servaes P, Verhagen S, Bleijenberg G. (2002c). Determinants of chronic fatigue in disease-free breast cancer patients: A cross-sectional study. *Annals of Oncology* 13(4):589-598.

Servatius RJ, Tapp WN, Bergen MT, Pollet CA, Drastal SD, Tiersky LA, Desai P, Natelson BH. (1998). Impaired associative learning in chronic fatigue syndrome. *Neuroreport* 9(6):1153-1157.

Sessa C, Aamdal S, Wolff I, Eppelbaum R, Smyth JF, Sulkes A, Ten Bokkel Huinink W, Vermorken J, Wanders J, Franklin H, et al. (1994). Gemcitabine in patients with advanced malignant melanoma or gastric cancer: Phase II studies of the EORTC Early Clinical Trials Group. *Annals of Oncology* 5(5):471-472.

Sessa C, Cuvier C, Caldiera S, Bauer J, Van Den Bosch S, Monnerat C, Semiond D, Perard D, Lebecq A, Besenval M, Marty M. (2002). Phase I clinical and pharmacokinetic studies of the taxoid derivative RPR 109881A administered as a 1-hour or a 3-hour infusion in patients with advanced solid tumors. *Annals of Oncology* 13(7):1140-1150.

Sessa C, Zucchetti M, Ghielmini M, Bauer J, D'Incalci M, de Jong J, Naegele H, Rossi S, Pacciarini MA, Domenigoni L, et al. (1999). Phase I clinical and pharmacological study of oral methoxymorpholinyl doxorubicin (PNU 152243). *Cancer Chemotherapy Pharmacology* 44(5):403-410.

Sessa C, Zucchetti M, Ginier M, Willems Y, D'Incalci M, Cavalli F. (1988). Phase I study of the antifolate N10-propargyl-5,8-dideazafolic acid, CB 3717. *European Journal of Cancer and Clinical Oncology* 24(4):769-775.

Sexauer J, Kass L, Schnitzer B. (1974). Subacute myelomonocytic leukemia: Clinical, morphologic and ultrastructural studies of 10 cases. *American Journal of Medicine* 57(6):853-861.

Seymour LW, Ferry DR, Anderson D, Hesslewood S, Julyan PJ, Poyner R, Doran J, Young AM, Burtles S, Kerr DJ. (2002). Hepatic drug targeting: Phase I evaluation of polymer-bound doxorubicin. *Journal of Clinical Oncology* 20(6):1668-1676.

Seymour MT, Dent JT, Papamichael D, Wilson G, Cresswell H, Slevin ML. (1999). Epirubicin, cisplatin and oral UFT with leucovorin ("ECU"): A phase I-II study in patients with advanced upper gastrointestinal tract cancer. *Annals of Oncology* 10(11):1329-1333.

Shade RJ, Pisters KM, Huber MH, Fossella F, Perez-Soler R, Shin DM, Kurie J, Glisson B, Lippman S, Lee JS. (1998-1999). Phase I study of paclitaxel administered by ten-day continuous infusion. *Investigative New Drugs* 16(3):237-243.

Shaheen H, Ghanghroo I, Malik I. (1999). Clinicopathological features and management of Pakistani patients with multiple myeloma. *Journal of the Pakistani Medical Association* 49(10):233-237.

Shaheen SO, Aaby P, Hall AJ, Barker DJ, Heyes CB, Shiell AW, Goudiaby A. (1996). Measles and atopy in Guinea-Bissau. *Lancet* 347:1792-1796.

Shamaan NA, Kadir KA, Rahmat A, Ngah WZ. (1998). Vitamin C and *Aloë vera* supplementation protects from chemical hepatocarcinogenesis in the rat. *Nutrition* 14(11/12):846-852.

Shamdas GJ, Alberts DS, Modiano M, Wiggins C, Power J, Kasunic DA, Elfring GL, Earhart RH. (1994). Phase I study of adozelesin (U-73,975) in patients with solid tumors. *Anticancer Drugs* 5(1):10-14.

Shapiro CM. (1998). Fatigue: How many types and how common? *Journal of Psychosomatic Research* 45:1-3.

Shapiro JD, Harold N, Takimoto C, Hamilton JM, Vaughn D, Chen A, Steinberg SM, Liewehr D, Allegra C, Monahan B, et al. (1999). A pilot study of interferon alpha-2a, fluorouracil, and leucovorin given with granulocyte-macrophage colony stimulating factor in advanced gastrointestinal adenocarcinoma. *Clinical Cancer Research* 5(9):2399-2408.

Shapiro JD, Millward MJ, Rischin D, Michael M, Walcher V, Francis PA, Toner GC. (1996). Activity of gemcitabine in patients with advanced ovarian cancer: Responses seen following platinum and paclitaxel. *Gynecological Oncology* 63(1):89-93.

Shapiro JD, Rothenberg ML, Sarosy GA, Steinberg SM, Adamo DO, Reed E, Ozols RF, Kohn EC. (1998). Dose intensive combination platinum and cyclophosphamide in the treatment of patients with advanced untreated epithelial ovarian cancer. *Cancer* 83(9):1980-1988.

Sharma S, Kemeny N, Kelsen DP, Ilson D, O'Reilly E, Zaknoen S, Baum C, Statkevich P, Hollywood E, Zhu Y, et al. (2002). A phase II trial of farnesyl protein transferase inhibitor SCH 66336, given by twice-daily oral administration, in patients with metastatic colorectal cancer refractory to 5-fluorouracil and irinotecan. *Annals of Oncology* 13(7):1067-1071.

Sharp E. (1993). Case management of the hospitalized patient receiving interleukin-2. *Seminars in Oncology Nursing* 9(3 Suppl 1):14-19.

Sharpe M, Clements A, Hawton K, Young AH, Sargent P, Cowen PJ. (1996). Increased prolactin response to buspirone in chronic fatigue syndrome. *Journal of Affective Disorders* 41(1):71-76.

Sharpe M, Hawton K, Clements A, Cowen PJ. (1997). Increased brain serotonin function in men with chronic fatigue syndrome. *British Medical Journal* 315 (7101):164-165.

Sharpe M, Hawton K, Seagroatt V, Pasvol G. (1992). Follow up of patients presenting with fatigue to an infectious diseases clinic. *British Medical Journal* 305: 147-152.

Sharpe M, Hawton K, Simkin S, Surawy C, Hackmann A, Klimes I, Peto T, Warrell D, Seagroatt V. (1997). Cognitive behaviour therapy for the chronic fatigue syndrome: A randomised controlled trial. *British Medical Journal* 312(7022): 22-26.

Sharpe M, Wessely S. (1998). Putting the rest cure to rest—again: Rest has no place in treating chronic fatigue. *British Journal of Medicine* 316:796.

Sharpley A, Clements A, Hawton K, Sharpe M. (1997). Do patients with "pure" chronic fatigue syndrome (neurasthenia) have abnormal sleep? *Psychosomatic Medicine* 59(6):592-596.

Shasha D, Harrison LB. (2001). Anemia treatment and the radiation oncologist: Optimizing patient outcomes. *Oncology* 15(11):1486-1491; discussion 1494-1496.

Shaskan EG, Brew BJ, Rosenblum M, Thompson RM, Price RW. (1992). Increased neopterin levels in brains of patients with human immunodeficiency virus type 1 infection. *Journal of Neurochemistry* 59(4):1541-1546.

Shaver JL, Lentz M, Landis CA, Heitkemper MM, Buchwald DS, Woods NF. (1997). Sleep, psychological distress, and stress arousal in women with fibromyalgia. *Research in Nursing and Health* 20(3):247-257.

Sheean GL, Murray NM, Rothwell JC, Miller DH, Thompson AJ. (1997). An electrophysiological study of the mechanism of fatigue in multiple sclerosis. *Brain* 120(Pt 2):299-315.

Sheean GL, Murray NM, Rothwell JC, Miller DH, Thompson AJ. (1998). An open-labelled clinical and electrophysiological study of 3,4-diaminopyridine in the treatment of fatigue in multiple sclerosis. *Brain* 121(Pt 5):967-975.

Sheehan DC, Forman WB. (1997). Symptomatic management of the older person with cancer. *Clinical Geriatric Medicine* 13(1):203-219.

Shefer A, Dobbins JG, Fukuda K, Steele L, Koo D, Nisembaum R, Rutherford GW. (1997). Fatiguing illness among employees in three large state office buildings, California, 1933: Was there an outbreak? *Journal of Psychiatric Research* 31(1):31-43.

Shelkovnikov IA, Krivoruchko BI. (1997). [Pathogenesis of fibromyalgia] Patogenez fibromyalgii. *Patol Fiziol Eksp Ter* (1):41-42.

Shen J, Glaspy J. (2001). Acupuncture: Evidence and implications for cancer supportive care. *Cancer Practice* 9(3):147-150.

Shephard RJ. (1986). Exercise and malignancy. *Sports Medicine* 3:235-241.

Shephard RJ. (1990). Physical activity and cancer. *International Journal of Sports Medicine* 11:413-420.

Shephard RJ (1992). Does exercise reduce all-cancer death rates? *British Journal of Sports Medicine* 23:11-22.

Shephard RJ. (1993). Exercise in the prevention and treatment of cancer. *Sports Medicine* 15:258-280.

Shephard RJ. (1995). Exercise and cancer: Linkages with obesity? *International Journal of Obesity* 19(Suppl 4):S63-S68.

Shephard RJ. (1996). Exercise and cancer: Linkages with obesity? *Critical Reviews of Food Science and Nutrition* 36:321-339.

Shephard RJ, Bouchard C. (1996). Associations between health behaviours and health-related fitness. *British Journal of Sports Medicine* 30:94-101.

Shephard RJ, Futcher R. (1997). Physical activity and cancer: How may protection be maximized? *Critical Reviews in Oncogenesis* 8(2&3):219-272.

Shephard RJ, Shek PN. (1995). Cancer, immune function and physical activity. *Canadian Journal of Applied Physiology* 20:1-25.

Shephard RJ, Shek PN. (1996a). Physical activity and immune changes: A potential model of subclinical inflammation and sepsis. *Critical Reviews of Physical Rehabilitation Medicine* 8:153-181.

Shephard RJ, Shek PN. (1996b). The risk of cancer in the international athlete. *Acta Academia Olympica Estoniae* 5:5-24.

Shepherd C, MacIntyre A. (1997). Graded exercise in chronic fatigue syndrome: Patients should have an initial period of rest before gradual increase in activity. *British Medical Journal* 315(7113):947-948.

Shepherd M, Cooper B, Brown AC, Kalton G. (1981). *Psychiatric Illness in General Practice,* Second Edition. Oxford: Oxford University Press.

Sherman ML, Spriggs DR, Arthur KA, Imamura K, Frei E III, Kufe DW. (1988). Recombinant human tumor necrosis factor administered as a five-day continuous infusion in cancer patients: Phase I toxicity and effects on lipid metabolism. *Journal of Clinical Oncology* 6(2):344-350.

Sherry BA, Gelin J, Fong Y. (1991). Anticachectin/tumor necrosis factor alpha antibodies attenuate development of cancer cachexia. *Cancer Research* 51:415-421.

Sherry DD. (1997). Musculoskeletal pain in children. *Curent Opinions in Rheumatology* 9(5):465-470.

Sherwin SA, Foon KA, Abrams PG, Heyman MR, Ochs JJ, Watson T, Maluish A, Oldham RK. (1984). A preliminary phase I trial of partially purified interferon-gamma in patients with cancer. *Journal of Biological Response Modifiers* 3(6): 599-607.

Sherwin SA, Knost JA, Fein S, Abrams PG, Foon KA, Ochs JJ, Schoenberger C, Maluish AE, Oldham RK. (1982). A multiple-dose phase I trial of recombinant leukocyte A interferon in cancer patients. *JAMA* 248(19):2461-2466.

Sherwin SA, Mayer D, Ochs JJ, Abrams PG, Knost JA, Foon KA, Fein S, Oldham RK. (1983). Recombinant leukocyte A interferon in advanced breast cancer: Results of a phase II efficacy trial. *Annals of Internal Medicine* 98(5 Pt 1):598-602.

Shimizu E, Saijo N, Eguchi K, Shinkai T, Tominaga K, Sasaki Y, Fujita J, Nomori H, Hoshi A. (1984). Phase II study of oral administration of 5'-deoxy-5-fluorouridine (5'-DFUR) for solid tumors. *Japanese Journal of Clinical Oncology* 14(4):679-683.

Shimooki O, Ishida K, Satoh N, Sugimura Y, Saitoh K, Uesugi N. (1995). [A case of so-called carcinosarcoma of the esophagus]. *Nippon Kyobu Geka Gakkai Zasshi* 43(12):1942-1947.

Shimoyama M, Tobinai K, Yamaguchi K, Hirashima K, Itoh S, Konishi H, Mikuni C, Togawa A, Hotta T, Toyoda N, et al. (1992). Treatment of hairy cell leukemia with deoxycoformycin (YK-176). The Deoxycoformycin (YK-176) Study Group. *Japanese Journal of Clinial Oncology* 22(6):406-410.

Shimozuma K, Ganz PA, Petersen L, Hirji K. (1999). Quality of life in the first year after breast cancer surgery: Rehabilitation needs and patterns of recovery. *Breast Cancer Research and Treatment* 56(1):45-57.

Shin DM, Glisson BS, Khuri FR, Clifford JL, Clayman G, Benner SE, Forastiere AA, Ginsberg L, Liu D, Lee JJ, et al. (2002). Phase II and biologic study of interferon alfa, retinoic acid, and cisplatin in advanced squamous skin cancer. *Journal of Clinical Oncology* 20(2):364-370.

Shin DM, Glisson BS, Khuri FR, Hong WK, Lippman SM. (1998). Role of paclitaxel, ifosfamide, and cisplatin in patients with recurrent or metastatic squamous cell carcinoma of the head and neck. *Seminars in Oncology* 25(2 Suppl 4):40-44; discussion 45-48.

Shin DM, Glisson BS, Khuri FR, Lippman SM, Ginsberg L, Diaz E, Papadimitrakopoulou V, Feng L, Francisco M, Garden A, et al. (2002). Phase II study of induction chemotherapy with paclitaxel, ifosfamide, and carboplatin (TIC) for patients with locally advanced squamous cell carcinoma of the head and neck. *Cancer* 95(2):322-330.

Shin DM, Khuri FR, Glisson BS, Ginsberg L, Papadimitrakopoulou VM, Clayman G, Lee JJ, Ang KK, Lippman SM, Hong WK. (2001). Phase II study of paclitaxel, ifosfamide, and carboplatin in patients with recurrent or metastatic head and neck squamous cell carcinoma. *Cancer* 91(7):1316-1323.

Shin DM, Khuri FR, Murphy B, Garden AS, Clayman G, Francisco M, Liu D, Glisson BS, Ginsberg L, Papadimitrakopoulou V, et al. (2001). Combined interferon-alfa, 13-cis-retinoic acid, and alpha-tocopherol in locally advanced head and neck squamous cell carcinoma: Novel bioadjuvant phase II trial. *Journal of Clinical Oncology* 19(12):3010-3017.

Shin E, Ishitobi M, Hiraoia M, Kazumasa F, Hideyuki M, Nishisho I, Toshiro S, Yasunori H, Tosimasa T. (2000). Phase I study of docetaxel administered by biweekly infusion to patients with metastatic breast cancer. *Anticancer Research* 20(6C):4721-4726.

Shinoda J, Sakai N, Hara A, Ueda T, Sakai H, Nakatani K. (1997). Clinical trial of external beam-radiotherapy combined with daily administration of low-dose cisplatin for supratentorial glioblastoma multiforme—A pilot study. *Journal of Neurooncology* 35(1):73-80.

Shoham S, Davenee D, Cady AB, Dinarello CA, Krueger JM. (1987). Recombinant tumor necrosis factor and interleukin-1 enhance slow-wave sleep. *American Journal of Physiology* 253:R142-R149.

Shojania K. (2000). Rheumatology: 2. What laboratory tests are needed? *Canadian Medical Association Journal* 162(8):1157-1163.

Sibbald B. (1998). Chronic fatigue syndrome comes out of the closet. *Canadian Medical Association Journal* 159(5):537-541.

Sibbald B. (1999). New federal office will spend millions to regulate herbal remedies, vitamins. *Canadian Medical Association Journal* 160(9):1355-1357.

Sieb JB, Dorfler P, Tolksdorf K, Jakschik J. (1997). Endplate ultrastructure in a case of primary fibromyalgia. *Clinical Rheumatology* 16(6):637-638.

Siegel DM, Janeway D, Baum J. (1998). Fibromyalgia syndrome in childen and adolescents: Clinical features at presentation and status at follow-up. *Pediatrics* 101(3 Pt 1):377-382.

Siegmeth W. (1999). [Panalgesia and the fibromyalgia concept] Panalgesie und das fibromyalgiekonzept. *Wien Medizin Wochenschrift* 149(19-20):558-560.

Sigurdardottir V, Bolund C, Brandberg Y, Sullivan M. (1993). The impact of generalized malignant melanoma on quality of life evaluated by the EORTC questionnaire technique. *Quality of Life Research* 2(3):193-203.

Sigurdsson B, Gudmundsson KR. (1956). Clinical findings six years after outbreak of Akureyri disease. *Lancet* 1:766.

Silberfarb PM, Holland JC, Anbar D, Bahna G, Maurer LH, Chahinian AP, Comis R. (1983). Psychological response of patients receiving two drug regimens for lung carcinoma. *American Journal of Psychiatry* 140(1):110-111.

Silgals RM, Ahlgren JD, Neefe JR, Rothman J, Rudnick S, Galicky FP, Schein PS. (1984). A phase II trial of high-dose intravenous interferon alpha-2 in advanced colorectal cancer. *Cancer* 54(10):2257-2261.

Silver HK, Connors JM, Salinas FA. (1985). Prospectively randomized toxicity study of high-dose versus low-dose treatment strategies for lymphoblastoid interferon. *Cancer Treatment Reports* 69(7-8):743-750.

Silver RT, Benn P, Verma RS, Coleman M, Soper L, Gutfriend A. (1990). Recombinant gamma-interferon has activity in chronic myeloid leukemia. *American Journal of Clinical Oncology* 13(1):49-54.

Silverman S, Gluck O, Silver D, Tesser J, Wallace D, Neumann K, Metzger A, Morris R. (1996). The prevalence of autoantibodies in symptomatic and asymptomatic patients with breast implants and patients with fibromyalgia. *Current Topics in Microbiology and Immunology* 210:277-282.

Silvestris F, Williams RC, Dammacco F. (1995). Autoreactivity in HIV-1 infection: The role of molecular mimicry. *Clinical Immunology and Immunopathology* 75:197-205.

Simmons SJ, Tjoa BA, Rogers M, Elgamal A, Kenny GM, Ragde H, Troychak MJ, Boynton AL, Murphy GP. (1999). GM-CSF as a systemic adjuvant in a phase II prostate cancer vaccine trial. *Prostate* 39(4):291-297.

Simms RW. (1996). Fibromyalgia syndrome: Current concepts in pathophysiology, clinical fetaures, and management. *Arthritis Care Research* 9(4):315-328.

Simms RW. (1998). Fibromyalgia is not a muscle disorder. *American Journal of Medical Sciences* 315(6):346-350.

Simon AM, Zittoun R. (1999). Fatigue in cancer patients. *Current Opinions in Oncology* 11(4):244-249.

Simonson N. (1996). [Can tamoxifen relieve fibromyalgia?] Kan tamoxifen lindra fibromyalgi? *Lakartidningen* 93(5):340.

Simopoulos AP. (1990). Energy imbalance and cancer of the breast, colon and prostate. *Medical Oncology and Tumor Pharmacotherapy* 7:109-120.

Simpson M. (1997). A body with chronic fatigue syndrome as a battleground for the fight to separate from the mother. *Journal of Analytical Psychology* 42(2):201-216.

Simpson M, Bennett A, Holland P. (1997). Chronic fatigue syndrome/myalgic encephalomyelitis as a twentieth-century disease: Analytic challenges. *Journal of Analytical Psychology* 42(2):191-199.

Singer S, Schwarz R. (2002). [Psychosocial aftercare of patients with endometrial or cervical cancer]. *Zentralblatt Gynakologie* 124(1):64-70.

Singh BB, Berman BM, Hadhazy VA, Creamer P. (1998). A pilot study of cognitive behavioral therapy in fibromyalgia. *Alternative Therapy, Health and Medicine* 4(2):67-70.

Singhal S, Mehta J. (2001). Thalidomide in cancer: Potential uses and limitations. *BioDrugs* 15(3):163-172.

Singhal S, Mehta J. (2002). Thalidomide in cancer. *Biomedical Pharmacotherapy* 56(1):4-12.

Singhal S, Mehta J, Desikan R, Ayers D, Roberson P, Eddlemon P, Munshi N, Anaissie E, Wilson C, Dhodapkar M, Zeddis J, Barlogie B. (1999). Antitumor activity of thalidomide in refractory multiple myeloma. *New England Journal of Medicine* 341(21):1565-1571.

Sinibaldi VJ, Carducci MA, Laufer M, Eisenberger M. (1999). Preliminary evaluation of a short course of estramustine phosphate and docetaxel (Taxotere) in the treatment of hormone-refractory prostate cancer. *Seminars in Oncology* 26 (5 Suppl 17):45-48.

Sinibaldi VJ, Carducci MA, Moore-Cooper S, Laufer M, Zahurak M, Eisenberger MA. (2002). Phase II evaluation of docetaxel plus one-day oral estramustine phosphate in the treatment of patients with androgen independent prostate carcinoma. *Cancer* 94(5):1457-1465.

Sinkovics JG. (1991). Kaposi's sarcoma: Its "oncogenes" and growth factors. *Critical Reviews in Oncology and Hematology* 11(2):87-107.

Sinnige HA, Buter J, de Vries EG, Uges DR, Roenhorst HW, Verschueren RC, Sleijfer DT, Willemse PH, Mulder NH. (1993). Phase I-II study of the addition of alpha-2a interferon to 5-fluorouracil/leucovorin: Pharmacokinetic interaction of alpha-2a interferon and leucovorin. *European Journal of Cancer* 29A(12): 1715-1720.

Sisto SA, LaManca JJ, Cordero DL, Bergen MT, Ellis SP, Drastal S, Boda WL, Tapp WN, Natelson BH. (1996). Metabolic and cardiovascular effects of a progressive exercise test in patients with chronic fatigue syndrome. *American Journal of Medicine* 100(6):634-640.

Sisto SA, Tapp WN, LaManca JJ, Ling W, Korn LR, Nelson AJ, Natelson BH. (1998). Physical activity before and after exercise in women with chronic fatigue syndrome. *Quarterly Journal of Medicine* 91(7):465-473.

Sitzia J, Huggins L. (1998). Side effects of cyclophosphamide, methotrexate, and 5-fluorouracil (CMF) chemotherapy for breast cancer. *Cancer Practice* 6(1): 13-21.

Sitzia J, Hughes J, Sobrido L. (1995). A study of patients' experiences of side-effects associated with chemotherapy: Pilot stage report. *International Journal of Nursing Studies* 32(6):580-600.

Sitzia J, North C, Stanley J, Winterberg N. (1997). Side effects of CHOP in the treatment of non-Hodgkin's lymphoma. *Cancer Nursing* 20(6):430-439.

Siu LL, Rowinsky EK, Hammond LA, Weiss GR, Hidalgo M, Clark GM, Moczygemba J, Choi L, Linnartz R, Barbet NC, et al. (2002). A phase I and pharmacokinetic study of SAM486A, a novel polyamine biosynthesis inhibitor, administered on a daily-times-five every-three-week schedule in patients with advanced solid malignancies. *Clinical Cancer Research* 8(7):2157-2166.

Sivula A, Ronni-Sivula H. (1984). The changing picture of primary hyperparathyroidism in the years 1956-1979. *Annales de Chirurgie Gynaecologie* 73(6): 319-324.

Sjostrom J, Blomqvist C, Mouridsen H, Pluzanska A, Ottosson-Lonn S, Bengtsson NO, Ostenstad B, Mjaaland I, Palm-Sjovall M, Wist E, et al. (1999). Docetaxel compared with sequential methotrexate and 5-fluorouracil in patients with advanced breast cancer after anthracycline failure: A randomised phase III study with crossover on progression by the Scandinavian Breast Group. *European Journal of Cancer* 35(8):1194-1201.

Skalla KA, Lacasse C. (1992). Patient education for fatigue. *Oncology Nursing Forum* 19(10):1537-1541.

Skillings J, Wierzbicki R, Eisenhauer E, Venner P, Letendre F, Stewart D, Weinerman B. (1992). A phase II study of recombinant tumor necrosis factor in renal cell carcinoma: A study of the National Cancer Institute of Canada Clinical Trials Group. *Journal of Immunotherapy* 11(1):67-70.

Sklar LS, Anisman H. (1981). Stress and cancer. *Psychological Bulletin* 89:369-406.

Sklarin NT, Lathia CD, Benson L, Grove WR, Thomas S, Roca J, Einzig AI, Wiernik PH. (1997). A phase I trial and pharmacokinetic evaluation of CI-980 in patients with advanced solid tumors. *Investigative New Drugs* 15(3):235-246.

Slabber CF, Falkson G, Burger W, Schoeman L. (1996). 13-cis-retinoic acid and interferon alpha-2a in patients with advanced esophageal cancer: A phase II trial. *Investigative New Drugs* 14(4):391-394.

Slavkin HC. (1997). Chronic disabling diseases and disorders: The challenges of fibromyalgia. *Journal of the American Dental Association* 128(11):1583-1589.

Small EJ, Figlin R, Petrylak D, Vaughn DJ, Sartor O, Horak I, Pincus R, Kremer A, Bowden C. (2000). A phase II pilot study of KW-2189 in patients with advanced renal cell carcinoma. *Investigative New Drugs* 18(2):193-197.

Smalley RV, Anderson SA, Tuttle RL, Connors J, Thurmond LM, Huang A, Castle K, Magers C, Whisnant JK. (1991). A randomized comparison of two doses of human lymphoblastoid interferon-alpha in hairy cell leukemia. Wellcome HCL Study Group. *Blood* 78(12):3133-3141.

Smeitink J, Verreussel M, Schröder C, Lippens R. (1988). Nephrotoxicity associated with ifosfamide. *European Journal of Pediatrics* 148:164-166.

Smetana Z, Leventon-Kriss S, Broide A, Jedwab M, Smetana SS. (1991). Varicella-zoster virus immune status in CAPD and chronic hemodialysis patients. *American Journal of Nephrology* 11:229-236.

Smets EMA, Garssen B, Bonke B, De Haes JCJM. (1995). The multidimensional fatigue inventory (MFI): Psychometric qualities of an instrument to assess fatigue. *Journal of Psychosomatic Research* 39:315-325.

Smets EMA, Garssen B, Cull A, De Haes JC. (1996). Application of the multidimensional fatigue inventory (MFI-20) in cancer patients receiving radiotherapy. *British Journal of Cancer* 73(2):241-245.

Smets EMA, Garssen B, Schuster-Uitterhoeve AL, de Haes JC. (1993). Fatigue in cancer patients. *British Journal of Cancer* 68(2):220-224.

Smets EMA, Visser MR, Garssen B, Frijda NH, Oosterveld P, De Haas JC. (1998). Understanding the level of fatigue in cancer patients undergoing radiotherapy. *Journal of Psychosomatic Research* 45(3):277-293.

Smets EMA, Visser MR, Willems-Groot AF, Garssen B, Oldenburger F, Van Tienhoven G, De Haes JC. (1998). Fatigue and radiotherapy: (A) Experience in patients undergoing treatment. *British Journal of Cancer* 78(7):899-906.

Smets EMA, Visser MR, Willems-Groot AF, Garssen B, Schuster-Uitterhoeve AL, de Haes JC. (1998). Fatigue and radiotherapy: (B) Experience in patients nine months following treatment. *British Journal of Cancer* 78(7):907-912.

Smit AA, Bolweg NM, Lenders JW, Wieling W. (1998). No strong evidence of disturbed regulation of blood pressure in chronic fatigue syndrome. *Nederlands Tijdschrift voor Geneeskunde* 142(12):625-658.

Smit JA, Stark JH, Myburgh JA. (1996). Induction of primate TH2 lymphokines to supress TH1 cells. *Transplantation Proceedings* 28(2):665-666.

Smith DR, Kunkel SL, Burdick MD, Wilke CA, Orringer MB, Whyte RI, Strieter RM. (1994). Production of interleukin-10 by human bronchogenic carcinoma. *American Journal of Pathology* 145:18-25.

Smith EM, Anderson B. (1985). The effects of symptoms and delay in seeking diagnosis on stage of disease at diagnosis among women with cancers of the ovary. *Cancer* 56(11):2727-2732.

Smith IE, O'Brien ME, Talbot DC, Nicolson MC, Mansi JL, Hickish TF, Norton A, Ashley S. (2001). Duration of chemotherapy in advanced non-small-cell lung cancer: A randomized trial of three versus six courses of mitomycin, vinblastine, and cisplatin. *Journal of Clinical Oncology* 19(5):1336-1343.

Smith JW II, Urba WJ, Clark JW, Longo DL, Farrell M, Creekmore SP, Conlon KC, Jaffe H, Steis RG. (1991). Phase I evaluation of recombinant tumor necrosis factor given in combination with recombinant interferon-gamma. *Journal of Immunotherapy* 10(5):355-362.

Smith KA. (1990a). Cytokines in the nineties. *European Cytokine Network* 1(1): 7-13.

Smith KA. (1990b). Interleukin-2. *Scientific American* 263(3):50-57.

Smith MD. (1998). The fibromyalgia problem. *Journal of Rheumatology* 25(5): 1027; discussion 1028-1030.

Smith MR, Kaufman D, Oh W, Guerin K, Seiden M, Makatsoris T, Manola J, Kantoff PW. (2000). Vinorelbine and estramustine in androgen-independent metastatic prostate cancer: A phase II study. *Cancer* 89(8):1824-1828.

Smith RE, Lew D, Rodriguez GI, Taylor SA, Schuller D, Ensley JF. (1996). Evaluation of topotecan in patients with recurrent metastatic squamous cell carcinoma of the head and neck: A phase II Southwest Oncology Group study. *Investigative New Drugs* 14(4):403-407.

Smith RE Jr, Jaiyesimi IA, Meza LA, Tchekmedyian NS, Chan D, Griffith H, Brosman S, Bukowski R, Murdoch M, Rarick M, et al. (2001). Novel erythropoiesis stimulating protein (NESP) for the treatment of anaemia of chronic disease associated with cancer. *British Journal of Cancer* 84(Suppl 1):24-30.

Smith SR, Boyd EL, Kirking DM. (1999). Nonprescription and alternative medication use by individuals with HIV disease. *Annals of Pharmacotherapy* 33(3): 294-300.

Smith WA. (1998). Fibromyalgia syndrome. *Nursing Clinics of North America* 33(4):653-669.

Smythe HA. (1995). Studies of sleep in fibromyalgia: Techniques, clinical significance, and future directions. *British Journal of Rheumatology* 34(10):897-899.

Smythe HA, Moldofsky H. (1977). Two contributions to understanding "fibrositis" syndrome. *Bulletin of Rheumatic Diseases* 28:928-931.

Sneeuw KC, Aaronson NK, Osoba D, Muller MJ, Hsu MA, Yung WK, Brada M, Newlands ES. (1997). The use of significant others as proxy raters of the quality of life of patients with brain cancer. *Medical Care* 35(5):490-506.

Snyder AC. (1998). Overtraining and glycogen depletion hypothesis. *Medicine and Science in Sports and Exercise* 30(7):1146-1150.

Snyderman R, Cianciolo GJ. (1984). Immunosuppressive activity of the retroviral envelope protein p15E and its possible relationship to neoplasia. *Immunology Today* 5:240-244.

Sobel RA, Hafler DA, Castro EE, Morimoto C, Weiner HL. (1988). The 2H4 (CD45R) antigen is selectively decreased in multiple sclerosis lesions. *Journal of Immunology* 140:2210-2214.

Sobol RE, Shawler DL, Carson C, Van Beveren C, Mercola D, Fakhrai H, Garrett MA, Barone R, Goldfarb P, Bartholomew RM, et al. (1999). Interleukin 2 gene therapy of colorectal carcinoma with autologous irradiated tumor cells and genetically engineered fibroblasts: A phase I study. *Clinical Cancer Research* 5(9): 2359-2365.

Sobrero A, Puglisi F, Guglielmi A, Belvedere O, Aprile G, Ramello M, Grossi F. (2001). Fatigue: A main component of anemia symptomatology. *Seminars in Oncology* 28(2 Suppl 8):15-18.

Soderberg S, Lundman B, Norberg A. (1997). Living with fibromyalgia: Sense of coherence, perception of well-being, and stress in daily life. *Research on Nursing and Health* 20(6):495-503.

Sodroski J, Patarca R, Perkins D, Briggs D, Lee T, Essex M, Colligan J, Wong-Staal F, Gallo RC, Haseltine WA. (1984). Sequence of the envelope glycoprotein gene of type II human T-lymphotropic virus. *Science* 225:421-423.

Sodroski J, Patarca R, Rosen C, Wong-Staal F, Haseltine WA. (1985). Location of the *trans*-activating region on the genome of human T-cell lymphotropic virus type III. *Science* 229:74-77.

Sodroski J, Trus M, Perkins D, Patarca R, Wong-Staal F, Gelman E, Gallo RC, Haseltine WA. (1984). Repetitive structure in the long terminal repeat element of a type II human T-cell leukemia virus. *Proceedings of the National Academy of Sciences of the United States of America* 81:4617-4621.

Solal-Celigny P, Lepage E, Brousse N, Reyes F, Haioun C, Leporrier M, Peuchmaur M, Bosly A, Parlier Y, Brice P, et al. (1993). Recombinant interferon alfa-2b combined with a regimen containing doxorubicin in patients with advanced follicular lymphoma. Groupe d'Etude des Lymphomes de l'Adulte. *New England Journal of Medicine* 329(22):1608-1614.

Solomon DH, Liang MH. (1997). Fibromyalgia: Scourge of humankind or bane of a rheumatologist's existence? *Arthritis and Rheumatism* 40(9):1553-1555.

Solomon G. (1994). A clinical and laboratory profile of symptomatic women with silicone breast implants. *Seminars in Arthritis and Rheumatism* 24(1 Suppl 1): 29-37.

Solomon GF. (1995). Psychoneuroimmunology and chronic fatigue syndrome: Toward new models of disease. *Journal of Chronic Fatigue Syndrome* 1(1):3-7.

Solomon V, Leckert SH, Goldberg AL. (1998). The N-end rule pathway catalyzes a major fraction of the protein degradation in skeletal muscle. *Journal of Biological Chemistry* 273:25216-25222.

Solves P, de la Rubia J, Jarque I, Cervera J, Sanz GF, Vera-Sempere FJ, Sanz MA. (1999). Liver disease as primary manifestation of multiple myeloma in a young man. *Leukemia Research* 23(4):403-405.

Sommer H, Prohl-Steimer B, Bajetta E, Haus U, Janni W, Kay A. (2001). [A randomized, double-blind, placebo-controlled, phase 3 trial comparing SMS 201-995 pa LAR plus tamoxifen versus tamoxifen plus placebo in women with locally recurrent or metastatic breast cancer]. *Zentralblatt Gynakologie* 123(10): 557-561.

Sondel PM, Kohler PC, Hank JA, Moore KH, Rosenthal NS, Sosman JA, Bechhofer R, Storer B. (1988). Clinical and immunological effects of recombinant interleukin 2 given by repetitive weekly cycles to patients with cancer. *Cancer Research* 48(9):2561-2567.

Sone A, Furukawa Y, Nakatsuka S, Tanaka H. (1989). [Primary choriocarcinoma of the bladder: A case report of autopsy]. *Nippon Hinyokika Gakkai Zasshi* 80(6): 902-906.

Song Z, Kharazmi A, Wu H, Faber V, Moser C, Krogh HK, Rygaard J, Hoiby N. (1998). Effects of ginseng treatment on neutrophil chemiluminescence and immunoglobulin G subclasses in a rat model of chronic *Pseudomonas aeruginosa* pneumonia. *Clinical Diagnostics and Laboratory Immunology* 5(6):882-887.

Soni N, Meropol NJ, Pendyala L, Noel D, Schacter LP, Gunton KE, Creaven PJ. (1997). Phase I and pharmacokinetic study of etoposide phosphate by protracted venous infusion in patients with advanced cancer. *Journal of Clinical Oncology* 15(2):766-772.

Sonnerborg A, Saaf J, Alexius B, Strannegard O, Wahlund LO, Wetterberg L. (1990). Quantitative detection of brain aberrations in human immunodeficiency virus type-1-infected individuals by magnetic resonance imaging. *Journal of Infectious Diseases* 162(6):1245-1251.

Soori GS, Dillman RO, Wiemann MC, Stark JJ, Tai F, DePriest CB, Church CK, Schulof R. (2002). Phase II trial of subcutaneous interleukin-2, subcutaneous interferon-alpha, 5-fluorouracil and cis-retinoic acid in the treatment of renal cell carcinoma: Final results of Cancer Biotherapy Research Group 94-10. *Cancer Biotherapy and Radiopharmacology* 17(2):165-173.

Soori GS, Oldham RK, Dobbs TW, Bury MJ, Church CK, DePriest C. (2000). Chemo-biotherapy with 5-fluorouracil, leucovorin, and alpha interferon in metastatic carcinoma of the colon—A Cancer Biotherapy Research Group [CBRG] phase II study. *Cancer Biotherapy and Radiopharmacology* 15(2):175-183.

Soori GS, Schulof RS, Stark JJ, Wiemann MC, Honeycutt PJ, Church CK, DePriest CB. (1999). Continuous-infusion floxuridine and alpha interferon in metastatic renal cancer: A national Biotherapy Study Group phase II study. *Cancer Investigation* 17(6):379-384.

Sorbe B, Hogberg T, Himmelmann A, Schmidt M, Raisanen I, Stockmeyer M, de Bruijn KM. (1994). Efficacy and tolerability of tropisetron in comparison with a combination of tropisetron and dexamethasone in the control of nausea and vomiting induced by cisplatin-containing chemotherapy. *European Journal of Cancer* 30A(5):629-634.

Sordillo PP, Magill GB, Welt S. (1985). Phase II trial of methylglyoxal-bis-guanylhydrazone (methyl-GAG) in patients with soft-tissue sarcomas. *American Journal of Clinical Oncology* 8(4):316-318.

Sorenson WG. (1999). Fungal spores: Hazardous to health? *Environmental Health Perspectives* 107(Suppl 3):469-472.

Sosman JA, Aronson FR, Sznol M, Atkins MB, Dutcher JP, Weiss GR, Isaacs RE, Margolin KA, Fisher RI, Ernest ML, et al. (1997). Concurrent phase I trials of intravenous interleukin 6 in solid tumor patients: Reversible dose-limiting neurological toxicity. *Clinical Cancer Research* 3(1):39-46.

Soucy MD. (1997). Fatigue and depression: Assessment in human immunodeficiency virus disease. *Nurse Practitioner Forum* 8(3):121-125.

Sparano JA, Robert N, Silverman P, Lazarus H, Malik U, Venkatraj U, Sarta C. (1996). Phase I trial of high-dose mitoxantrone plus cyclophosphamide and filgrastim in patients with advanced breast carcinoma. *Journal of Clinical Oncology* 14(9):2576-2583.

Sparano JA, Wadler S, Diasio RB, Zhang R, Lu Z, Schwartz EL, Einzig A, Wiernik PH. (1993). Phase I trial of low-dose, prolonged continuous infusion fluorouracil plus interferon-alfa: Evidence for enhanced fluorouracil toxicity without pharmacokinetic perturbation. *Journal of Clinical Oncology* 11(8):1609-1617.

Spiegel D, Bloom JR. (1983). Group therapy and hypnosis reduce metastatic breast carcinoma pain. *Psychosomatic Medicine* 45(4):333-339.

Spiegel D, Sands S, Koopman C. (1994). Pain and depression in patients with cancer. *Cancer* 74(9):2570-2578.

Spivak JL. (2000). The blood in systemic disorders. *Lancet* 355:1707-1712.

Sprangers MA, Van Dam FS, Broersen J, Lodder L, Wever L, Visser MR, Oosterveld P, Smets EM. (1999). Revealing response shift in longitudinal research on fatigue—The use of the thentest approach. *Acta Oncologica* 38(6):709-718.

Spriggs DR, Sherman ML, Michie H, Arthur KA, Imamura K, Wilmore D, Frei E III, Kufe DW. (1988). Recombinant human tumor necrosis factor administered as a 24-hour intravenous infusion: A phase I and pharmacologic study. *Journal of the National Cancer Institutes* 80(13):1039-1044.

Spronk PE, Ter Borg EJ, Limburg PC, Kallenberg CGM. (1992). Plasma concentration of IL-6 in systemic lupus erythematosus: An indicator of disease activity? *Clinical and Experimental Immunology* 90:106-160.

Sprott H, Franke S, Kluge H, Hein G. (1998). Pain treatment of fibromyalgia by acupuncture. *Rheumatology International* 18(1):35-36.

Sriskandan K, Garner P, Watkinson J, Pettingale KW, Brinkley D, Calman FM, Tee DE. (1986). A toxicity study of recombinant interferon-gamma given by intravenous infusion to patients with advanced cancer. *Cancer Chemotherapy Pharmacology* 18(1):63-68.

Stacey D. (1998). Coping with fatigue: An education session for cancer patients. *Canadian Oncology Nursing Journal* 8(S1):S15.

Stadler WM, Kuzel T, Dumas M, Vogelzang NJ. (1998). Multicenter phase II trial of interleukin-2, interferon-alpha, and 13-cis-retinoic acid in patients with metastatic renal-cell carcinoma. *Journal of Clinical Oncology* 16(5):1820-1825.

Stadler WM, Kuzel T, Shapiro C, Sosman J, Clark J, Vogelzang NJ. (1999). Multi-institutional study of the angiogenesis inhibitor TNP-470 in metastatic renal carcinoma. *Journal of Clinical Oncology* 17(8):2541-2545.

Stadler WM, Rybak ME, Vogelzang NJ. (1995). A phase II study of subcutaneous recombinant human interleukin-4 in metastatic renal cell carcinoma. *Cancer* 76(9):1629-1633.

Staedt J, Windt H, Hajaki G, Stoppe G, Rudolph G, Ensink FBM. (1993). Cluster arousal analysis in chronic pain-disturbed sleep. *Journal of Sleep Research* 2:134-137.

Stancu M, Jones D, Vega F, Medeiros LJ. (2002). Peripheral T-cell lymphoma arising in the liver. *American Journal of Clinical Pathology* 118(4):574-581.

Stanley-Brown EG, Dargeon HW. (1966). Presenting symptoms of neuroblastomas and Wilms' tumors. *Clinical Pediatrics* 5(11):681-682.

Stanton AL, Snider PR. (1993). Coping with a breast cancer diagnosis: A prospective study. *Health and Psychology* 12(1):16-23.

Stanton T. (1999). Coping with stress on the job. *Nursing in New Zealand* 4(11): 17-18.

Stea B, Halpern RM, Smith RA. (1981). Urinary excretion levels of unconjugated pterins in cancer patients and normal individuals. *Clinica Chimica Acta* 113: 231-242.

Steginga SK, Dunn J. (1997). Women's experiences following treatment for gynecologic cancer. *Oncology Nursing Forum* 24(8):1403-1408.

Stein KD, Jacobsen PB, Hann DM, Greenberg H, Lyman G. (2000). Impact of hot flashes on quality of life among postmenopausal women being treated for breast cancer. *Journal of Pain Symptomatology and Management* 19(6):436-445.

Stein KD, Martin SC, Hann DM, Jacobsen PB. (1998). A multidimensional measure of fatigue for use with cancer patients. *Cancer Practice* 6(3):143-152.

Stein MT, First LR, Friedman SB. (1998). Twelve-year-old girl with chronic fatigue, school absence, and fluctuating somatic symptoms. *Journal of Developmental and Behavioral Pediatrics* 19(3):196-201.

Stein MT, First LR, Friedman SB. (2001). Twelve-year-old girl with chronic fatigue, school absence, and fluctuating somatic symptoms. *Journal of Developmental and Behavioral Pediatrics* 22(2 Suppl):S151-S156.

Steinberg P, McNutt BE, Marshall P, Schenck C, Lurie N, Pheley A, Peterson PK. (1996). Double-blind placebo-controlled study of the efficacy of oral terfenadine in the treatment of chronic fatigue syndrome. *Journal of Allergy and Clinical Immunology* 97(1 Pt 1):119-126.

Steinberg P, Pheley A, Peterson PK. (1996). Influence of immediate hypersensitivity skin reaction on delayed reactions in patients with chronic fatigue syndrome. *Journal of Allergy and Clinical Immunology* 98(6 Pt. 1):1126-1128.

Steiner A, Wolf C, Pehamberger H. (1987). Comparison of the effects of three different treatment regimens of recombinant interferons (r-IFN alpha, r-IFN gamma, and r-IFN alpha + cimetidine) in disseminated malignant melanoma. *Journal of Cancer Research and Clinical Oncology* 113(5):459-465.

Steins MB, Padro T, Bieker R, Ruiz S, Kropff M, Kienast J, Kessler T, Buechner T, Berdel WE, Mesters RM. (2002). Efficacy and safety of thalidomide in patients with acute myeloid leukemia. *Blood* 99(3):834-839.

Stephan JL, Jeannoel P, Chanoz J, Gentil-Perret A. (2001). Epstein-Barr virus-associated Kikuchi disease in two children. *Journal of Pediatric Hematology-Oncology* 23(4):240-243.

Sternfeld B. (1992). Cancer and the protective effect of physical activity: The epidemiological evidence. *Medical Science, Sports, and Exercise* 24:1195-1209.

Sterzl I, Zamrazil V. (1996). Endocrinopathy in the differential diagnosis of chronic fatigue syndrome. *Vnitrni Lekarstvi* 42(9):624-626.

Stevenson HC, Abrams PG, Schoenberger CS, Smalley RB, Herberman RB, Foon KA. (1985). A phase I evaluation of poly(I,C)-LC in cancer patients. *Journal of Biological Response Modifiers* 4(6):650-655.

Stevenson JP, DeMaria D, Sludden J, Kaye SB, Paz-Ares L, Grochow LB, McDonald A, Selinger K, Wissel P, O'Dwyer PJ, et al. (1999). Phase I/pharmacokinetic study of the topoisomerase I inhibitor GG211 administered as a 21-day continuous infusion. *Annals of Oncology* 10(3):339-344.

Stevenson JP, Redlinger M, Kluijtmans LA, Sun W, Algazy K, Giantonio B, Haller DG, Hardy C, Whitehead AS, O'Dwyer PJ. (2001). Phase I clinical and pharmacogenetic trial of irinotecan and raltitrexed administered every 21 days to patients with cancer. *Journal of Clinical Oncology* 19(20):4081-4087.

Stevenson P. (1999). Pharmaceutical companies target plant products for drugs of the future. *Lancet* 354(9177):490.

Stewart D, Abbey S, Meana M, Boydell JM. (1998). What makes women tired? A community sample. *Journal of Women's Health* 7(1):69-76.

Stewart DJ, Goel R, Gertler SZ, Huan S, Tomiak EM, Yau J, Cripps C, Evans WK. (1999). Concurrent use of multiple low dose chemotherapy agents with differing mechanisms of action as a strategy vs. passive resistance: A pilot study. *International Journal of Oncology* 15(4):693-699.

Stewart DJ, Tomiak EM, Goss G, Gertler SZ, Logan D, Huan S, Yau J, Dulude H, Evans WK. (1996). Paclitaxel plus hydroxyurea as second line therapy for nonsmall cell lung cancer. *Lung Cancer* 15(1):115-123.

Stewart J, Weldon A, Arlievsky N, Li K, Munoz J. (1998). Neurally mediated hypotension and autonomic dysfunction measured by heart rate variability during head up tilt testing in children with chronic fatigue syndrome. *Clinical Autonomic Research* 8(4):221-230.

Stewart MJ, Steenkamp V, Zuckerman M. (1998). The toxicology of African herbal remedies. *Therapeutic Drug Monitoring* 20(5):510-516.

Stewart SH. (2002). Alcohol and inflammation: A possible mechanism for protection against ischemic heart disease. *Nutrition, Metabolism and Cardiovascular Disease* 12(3):148-151.

St. George IM. (1996). Did Cook's sailors have Tapanui flu?—Chronic fatigue syndrome on the resolution. *New Zealand Medical Journal* 109(1014):15-17.

Stimpel M, Steinmann U, Siegenthaler-Zuber G, Vetter W. (1985). [Fatigue, muscle weakness]. *Schweizerische Rundschau fur Medizin Praxis* 74(15):384-387.

Stitz L, Bilzer T, Tich JA, Rott R. (1993). Pathogenesis of Borna disease. *Archives of Virology* 7:135-151.

Stöger H, Wilders-Truscnig M, Samonigg H, Schmid M, Bauernhofer T, Tiran A, Tas M, Drexhage HA. (1993). The presence of immunosuppressive "p15E-like" factor in the serum and urine of patients suffering from malign and benign breast tumors. *Clinical and Experimental Immunology* 93:437-441.

Stoll AL. (2000). Fibromyalgia symptoms relieved by flupirtine: An open-label case series. *Psychosomatics* 41(4):371-372.

Stone AA, Broderick JE, Porter LS, Kaell AT. (1997). The experience of rheumatoid arthritis pain and fatigue: Examining momentary reports and correlates over one week. *Arthritis Care and Research* 10(3):185-193.

Stone P. (2002). The measurement, causes and effective management of cancer-related fatigue. *International Journal of Palliative Nursing* 8(3):120-128.

Stone P, Hardy J, Broadley K, Tookman AJ, Kurowska A, A'Hern R. (1999). Fatigue in advanced cancer: A prospective controlled cross-sectional study. *British Journal of Cancer* 79(9-10):1479-1486.

Stone P, Hardy J, Huddart R, A'Hern R, Richards M. (2000). Fatigue in patients with prostate cancer receiving hormone therapy. *European Journal of Cancer* 36(9):1134-1141.

Stone P, Richards M, A'Hern R, Hardy J. (2000). A study to investigate the prevalence, severity and correlates of fatigue among patients with cancer in comparison with a control group of volunteers without cancer. *Annals of Oncology* 11(5):561-567.

Stone P, Richards M, A'Hern R, Hardy J. (2001). Fatigue in patients with cancers of the breast or prostate undergoing radical radiotherapy. *Journal of Pain Symptomatology Management* 22(6):1007-1015.

Stone P, Richards M, Hardy J. (1998). Fatigue in patients with cancer. *European Journal of Cancer Care* 34(11):1670-1676.

Stone P, Richardson A, Ream E, Smith AG, Kerr DJ, Kearney N. (2000). Cancer-related fatigue: Inevitable, unimportant and untreatable? Results of a multi-centre patient survey. Cancer Fatigue Forum. *Annals of Oncology* 11(8):971-975.

Stopeck A, Sheldon M, Vahedian M, Cropp G, Gosalia R, Hannah A. (2002). Results of a phase I dose-escalating study of the antiangiogenic agent, SU5416, in patients with advanced malignancies. *Clinical Cancer Research* 8(9):2798-2805.

Stores G, Fry A, Crawford C. (1998). Sleep abnormalities demonstrated by home polysomnography in teenagers with chronic fatigue syndrome. *Journal of Psychosomatic Research* 45(1 Spec. No.):85-91.

Stormorken H, Brosstad F. (1999). [The "diffuse" health problems of women] Kvinners "ubestemte" helseplager. *Tidsskr Nor Laegeforen* 119(20):3043.

Stoter G, Aamdal S, Rodenhuis S, Cleton FJ, Iacobelli S, Franks CR, Oskam R, Shiloni E. (1991). Sequential administration of recombinant human interleukin-2 and dacarbazine in metastatic melanoma: A multicenter phase II study. *Journal of Clinical Oncology* 9(9):1687-1691.

Stoter G, Shiloni E, Aamdal S, Cleton FJ, Iacobelli S, Bijman JT, Palmer P, Franks CR, Rodenhuis S. (1989). Sequential administration of recombinant human interleukin-2 and dacarbazine in metastatic melanoma: A multicentre phase II study. *European Journal of Cancer and Clinical Oncology* 25(Suppl 3):S41-S43.

Stovall TG. (2001). Clinical experience with epoetin alfa in the management of hemoglobin levels in orthopedic surgery and cancer: Implications for use in gynecologic surgery. *Journal of Reproductive Medicine* 46(5 Suppl):531-538.

St. Pierre BA, Kasper CE, Lindsey AM. (1992). Fatigue mechanisms in patients with cancer: Effects of tumor necrosis factor and exercise on skeletal muscle. *Oncology Nursing Forum* 19(3):419-425.

Strang P. (1997). The effect of megestrol acetate on anorexia, weight loss and cachexia in cancer and AIDS patients (review). *Anticancer Research* 17(1B):657-662.

Strannegård IL, Larsson LO, Wennergren G, Strannegård O. (1998). Prevalence of allergy in children in relation to prior BCG vaccination and infection with atypical mycobacteria. *Allergy* 53:249-254.

Strassmann G, Fong M, Kenney JS, Jacob CO. (1992). Evidence for the involvement of interleukin-6 in experimental cancer cachexia. *Journal of Clinical Investigation* 89:1681-1684.

Strassmann G, Jacob CO, Evans R, Beall D, Fong M. (1992). Mechanisms of experimental cancer cachexia: Interaction between mononuclear phagocytes and colon-26 carcinoma and its relevance to IL-6-mediated cancer cachexia. *Journal of Immunology* 148(11):3674-3678.

Straus DJ. (2002). Epoetin alfa as a supportive measure in hematologic malignancies. *Seminars in Hematology* 39(4 Suppl 3):25-31.

Straus SE, Dale JK, Peter JB, Dinarello CA. (1989). Circulating lymphokine levels in the chronic fatigue syndrome. *Journal of Infectious Diseases* 160(6):1085-1086.

Straus SE, Tosato G, Armstrong G, Lawley T, Preble OT, Henle W, Davey R, Pearson G, Epstein J, Brus I. (1985). Persisting illness and fatigue in adults with evidence of Epstein-Barr virus infection. *Annals of Internal Medicine* 102:7-16.

Streeten DH. (1998). The nature of chronic fatigue. *JAMA* 280(12):1094-1095.

Streeten DH, Anderson GH Jr. (1998). The role of delayed orthostatic hypotension in the pathogenesis of chronic fatigue syndrome. *Clinical Autonomic Research* 8(2):119-124.

Streeten DHP, Bell DS. (1998). Circulating blood volume in chronic fatigue syndrome. *Journal of Chronic Fatigue Syndrome* 4(1):3-12.

Strickland FM, Darvill A, Albersheim P, Eberhard S, Pauly M, Pelley RP. (1999). Inhibition of UV-induced immune suppression and interleukin-10 production by plant oligosaccharides and polysaccharides. *Photochemistry and Photobiology* 69(2):141-147.

Strickland P, Morriss R, Wearden A, Deakin B. (1998). A comparison of salivary cortisol in chronic fatigue syndrome, community depression and healthy controls. *Journal of Affective Disorders* 47(1-3):191-194.

Strickland PS, Levine PH, Peterson DL, O'Brien K, Fears T. (2001). Neuromyasthenia and chronic fatigue syndrome (CFS) in Northern Nevada/California: A ten-year follow-up of an outbreak. *Journal of Chronic Fatigue Syndrome* 9(3/4):3-14.

Strohl RA. (1988). The nursing role in radiation oncology: Symptom management of acute and chronic reactions. *Oncology Nursing Forum* 15(4):429-434.

Strombeck B, Ekdahl C, Manthorpe R, Wikstrom I, Jacobsson L. (2000). Health-related quality of life in primary Sjögren's syndrome, rheumatoid arthritis and fibromyalgia compared to normal population data using SF-36. *Scandinavian Journal of Rheumatology* 29(1):20-28.

Stromgren AS, Goldschmidt D, Groenvold M, Petersen MA, Jensen PT, Pedersen L, Hoermann L, Helleberg C, Sjogren P. (2002). Self-assessment in cancer patients referred to palliative care: A study of feasibility and symptom epidemiology. *Cancer* 94(2):512-520.

Struder HK, Hollmann W, Platen P, Donike M, Gotzmann A, Weber K. (1998). Influence of paroxetine, branched-chain amino acids and tyrosine on neuroendocrine system responses and fatigue in humans. *Hormone and Metabolic Research* 30(4):188-194.

Strum WB. (1987). Excessive fatigue in a young man with refractory ulcerative colitis. *Hospital Practice* 22(9):102, 105-106.

Strupp C, Germing U, Aivado M, Misgeld E, Haas R, Gattermann N. (2002). Thalidomide for the treatment of patients with myelodysplastic syndromes. *Leukemia* 16(1):1-6.

Struthers CS. (1994). Lambert-Eaton myasthenic syndrome in small cell lung cancer: Nursing implications. *Oncology Nursing Forum* 21(4):677-683.

Studer H, Staub JJ, Wyss F. (1971). [Late clinical and metabolic effects of malignant tumors]. *Schweize Medizinische Wochenschrift* 101(13):446-451.

Stuifbergen AK, Rogers S. (1997). The experience of fatigue and strategies of self-care among persons with multiple sclerosis. *Applied Nursing Research* 10(1): 2-10.

Stupp R, Bodmer A, Duvoisin B, Bauer J, Perey L, Bakr M, Ketterer N, Leyvraz S. (2001). Is cisplatin required for the treatment of non-small-cell lung cancer? Experience and preliminary results of a phase I/II trial with topotecan and vinorelbine. *Oncology* 61(Suppl 1):35-41.

Suarez-Lozano I. (1996). Isolated general malaise of unknown origin: A new syndrome. *Anales de Medicina Interna* 14(4):209-210.

Subira ML, Castilla A, Civeira MP, Prieto J. (1989). Deficient display of CD3 on lymphocytes of patients with chronic fatigue syndrome. *Journal of Infectious Diseases* 160(1):165-166.

Subramanyan S, Abeloff MD, Bond SE, Davidson NE, Fetting JH, Gordon GB, Kennedy MJ. (1999). A phase I/II study of vinorelbine, doxorubicin, and methotrexate with leucovorin rescue as first-line treatment for metastatic breast cancer. *Cancer Chemotherapy Pharmacology* 43(6):497-502.

Sudakin DL. (1998). Toxigenic fungi in a water-damaged building: An intervention study. *American Journal of Industrial Medicine* 34(2):183-190.

Sugawara Y, Akechi T, Shima Y, Okuyama T, Akizuki N, Nakano T, Uchitomi Y. (2002). Efficacy of methylphenidate for fatigue in advanced cancer patients: A preliminary study. *Palliative Medicine* 16(3):261-263.

Sugie Y, Tsuji H, Nomiyama K, Ishitsuka T, Akagi K, Fujishima M, Shibuya T, Okamura T. (1992). [A case of idiopathic hemochromatosis associated with gastric cancer]. *Fukuoka Igaku Zasshi* 83(9):357-361.

Sugita K, Kaneko T, Sekine Y, Taguchi N, Miyauchi J. (1996). [Mast cell leukemia evolved from RAEB-T (5q-syndrome) in a 12 year-old girl]. *Rinsho Ketsueki* 37(5):430-436.

Suhadolnik RJ, Peterson DL, Cheney PR, Horvath SE, Reichenbach NL, O'Brien K, Lombardi V, Welsh S, Furr EG, Charubala R, et al. (1999). Biochemical dysregulation of the 2-5A synthetase/RNase L antiviral defense pathways in chronic fatigue syndrome. *Journal of Chronic Fatigue Syndrome* 5(3/4):223-242.

Suhadolnik RJ, Peterson DL, O'Brien K, Cheney PR, Herst CV, Reichenbach NL, Kon N, Horrath SE, Iacono KT, Adelson ME, et al. (1997). Biochemical evidence for a novel low molecular weight 2-5-A-dependent RNase L in chronic fatigue syndrome. *Journal of Interferon and Cytokine Research* 17(7):377-385.

Suhadolnik RJ, Reichenbach NL, Hitzges P, Adelson ME, Peterson DL, Cheney P, Salvato P, Thompson C, Loveless M, Muller WE, et al. (1994). Changes in the 2-5A synthetase/RNase L antiviral pathway in a controlled clinical trial with poly(I)-Poly(C$_{12}$U) in chronic fatigue syndrome. *In Vivo* 8(4):599-604.

Suhadolnik RJ, Reichenbach NL, Hitzges P, Sobol RW, Peterson DL, Henry B, Ablashi DV, Muller WE, Schroder HC, Carter WA, et al. (1994). Upregulation of the 2-5A synthetase/RNase L antiviral pathway associated with chronic fatigue syndrome. *Clinical Infectious Diseases* 18:S96-S104.

Sulkes A, Beller U, Peretz T, Shacter J, Hornreich G, McDaniel C, Winograd B. (1994). Taxol: Initial Israeli experience with a novel anticancer agent. *Israeli Journal of Medical Sciences* 30(1):70-78.

Sulkes A, Benner SE, Canetta RM. (1998). Uracil-ftorafur: An oral fluoropyrimidine active in colorectal cancer. *Journal of Clinical Oncology* 16(10):3461-3475.

Surawy C, Hackman A, Hawton K, Sharpe M. (1995). Chronic fatigue syndrome: A cognitive approach. *Behavioural Research and Therapy* 33(5):535-544.

Sutton GC. (1996). "Too tired to go to the support group": A health needs assessment of myalgic encephalomyelitis. *Journal of Public Health Medicine* 18(3): 343-349.

Suzuki A, Iwase O, Ohkubo T, Nakano M, Toyama K. (1991). [The successful use of natural alpha-interferon single therapy in multiple myeloma of IgD (lambda)-type]. *Rinsho Ketsueki* 32(1):47-51.

Suzuki H, Yasui A, Nishida Y, Kumagai K, Nakajima M, Watanabe T, Suzuki S. (1987). [Esophageal adenocarcinoma in an 81-year-old man]. *Gan No Rinsho* 33(1):70-75.

Suzuki K. (1986). [Phase II study of etoposide (VP-16-213) in genitourinary tumors. VP-16-213 Genitourinary Study Group]. *Gan To Kagaku Ryoho* 13(9): 2772-2779.

Suzuki R, Hirao M, Miyo T, Nagashima G, Fujimoto T, Ooshima A, Higuchi T. (1998). [Changes in QOL in patients with brain tumors measured by mood changes during and after treatment]. *No Shinkei Geka* 26(9):795-801.

Suzuki T, Suzuki N, Daynes RA, Engleman EG. (1991). Dehydroepiandrosterone enhances IL2 production and cytotoxic effector function of human T cells. *Clinical Immunology and Immunopathology* 61(2):202-211.

Swanink CM, Stolk-Engelaar VM, Van der Meer JW, Vercoulen JH, Bleijenberg G, Fennis JM, Galama JM, Hoogkamp-Korstanje JA. (1998). *Yersinia enterocolitica* and the chronic fatigue syndrome. *Journal of Infection* 36(3):269-272.

Swanink CM, Vercoulen JH, Galama JM, Roos MT, Meyaard L, Van der Ven-Jongekrijg J, De Nijs R, Bleijenberg G, Fennis JF, Miedema F, et al. (1996). Lymphocyte subsets, apoptosis, and cytokines in patients with chronic fatigue syndrome. *Journal of Infectious Diseases* 173(2):460-463.

Sweeney CW. (2002). Understanding peripheral neuropathy in patients with cancer: Background and patient assessment. *Clinical Journal of Oncology Nursing* 6(3):163-166.

Sweeney J. (2000). Fatigue: Online resources and advice. *International Journal of Palliative Nursing* 6(4):205.

Syed TA, Ahmad SA, Holt AH, Ahmad SA, Ahmad SH, Afzal M. (1996). Management of psoriasis with *Aloë vera* extract in a hydrophilic cream: A placebo-controlled double-blind study. *Tropical Medicine and International Health* 1(4): 505-509.

Szarka CE, Yao KS, Pfeiffer GR, Balshem AM, Litwin S, Frucht H, Goosenberg EB, Engstrom PF, Clapper ML, O'Dwyer PJ. (2001). Chronic dosing of oltipraz in people at increased risk for colorectal cancer. *Cancer Detection and Prevention* 25(4):352-361.

Sznol M, Mier JW, Sparano J, Gaynor ER, Weiss GR, Margolin KA, Bar MH, Hawkins MJ, Atkins MB, Dutcher JP, et al. (1990). A phase I study of high-dose interleukin-2 in combination with interferon-alpha 2b. *Journal of Biological Response Modifiers* 9(6):529-537.

Tabeeva GR, Korotkova SB, Vein AM. (2000). [Fibromyalgia] Fibromialgiia. *Zh Nevrol Psikhiatr Im S S Korsakova* 100(4):69-77.

Tada T, Ono S, Fukuta H, Tomichi N, Katoh R, Yagawa K, Hirota Y, Sugawara H, Baba H, Yaegashi Y, et al. (1989). [A case of leiomyoblastoma of the jejunum]. *Gan No Rinsho* 35(9):1081-1086.

Taddei-Bringas GA, Santillana-Macedo MA, Romero-Cancio JA, Romero-Tellez MB. (1999). Aceptación y uso de heblaria en medicina familiar. *Salud Publica Mexicana* 41(3):216-220.

Taguchi T. (1984). [Effects of interferon on various malignancies]. *Gan To Kagaku Ryoho* 11(2):194-204.

Taguchi T. (1985). [Phase I study of recombinant human interferon alpha A (Ro 22-8181) in patients with malignant tumors]. *Gan To Kagaku Ryoho* 12(3 Pt 1):456-464.

Taguchi T. (1986). [A phase I study of recombinant human tumor necrosis factor (rHu-TNF: PT-050). The PT-050 Study Group]. *Gan To Kagaku Ryoho* 13(12): 3491-3497.

Taguchi T. (1987). Clinical efficacy of lentinan on patients with stomach cancer: End point results of a four-year follow-up survey. *Cancer Detection and Prevention Supplement* 1:333-349.

Taguchi T. (1994). [An early phase II clinical study of RP56976 (docetaxel) in patients with cancer of the gastrointestinal tract]. *Gan To Kagaku Ryoho* 21(14): 2431-2437.

Taguchi T, Furue H, Niitani H, Ishitani K, Kanamaru R, Hasegawa K, Ariyoshi Y, Noda K, Furuse K, Fukuoka M, et al. (1994). [Phase I clinical trial of RP 56976 (docetaxel) a new anticancer drug]. *Gan To Kagaku Ryoho* 21(12):1997-2005.

Taguchi T, Furuse K, Fukuoka M, Shimoyama T, Morimoto K, Nakamura T, Furue H, Majima H, Niitani H, Ohta K, et al. (1996). [LY188011 phase I study. Research Group of Gemcitabine (LY188011)]. *Gan To Kagaku Ryoho* 23(8):1011-1018.

Taguchi T, Hirata K, Kunii Y, Tabei T, Suwa T, Kitajima M, Adachi I, Tominaga T, Shimada H, Sano M, et al. (1994). [An early phase II clinical study of RP56976 (docetaxel) in patients with breast cancer]. *Gan To Kagaku Ryoho* 21(14):2453-2460.

Taguchi T, Mori S, Abe R, Hasegawa K, Morishita Y, Tabei T, Sasaki Y, Fujita M, Enomoto K, Hamano K, et al. (1994). [Late phase II clinical study of RP56976 (docetaxel) in patients with advanced/recurrent breast cancer]. *Gan To Kagaku Ryoho* 21(15):2625-2632.

Taguchi T, Morimoto K, Horikoshi N, Takashima S, Toge T, Kimura M, Sano M, Aoyama H, Ota J, Noguchi S. (1998). [An early phase II clinical study of S-1 in patients with breast cancer. S-1 Cooperative Study Group (Breast Cancer Working Group)]. *Gan To Kagaku Ryoho* 25(7):1035-1043.

Taguchi T, Sakata Y, Kanamaru R, Kurihara M, Suminaga M, Ota J, Hirabayashi N. (1998). [Late phase II clinical study of RP56976 (docetaxel) in patients with advanced/recurrent gastric cancer: A Japanese Cooperative Study Group trial (group A)]. *Gan To Kagaku Ryoho* 25(12):1915-1924.

Tait N, Aisner J. (1989). Nutritional concerns in cancer patients. *Seminars in Oncology Nursing* 5(2 Suppl 1):58-62.

Takada M, Negoro S, Kudo S, Furuse K, Nishikawa H, Takada Y, Kamei T, Niitani H, Fukuoka M. (1998). Activity of gemcitabine in non-small-cell lung cancer: Results of the Japan gemcitabine group (A) phase II study. *Cancer Chemotherapy Pharmacology* 41(3):217-222.

Takechi A, Uozumi T, Mukada K, Kurisu K, Arita K, Yano T, Hirohata T, Ogasawara H, Ondo J, Hanaya R, et al. (1991). [A case of pituitary adenoma with simultaneous secretion of TSH and GH detected by double immunostaining method]. *No To Shinkei* 43(8):775-779.

Takei A, Nagashima G, Suzuki R, Hokaku H, Takahashi M, Miyo T, Asai J, Sanada Y, Fujimoto T. (1997). Meningoencephalocele associated with *Tripterygium wildorfii* treatment. *Pediatric Neurosurgery* 27(1):45-48.

Takeuchi J, Kawamura M, Sawada U, Ohshima T, Horie T, Horikoshi A, Abe T. (1995). [Natural interferon alpha for chronic myelogenous leukemia in the chronic phase: Hematologic, cytogenetic and molecular response]. *Rinsho Ketsueki* 36(10):1149-1156.

Talal N, Dauphinée MJ, Dang H, Alexander SS, Hart DJ, Garry RF. (1990). Detection of serum antibodies to retroviral proteins in patients with primary Sjögren's syndrome (autoimmune exocrinopathy). *Arthritis and Rheumatism* 33(6):774-781.

Talal N, Garry RF, Schur PH, Alexander S, Dauphinée MJ, Livas IH, Ballester A, Takei M, Dang H. (1990). A conserved idiotype and antibodies to retroviral proteins in systemic lupus erythematosus. *Journal of Clinical Investigation* 85(6):1866-1887.

Talpaz M, O'Brien S, Rose E, Gupta S, Shan J, Cortes J, Giles FJ, Faderl S, Kantarjian HM. (2001). Phase 1 study of polyethylene glycol formulation of interferon alpha-2B (Schering 54031) in Philadelphia chromosome-positive chronic myelogenous leukemia. *Blood* 98(6):1708-1713.

Tamburini M, Brunelli C, Rosso S, Ventafridda V. (1996). Prognostic value of quality of life scores in terminal cancer patients. *Journal of Pain Symptomatology and Management* 11(1):32-41.

Tamulevicius P, Streffer C. (1995). Metabolic imaging in tumours by means of bioluminiscence. *British Journal of Cancer* 72:1102-1112.

Tamura K, Tashiro H, Kondoh S, Kisanuki A, Sumiyoshi A, Suzumiya J, Takeshita M. (1994). Ki-1 (CD30)-positive large cell lymphoma presented with leukemia: A case report. *Fukuoka Igaku Zasshi* 85(12):366-371.

Tamura T, Sasaki Y, Shinkai T, Eguchi K, Sakurai M, Fujiwara Y, Nakagawa K, Minato K, Bungo M, Saijo N. (1989). Phase I study of combination therapy with interleukin 2 and beta-interferon in patients with advanced malignancy. *Cancer Research* 49(3):730-735.

Tan AR, Headlee D, Messmann R, Sausville EA, Arbuck SG, Murgo AJ, Melillo G, Zhai S, Figg WD, Swain SM, Senderowicz AM. (2002). Phase I clinical and pharmacokinetic study of flavopiridol administered as a daily 1-hour infusion in patients with advanced neoplasms. *Journal of Clinical Oncology* 20(19):4074-4082.

Tanabe H, Imai N, Takechi K. (1990). Studies on usefulness of postoperative adjuvant chemotherapy with lentinan in patients with gastrointestinal cancer. *Journal of the Japanese Society for Cancer Therapy* 25:1657.

Tanabe K, Yamamoto A, Suzuki N, Osada N, Yokoyama Y, Samejima H, Seki A, Oya M, Murabayashi T, Nakayama M, et al. (1998). Efficacy of oral magnesium administration on decreased exercise tolerance in a state of chronic sleep deprivation. *Japanese Circulation Journal* 62(5):341-346.

Tanaka H, West KA, Duncan GE, Bassett DR Jr. (1997). Changes in plasma tryptophan/branched amino acid ratio in responses to training volume variation. *International Journal of Sports Medicine* 18(4):270-275.

Tanaka K, Akechi T, Okuyama T, Nishiwaki Y, Uchitomi Y. (2002). Impact of dyspnea, pain, and fatigue on daily life activities in ambulatory patients with advanced lung cancer. *Journal of Pain Symptomatology Management* 23(5): 417-423.

Tanaka M, Iizuka Y, Sudou N, Kikuchi T, Oyama A, Takiguchi Y, Onikura S, Kajiwara N. (1990). [Smoldering leukemia with pyoderma gangrenosum]. *Rinsho Ketsueki* 31(10):1680-1683.

Tantucci C, Massucci M, Piperno R, Grassi V, Sobirni CA. (1996). Energy cost of exercise in multiple sclerosis patients with low degree of disability. *Multiple Sclerosis* 2(3):161-167.

Taphoorn MJ, Schiphorst AK, Snoek FJ, Lindeboom J, Wolbers JG, Karim AB, Huijgens PC, Heimans JJ. (1994). Cognitive functions and quality of life in patients with low-grade gliomas: The impact of radiotherapy. *Annals of Neurology* 36(1):48-54.

Taplin SC, Blanke CD, Baughman C. (1997). Nursing care strategies for the management of side effects in patients treated for colorectal cancer. *Seminars in Oncology* 24(5 Suppl 18):S18-64-S18-70.

Tarbleton P. (1995). To whom it may concern. Affidavit to the Southern Association Medical Council, January.

Targan S, Stebbing N. (1982). In vitro interactions of purified cloned human interferons on NK cells: Enhanced activation. *Journal of Immunology* 129:934-935.

Tari K, Satake I, Nakagomi K, Ozawa K, Oowada F, Higashi Y, Negishi T, Yamada T, Saito H, Yoshida K. (1994). Effect of lentinan for advanced prostate carcinoma. *Acta Urologica Japonica* 40:119.

Tate J, Olencki T, Finke J, Kottke-Marchant K, Rybicki LA, Bukowski RM. (2001). Phase I trial of simultaneously administered GM-CSF and IL-6 in patients with renal-cell carcinoma: Clinical and laboratory effects. *Annals of Oncology* 12(5): 655-659.

Tavio M, Milan I, Tirelli U. (2002). Cancer-related fatigue (review). *International Journal of Oncology* 21(5):1093-1099.

Tayag-Kier CE, Keenan GF, Scalzi LV, Schultz B, Elliott J, Zhao RH, Arens R. (2000). Sleep and periodic limb movement in sleep in juvenile fibromyalgia. *Pediatrics* 106(5):E70.

Taylor A, Taylor RS. (1998). Neuropsychologic aspects of multiple sclerosis. *Physical Medicine and Rehabilitation Clinics of North America* 9(3):643-657.

Taylor CW, Chase EM, Whitehead RP, Rinehart JJ, Neidhart JA, Gonzalez R, Bunn PA, Hersh EM. (1992). A Southwest Oncology Group phase I study of the sequential combination of recombinant interferon-gamma and recombinant interleukin-2 in patients with cancer. *Journal of Immunotherapy* 11(3):176-183.

Taylor CW, Dorr RT, Fanta P, Hersh EM, Salmon SE. (2001). A phase I and pharmacodynamic evaluation of polyethylene glycol-conjugated L-asparaginase in patients with advanced solid tumors. *Cancer Chemotherapy Pharmacology* 47(1):83-88.

Taylor CW, LeBlanc M, Fisher RI, Moore DF Sr, Roach RW, Elias L, Miller TP. (2000). Phase II evaluation of interleukin-4 in patients with non-Hodgkin's lymphoma: A Southwest Oncology Group trial. *Anticancer Drugs* 11(9):695-700.

Taylor CW, Modiano MR, Woodson ME, Marcus SG, Alberts DS, Hersh EM. (1992). A phase I trial of fluorouracil, leucovorin, and recombinant interferon alpha-2b in patients with advanced malignancy. *Seminars in Oncology* 19(2 Suppl 3):185-190.

Taylor RR, Jason LA, Kennedy CL, Friedberg F. (2001). Evaluating attributions for chronic fatigue syndrome based upon type of treatment recommended. *Rehabilitation Psychology* 46:165-177.

Taylor RS. (1998). Multiple sclerosis potpourri: Paroxysmal symptoms, seizures, fatigue, pregnancy, and more. *Physical Medicine and Rehabilitation Clinics of North America* 9(3):551-559.

Tchekmedyian NS. (1995). Costs and benefits of nutrition support in cancer. *Oncology* 9(11 Suppl):79-84.

Tedeschi R, Foong YT, Cheng HM, dePaoli P, Lehtinen T, Elfborg T, Dillner J. (1995). The disease associations of the antibody response against the Epstein-Barr virus transactivator protein ZEBRA can be separated into different epitopes. *Journal of General Virology* 76(Pt 6):1393-1400.

Tedla N, Dwyer J, Truskett P, Taub D, Wakefield D, Lloyd A. (1999). Phenotypic and functional characterization of lymphocytes derived from normal and HIV-1-infected human lymph nodes. *Clinical and Experimental Immunology* 117(1): 92-99.

Teel CS, Press AN. (1999). Fatigue among elders in caregiving and noncaregiving roles. *Western Journal of Nursing Research* 21(4):498-514; discussion 514-520.

Tefferi A, Witzig TE, Reid JM, Li CY, Ames MM. (1994). Phase I study of combined 2-chlorodeoxyadenosine and chlorambucil in chronic lymphoid leukemia and low-grade lymphoma. *Journal of Clinical Oncology* 12(3):569-574.

Teh BS, Aguilar-Cordova E, Kernen K, Chou CC, Shalev M, Vlachaki MT, Miles B, Kadmon D, Mai WY, Caillouet J, et al. (2001). Phase I/II trial evaluating combined radiotherapy and in situ gene therapy with or without hormonal therapy in the treatment of prostate cancer—A preliminary report. *International Journal of Radiation Oncology, Biology and Physics* 51(3):605-613.

Telenius-Berg M, Ponder MA, Berg B, Ponder BA, Werner S. (1989). Quality of life after bilateral adrenalectomy in MEN 2. *Henry Ford Hospital Medical Journal* 37(3-4):160-163.

Tepler I, Elias A, Kalish L, Shulman L, Strauss G, Skarin A, Lynch T, Levitt D, Resta D, Demetri G, et al. (1994). Effect of recombinant human interleukin-3 on haematological recovery from chemotherapy-induced myelosuppression. *British Journal of Haematology* 87(4):678-686.

Tepler I, Elias L, Smith JW II, Hussein M, Rosen G, Chang AY, Moore JO, Gordon MS, Kuca B, Beach KJ, et al. (1996). A randomized placebo-controlled trial of recombinant human interleukin-11 in cancer patients with severe thrombocytopenia due to chemotherapy. *Blood* 87(9):3607-3614.

Teran Diaz E. (1996). Isolated general malaise of unknown origin: A new syndrome. *Anales de Medicina Interna* 13(10):467-470.

Terao I. (2002). [Phase I study of gemcitabine (GEM) and docetaxel (TXT) combination chemotherapy for unresectable non-small-cell lung cancer]. *Gan To Kagaku Ryoho* 29(11):1929-1933.

Terman M, Levine SM, Terman JS, Doherty S. (1998). Chronic fatigue syndrome and seasonal affective disorder: Comorbidity, diagnostic overlap, and implications for treatment. *American Journal of Medicine* 105(3A):115S-124S.

Tezelman S, Rodriguez JM, Shen W, Siperstein AE, Duh QY, Clark OH. (1995). Primary hyperparathyroidism in patients who have received radiation therapy and in patients who have not received radiation therapy. *Journal of the American College of Surgery* 180(1):81-87.

Tezelman S, Shen W, Shaver JK, Siperstein AE, Duh QY, Klein H, Clark OH. (1993). Double parathyroid adenomas: Clinical and biochemical characteristics before and after parathyroidectomy. *Annals of Surgery* 218(3):300-307; discussion 307-309.

Thacker HL, Booher DL. (1999). Management of perimenopause: Focus on alternative therapies. *Cleveland Clinic Journal of Medicine* 66(4):213-218.

Thase MF. (1991). Assessment of depression in patients with chronic fatigue syndrome. *Reviews of Infectious Diseases* 13(Suppl):S114-S118.

Theophrastus (370-285BC). (1916). *Enquiry into Plants,* Volumes 1 and 2. Translated by Hort A. London: W. Heinemann.

Thodtmann R, Depenbrock H, Blatter J, Johnson RD, van Oosterom A, Hanauske AR. (1999). Preliminary results of a phase I study with MTA (LY231514) in combination with cisplatin in patients with solid tumors. *Seminars in Oncology* 26(2 Suppl 6):89-93.

Thodtmann R, Depenbrock H, Dumez H, Blatter J, Johnson RD, van Oosterom A, Hanauske AR. (1999). Clinical and pharmacokinetic phase I study of multi-targeted antifolate (LY231514) in combination with cisplatin. *Journal of Clinical Oncology* 17(10):3009-3016.

Thomas JP, Arzoomanian R, Alberti D, Feierabend C, Binger K, Tutsch KD, Steele T, Marnocha R, Smith C, Smith S, et al. (2001). Phase I clinical and pharmacokinetic trial of irofulven. *Cancer Chemotherapy Pharmacology* 48(6):467-472.

Thomas ML. (1998a). Impact of anemia and fatigue on quality of life in cancer patients: A brief review. *Medical Oncology* 15(Suppl 1):S3-S7.

Thomas ML. (1998b). Quality of life and psychosocial adjustment in patients with myelodysplastic syndromes. *Leukemia Research* 22(Suppl 1):S41-S47.

Thomas RR, Dahut W, Harold N, Grem JL, Monahan BP, Liang M, Band RA, Cottrell J, Llorens V, Smith JA, et al. (2001). A phase I and pharmacologic study of 9-aminocamptothecin administered as a 120-h infusion weekly to adult cancer patients. *Cancer Chemotherapy Pharmacology* 48(3):215-222.

Thomas WO III, Harper LL, Wong SW, Michalski JP, Harris CN, Moore JT, Rodning CB. (1997). Explanation of silicone breast implants. *American Surgery* 63(5):421-429.

Thompson EA. (1999). Using homoeopathy to offer supportive cancer care, in a National Health Service outpatient setting. *Complementary Therapy and Nursing Midwifery* 5(2):37-41.

Thompson EA, Reilly D. (2002). The homeopathic approach to symptom control in the cancer patient: A prospective observational study. *Palliation Medicine* 16 (3):227-233.

Thompson JA, Rubin E, Fefer A. (1987). The treatment of hairy cell leukemia with alpha 2b-interferon: Experience with 27 patients treated more than one year. *Leukemia* 1(4):328-330.

Thompson TC. (1990). Growth factors and oncogenes in prostate cancer. *Cancer Cells* 2:345-354.

Thomson DB, Adena M, McLeod GR, Hersey P, Gill PG, Coates AS, Olver IN, Kefford RF, Lowenthal RM, Beadle GF, et al. (1993). Interferon-alpha 2a does not improve response or survival when combined with dacarbazine in metastatic malignant melanoma: Results of a multi-institutional Australian randomized trial. *Melanoma Research* 3(2):133-138.

Thorn J, Kerekes E. (2001). Health effects among employees in sewage treatment plants: A literature survey. *American Journal of Indian Medicine* 40(2):170-179.

Thorson K. (1998). The fibromyalgia problem. *Journal of Rheumatology* 25(5): 1023, discussion 1028-1030.

Thorson K. (1999). Is fibromyalgia a distinct clinical entity? The patient's evidence. *Baillieres Best Practice Research in Clinical Rheumatology* 13(3):463-467.

Thorsteinsson G. (1997). Management of post-polio syndrome. *Mayo Clinic Proceedings* 72(7):627-638.

Thune I, Smeland S. (2000). [Is physical activity important in treatment and rehabilitation of cancer patients?] *Tidsskr Nor Laegeforen* 120(27):3302-3304.

Tian J, Lehmann PV, Kaufman DL. (1994). T cell cross-reactivity between coxsackievirus and glutamate decarboxylase is associated with a murine diabetes susceptibility allele. *Journal of Experimental Medicine* 180:1979-1984.

Tiersky LA, Johnson SK, Lange G, Natelson BH, DeLuca J. (1997). Neuropsychology of chronic fatigue syndrome: A critical review. *Journal of Clinical and Experimental Neuropsychology* 19(4):560-586.

Tiesinga LJ, Dassen TW, Halfens RJ. (1996). Fatigue: A summary of the definitions, dimensions, and indicators. *Nursing Diagnosis* 7(2):51-62.

Tinsley JA. (1999). The hazards of psychotropic herbs. *Minnesota Medicine* 82(5): 29-31.

Tirelli U, Chierichetti F, Tavio M, Simonelli C, Bianchin G, Zanco P, Ferlin G. (1998). Brain positron emission tomography (PET) in chronic fatigue syndrome: Preliminary data. *American Journal of Medicine* 105(3A):54S-58S.

Tirelli U, Marotta G, Improta S, Pinto A. (1994). Immunological abnormalities in patients with chronic fatigue syndrome. *Scandinavian Journal of Immunology* 40(6):601-608.

Tisdale MJ. (1997a). Biology of cachexia. *Journal of the National Cancer Institute* 89:1763-1773.

Tisdale MJ. (1997b). Cancer cachexia: Metabolic alterations and clinical manifestations. *Nutrition* 13:1-7.

Tishelman C, Degner LF, Mueller B. (2000). Measuring symptom distress in patients with lung cancer: A pilot study of experienced intensity and importance of symptoms. *Cancer Nursing* 23(2):82-90.

Tishler M, Barak Y, Paran D, Yaron M. (1997). Sleep disturbances, fibromyalgia and primary Sjögren's syndrome. *Clinical and Experimental Rheumatology* 15 (1):71-74.

Tiwari RK, Geliebter J, Garikapaty VP, Yedavelli SP, Chen S, Mittelman A. (1999). Anti-tumor effects of PC-SPES, an herbal formulation, in prostate cancer. *International Journal of Oncology* 14(4):713-719.

Tobi M, Morag A, Ravid Z, Chowers I, Feldman-Weiss V, Michaeli Y, Ben-Chetrit E, Shalit M, Knobler H. (1982). Prolonged atypical illness associated with serological evidence of persistent Epstein-Barr virus infection. *Lancet* 1(8263): 61-64.

Tokunaga M, Kinoshita Y, Kawano F, Hashimoto Y, Uchino M. (2000). [Malignant lymphoma at the cavernous sinus]. *No To Shinkei* 52(2):173-177.

Tola MA, Yugueros MI, Fernandez-Buey N, Fernandez-Herranz R. (1998). Impact of fatigue in multiple sclerosis: Study of a population-based series in Valladolid. *Revista de Neurología* 26(154):930-933.

Tolcher AW, Gelmon KA. (1995). Interim results of a phase I/II study of biweekly paclitaxel and cisplatin in patients with metastatic breast cancer. *Seminars in Oncology* 22(4 Suppl 8):28-32.

Toma S, Palumbo R, Vincenti M, Aitini E, Paganini G, Pronzato P, Grimaldi A, Rosso R. (1994). Efficacy of recombinant alpha-interferon 2a and 13-cis-retinoic acid in the treatment of squamous cell carcinoma. *Annals of Oncology* 5(5):463-465.

Tominaga T, Abe O, Izuo M, Nomura Y. (1993). [Phase II study of NK 622 (toremifene citrate) in advanced breast cancer, a multicentral cooperative dose finding study]. *Gan To Kagaku Ryoho* 20(1):79-90.

Tominaga T, Hayashi K, Hayasaka A, Asaishi K, Abe R, Kimishima I, Izuo M, Iino Y, Yokoe T, Abe O, et al. (1992). [Phase I study of NK 622 (toremifene citrate)]. *Gan To Kagaku Ryoho* 19(14):2363-2372.

Tominaga T, Nomura Y, Adachi I, Aoyama H, Nagao K, Mitsuyama S, Nakamura Y, Ogita M, Sano M, Takashima S, et al. (1994). [Late phase II study of KW-2307 in advanced or recurrent breast cancer. KW-2307 Cooperative Study Group (Breast Cancer Section)]. *Gan To Kagaku Ryoho* 21(6):809-816.

Tominaga T, Nomura Y, Adachi I, Takashima S, Kimura M, Koyama H, Toge T, Tamura K, Hayasaka H, Kunii Y, et al. (1994). [Early phase II study of KW-2307 in advanced or recurrent breast cancer. KW-2307 Cooperative Study Group (Breast Cancer Section)]. *Gan To Kagaku Ryoho* 21(6):801-808.

Torii T, Takasuga H, Mizushima M, Ito J, Kanaya T, Matsushima T. (1989). [Primary malignant mesothelioma of the pericardium masquerading as malignant pleural mesothelioma: Report of an autopsy case and review of the reported cases in Japan as to its invasion to neighboring organs]. *Kokyu To Junkan* 37(9):1027-1032.

Torpy DJ, Chrousos GP. (1996). The three-way interactions between the hypothalamic-pituitary-adrenal and gonadal axes and the immune system. *Baillieres Clinical Rheumatology* 10(2):181-198.

Torpy DJ, Papanicolaou DA, Lotsikas AJ, Wilder RL, Chrousos GP, Pillemer SR (2000). Responses of the sympathetic nervous system and the hypothalamic-pituitary-adrenal axis to interleukin-6: A pilot study in fibromyalgia. *Arthritis and Rheumatism* 43(4):872-880.

Tosato G, Straus S, Henle W, Pike SE, Blaese RM. (1985). Characteristic T cell dysfunction in patients with chronic active Epstein-Barr virus infection (chronic infectious mononucleosis). *Journal of Immunology* 134(5):3082-3088.

Touchon J. (1995). [Use of antidepressants in sleep disorders: Practical considerations] Utilisation des antidepresseurs dans les troubles du sommeil: Considerations pratiques. *Encephale* 21(Spec. No. 7):41-47.

Touchon J, Besset A, Billiard M, Simon L, Herrison C, Cadihac J. (1988). Fibrositis syndrome: Polysomnographic and psychological aspects. In *Sleep '86,* Koella WP, Obai F, Schulz H, Visser P, eds. New York: Gustav Fischer Verlag, pp. 445-447.

Tougas G. (1999). The autonomic nervous system in functional bowel disorders. *Canadian Journal of Gastroenterology* 13(Suppl A):15A-17A.

Touroutoglou N, Gravel D, Raber MN, Plunkett W, Abbruzzese JL. (1998). Clinical results of a pharmacodynamically-based strategy for higher dosing of gemcitabine in patients with solid tumors. *Annals of Oncology* 9(9):1003-1008.

Trabacchi G. (1997). [A poorly understood symptom: Fatigue in oncology]. *Revue de Infirmiere* 30:10-13.

Treat J, Greenberg R, Bratschi J, Gorman G, Meehan L, Friedland D. (1994). First hints in non-small cell lung cancer (NSCLC). *Leukemia* 8(Suppl 3):S55-S58.

Treat J, Johnson E, Langer C, Belani C, Haynes B, Greenberg R, Rodriquez R, Drobins P, Miller W Jr, Meehan L, et al. (1998). Tirapazamine with cisplatin in patients with advanced non-small-cell lung cancer: A phase II study. *Journal of Clinical Oncology* 16(11):3524-3527.

Treib J, Grauer MT, Haas A, Langenbach J, Holzer G, Woessner R. (2000). Chronic fatigue syndrome in patients with Lyme borreliosis. *European Journal of Neurology* 43(2):107-109.

Trijsburg RW, van Knippenberg FC, Rijpma SE. (1992). Effects of psychological treatment on cancer patients: A critical review. *Psychosomatic Medicine* 54(4): 489-517.

Triozzi PL, Walker MJ, Pellegrini AE, Dayton MA. (1996). Isotretinoin and recombinant interferon alfa-2a therapy of metastatic malignant melanoma. *Cancer Investigation* 14(4):293-298.

Tripathy D. (2002). Overview: Gemcitabine as single-agent therapy for advanced breast cancer. *Clinical Breast Cancer* 3(Suppl 1):8-11.

Trojan DA, Cashman NR. (1995). Fibromyalgia is common in a postpoliomyelitis clinic. *Archives of Neurology* 52(6):620-624.

Trudeau, M, Stuart G, Hirte H, Drouin P, Plante M, Bessette P, Dulude H, Lebwohl D, Fisher B, Seymour L. (2002). A phase II trial of JM-216 in cervical cancer: An NCIC CTG study. *Gynecological Oncology* 84(2):327-331.

Trudeau M, Zukiwski A, Langleben A, Boos G, Batist G. (1995). A phase I study of recombinant human interferon alpha-2b combined with 5-fluorouracil and cisplatin in patients with advanced cancer. *Cancer Chemotherapy Pharmacology* 35(6):496-500.

Trudeau M, Zukiwski A, Langleben A, Boos G, Hayden K, Batist G. (1993). A phase I study of escalating interferon alpha-2a combined with 5-fluorouracil and leucovorin in patients with gastrointestinal malignancies. *Acta Oncologica* 32 (5):537-539.

Trujillo JR, McLane MF, Lee T-H, Essex M. (1993). Molecular mimicry between the human immunodeficiency virus type 1 gp120 V3 loop and human brain proteins. *Journal of Virology* 67:7711-7715.

Trump DL, Ravdin PM, Borden EC, Magers CF, Whisnant JK. (1990). Interferon-alpha-n1 and continuous infusion vinblastine for treatment of advanced renal cell carcinoma. *Journal of Biological Response Modifiers* 9(1):108-111.

Tsavaris N, Foutzilas G, Markantonakis P, Mylonakis N, Bacoyannis C, Zisiadis A, Basdanis G, Karvounis N, Sobolos K, Kosmidis P. (1995). A comparative study with two administration schedules of leucovorin and 5-fluorouracil in advanced colorectal cancer. *Journal of Chemotherapy* 7(1):71-77.

Tsavaris N, Kosmas C, Polyzos A, Genatas K, Vadiaka M, Paliaros P, Dimitrakopoulos A, Rokana S, Karatzas G, Vachiotis P, et al. (2001). Leucovorin + 5-fluorouracil plus dipyridamole in leucovorin + 5-fluorouracil-pretreated patients with advanced colorectal cancer: A pilot study of three different dipyridamole regimens. *Tumori* 87(5):303-307.

Tsavaris N, Mylonakis N, Bacoyiannis C, Tsoutsos H, Karabelis A, Kosmidis P. (1993). Treatment of renal cell carcinoma with escalating doses of alpha-interferon. *Chemotherapy* 39(5):361-366.

Tsavaris N, Primikirios N, Mylonakis N, Varouchakis G, Dosios T, Pavlidis N, Skarlos D, Tasopoulos T, Dritsas J, Kosmidis P. (1997). Combination chemotherapy with cisplatin and/or doxorubicin in malignant mesothelioma: A retrospective study [corrected from prospective]. *Anticancer Research* 17(5B):3799-3802.

Tsavaris N, Skarlos D, Bacoyiannis C, Aravantinos G, Kosmas C, Retalis G, Panopoulos C, Vadiaka M, Dimitrakopoulos A, Kostantinidis K, et al. (2000). Combined treatment with low-dose interferon plus vinblastine is associated with less toxicity than conventional interferon monotherapy in patients with metastatic renal cell carcinoma. *Journal of Interferon and Cytokine Research* 20(8): 685-690.

Tsavaris NB, Tentas K, Kosmidis P, Mylonakis N, Sakelaropoulos N, Kosmas C, Lisaios B, Soumilas A, Mandrekois D, Tsetis A, et al. (1996). 5-Fluorouracil, epirubicin, and mitomycin C versus 5-fluorouracil, epirubicin, mitomycin C, and leucovorin in advanced gastric carcinoma: A randomized trial. *American Journal of Clinical Oncology* 19(5):517-521.

Tsiodras S, Shin RK, Christian M, Shaw LM, Sass DA. (1999). Anticholinergic toxicity associated with lupine seeds as a home remedy for diabetes mellitus. *Annals of Emergency Medicine* 33(6):715-717.

Tsudo M, Ichiyama T, Uchino H. (1984). Expression of Tac antigen on activated human B cells. *Journal of Experimental Medicine* 160:612-617.

Tsuji Y, Okada K, Fukuoka M, Watanabe Y, Ataka K, Minami R, Hanioka K, Tachibana S, Saito H, Sasada A, Okita Y. (2001). Hepatocellular carcinoma with a sarcomatous appearance: Report of a case. *Surgery Today* 31(8):735-739.

Tsukagoshi S. (1987). [Introduction of natural interferon-alpha "Sumiferon"]. *Gan To Kagaku Ryoho* 14(9):2800-2803.

Tsukagoshi S. (1995). [Introduction of a new aromatase inhibitor fadrozole hydrochloride hydsate]. *Gan To Kagaku Ryoho* 22(13):1991-1997.

Tsushima H, Kawata S, Tamura S, Ito N, Shirai Y, Kiso S, Imai Y, Shimomukai H, Nomura Y, Matsuda Y, et al. (1996). High levels of transforming growth factor beta 1 in patients with colorectal cancer: Association with disease progression. *Gastroenterology* 110:375-382.

Tsutsumi M, Yamauchi A, Tsukamoto S, Ishikawa S. (2001). A case of angiomyolipoma presenting as a huge retroperitoneal mass. *International Journal of Urology* 8(8):470-471.

Tuck I, Human N. (1998). The experience of living with chronic fatigue syndrome. *Journal of Psychosocial Nursing and Mental Health Services* 36(2):15-19.

Tucker TJ, Bardales RH, Miranda RN. (1999). Intravascular lymphomatosis with bone marrow involvement. *Archives of Pathology and Laboratory Medicine* 123(10):952-956.

Tuckey JA, Parry BR, McCall JL. (1993). Pentoxifylline and wellbeing in cancer. *Lancet* 342(8871):617.

Tulpule A, Rarick MU, Kolitz J, Bernstein J, Myers A, Buchanan LA, Espina BM, Traynor A, Letzer J, Justice GR, et al. (2001). Liposomal daunorubicin in the treatment of relapsed or refractory non-Hodgkin's lymphoma. *Annals of Oncology* 12(4):457-462.

Tulpule A, Schiller G, Harvey-Buchanan LA, Lee M, Espina BM, Khan AU, Boswell W, Nathwani B, Levine AM. (1998). Cladribine in the treatment of advanced relapsed or refractory low and intermediate grade non-Hodgkin's lymphoma. *Cancer* 83(11):2370-2376.

Tummino PJ, Prasad JVNV, Ferguson D, Nouhan C, Graham N, Dormagala JM, Ellsworth E, Gajda C, Hagen SE, Lunney EA, et al. (1996). Discovery and optimization of nonpeptide HIV-1 protease inhibitors. *Bioorganic Medicine Chemistry Letters* 4(9):1401-1410.

Tur E, Brenner S. (1998). Classic Kaposi's sarcoma: Low-dose interferon alfa treatment. *Dermatology* 197(1):37-42.

Turek FW, Czeisler CA. (1999). Role of melatonin in the regulation of sleep. In *Regulation of Sleep and Circadian Rhythms,* Turek FW, Zee PC, eds. New York: Marcel Dekker, pp. 181-195.

Turk DC, Okifuji A, Sinclair JD, Starz TW. (1996). Pain, disability, and physical functioning in subgroups of patients with fibromyalgia. *Journal of Rheumatology* 23(7):1255-1262.

Turk DC, Okifuji A, Sinclair JD, Starz TW. (1998). Differential responses by psychosocial subgroups of fibromyalgia syndrome patients to an interdisciplinary treatment. *Arthritis Care Research* 11(5):397-404.

Turnbull A, Rivier C. (1995a). Brain-periphery connections: Do they play a role in mediating the effect of centrally injected interleukin-1 beta on gonadal function? *Neuroimmunomodulation* 2:224.

Turnbull A, Rivier C. (1995b). Regulation of the HPA axis by cytokines. *Brain, Behavior and Immunity* 9:153.

Turner R, Anglin P, Burkes R, Couture F, Evans W, Goss G, Grimshaw R, Melosky B, Paterson A, Quirt I, Canadian Cancer and Anemia Guidelines Development Group. (2001). Epoetin alfa in cancer patients: Evidence-based guidelines. *Journal of Pain Symptomatology and Management* 22(5):954-965.

Turner S, Maher EJ, Young T, Young J, Vaughan Hudson G. (1996). What are the information priorities for cancer patients involved in treatment decisions? An experienced surrogate study in Hodgkin's disease. *British Journal of Cancer* 73(2):222-227.

Tursz T, Dorval T, Berthaud P, Jouve M, Avril MF, Garcia-Giralt E, Le Chevalier T, Spielmann M, Sevin D, Palangie T, et al. (1991). [Phase I trial of a recombinant human interleukin 2: Results in patients with disseminated solid tumors]. *Presse Medicale* 20(6):250-254.

Twelves CJ, Dobbs NA, Curnow A, Coleman RE, Stewart AL, Tyrrell CJ, Canney P, Rubens RD. (1994). A phase II, multicentre, UK study of vinorelbine in advanced breast cancer. *British Journal of Cancer* 70(5):990-993.

Uchita S, Hata T, Tsushima Y, Matsumoto M, Hina K, Moritani T. (1998). Primary cardiac angiosarcoma with superior vena caval syndrome: Review of surgical resection and interventional management of venous inflow obstruction. *Canadian Journal of Cardiology* 14(10):1283-1285.

Udoh FV, Lot TY, Braide VB. (1999). Effects of extracts of seed and leaf of *Piper guineense* on skeletal muscle activity in rat and frog. *Phytotherapy Research* 13(2):106-110.

Uehara N, Iwahori Y, Asamoto M, Baba-Toriyama H, Iigo M, Ochiai M, Nagao M, Nakayama M, Degawa M, Matsumoto K, et al. (1996). Decreased levels of 2-amino-3-methylimidazol[4,5-f]quinoline-DNA adducts in rats treated with beta-carotene, alpha-tocopherol and freeze-dried aloe. *Japanese Journal of Cancer Research* 87(4):342-348.

Uemura A, Okano A, Sato A. (1992). [A case of secondary lung cancer of cystadenocarcinoma showing multiple thin-walled cavities]. *Nihon Kyobu Shikkan Gakkai Zasshi* 30(11):1986-1990.

Ueno N, Sano T, Kanamaru T, Tanaka K, Nishihara T, Idei Y, Yamamoto M, Okuno T, Kawaguchi K. (2002). Adenosquamous cell carcinoma arising from the papilla major. *Oncology Reports* 9(2):317-320.

Uetsuji S, Yamamura M, Hamada Y, Minoura T, Okuda Y, Yamamichi K, Yamada O, Yamamoto M. (1990). [A double cancer of the gallbladder and common bile duct associated with an anomalous arrangement of the choledocho-pancreatic ductal junction—A case report and a review of the literature]. *Gan No Rinsho* 36(6):752-757.

Unger J. (1996). Fibromyalgia. *Journal of the American Academy of Nurse Practitioners* 8(1):27-29.

Uppgaard RO. (2000). Definition of myofascial face pain. *Journal of the American Dental Association* 131(7):854, 856, 858.

Urba SG, Forastiere AA, Wolf GT, Amrein PC. (1993). Intensive recombinant interleukin-2 and alpha-interferon therapy in patients with advanced head and neck squamous carcinoma. *Cancer* 71(7):2326-2331.

Urba WJ, Longo DL. (1986). Alpha-interferon in the treatment of nodular lymphomas. *Seminars in Oncology* 13(4 Suppl 5):40-47.

Uter W. (2000). Chronic fatigue syndrome and nickel allergy. *Contact Dermatitis* 42(1):56-57.

Vadhan-Raj S, Al-Katib A, Bhalla R, Pelus L, Nathan CF, Sherwin SA, Oettgen HF, Krown SE. (1986). Phase I trial of recombinant interferon gamma in cancer patients. *Journal of Clinical Oncology* 4(2):137-146.

Vadhan-Raj S, Papadopoulos NE, Burgess MA, Linke KA, Patel SR, Hays C, Arcenas A, Plager C, Kudelka AP, Hittelman WN, et al. (1994). Effects of PIXY321, a granulocyte-macrophage colony-stimulating factor/interleukin-3 fusion protein, on chemotherapy-induced multilineage myelosuppression in patients with sarcoma. *Journal of Clinical Oncology* 12(4):715-724.

Vaishampayan UN, Ben-Josef E, Philip PA, Vaitkevicius VK, Du W, Levin KJ, Shields AF. (2002). A single-institution experience with concurrent capecitabine and radiation therapy in gastrointestinal malignancies. *International Journal of Radiation Oncology, Biology, and Physics* 53(3):675-679.

Valdini AF. (1985). Fatigue of unknown aetiology—A review. *Family Practice* 2(1):48-53.

Valdres RU, Escalante C, Manzullo E. (2001). Fatigue: A debilitating symptom. *Nursing Clinics of North America* 36(4):685-694.

Valentine AD, Meyers CA. (2001). Cognitive and mood disturbance as causes and symptoms of fatigue in cancer patients. *Cancer* 92(6 Suppl):1694-1698.

Valero V, Buzdar AU, Theriault RL, Azarnia N, Fonseca GA, Willey J, Ewer M, Walters RS, Mackay B, Podoloff D, et al. (1999). Phase II trial of liposome-encapsulated doxorubicin, cyclophosphamide, and fluorouracil as first-line therapy in patients with metastatic breast cancer. *Journal of Clinical Oncology* 17(5):1425-1434.

Valley AW. (2002). Overview of cancer-related anemia: Focus on the potential role of darbepoetin alfa. *Pharmacotherapy* 22(9 Pt 2):150S-159S.

Van Andel G, Kurth KH, de Haes JC. (1997). Quality of life in patients with prostatic carcinoma: A review and results of a study in N+ disease. Prostate-specific antigen as predictor of quality of life. *Urology Research* 25(Suppl 2):S79-S88.

Van Basten JP, van Driel MF, Jonker-Pool G, Sleijfer DT, Schraffordt Koops H, van de Wiel HB, Hoekstra HJ. (1997). Sexual functioning in testosterone-supplemented patients treated for bilateral testicular cancer. *British Journal of Urology* 79(3):461-467.

Van Besien K, Margolin K, Champlin R, Forman S. (1997). Activity of interleukin-2 in non-Hodgkin's lymphoma following transplantation of interleukin-2-activated autologous bone marrow or stem cells. *Cancer Journal Scientific American* 3(Suppl 1):S54-S58.

Van Dam FS, Linssen AC, Engelsman E, van Benthem J, Hanewald GJ. (1980). Life with cytostatic drugs. *European Journal of Cancer* 1:229-233.

Van de Luit L, Van der Meulen J, Cleophas TJ, Zwinderman AH. (1998). Amplified amplitudes of circadian rhythms and nighttime hypotension in patients with chronic fatigue syndrome: Improvement by inomapil but not by melatonin. *Angiology* 49(11):903-908.

Van de Pol M, ten Velde GP, Wilmink JT, Volovics A, Twijnstra A. (1997). Efficacy and safety of prophylactic cranial irradiation in patients with small cell lung cancer. *Journal of Neurooncology* 35(2):153-160.

Van der Bruggen P, Travesari C, Chomez P, Lurquin C, De Plaen E, Van den Endye B, Knuth A, Boon T. (1991). A gene encoding an antigen recognized by cytolytic T lymphocytes on a human melanoma. *Science* 254:1643-1647.

Van der Burg M, Edelstein M, Gerlis L, Liang CM, Hirschi M, Dawson A. (1985). Recombinant interferon-gamma (immuneron): Results of a phase I trial in patients with cancer. *Journal of Biological Response Modifiers* 4(3):264-272.

Van der Lely AJ, Brownell J, Lamberts SW. (1991). The efficacy and tolerability of CV 205-502 (a nonergot dopaminergic drug) in macroprolactinoma patients and in prolactinoma patients intolerant to bromocriptine. *Journal of Clinical Endocrinology and Metabolism* 72(5):1136-1141.

Van der Meer JW, Elving LD. (1997). [Chronic fatigue—"tired with 23 i's"]. *Nederlander Tijdschrift Geneeskunde* 141(31):1505-1507.

Van der Meer JW, Rijken PM, Bleijenberg G, Thomas S, Hinloopen RJ, Bensing JM. (1997). Indications for management in long-term, physically unexplained fatigue symptoms. *Nederlands Tijdschrift voor Geneeskunde* 141(31):1516-1519.

Van de Wal HJ, Fritschy WM, Skotnicki SH, Lacquet LK. (1988). Primary cardiac tumors. *Acta Chirurgica Belgica* 88(2):74-78.

Van Dijk JM, Sonnenblick M, Kornberg A, Rosin AJ. (1985). Preleukemic syndrome in elderly patients—Report of 11 cases. *Israeli Journal of Medical Sciences* 21(3):292-295.

Vanel D, Couanet D, Piekarski JD, Masselot J. (1983). Radiological findings in 23 pediatric cases of malignant histiocytosis (MH). *European Journal of Radiology* 3(1):60-62.

Van Eldik LJ, Zimmer DB. (1987). Secretion of S-100 from rat C6 glioma cells. *Brain Research* 436:367-370.

Van Ert G, Foss JF, Barlow JF. (1981). Fifty-four year old caucasian male with progressive fatigability. *South Dakota Journal of Medicine* 34(9):29-33.

van Groeningen CJ, Leyva A, O'Brien AM, Gall HE, Pinedo HM. (1986). Phase I and pharmacokinetic study of 5-aza-2'-deoxycytidine (NSC 127716) in cancer patients. *Cancer Research* 46(9):4831-4836.

Van Harten WH, van Noort O, Warmerdam R, Hendricks H, Seidel E. (1998). Assessment of rehabilitation needs in cancer patients. *International Journal of Rehabilitation Research* 21(3):247-257.

Van Herpen CM, Jansen RL, Kruit WH, Hoekman K, Groenewegen G, Osanto S, De Mulder PH. (2000). Immunochemotherapy with interleukin-2, interferon-alpha and 5-fluorouracil for progressive metastatic renal cell carcinoma: A multicenter phase II study. Dutch Immunotherapy Working Party. *British Journal of Cancer* 82(4):772-776.

Vanky F, Nagy N, Hising C, Sjovall K, Larson B, Klein E. (1997). Human ex vivo carcinoma cells produce transforming growth factor beta and thereby can inhibit lymphocyte functions in vitro. *Cancer Immunology and Immunotherapy* 43:317-323.

Van Mens-Verhulst J, Bensing JM. (1997). Sex differences in persistent fatigue. *Women and Health* 26(3):51-70.

Van Mens-Verhulst J, Bensing JM. (1998). Distinguishing between chronic and non-chronic fatigue, the role of gender and age. *Social Science and Medicine* 47(5): 621-634.

Van Poznak C, Seidman AD, Reidenberg MM, Moasser MM, Sklarin N, Van Zee K, Borgen P, Gollub M, Bacotti D, Yao TJ, et al. (2001). Oral gossypol in the treatment of patients with refractory metastatic breast cancer: A phase I/II clinical trial. *Breast Cancer Research and Treatment* 66(3):239-248.

Van Santen-Hoeufft M. (1996). Typical fibromyalgia. *Clinical Rheumatology* 15(3): 233-235.

Van Snick J. (1990). Interleukin-6: An overview. *Annual Reviews in Immunology* 8:253-278.

Vansteenkiste J, Pirker R, Massuti B, Barata F, Font A, Fiegl M, Siena S, Gateley J, Tomita D, Colowick AB, et al. (2002). Double-blind, placebo-controlled, randomized phase III trial of darbepoetin alfa in lung cancer patients receiving chemotherapy. *Journal of the National Cancer Institutes* 94(16):1211-1220.

Van Waveren EK. (1996). The rise and fall of the chronic fatigue syndrome as defined by Holmes et al. *Medical Hypotheses* 46(2):63-66.

Van Wegberg B, Bacchi M, Heusser P, Helwig S, Schaad R, von Rohr E, Bernhard J, Hurny C, Castiglione M, Cerny T. (1998). The cognitive-spiritual dimension—an important addition to the assessment of quality of life: Validation of a questionnaire (SELT-M) in patients with advanced cancer. *Annals of Oncology* 9(10):1091-1096.

Van Zandwijk N, Jassem E, Dubbelmann R, Braat MC, Rumke P. (1990). Aerosol application of interferon-alpha in the treatment of bronchioloalveolar carcinoma. *European Journal of Cancer* 26(6):738-740.

Vara-Thorbeck R, Guerrero JA, Ruiz-Requena E, Garcia-Carriazo M. (1996). Can the use of growth hormone reduce the postoperative fatigue syndrome? *World Journal of Surgery* 20(1):81-86; discussion 86-87.

Varga E, Hadju Z, Veres K, Mathe I, Nemeth E, Pluhar Z, Bernath J. (1998). Investigation of variation of the production of biological and chemical compounds of *Hyssopus officinalis* L. *Acta Pharmaceutica Hungarica* 68(3):183-188.

Varni JW, Burwinkle TM, Katz ER, Meeske K, Dickinson P. (2002). The PedsQL in pediatric cancer: Reliability and validity of the Pediatric Quality of Life Inventory Generic Core Scales, Multidimensional Fatigue Scale, and Cancer Module. *Cancer* 94(7):2090-2106.

Varterasian ML, Mohammad RM, Eilender DS, Hulburd K, Rodriguez DH, Pemberton PA, Pluda JM, Dan MD, Pettit GR, Chen BD, et al. (1998). Phase I study of bryostatin 1 in patients with relapsed non-Hodgkin's lymphoma and chronic lymphocytic leukemia. *Journal of Clinical Oncology* 16(1):56-62.

Varterasian ML, Mohammad RM, Shurafa MS, Hulburd K, Pemberton PA, Rodriguez DH, Spadoni V, Eilender DS, Murgo A, Wall N, et al. (2000). Phase II trial of bryostatin 1 in patients with relapsed low-grade non-Hodgkin's lymphoma and chronic lymphocytic leukemia. *Clinical Cancer Research* 6(3):825-828.

Varveris H, Mazonakis M, Vlachaki M, Kachris S, Lyraraki E, Zoras O, Maris T, Froudarakis M, Velegrakis J, Perysinakis C, et al. (2003). A phase I trial of weekly docetaxel and cisplatinum combined to concurrent hyperfractionated radiotherapy for non-small cell lung cancer and squamous cell carcinoma of head and neck. *Oncology Reports* 10(1):185-195.

Vasey FB. (1997). Clinical experience with systemic illness in women with silicone breast implants: Comment on the editorial by Rose. *Arthritis and Rheumatism* 40(8):1545.

Vasey FB, Aziz N. (1995). Breast implants and connective-tissue diseases. *New England Journal of Medicine* 333(21):1423; discussion 1424.

Vasey PA, Atkinson R, Coleman R, Crawford M, Cruickshank M, Eggleton P, Fleming D, Graham J, Parkin D, Paul J, et al. (2001). Docetaxel-carboplatin as first line chemotherapy for epithelial ovarian cancer. *British Journal of Cancer* 84(2):170-178.

Vasey PA, Bissett D, Strolin-Benedetti M, Poggesi I, Breda M, Adams L, Wilson P, Pacciarini MA, Kaye SB, Cassidy J. (1995). Phase I clinical and pharmacokinetic study of 3'-deamino-3'-(2-methoxy-4-morpholinyl)doxorubicin (FCE 23762). *Cancer Research* 55(10):2090-2096.

Vastag B, Bleider N. (1998). Tired out: Patients find easy answers for cancer-related fatigue. *Journal of the National Cancer Institute* 90(21):1591-1594.

Vazquez B, Avila G, Segura D, Escalante B. (1996). Anti-inflammatory activity of extracts from *Aloë vera* gel. *Journal of Ethnopharmacology* 55(1):69-75.

Vecchiet L, Montanari G, Pizzigallo E, Iezzi S, De Bigontina P, Dragani L, Vecchiet J, Giamberardino MA. (1996). Sensory characterization of somatic parietal tissues in humans with chronic fatigue syndrome. *Neuroscience Letters* 208(2):117-120.

Veldhuis GJ, Willemse PH, Mulder NH, Limburg PC, De Vries EG. (1996). Potential use of recombinant human interleukin-6 in clinical oncology. *Leukemia and Lymphoma* 20(5-6):373-379.

Velikova G, Wright EP, Smith AB, Cull A, Gould A, Forman D, Perren T, Stead M, Brown J, Selby PJ. (1999). Automated collection of quality-of-life data: A comparison of paper and computer touch-screen questionnaires. *Journal of Clinical Oncology* 17(3):998-1007.

Velikova G, Wright P, Smith AB, Stark D, Perren T, Brown J, Selby P. (2001). Self-reported quality of life of individual cancer patients: Concordance of results with disease course and medical records. *Journal of Clinical Oncology* 19(7):2064-2073.

Venetsanakos E, Beckman I, Bradley J, Skinner JM. (1997). High incidence of interleukin 10 mRNA but not interleukin-2 mRNA detected in human breast tumors. *British Journal of Cancer* 75(12):1826-1830.

Vercoulen JH, Bazelmans E, Swanink CM, Galama JM, Fennis JF, Van der Meer JW, Bleijenberg G. (1998). Evaluating neuropsychological impairment in chronic fatigue syndrome. *Journal of Clinical and Experimental Neuropsychology* 20(2):144-156.

Vercoulen JH, Hommes OR, Swanink CM, Jongen PJ, Fennis JF, Galama JM, Van der Meer JW, Bleijenberg G. (1996). The measurement of fatigue in patients with multiple sclerosis: A multidimensional comparison with patients with chronic fatigue syndrome and healthy subjects. *Archives of Neurology* 53(7):642-649.

Vercoulen JH, Swanink CM, Fennis JF, Galama JM, Van der Meer JW, Bleijenberg G. (1996). Prognosis in chronic fatigue syndrome: A prospective study on the natural course. *Journal of Neurology, Neurosurgery and Psychiatry* 60(5):489-494.

Vercoulen JH, Swanink CM, Zitman FG, Vreden SGS, Hoofs MPE, Fennis JFM, Galama JMD, van der Meer JWM, Bleijenberg G. (1996). Randomized, double-blind, placebo-controlled study of fluoxetine in chronic fatigue syndrome. *Lancet* 347(9005):858-861.

Verdi CJ, Taylor CW, Croghan MK, Dalke P, Meyskens FL, Hersh EM. (1992). Phase I study of low-dose cyclophosphamide and recombinant interleukin-2 for the treatment of advanced cancer. *Journal of Immunotherapy* 11(4):286-291.

Verschraegen CF, Kavanagh JJ, Loyer E, Bodurka-Bevers D, Kudelka AP, Hu W, Vincent M, Nelson T, Levenback C, Community Clinical Oncology Program. (2001). Phase II study of carboplatin and liposomal doxorubicin in patients with recurrent squamous cell carcinoma of the cervix. *Cancer* 92(9):2327-2333.

Verschraegen CF, Levy T, Kudelka AP, Llerena E, Ende K, Freedman RS, Edwards CL, Hord M, Steger M, Kaplan AL, et al. (1997). Phase II study of irinotecan in prior chemotherapy-treated squamous cell carcinoma of the cervix. *Journal of Clinical Oncology* 15(2):625-631.

Versluis RG, De Waal MW, Opmeer C, Petri H, Springer MP. (1997). Prevalence of chronic fatigue syndrome in 4 family practices in Leiden. *Nederlands Tijdschrift voor Geneeskunde* 141(31):1523-1526.

Vest S, Bork E, Hansen HH. (1988). A phase I evaluation of N10-propargyl-5,8-dideazafolic acid. *European Journal of Cancer and Clinical Oncology* 24(2): 201-204.

Villa ML, Ferrario E, Bergamasco E, Bozzetti F, Cozzaglio L, Clerici E. (1991). Reduced natural killer cell activity and IL-2 production in malnourished cancer patients. *British Journal of Cancer* 63:1010-1014.

Villemain F, Chatenoud L, Galinowski A, Homo-Delarche F, Ginestet D, Loo H, Zarifian E, Bach JF. (1989). Aberrant T-cell-mediated immunity in untreated schizophrenic patients: Deficient interleukin-2 production. *American Journal of Psychiatry* 146(5):609-616.

Virik K, Glare P. (2002). Requests for euthanasia made to a tertiary referral teaching hospital in Sydney, Australia in the year 2000. *Support Care in Cancer* 10(4): 309-313.

Visser J, Blauw B, Hinloopen B, Brommer E, De Kloet ER, Kluft C, Nagelkerken L. (1998). CD4 T lymphocytes from patients with chronic fatigue syndrome have decreased interferon-gamma production and increased sensitivity to dexamethasone. *Journal of Infectious Diseases* 177(2):451-454.

Visser MR, Smets EM. (1998). Fatigue, depression and quality of life in cancer patients: How are they related? *Support Care in Cancer* 6(2):101-108.

Visser MR, Smets EM, Sprangers MA, de Haes HJ. (2000). How response shift may affect the measurement of change in fatigue. *Journal of Pain Symptomatology and Management* 20(1):12-18.

Vitale G, Tagliaferri P, Caraglia M, Rampone E, Ciccarelli A, Bianco AR, Abbruzzese A, Lupoli G. (2000). Slow release lanreotide in combination with interferon-alpha2b in the treatment of symptomatic advanced medullary thyroid carcinoma. *Journal of Clinical Endocrinology and Metabolism* 85(3):983-988.

Vlaeyen JW, Teeken-Gruben NJ, Goosens ME, Rutten-van Molken MP, Pelt RA, Van Eek H, Heuts PH. (1996). Cognitive-educational treatment of fibromyalgia: A randomized clinical trial. I. Clinical effects. *Journal of Rheumatology* 23(7): 1237-1245.

Vlasveld LT, Rankin EM, Hekman A, Rodenhuis S, Beijnen JH, Hilton AM, Dubbelman AC, Vyth-Dreese FA, Melief CJ. (1992). A phase I study of prolonged continuous infusion of low dose recombinant interleukin-2 in melanoma and renal cell cancer: Part I. Clinical aspects. *British Journal of Cancer* 65(5): 744-750.

Vogelzang NJ, Breitbart W, Cella D, Curt GA, Groopman JE, Horning SJ, Itri LM, Johnson DH, Scherr SL, Portenoy RK. (1997). Patient, caregiver, and oncologist perceptions of cancer-related fatigue: Results of a tripart assessment survey. The Fatigue Coalition. *Seminars in Hematology* 34(3 Suppl 2):4-12.

Vogelzang NJ, Lipton A, Figlin RA. (1993). Subcutaneous interleukin-2 plus interferon alfa-2a in metastatic renal cancer: An outpatient multicenter trial. *Journal of Clinical Oncology* 11(9):1809-1816.

Vogl SE, Pagano M, Horton J. (1984). Phase II study of methyl-glyoxal bis-guanylhydrazone (NSC 3296) in advanced ovarian cancer. *American Journal of Clinical Oncology* 7(6):733-736.

Vojdani A, Choppa PC, Tagle C, Andrin R, Samimi B, Lapp CW. (1998). Detection of *Mycoplasma* genus and *Mycoplasma fermentans* by PCR in patients with chronic fatigue syndrome. *FEMS Immunology and Medical Microbiology* 22: 355-365.

Vojdani A, Franco AR. (1999). Multiplex PCR for the detection of *Mycoplasma fermentans, M. hominis* and *M. penetrans* in patients with chronic fatigue syndrome, fibromyalgia, rheumatoid arthritis and Gulf War illness. *Journal of Chronic Fatigue Syndrome* 5:187-197.

Vojdani A, Ghoneum M, Choppa PC, Magtoto L, Lapp CW. (1997). Elevated apoptotic cell population in patients with chronic fatigue syndrome: The pivotal role of protein kinase RNA. *Journal of Internal Medicine* 242(6):465-478.

Vojdani A, Lapp CW. (1999). The relationship between chronic fatigue syndrome and chemical exposure. *Journal of Chronic Fatigue Syndrome* 5(3/4):207-221.

Vokes EE, Figlin R, Hochster H, Lotze M, Rybak ME. (1998). A phase II study of recombinant human interleukin-4 for advanced or recurrent non-small cell lung cancer. *Cancer Journal Scientific American* 4(1):46-51.

Vokes EE, Gordon GS, Rudin CM, Mauer AM, Watson S, Krauss S, Arrieta R, Golomb HM, Hoffman PC. (2001). A phase II trial of 9-aminocaptothecin (9-AC) as a 120-h infusion in patients with non-small cell lung cancer. *Investigative New Drugs* 19(4):329-333.

Vollmer-Conna U, Wakefield D, Lloyd A, Hickie I, Lemon J, Bird KD, Westbrook RF. (1997). Cognitive deficits in patients suffering from chronic fatigue syndrome, acute infective illness or depression. *British Journal of Psychiatry* 171: 377-381.

Von der Maase H, Geertsen P, Thatcher N, Jasmin C, Mercatello A, Fossa SD, Symann M, Stoter G, Nagel G, Israel L, et al. (1991). Recombinant interleukin-2 in metastatic renal cell carcinoma—A European multicentre phase II study. *European Journal of Cancer* 27(12):1583-1589.

Von der Maase H, Hansen SW, Roberts JT, Dogliotti L, Oliver T, Moore MJ, Bodrogi I, Albers P, Knuth A, Lippert CM, et al. (2000). Gemcitabine and cisplatin versus methotrexate, vinblastine, doxorubicin, and cisplatin in advanced or metastatic bladder cancer: Results of a large, randomized, multinational, multicenter, phase III study. *Journal of Clinical Oncology* 18(17):3068-3077.

Von Mehren M, Giantonio BJ, McAleer C, Schilder R, McPhillips J, O'Dwyer PJ. (1995). Phase I trial of ilmofosine as a 24 hour infusion weekly. *Investigative New Drugs* 13(3):205-210.

Von Mikecz A, Konstantinov K, Buchwald DS, Gerace L, Tan EM. (1997). High frequency of autoantibodies in patients with chronic fatigue syndrome. *Arthritis and Rheumatism* 40(2):295-305.

Von Pawel J, Schiller JH, Shepherd FA, Fields SZ, Kleisbauer JP, Chrysson NG, Stewart DJ, Clark PI, Palmer MC, Depierre A, et al. (1999). Topotecan versus cyclophosphamide, doxorubicin, and vincristine for the treatment of recurrent small-cell lung cancer. *Journal of Clinical Oncology* 17(2):658-667.

Von Petrykowski W, Jobke A, Keefer I, Kuhn FP. (1983). [Asymptomatic, excessive hypercalcemia in a 12-year-old boy]. *Monatsschrift Kinderheilkunde* 131(3): 166-168.

Voravud N, Lippman SM, Weber RS, Rodriquez GI, Yee D, Dimery IW, Earley CL, Von Hoff DD, Hong WK. (1993). Phase II trial of 13-cis-retinoic acid plus interferon-alpha in recurrent head and neck cancer. *Investigative New Drugs* 11(1):57-60.

Vordermark D, Schwab M, Flentje M, Sailer M, Kolbl O. (2002). Chronic fatigue after radiotherapy for carcinoma of the prostate: Correlation with anorectal and genitourinary function. *Radiotherapy and Oncology* 62(3):293-297.

Vree R. (1997). Fireworks over fibromyalgia, CFS, and IBS. *Postgraduate Medicine* 102(6):44.

Vroegop P, Burghouts JT. (1989). [Prolonging of life with cytostatic agents: Is it worthwhile? A questionnaire survey of relatives]. *Nederlander Tijdschrift Geneeskunde* 133(44):2173-2177.

Vugrin D, Hood L, Laszlo J. (1986). A phase II trial of high-dose human lymphoblastoid alpha interferon in patients with advanced renal carcinoma. *Journal of Biological Response Modifiers* 5(4):309-312.

Vujosevic M, Gvozdenovic E. (1994). [The role of Epstein-Barr virus infections in human pathology]. *Med Pregl* 47(11-12):393-397.

Vuoristo M, Jantunen I, Pyrhonen S, Muhonen T, Kellokumpu-Lehtinen P. (1994). A combination of subcutaneous recombinant interleukin-2 and recombinant interferon-alpha in the treatment of advanced renal cell carcinoma or melanoma. *European Journal of Cancer* 30A(4):530-532.

Wada S, Kurihara S, Imamaki K, Yokota K, Kitahama S, Yamanaka K, Itabashi A, Iitaka M, Katayama S. (1999). Hypercalcemia accompanied by hypothalamic hypopituitarism, central diabetes insipidus and hyperthyroidism. *Internal Medicine* 38(6):486-490.

Wadler S, Brain C, Catalano P, Einzig AI, Cella D, Benson AB III. (2002). Randomized phase II trial of either fluorouracil, parenteral hydroxyurea, interferon-alpha-2a, and filgrastim or doxorubicin/docetaxel in patients with advanced gastric cancer with quality-of-life assessment: Eastern Cooperative Oncology Group study E6296. *Cancer Journal* 8(3):282-286.

Wadler S, Einzig AI, Dutcher JP, Ciobanu N, Landau L, Wiernik PH. (1988). Phase II trial of recombinant alpha-2b-interferon and low-dose cyclophosphamide in advanced melanoma and renal cell carcinoma. *American Journal of Clinical Oncology* 11(1):55-59.

Wadler S, Gleissner B, Hilgenfeld RU, Thiel E, Haynes H, Kaleya R, Rozenblit A, Kreuser ED. (1996). Phase II trial of *N*-(phosphonacetyl)-L-aspartate (PALA), 5-fluorouracil and recombinant interferon-alpha-2b in patients with advanced gastric carcinoma. *European Journal of Cancer* 32A(7):1254-1256.

Wadler S, Goldman M, Lyver A, Wiernik PH. (1990). Phase I trial of 5-fluorouracil and recombinant alpha 2a-interferon in patients with advanced colorectal carcinoma. *Cancer Research* 50(7):2056-2059.

Wadler S, Haynes H, Rozenblit A, Hu X, Kaleya R, Wiernik PH. (1998). Sequential phase II trials of fluorouracil and interferon beta ser with or without sargramostim in patients with advanced colorectal carcinoma. *Cancer Journal Scientific American* 4(5):331-337.

Wadler S, Lembersky B, Atkins M, Kirkwood J, Petrelli N. (1991). Phase II trial of fluorouracil and recombinant interferon alfa-2a in patients with advanced colorectal carcinoma: An Eastern Cooperative Oncology Group study. *Journal of Clinical Oncology* 9(10):1806-1810.

Wadler S, Wiernik PH. (1990). Clinical update on the role of fluorouracil and recombinant interferon alfa-2a in the treatment of colorectal carcinoma. *Seminars in Oncology* 17(1 Suppl 1):16-21; discussion 38-41.

Wagner GJ, Rabkin JG. (1998). Testosterone, illness progression, and megestrol use in HIV-positive men. *Journal of AIDS and Human Retrovirology* 17(2):179-180.

Wagner GJ, Rabkin JG, Rabkin R. (1998). Testosterone as a treatment for fatigue in HIV+ men. *General Hospital Psychiatry* 20(4):209-213.

Wagstaff J, Chadwick G, Howell A, Thatcher N, Scarffe JH, Crowther D. (1984). A phase I toxicity study of human rDNA interferon in patients with solid tumours. *Cancer Chemotherapy Pharmacology* 13(2):100-105.

Wakui A, Konno K, Abe R, Kanamaru R, Takahashi K, Nakai Y, Yoshida Y, Koie H, Masuda H, et al. (1986). Randomized study of lentinan on patients with advanced gastric and colorectal cancer. Tohoku Lentinan Study Group. *Japanese Journal of Cancer Chemotherapy* 13:1050.

Walger P, Baumgart P, Adams U, Vetter H. (1992). [Adrenal cortex carcinoma: Diagnosis, therapy and course in 10 cases]. *Schweizerische Rundschau fur Medizin Praxis* 81(25):824-833.

Walker BL, Nail LM, Larsen L, Magill J, Schwartz A. (1996). Concerns, affect, and cognitive disruption following completion of radiation treatment for localized breast or prostate cancer. *Oncology Nursing Forum* 23(8):1181-1187.

Walker EA, Katon WJ, Keegan D, Gardner G, Sullivan M. (1997). Predictors of physician frustration in the care of patients with rheumatological complaints. *General Hospital Psychiatry* 19(5):315-323.

Walker EA, Keegan D, Gardner G, Sullivan M, Katon WJ, Bernstein D. (1997). Psychosocial factors in fibromyalgia compared with rheumatoid arthritis: I. Psychiatric diagnoses and functional disability. *Psychosomatic Medicine* 59(6):565-571.

Walker K, McGown A, Jantos M, Anson J. (1997). Fatigue, depression, and quality of life in HIV-positive men. *Journal of Psychosocial Nursing and Mental Health Services* 35(9):32-40.

Wallace DJ. (1997). The fibromyalgia syndrome. *Annals of Medicine* 29(1):9-21.

Wallace DJ. (1999). What constitutes a fibromyalgia expert? *Arthritis Care Research* 12(2):82-84.

Wallace DJ, Shapiro S, Panush RS. (1999). Update on fibromyalgia syndrome. *Bulletin of Rheumatic Diseases* 48(5):1-4.

Walsh D, Donnelly S, Rybicki L. (2000). The symptoms of advanced cancer: Relationship to age, gender, and performance status in 1,000 patients. *Support Care in Cancer* 8(3):175-179.

Walsh JK, Hartman PG, Schweitzer PK. (1994). Slow wave sleep deprivation and waking function. *Journal of Sleep Research* 3:16-25.

Walston J, McBurnie MA, Newman A, Tracy RP, Kop WJ, Hirsch CH, Gottdiener J, Fried LP. (2002). Frailty and activation of the inflammation and coagulation systems with and without clinical comorbidities: Results from the Cardiovascular Health Study. *Archives of Internal Medicine* 162(20):2333-2341.

Walter G, Rey JM. (1999). The relevance of herbal treatments for psychiatric practice. *Australian and New Zealand Journal of Psychiatry* 33(4):482-489; discussion 490-493.

Walters RS, Holmes FA, Valero V, Esparza-Guerra L, Hortobagyi GN. (1998). Phase II study of ifosfamide and mesna in patients with metastatic breast cancer. *American Journal of Clinical Oncology* 21(4):413-415.

Wander HE, Nagel GA, Blossey HC, Kleeberg U. (1986). Aminoglutethimide and medroxyprogesterone acetate in the treatment of patients with advanced breast cancer: A phase II study of the Association of Medical Oncology of the German Cancer Society (AIO). *Cancer* 58(9):1985-1989.

Wang B, Gladman DD, Urowitz MB. (1998). Fatigue in lupus is not correlated with disease activity. *The Journal of Rheumatology* 25(5):892-895.

Wang L. (2002). Cancer care should include symptom management, panel says. *Journal of the National Cancer Institutes* 94(15):1123-1124.

Wang QL, Sun Y, Zhou JC, Song SZ, Feng FY, Lu L, Yie ZS. (1988). [High-dose methotrexate with citrovorum factor rescue (HD-MTX-CFR) in the treatment of malignant solid tumors—Clinical analysis of 62 patients]. *Zhonghua Zhong Liu Za Zhi* 10(2):152-154.

Wang XS, Giralt SA, Mendoza TR, Engstrom MC, Johnson BA, Peterson N, Broemeling LD, Cleeland CS. (2002). Clinical factors associated with cancer-related fatigue in patients being treated for leukemia and non-Hodgkin's lymphoma. *Journal of Clinical Oncology* 20(5):1319-1328.

Wang XS, Janjan NA, Guo H, Johnson BA, Engstrom MC, Crane CH, Mendoza TR, Cleeland CS. (2001). Fatigue during preoperative chemoradiation for resectable rectal cancer. *Cancer* 92(6 Suppl):1725-1732.

Wank R, Thomsen C. (1991). High risk of squamous-cell carcinoma of the cervix for women with HLA-DQ3. *Nature* 352:723-725.

Ward MH, DeLisle H, Shores JH, Slocum PC, Foresman BH. (1996). Chronic fatigue complaints in primary care: Incidence and diagnostic patterns. *Journal of the American Osteopathic Association* 96(1):34-46.

Ware JC, Russell IJ, Campos E. (1986). Alpha intrusions into the sleep of depression and fibromyalgia syndrome (fibrositis) patients. *Sleep Research* 15:210.

Ware JE, Sherbourne CD. (1992). The MOS 36-item Short-Form Health Survey (SF-36): Conceptual framework and item selection. *Medical Care* 6:473-483.

Ware NC. (1998). Sociosomatics and illness in chronic fatigue syndrome. *Psychosomatic Medicine* 60(4):394-401.

Warner E, Keshavjee al-N, Shupack R, Bellini A. (1997). Rheumatic symptoms following adjuvant therapy for breast cancer. *American Journal of Clinical Oncology* 20(3):322-326.

Warrell RP Jr, Coonley CJ, Burchenal JH. (1983). Sequential inhibition of polyamine synthesis: A phase I trial of DFMO (alpha-difluoromethylornithine) and methyl-GAG [methylglyoxal-bis(guanylhydrazone)]. *Cancer Chemotherapy Pharmacology* 11(2):134-136.

Watanabe K. (2001). [Presentation of a case of hematological malignancy in reversed C.P.C.]. *Rinsho Byori* 115:129-134.

Watanabe M, Watanabe A, Noguchi M, Nishiwaki K. (1997). [Invasive thymoma in patient with pernicious anemia and pericardial effusion]. *Nihon Kyobu Shikkan Gakkai Zasshi* 35(6):665-669.

Watanabe N, Yamauchi N, Maeda M, Neda H, Tsuji Y, Okamoto T, Tsuji N, Akiyama S, Sasaki H, Niitsu Y. (1994). Recombinant human tumor necrosis factor causes regression in patients with advanced malignancies. *Oncology* 51(4): 360-365.

Wataya H, Ogata K, Morooka M, Nakahashi H, Hara N. (1998). [T 0 N 2 M 0 small cell lung cancer in a patient with Lambert-Eaton myasthenic syndrome]. *Nihon Kokyuki Gakkai Zasshi* 36(4):389-393.

Watson J, Mochizuki D. (1980). Interleukin-2: A class of T cell growth factor. *Immunological Reviews* 51:257-278.

Watson WS, McMillan DC, Chaudhuri A, Behan PO. (1998). Increased resting energy expenditure in the chronic fatigue syndrome. *Journal of Chronic Fatigue Syndrome* 4(4):3-14.

Watt-Watson J, Graydon J. (1995). Impact of surgery on head and neck cancer patients and their caregivers. *Nursing Clinics of North America* 30(4):659-671.

Wearden AJ, Appleby L. (1996). Research on cognitive complaints and cognitive functioning in patients with chronic fatigue syndrome (CFS): What conclusions can we draw? *Journal of Psychosomatic Research* 41(3):197-211.

Wearden AJ, Appleby L. (1997). Cognitive performance and complaints of cognitive impairment in chronic fatigue syndrome (CFS). *Psychological Medicine* 27(1):81-90.

Wearden AJ, Morriss RK, Mullis R, Strickland PL, Pearson DJ, Appleby L, Campbell IT, Morris JA. (1998). Randomised, double-blind, placebo-controlled treatment trial of fluoxetine and graded exercise for chronic fatigue syndrome. *British Journal of Psychiatry* 172(June):485-490.

Weaver D. (1999). Melatonin and circadian rhythmicity in vertebrates: Physiological roles and pharmacological effects. In *Regulation of Sleep and Circadian Rhythms,* Turek FW, Zee PC, eds. New York: Marcel Dekker, pp. 197-262.

Webb SM. (1998). Fibromyalgia and melatonin: Are they related? *Clinical Endocrinology* (Oxford) 49(2):161-162.

Weber J, Yang JC, Topalian SL, Parkinson DR, Schwartzentruber DS, Ettinghausen SE, Gunn H, Mixon A, Kim H, Cole D, et al. (1993). Phase I trial of subcutaneous interleukin-6 in patients with advanced malignancies. *Journal of Clinical Oncology* 11(3):499-506.

Weber U. (1998). [Fibromyalgia (generalized tendomyopathy) expert assessment practice] Die fibromyalgie (generalisierte tendomyopathie) in der begutachtungssituation. *Schweize Rundschift Medizin Praxis* 87(24):856.

Webster T, Patarca R, Lathrop R, Smith TF. (1989). Potential structural motifs for reverse transcriptases. *Molecular Biology and Evolution* 6:317-320.

Weglicki WB, Stafford RE, Dickens BF, Mak IT, Cassidy MM, Phillips TM. (1993). Inhibition of tumor necrosis factor-alpha by thalidomide in magnesium deficiency. *Molecular and Cellular Biochemistry* 129(2):195-200.

Wei T, Lightman SL. (1997). The neuroendocrine axis in patients with multiple sclerosis. *Brain* 120(Pt 6):1067-1076.

Weibel RE, Benor DE. (1996). Chronic arthropathy and musculoskeletal symptoms associated with rubella vaccines: A review of 124 claims submitted to the National Vaccine Injury Compensation Program. *Arthritis and Rheumatism* 39(9): 1529-1534.

Weiner LM, Padavic-Shaller K, Kitson J, Watts P, Krigel RL, Litwin S. (1991). Phase I evaluation of combination therapy with interleukin 2 and gamma-interferon. *Cancer Research* 51(15):3910-3918.

Weinstein L. (1987). Thyroiditis and "chronic infectious mononucleosis." *New England Journal of Medicine* 317:1225-1226.

Weintraub MI. (1999). Legal implications of practicing alternative medicine. *JAMA* 281(18):1698-1699.

Weisburger JH, Wynder EL. (1987). Etiology of colorectal cancer with emphasis on mechanism of action and prevention. *Important Advances in Oncology* 15:197-220.

Weisdorf D, Katsanis E, Verfaillie C, Ramsay NK, Haake R, Garrison L, Blazar BR. (1994). Interleukin-1 alpha administered after autologous transplantation: A phase I/II clinical trial. *Blood* 84(6):2044-2049.

Weiss B. (1998). Neurobehavioral properties of chemical sensitivity syndromes. *Neurotoxicology* 19(2):259-268.

Weiss GR, Garnick MB, Osteen RT, Steele GD Jr, Wilson RE, Schade D, Kaplan WD, Boxt LM, Kandarpa K, Mayer RJ, et al. (1983). Long-term hepatic arterial infusion of 5-fluorodeoxyuridine for liver metastases using an implantable infusion pump. *Journal of Clinical Oncology* 1(5):337-344.

Weiss GR, Kuhn JG, Rizzo J, Smith LS, Rodriguez GI, Eckardt JR, Burris HA III, Fields S, VanDenBerg K, von Hoff DD. (1995). A phase I and pharmacokinetics study of 2-chlorodeoxyadenosine in patients with solid tumors. *Cancer Chemotherapy Pharmacology* 35(5):397-402.

Weiss GR, Liu PY, Alberts DS, Peng YM, Fisher E, Xu MJ, Scudder SA, Baker LH Jr, Moore DF, Lippman SM. (1998). 13-cis-retinoic acid or all-trans-retinoic acid plus interferon-alpha in recurrent cervical cancer: A Southwest Oncology Group phase II randomized trial. *Gynecological Oncology* 71(3):386-390.

Weiss GR, McGovren JP, Schade D, Kufe DW. (1982). Phase I and pharmacological study of acivicin by 24-hour continuous infusion. *Cancer Research* 42(9): 3892-3895.

Weiss RB, Greene RF, Knight RD, Collins JM, Pelosi JJ, Sulkes A, Curt GA. (1988). Phase I and clinical pharmacology study of intravenous flavone acetic acid (NSC 347512). *Cancer Research* 48(20):5878-5882.

Weitzner MA, Moncello J, Jacobsen PB, Minton S. (2002). A pilot trial of paroxetine for the treatment of hot flashes and associated symptoms in women with breast cancer. *Journal of Pain Symptom and Management* 23(4):337-345.

Wells JN, Fedric T. (2001). Helping patients manage cancer-related fatigue. *Home Healthcare Nurse* 19(8):486-493.

Wells V, Mallucci L. (1985). Expression of the 2-5A system during the cell cycle. *Experimental Cell Research* 159:27-36.

Wenzel L, Berkowitz R, Robinson S, Bernstein M, Goldstein D. (1992). The psychological, social, and sexual consequences of gestational trophoblastic disease. *Gynecological Oncology* 46(1):74-81.

Werner ER, Werner-Felmayer G, Fuchs D, Hausen A, Reibnegger G, Yim JJ, Pfeiderer W, Wachter H. (1990). Tetrahydrobiopterin biosynthetic activities in human macrophages, fibroblasts, THP-1, and T24 cells: GTP-cyclohydrolase I is stimulated by interferon-gamma, and 6-pyruvoyl tetrahydopterin synthase and sepiapterin reductase are constitutively present. *Journal of Biological Chemistry* 265(6):3189-3192.

Werner R. (1974). [Primary reticulum cell sarcomas of the small intestine]. *Zentralblatt Allergie Pathologie* 118(4):390-392.

Werner S, Jacobsson B, Bostrom L, Curstedt T, Weger A, Biberfeld P. (1985). Cushing's syndrome due to an ACTH-producing neuroendocrine tumour in the nasal roof. *Acta Medica Scandinavica* 217(2):235-240.

Werter M, de Witte R, Janssen J, de Pauw B, Haanen C. (1988). Recombinant human interferon-alpha induced cytoreduction in chronic myelogenous leukemia: Results of a multicenter study. *Blut* 56(5):209-212.

Wessely S. (1990). Old wine in new bottles: Neurasthenia and "ME." *Psychological Medicine* 20:35-53.

Wessely S. (1991). History of postviral fatigue syndrome. *British Medical Bulletin* 47(4):919-941.

Wessely S. (1996). Chronic fatigue syndrome: Summary of a report of a joint committee of the Royal College of Physicians, Psychiatrists and General Practitioners. *Journal of the Royal College of Physicians of London* 30(6):497-504.

Wessely S. (1997). Chronic fatigue syndrome: A 20th century illness? *Scandinavian Journal of Work, Environment and Health* 23(Suppl. 3):17-34.

Wessely S. (1998). The epidemiology of chronic fatigue syndrome. *Epidemiologia E. Psichiatria Sociale* 7(1):10-24.

Wessely S. (2001). Chronic fatigue: Symptom and syndrome. *Annals of Internal Medicine* 134(9 Pt 2):838-843.

Wessely S, Chalder T, Hirsch S, Wallace P, Wright D. (1996). Psychological symptoms, somatic symptoms, and psychiatric disorder in chronic fatigue and chronic fatigue syndrome. *American Journal of Psychiatry* 153(8):1050-1059.

Wessely S, Chalder T, Hirsch S, Wallace P, Wright D. (1997). The prevalence and morbidity of chronic fatigue and chronic fatigue syndrome: A prospective primary care study. *American Journal of Public Health* 87(9):1449-1455.

Wessely S, Hotopf M. (1999). Is fibromyalgia a distinct clinical entity? Historical and epidemiological evidence. *Baillieres Best Practice Research in Clinical Rheumatology* 13(3):427-436.

Wessely S, Powell R. (1989). Fatigue syndromes: A comparison of chronic post-viral fatigue with neuromuscular and affective disorders. *Journal of Neurology, Neurosurgery and Psychiatry* 52:940-948.

Westemann J, Pabst R. (1996). How organ specific is the migration of "naïve" and "memory" T cells? *Immunology Today* 17:278-282.

Westendorf J, Pfau W, Schulte A. (1998). Carcinogenicity and DNA adduct formation observed in ACI rats after long-term treatment with madder root, *Rubia tinctorum* L. *Carcinogenesis* 19(12):2163-2168.

Westermann AM, Taal BG, Swart M, Boot H, Craanen M, Gerritsen WR. (2000). Sequence-dependent toxicity profile in modified FAMTX (fluorouracil-adriamycin-methotrexate) chemotherapy with lenograstim support for advanced gastric cancer: A feasibility study. *Pharmacology Research* 42(2):151-156.

Westin J, Rodjer S, Turesson I, Cortelezzi A, Hjorth M, Zador G. (1995). Interferon alfa-2b versus no maintenance therapy during the plateau phase in multiple myeloma: A randomized study. Cooperative Study Group. *British Journal of Haematology* 89(3):561-568.

Wharton RH. (2002). Sleeping with the enemy: Treatment of fatigue in individuals with cancer. *Oncologist* 7(2):96-99.

Whedon M, Stearns D, Mills LE. (1995). Quality of life of long-term adult survivors of autologous bone marrow transplantation. *Oncology Nursing Forum* 22(10): 1527-1535; discussion 1535-1537.

Whelan TJ, Mohide EA, Willan AR, Arnold A, Tew M, Sellick S, Gafni A, Levine MN. (1997). The supportive care needs of newly diagnosed cancer patients attending a regional cancer center. *Cancer* 80(8):1518-1524.

Whelton CL, Salit I, Moldofsky H. (1992). Sleep, Epstein-Barr virus infection, musculoskeletal pain, and depressive symptoms in chronic fatigue syndrome. *Journal of Rheumatology* 19(6):939-943.

White A. (1995). The fibromyalgia syndrome: Electroacupuncture is a potentially valuable treatment. *British Medical Journal* 310(6991):1406.

White AM. (2001). Clinical applications of research on fatigue in children with cancer. *Journal of Pediatric Oncology Nursing* 18(2 Suppl 1):17-20.

White KP, Harth M. (1998). The fibromyalgia problem. *Journal of Rheumatology* 25(5):1022-1023; discussion 1028-1030.

White NJ, Given BA, Devoss DN. (1996). The advanced practice nurse: Meeting the information needs of the rural cancer patient. *Journal of Cancer Education* 11(4):203-209.

White PD. (1997). The relationship between infection and fatigue. *Journal of Psychosomatic Research* 43(4):345-350.

White PD, Dash AR, Thomas JM. (1998). Poor concentration and the ability to process information after glandular fever. *Journal of Psychosomatic Research* 44(2):269-278.

White PD, Thomas JM, Amess J, Crawford DH, Grover SA, Kangro HO, Clare AW. (1998). Incidence, risk, and prognosis of acute and chronic fatigue syndromes and psychiatric disorders after glandular fever. *British Journal of Psychiatry* 173:475-481.

White SC, Cheeseman S, Thatcher N, Anderson H, Carrington B, Hearn S, Ross G, Ranson M. (2000). Phase II study of oral topotecan in advanced non-small cell lung cancer. *Clinical Cancer Research* 6(3):868-873.

Whitehead RP, Figlin R, Citron ML, Pfile J, Moldawer N, Patel D, Jones G, Levitt D, Zeffren J. (1993). A phase II trial of concomitant human interleukin-2 and interferon-alpha-2a in patients with disseminated malignant melanoma. *Journal of Immunotherapy* 13(2):117-121.

Whitehead RP, Friedman KD, Clark DA, Pagani K, Rapp L. (1995). Phase I trial of simultaneous administration of interleukin 2 and interleukin 4 subcutaneously. *Clinical Cancer Research* 1(10):1145-1152.

Whitehead RP, Jacobson J, Brown TD, Taylor SA, Weiss GR, Macdonald JS. (1997). Phase II trial of paclitaxel and granulocyte colony-stimulating factor in patients with pancreatic carcinoma: A Southwest Oncology Group study. *Journal of Clinical Oncology* 15(6):2414-2419.

Whitehead RP, Unger JM, Flaherty LE, Eckardt JR, Taylor SA, Didolkar MS, Samlowski W, Sondak VK. (2001). Phase II trial of CI-980 in patients with disseminated malignant melanoma and no prior chemotherapy. A Southwest Oncology Group study. *Investigative New Drugs* 19(3):239-243.

Whitehead RP, Unger JM, Flaherty LE, Kraut EH, Mills GM, Klein CE, Chapman RA, Doolittle GC, Hammond N, Sondak VK; Southwest Oncology Group. (2002). A phase II trial of pyrazine diazohydroxide in patients with disseminated malignant melanoma and no prior chemotherapy—Southwest Oncology Group study. *Investigative New Drugs* 20(1):105-111.

Whitehead RP, Unger JM, Goodwin JW, Walker MJ, Thompson JA, Flaherty LE, Sondak VK. (1998). Phase II trial of recombinant human interleukin-4 in patients with disseminated malignant melanoma: A Southwest Oncology Group study. *Journal of Immunotherapy* 21(6):440-446.

Whitehead RP, Ward D, Hemingway L, Hemstreet GP III, Bradley E, Konrad M. (1990). Subcutaneous recombinant interleukin 2 in a dose escalating regimen in patients with metastatic renal cell adenocarcinoma. *Cancer Research* 50(20): 6708-6715.

Whitehead RP, Wolf MK, Solanki DL, Hemstreet GP III, Benedetto P, Richman SP, Flanigan RC, Crawford ED. (1995). A phase II trial of continuous-infusion recombinant interleukin-2 in patients with advanced renal cell carcinoma: A Southwest Oncology Group study. *Journal of Immunotherapy. Emphasis on Tumor Immunology* 18(2):104-114.

Whiteside TL. (1994). Cytokine measurements and interpretation in human disease. *Journal of Clinical Immunology* 14:327-339.

Whiteside TL, Friberg D. (1998). Natural killer cells and natural killer cell activity in chronic fatigue syndrome. *American Journal of Medicine* 105(3A):27S-34S.

Whiteside TL, Herberman RB. (1989). The role of natural killer cells in human disease. *Clinical Immunology and Immunopathology* 53(1):1-23.

Whitmer K, Barsevick A. (2001). Patient resources for cancer-related fatigue. *Cancer Practice* 9(6):311-313.

Whitmer KR, Jakubek PR, Barsevick AM. (1998). Use of a daily journal for fatigue management. *Oncology Nursing Forum* 25(6):987-988.

Whynes DK, Neilson AR. (1993). Convergent validity of two measures of the quality of life. *Health Economics* 2(3):229-235.

Wichers M, Maes M. (2002). The psychoneuroimmuno-pathophysiology of cytokine-induced depression in humans. *International Journal of Neuropsychopharmacology* 5(4):375-388.

Widdicombe JG. (1998). Afferent receptors in the airways and cough. *Respiratory Physiology* 114:5-15.

Wiebe E. (1996). N of 1 trials: Managing patients with chronic fatigue syndrome, two case reports. *Canadian Family Physician* 42:2214-2217.

Wiedenmann B, Reichardt P, Rath U, Theilmann L, Schule B, Ho AD, Schlick E, Kempeni J, Hunstein W, Kommerell B. (1989). Phase-I trial of intravenous continuous infusion of tumor necrosis factor in advanced metastatic carcinomas. *Journal of Cancer Research and Clinical Oncology* 115(2):189-192.

Wigers SH, Stiles TC, Vogel PA. (1996). Effects of aerobic exercise versus stress management treatment in fibromyalgia: A 4.5 year prospective study. *Scandinavian Journal of Rheumatology* 25(2):77-86.

Wigley R. (1999). Can fibromyalgia be separated from regional pain syndrome affecting the arm? *Journal of Rheumatology* 26(3):515-516.

Wikner J, Hirsch U, Wetterberg L, Rojdmark S. (1998). Fibromyalgia—A syndrome associated with decreased nocturnal melatonin secretion. *Clinical Endocrinology* (Oxford) 49(2):179-183.

Wilke WS. (1996a). Fibromyalgia: More than a label. *Cleveland Clinic Journal of Medicine* 63(2):87-89.

Wilke WS. (1996b). Fibromyalgia: Recognizing and addressing the multiple interrelated factors. *Postgraduate Medicine* 100(1):153-156, 163-166.

Wilke WS, Fouad-Tarazi FM, Cash JM, Calabrese LH. (1998). The connection between chronic fatigue syndrome and neurally mediated hypotension. *Cleveland Clinic Journal of Medicine* 65(5):261-266.

Wilkie DJ, Huang HY, Berry DL, Schwartz A, Lin YC, Ko NY, Chen A, Gralow J, Lindsley SK, Fitzgibbon D. (2001). Cancer symptom control: Feasibility of a tailored, interactive computerized program for patients. *Family Community Health* 24(3):48-62.

Williams DR, Rucker TD. (2000). Understanding and addressing racial disparities in health care. *Health Care Financial Reviews* 21:75-90.

Williams G, Pirmohamed J, Minors D, Waterhouse J, Buchan I, Arendt J. (1996). Dissociation of body temperature and melatonin secretion circadian rhythms in patients with chronic fatigue syndrome. *Clinical Physiology* 16(4):327-337.

Williams MS, Burk M, Loprinzi CL, Hill M, Schomberg PJ, Nearhood K, O'Fallon JR, Laurie JA, Shanahan TG, Moore RL, et al. (1996). Phase III double-blind evaluation of an *Aloë vera* gel as a prophylactic agent for radiation-induced skin toxicity. *International Journal of Radiation Oncology, Biology, and Physics* 36(2):345-349.

Williams PD, Ducey KA, Sears AM, Williams AR, Tobin-Rumelhart SE, Bunde P. (2001). Treatment type and symptom severity among oncology patients by self-report. *International Journal of Nursing Studies* 38(3):359-367.

Wilson A, Hickie I, Lloyd A, Hadzi-Pavlovic D, Boughton C, Dwyer J, Wakefield D. (1994). Longitudinal study of outcome of chronic fatigue syndrome. *British Medical Journal* 308:756-759.

Wilson A, Hickie I, Lloyd A, Wakefield D. (1994). The treatment of chronic fatigue syndrome: Science and speculation. *American Journal of Medicine* 96:544-550.

Wilson JT, Wald SL, Aitken PA, Mastromateo J, Vieco PT. (1995). Primary diffuse chiasmatic germinomas: Differentiation from optic chiasm gliomas. *Pediatric Neurosurgery* 23(1):1-5; discussion 6.

Wilt SG, Milward E, Zhou JM, Nagasato K, Patton H, Rusten R, Griffin DE, O'Connor M, Dubois-Dalag M. (1995). In vitro evidence for a dual role of tumor necrosis factor in human immunodeficiency virus type 1 encephalopathy. *Annals of Neurology* 37(3):381-394.

Winer EP, Lindley C, Hardee M, Sawyer WT, Brunatti C, Borstelmann NA, Peters W. (1999). Quality of life in patients surviving at least 12 months following high dose chemotherapy with autologous bone marrow support. *Psychooncology* 8(2):167-176.

Winfield JB. (1997). Fibromyalgia: What's next? *Arthritis Care Research* 10(4):219-221.

Winfield JB. (1999). Pain in fibromyalgia. *Rheumatic Diseases Clinics of North America* 25(1):55-79.

Winfield JB. (2000). Psychological determinants of fibromyalgia and related syndromes. *Current Reviews in Pain* 4(4):276-286.

Winkelaar PG. (1999). Medicolegal file: Tacit approval of alternative therapy. *Canadian Family Physician* 45:905.

Winningham ML. (1991). Walking program for people with cancer: Getting started. *Cancer Nursing* 14(5):270-276.

Winningham ML. (2000). Reader clarifies concepts of structured exercise programs in managing fatigue. *Oncology Nursing Forum* 27(3):425-426.

Winningham ML. (2001). Strategies for managing cancer-related fatigue syndrome: A rehabilitation approach. *Cancer* 92(4 Suppl):988-997.

Winningham ML, Nail LM, Burke MB, Brophy L, Cimprich B, Jones LS, Pickard-Holley S, Rhodes V, St Pierre B, Beck S, et al. (1994). Fatigue and the cancer experience: The state of the knowledge. *Oncology Nursing Forum* 21(1):23-36.

Winslow LC, Kroll DJ. (1998). Herbs as medicines. *Archives of Internal Medicine* 158(20):2192-2199.

Winstead-Fry P. (1998). Psychometric assessment of four fatigue scales with a sample of rural cancer patients. *Journal of Nursing Measurements* 6(2):111-122.

Winston D, Dattner AM. (1999). The American system of medicine. *Clinical Dermatology* 17(1):53-56.

Winterholler M, Erbguth F, Neundorfer B. (1997). Verwendung para-medizinischer Verfahren durch MS-Patienten—Patientencharakterisierung und Anwendungsgewohnheiten. *Fortschrift Neurologie Psychiatrie* 65(12):555-561.

Wiseman LR, Spencer CM. (1997). Mitoxantrone: A review of its pharmacology and clinical efficacy in the management of hormone-resistant advanced prostate cancer. *Drugs and Aging* 10(6):473-485.

Wisloff F, Gulbrandsen N. (2000). Health-related quality of life and patients' perceptions in interferon-treated multiple myeloma patients. Nordic Myeloma Study Group. *Acta Oncologica* 39(7):809-813.

Wisloff F, Hjorth M. (1997). Health-related quality of life assessed before and during chemotherapy predicts for survival in multiple myeloma. Nordic Myeloma Study Group. *British Journal of Haematology* 97(1):29-37.

Wisloff F, Hjorth M, Kaasa S, Westin J. (1996). Effect of interferon on the health-related quality of life of multiple myeloma patients: Results of a Nordic randomized trial comparing melphalan-prednisone to melphalan-prednisone + alpha-interferon. The Nordic Myeloma Study Group. *British Journal of Haematology* 94(2):324-332.

Witt J, Murray-Edwards D. (2002). Living with fatigue: Managing cancer-related fatigue at home and in the workplace. *American Journal of Nursing* 102(Suppl 4): 28-31.

Witt PL, Zahir S, Ritch PS, McAuliffe TM, Ewel CH, Borden EC. (1996). Phase I/IB study of polyadenylic-polyuridylic acid in patients with advanced malignancies: Clinical and biologic effects. *Journal of Interferon and Cytokine Research* 16(8):631-635.

Wittig RM, Zorick FJ, Blumer D, Heilbronn M, Roth T. (1982). Disturbed sleep in patients complaining of chronic pain. *Journal of Nerve and Mental Diseases* 170:429-431.

Wlodawer A, Erickson JW. (1993). Structure-based inhibitors of HIV-1 protease. *Annual Reviews of Biochemistry* 62:543-585.

Woldehiwe T. (1991). Lymphocytic subpopulations in peripheral blood of sheep experimentally infected with tick-borne disease. *Research Veterinary Scientist* 7:20-25.

Wolfe F. (1997). The fibromyalgia problem. *Journal of Rheumatology* 24(7):1247-1249.

Wolfe F. (1999). "Silicone-related symptoms" are common in patients with fibromyalgia: No evidence for a new disease. *Journal of Rheumatology* 26(5):1172-1175.

Wolfe F, Anderson J. (1999). Silicone-filled breast implants and the risk of fibromyalgia and rheumatoid arthritis. *Journal of Rheumatology* 26(9):2025-2028.

Wolfe F, Anderson J, Harkness D, Bennett RM, Caro XJ, Goldenberg DL, Russell IJ, Yunus MB. (1997). A prospective, longitudinal, multicenter study of service utilization and costs in fibromyalgia. *Arthritis and Rheumatism* 40(9):1560-1570.

Wolfe F, Cathey MA. (1983). Prevalence of primary and secondary fibrositis. *Journal of Rheumatology* 10:965-968.

Wolfe F, Hawley DJ. (1997). Measurement of the quality of life in rheumatic disorders using the EuroQol. *British Journal of Rheumatology* 36(7):786-793.

Wolfe F, Hawley DJ. (1998). Psychosocial factors and the fibromyalgia syndrome. *Zeitschrift Rheumatologie* 57(Suppl 2):88-91.

Wolfe F, Hawley DJ, Wilson K. (1996). The prevalence and meaning of fatigue in rheumatic disease. *The Journal of Rheumatology* 23(8):1407-1417.

Wolfe F, Smythe HA, Yunus MB, Bennett RM, Bombardier C, Goldenberg DL, Tugwell P, Campbell SM, Abeles M, Clark P. (1990). The American College of Rheumatology 1990 criteria for the classification of fibromyalgia: Report of the multicenter criteria committee. *Arthritis and Rheumatism* 33:160-172.

Wolfe G. (2000). Fatigue: The most important consideration for the patient with cancer. *Caring* 19(4):46-47.

Wolfe J, Grier HE, Klar N, Levin SB, Ellenbogen JM, Salem-Schatz S, Emanuel EJ, Weeks JC. (2000). Symptoms and suffering at the end of life in children with cancer. *New England Journal of Medicine* 342(5):326-333.

Wolff RA, Evans DB, Gravel DM, Lenzi R, Pisters PW, Lee JE, Janjan NA, Charnsangavej C, Abbruzzese JL. (2001). Phase I trial of gemcitabine combined with radiation for the treatment of locally advanced pancreatic adenocarcinoma. *Clinical Cancer Research* 7(8):2246-2253.

Wolf-Klein GP, Jason MK, Desner M, Fish B, Silvergleid R. (1989). A new onset of fatigue in an active elderly man. *Geriatrics* 44(9):85-86.

Wong HCG. (1999). Probable false authentication of herbal plants: Ginseng. *Archives of Internal Medicine* 159(10):11142.

Wong HCG, Wong NYY, Wong JKT, Wong AMY. (1999). Chinese proprietary and herbal medicines used in three allergic diseases [abstract]. *Journal of Allergy and Clinical Immunology* 103(1 Pt 2):A771.

Wong LK, Jue P, Lam A, Yeung W, Cham-Yah Y, Birtwhistle R. (1998). Chinese herbal medicine and acupuncture: How do patients who consult family physicians use these therapies? *Canadian Family Physician* 44:1009-1015.

Wong RK, Franssen E, Szumacher E, Connolly R, Evans M, Page B, Chow E, Hayter C, Harth T, Andersson L, et al. (2002). What do patients living with advanced cancer and their carers want to know?—A needs assessment. *Support Care in Cancer* 10(5):408-415.

Woo B, Dibble SL, Piper BF, Keating SB, Weiss MC. (1998). Differences in fatigue by treatment methods in women with breast cancer. *Oncology Nursing Forum* 25(5):915-920.

Wood B, Wessely S, Papadopoulos A, Poon L, Checkley S. (1998). Salivary cortisol profiles in chronic fatigue syndrome. *Neuropsychobiology* 37(1):1-4.

Wood C, Magnello ME. (1992). Diurnal changes in perceptions of energy and mood. *Journal of the Royal Scociety of Medicine* 85:191-194.

Wood GC, Bentall RP, Gopfert M, Dewey ME, Edwards RHT. (1994). The differential response of chronic fatigue, neurotic and muscular dystrophy patients to experimental psychological stress. *Psychological Medicine* 24:357-364.

Woolley PV, Schultz CJ, Rodriguez GI, Gams RA, Rowe KW Jr, Dadey ML, Von Hoff DD, McPhillips JJ. (1996). A phase II trial of ilmofosine in non-small cell bronchogenic carcinoma. *Investigative New Drugs* 14(2):219-222.

Wootton JC. (2000). Fibromyalgia. *Journal of Women's Health and Gender Based Medicine* 9(5):571-573.

Wright JB, Beverly DW. (1998). Chronic fatigue syndrome. *Archives of Disease in Childhood* 79(4):368-374.

Wu CW, Lo SS, Shen KH, Hsieh MC, Lui WY, P'eng FK. (2000). Surgical mortality, survival, and quality of life after resection for gastric cancer in the elderly. *World Journal of Surgery* 24(4):465-472.

Wu CY, Sarfati M, Heusser C, Fournier S, Rubio-Trujillo M, Peleman R, Delespesse G. (1991). Glucocorticoids increase the synthesis of immunoglobulin E by interleukin 4-stimulated human lymphocytes. *Journal of Clinical Investigation* 87(3):870-877.

Wu HS, McSweeney M. (2001). Measurement of fatigue in people with cancer. *Oncology Nursing Forum* 28(9):1371-1384.

Wu Y, Zhang Y, Wu JA, Lowell T, Gu M, Yuan CS. (1998). Effects of Erkang, a modified formulation of Chinese folk medicine Shi-Quan-Da-Bu-Tang, on mice. *Journal of Ethnopharmacology* 61(2):153-159.

Wyatt GK, Friedman LL. (1998). Physical and psychosocial outcomes of midlife and older women following surgery and adjuvant therapy for breast cancer. *Oncology Nursing Forum* 25(4):761-768.

Wydra EW. (2001). The effectiveness of a self-care management interactive multimedia module. *Oncology Nursing Forum* 28(9):1399-1407.

Wymenga AN, Eriksson B, Salmela PI, Jacobsen MB, Van Cutsem EJ, Fiasse RH, Valimaki MJ, Renstrup J, de Vries EG, Oberg KE. (1999). Efficacy and safety of prolonged-release lanreotide in patients with gastrointestinal neuroendocrine tumors and hormone-related symptoms. *Journal of Clinical Oncology* 17(4):1111.

Xia Y, Ross GD. (1999). Generation of recombinant fragments of CD11b expressing the functional ß-glucan-binding lectin site of CR3 (CD11b/CD18). *Journal of Immunology* 162:7285-7293.

Xia Y, Vetvicka V, Yan J, Hanikyrova M, Mayadas T, Ross GD. (1999). The ß-glucan-binding lectin site of mouse CR3 (CD11b/CD18) and its function in generating a primed state of the receptor that mediates cytotoxic activation in response to iC3b-opsonized target cells. *Journal of Immunology* 162:2281-2290.

Xie X, Ye C. (1997). [Clinical analysis of 120 patients with fibromyalgia]. *Hunan I Ko Ta Hsueh Hsueh Pao* 22(2):167-170.

Yagi A, Egusa T, Arase M, Tanabe M, Tsuji H. (1997). Isolation and characterization of the glycoprotein fraction with a proliferation-promoting activity on human and hamster cells in vitro from *Aloë vera* gel. *Planta Medica* 63(1):18-21.

Yagi A, Nakamori J, Yamada T, Iwase H, Tanaka T, Kaneo Y, Qiu J, Orndorff S. (1999). In vivo metabolism of aloemannan. *Planta Medica* 65(5):417-420.

Yahchouchi E, Cherqui D. (2000). [Biliary tract cancers]. *Rev Prat* 50(19):2130-2135.

Yamada H. (1989). [Chemical characterization and biological activity of the immunologically active substances in Juzen-taiho-to (Japanese kampo prescription)]. *Gan To Kagaku Ryoho* 16(4 Pt 2-2):1500-1505.

Yamaguchi M, Oka K, Ohno T, Kageyama S, Kita K, Shirakawa S. (1993). [Intermediate lymphocytic lymphoma with multiple lymphomatous polyposis of the gastrointestinal tract]. *Rinsho Ketsueki* 34(1):44-49.

Yamaguchi S, Fukuda M, Ota T, Nakayama Y, Ogata H, Shimizu K, Nishikawa T, Adachi Y, Fukuma E. (1999). [A study on the efficacy of combination chemo-endocrine therapy consisting of cyclophosphamide, adriamycin, UFT, and tamoxifen for advanced or recurrent breast cancer]. *Gan To Kagaku Ryoho* 26(8): 1145-1152.

Yamamoto J, Abe Y, Nishihara K, Katsumoto F, Takeda S, Abe R, Toyoshima S. (1998). Composite glandular-neuroendocrine carcinoma of the hilar bile duct: Report of a case. *Surgery Today* 28(7):758-762.

Yamamoto K, Masuyama T, Hori M. (1999). [A 49-year-old man with general fatigue and an increase in cardiothoracic ratio]. *Journal of Cardiology* 34(3):157-158.

Yamamoto K, Yajima A, Terashima Y, Nozawa S, Taketani Y, Yakushiji M, Noda K. (1999). Phase II clinical study on the effects of recombinant human interleukin-3 on thrombocytopenia after chemotherapy for advanced ovarian cancer. SDZ ILE 964 [IL-3] Study Group. *Journal of Immunotherapy* 22(6):539-545.

Yamamoto N, Zou JP, Li XF, Takenaka H, Noda S, Fujii T, Ono S, Kobayashi Y, Mukaida N, Matsushima K, et al. (1995). Regulatory mechanisms for production of IFN-gamma and TNF by antitumor T cells or macrophages in the tumor-bearing state. *Journal of Immunology* 154:2281-2290.

Yamamoto T, Castell LM, Botella J, Powell H, Hall GM, Young A, Newsholme EA. (1997). Changes in the albumin binding of tryptophan during postoperative recovery: A possible link wuth central fatigue? *Brain Research Bulletin* 43(1): 43-46.

Yamamura M, Modlin RL, Ohmen JD, Moy RL. (1993). Local expression of anti-inflammatory cytokines in cancer. *Journal of Clinical Investigation* 91:1005-1010.

Yamashiki M, Nishimura A, Nobori T, Nakabayashi S, Takagi T, Inoue K, Ito M, Matsushita K, Ohtaki H, Kosaka Y. (1997). In vitro effects of Sho-saiko-to on production of granulocyte colony-stimulating factor by mononuclear cells from patients with chronic hepatitis C. *International Journal of Immunopharmacology* 19(7):381-385.

Yan J, Vetvicka V, Xia Y, Coxon A, Carroll MC, Mayadas TN, Ross GD. (1999). ß-glucan, a "specific" biologic response modifier that uses antibodies to target tumors for cytotoxic recognition by leukocyte complement receptor 3 (CD11b/ CD18). *Journal of Immunology* 163:3045-3052.

Yang G, Hellstrom KE, Mizuno MT, Chen L. (1995). In vitro priming of tumor-reactive cytolytic T lymphocytes by combining IL-10 with B7-CD28 costimulation. *Journal of Immunology* 155:3897-3903.

Yang TS, Hsu KC, Chiang JM, Tang R, Chen JS, Changchien CR, Wang JY. (1999). A simplified regimen of weekly high dose 5-fluorouracil and leucovorin as a 24-hour infusion in patients with advanced colorectal carcinoma. *Cancer* 85(9):1925-1930.

Yano T, Ishida T, Yoshino I, Murata M, Yasumoto K, Kimura G, Nomoto K, Sugimachi K. (1991). A regimen of surgical adjuvant immunotherapy for cancer with interleukin 2 and lymphokine-activated killer cells: Basis, clinical toxicity, and immunomodulatory effects. *Biotherapy* 3(3):245-251.

Yap BS, Plager C, Benjamin RS, Murphy WK, Legha SS, Bodey GP. (1981). Phase II evaluation of AMSA in adult sarcomas. *Cancer Treatment Reports* 65(3-4): 341-343.

Yarbro CH. (1996). Interventions for fatigue. *European Journal of Cancer Care* (English Language Edition) 5(2 Suppl):35-38.

Yarchoan R, Pluda JM, Perno CF, Mitsuya H, Broder S. (1991). Antiretroviral therapy of human immunodeficiency virus infection: Current strategies and challenges for the future. *Blood* 78(4):859-884.

Yasko JM, Greene P. (1987). Coping with problems related to cancer and cancer treatment. *CA Cancer Journal for Clinicians* 37(2):106-125.

Yasumoto R, Asakawa M, Hayahara N, Maekawa T, Wada S, Kishimoto T, Maekawa M, Morikawa Y, Kawakita J, Umeda M, et al. (1992). [Clinical study of prophylactic therapy of interferon on postoperative renal cell carcinoma]. *Hinyokika Kiyo* 38(3):267-275.

Yasumoto S. (1995). Human papilloma virus type 16 gene functions relevant to molecular human carcinogenesis. *Nippon Rinski* 53(11):2858-2867.

Yata K, Wada H, Otsuki T, Sadahira Y, Sugihara T, Yamada O, Yawata Y. (1999). [Primary splenic lymphoma with t(3;14)(q27;q32) chromosomal abnormality and rearrangement of BCL-6 gene]. *Rinsho Ketsueki* 40(7):587-592.

Yataco A, Talo H, Rowe P, Kass DA, Berger D, Calkins H. (1997). Comparison of heart rate variability in patients with chronic fatigue syndrome and controls. *Clinical Autonomic Research* 7(6):293-297.

Yatham LN, Morehouse RL, Chisholm T, Haase DA, MacDonald DD, Marrie TJ. (1995). Neuroendocrine assessment of serotonin (5-HT) function in chronic fatigue syndrome. *Canadian Journal of Psychiatry* 40(2):93-96.

Yellen SB, Cella DF, Webster K, Blendowski C, Kaplan E. (1997). Measuring fatigue and other anemia-related symptoms with the Functional Assessment of Cancer Therapy (FACT) measurement system. *Journal of Pain Symptomatology and Management* 13(2):63-74.

Yoder LH, O'Rourke TJ, Etnyre A, Spears DT, Brown TD. (1997). Expectations and experiences of patients with cancer participating in phase I clinical trials. *Oncology Nursing Forum* 24(5):891-896.

Yoshida K, Aida K, Horibe T, Kashimura T, Handa A, Matsuda A, Murohashi I, Jinnai I, Ino H, Bessho M, et al. (1997). [Plasma cell leukemia associated with monocytosis]. *Rinsho Ketsueki* 38(7):604-609.

Yoshida M. (2001). [Management of complications in patients with chronic myelogenous leukemia]. *Nippon Rinsho* 59(12):2410-2415.

Yoshida T, Takagi T, Shimoyama M, Mikuni C, Suzuki K, Egami K, Furusawa S, Nomura T, Mori M, Sugimoto T, et al. (1994). [Late phase II study with 21-consecutive-day oral administration of etoposide for malignant lymphoma]. *Gan To Kagaku Ryoho* 21(16):2793-2801.

Yoshimoto J, Nasu Y, Akagi T, Obama T, Tsushima T, Ozaki Y, Matsumura Y, Ohmori H, Asahi T, Ohkita K, et al. (1985). [Combination chemotherapy with cisplatin, ifosfamide and adriamycin in patients with advanced transitional cell carcinoma of the urinary tract]. *Gan To Kagaku Ryoho* 12(6):1312-1317.

Yoshimoto J, Tsushima T, Matsumura Y, Ohmori H, Saito N, Tanaka H, Asahi T, Ohkita K, Tanahashi T, Nanba K, et al. (1985). [Phase II study of recombinant human leukocyte A interferon on urogenital cancer patients]. *Gan To Kagaku Ryoho* 12(3 Pt 1):465-470.

Yoshino I, Goedegebuure PS, Peoples GE, Parikh AS, DiMaio JM, Lyerly HK, Gazdar AF, Eberlein TJ. (1994). HER 2/neu-derived peptides are shared antigens among human non-small cell lung cancer and ovarian cancer. *Cancer Research* 54:3387.

Yoshino S, Oka M, Hazama S, Suzuki T. (1989). Effect of intrapleural and/or intraperitoneal Lentinan therapy on carcinomatous pleuritis with special reference to immunological evaluation. *Nippon Geka Hokan* 58:310-319.

Yoshioka M, Ihara H, Shima H, Mori Y, Ikoma F, Ueno Y, Uematsu K. (1994). [Adrenal hepatoid carcinoma producing alpha-fetoprotein: A case report]. *Hinyokika Kiyo* 40(5):411-414.

Younes A, Sarris A, Consoli U, Rodriguez A, McLaughlin P, Huh Y, Starry S, Cabanillas F, Andreeff M. (1996). A pilot study of high-dose interleukin-3 treatment of relapsed follicular small cleaved-cell lymphoma: Hematologic, immunologic, and clinical results. *Blood* 87(5):1698-1703.

Young AH, Sharpe M, Clements A, Dowling B, Hawton KE, Cowen PJ. (1998). Basal activity of the hypothalamic-pituitary-adrenal axis in patients with the chronic fatigue syndrome (neurasthenia). *Biological Psychiatry* 43(3):236-237.

Young MR, Wright MA, Lozano Y, Matthews JP, Benefiedl J, Prechel MM. (1996). Mechanisms of immune suppression in patients with head and neck cancer: Influence on the immune infiltrate of the cancer. *International Journal of Cancer* 67:333-338.

Young VL, Nemecek JR, Schwartz BD, Phelan DL, Schorr MW. (1995). HLA typing in women with breast implants. *Plastic and Reconstructive Surgery* 96(7): 1497-1519, discussion 1520.

Yount S, Cella D, Webster K, Heffernan N, Chang C, Odom L, Van Gool R. (2002). Assessment of patient-reported clinical outcome in pancreatic and other hepatobiliary cancers: The FACT Hepatobiliary Symptom Index. *Journal of Pain Symptom Management* 24(1):32-44.

Yount S, Lai JS, Cella D. (2002). Methods and progress in assessing the quality of life effects of supportive care with erythropoietin therapy. *Current Opinions in Hematology* 9(3):234-240.

Yron I, Wood TA Jr, Spiess PJ, Rosenberg SA. (1980). In vitro growth of murine T cells: V. The isolation and growth of lymphoid cells infiltrating syngeneic solid tumors. *Journal of Immunology* 125:238-245.

Yu Z, Zhang M, Shi Q. (1997). [Hodgkin's disease with concurrent infection of toxoplasmosis]. *Zhonghua Wai Ke Za Zhi* 35(1):33-34.

Yunus MB, Aldag JC. (1996). Restless legs syndrome and leg cramps in fibromyalgia syndrome: A controlled study. *British Medical Journal* 312(7042): 1339.

Yunus MB, Inanici F, Aldag JC, Mangold RF. (2000). Fibromyalgia in men: Comparison of clinical features with women. *Journal of Rheumatology* 27(2):485-490.

Yunus MB, Masi AT, Calabro JJ, Miller KA, Feigenbaum SI. (1981). Primary fibromyalgia (fibrositis): Clinical study of 50 patients with matched controls. *Seminars in Arthritis and Rheumatism* 11:151-172.

Zachrisson O, Regland B, Jahreskog M, Jonsson M, Kron M, Gottfries CG. (2002). Treatment with staphylococcus toxoid in fibromyalgia/chronic fatigue syndrome—A randomised controlled trial. *European Journal of Pain* 6(6):455-466.

Zachrisson O, Regland B, Jahreskog M, Kron M, Gottfries CG. (2002). A rating scale for fibromyalgia and chronic fatigue syndrome (the FibroFatigue Scale). *Journal of Psychosomatic Research* 52(6):501-509.

Zahner J. (2000). [Fatigue and exhaustion in tumor patients: Etiology, diagnosis and treatment possibilities]. *Medizinische Klinik* 95(11):613-617.

Zahner J, Meran J, Karthaus M. (2001). [Exhaustion and fatigue—A neglected problem in hematologic oncology]. *Wien Medizinische Wochenschrift* 151(3-4): 89-93.

Zaloga GP, Eil C, Medbery CA. (1985). Humoral hypercalcemia in Hodgkin's disease: Association with elevated 1,25-dihydroxycholecalciferol levels and subperiosteal bone resorption. *Archives of Internal Medicine* 145(1):155-157.

Zamagni C, Martoni A, Cacciari N, Gentile A, Pannuti F. (1998). The combination of paclitaxel and carboplatin as first-line chemotherapy in patients with stage III and stage IV ovarian cancer: A phase I-II study. *American Journal of Clinical Oncology* 21(5):491-497.

Zaoui P, Green W, Hakim RM. (1991). Hemodialysis with cuprophane membrane modulates interleukin-2 receptor expression. *Kidney International* 39:1020-1026.

Zaridze DG, Boyle P. (1987). Cancer of the prostate: Epidemiology and aetiology. *British Journal of Urology* 59:493-502.

Zarogoulidis K, Ziogas E, Papagiannis A, Charitopoulos K, Dimitriadis K, Economides D, Maglaveras N, Vamvalis C. (1996). Interferon alpha-2a and combined chemotherapy as first line treatment in SCLC patients: A randomized trial. *Lung Cancer* 15(2):197-205.

Zborovskii AB, Babaeva AR. (1998). [Diagnosis of primary fibromyalgia: Clinical criteria] Klinicheskie kriterii diagnoza pervichnoi fibromialgii. *Klinik Medizin* (Mosk) 76(8):18-21.

Zebrack BJ, Chesler MA. (2002). Quality of life in childhood cancer survivors. *Psychooncology* 11(2):132-141.

Zee-Cheng RK. (1992). Shi-quan-da-bu-tang (ten significant tonic decoction), SQT: A potent Chinese biological response modifier in cancer immunotherapy, potentiation and detoxification of anticancer drugs. *Methods and Findings in Experimental and Clinical Pharmacology* 14(9):725-736.

Zelefsky MJ, Kelly WK, Scher HI, Lee H, Smart T, Metz E, Schwartz L, Fuks Z, Leibel SA. (2000). Results of a phase II study using estramustine phosphate and vinblastine in combination with high-dose three-dimensional conformal radiotherapy for patients with locally advanced prostate cancer. *Journal of Clinical Oncology* 18(9):1936-1941.

Zeltzer LK, Chen E, Weiss R, Guo MD, Robison LL, Meadows AT, Mills JL, Nicholson HS, Byrne J. (1997). Comparison of psychologic outcome in adult survivors of childhood acute lymphoblastic leukemia versus sibling controls: A cooperative Children's Cancer Group and National Institutes of Health study. *Journal of Clinical Oncology* 15(2):547-556.

Zenone T. (1992). Autoimmunity and cancer: Paraneoplastic neurological syndromes associated with small cell lung cancer. *Cancer Bulletin* 79:837-853.

Zhai S, Senderowicz AM, Sausville EA, Figg WD. (2002). Flavopiridol, a novel cyclin-dependent kinase inhibitor, in clinical development. *Annals of Pharmacotherapy* 36(5):905-911.

Zhang L, Tizard IR. (1996). Activation of a mouse macrophage cell line by acemannan: The major carbohydrate fraction from *Aloë vera* gel. *Immunopharmacology* 35(2):119-128.

Zheng Z, Liu D, Song C, Chang C, Hu Z. (1998). Studies on chemical constituents and immunological function activity of hairy root of *Astragalus membranaceus*. *Chinese Journal of Biotechnology* 14(2):93-97.

Zhu M, Wong PY, Li RC. (1999). Influence of *Sanguisorba officinalis,* a mineral-rich plant drug, on the pharmacokinetics of ciprofloxacin in the rat. *Journal of Antimicrobial Chemotherapy* 44(1):125-128.

Zhu XP. (1988). [Adrenal cortical carcinoma (ACC)—Report of 10 cases]. *Zhonghua Zhong Liu Za Zhi* 10(6):462-464.

Zieren HU, Jacobi CA, Zieren J, Muller JM. (1996). Quality of life following resection of oesophageal carcinoma. *British Journal of Surgery* 83(12):1772-1775.

Zimmerman S, Adkins D, Graham M, Petruska P, Bowers C, Vrahnos D, Spitzer G. (1994). Irreversible, severe congestive cardiomyopathy occurring in association with interferon alpha therapy. *Cancer Biotherapy* 9(4):291-299.

Zittoun R, Achard S, Ruszniewski M. (1999). Assessment of quality of life during intensive chemotherapy or bone marrow transplantation. *Psychooncology* 8(1):64-73.

Zlotnik A, Shimonkewitz P, Gefter ML, Kappler J, Marrack P. (1983). Characterization of the gamma interferon-mediated induction of antigen-presenting ability in P388D cells. *Journal of Immunology* 131(6):2814-2820.

Zorat F, Pozzato G. (2002). Thalidomide in myelodysplastic syndromes. *Biomedical Pharmacotherapy* 56(1):20-30.

Zujewski J, Horak ID, Bol CJ, Woestenborghs R, Bowden C, End DW, Piotrovsky VK, Chiao J, Belly RT, Todd A, et al. (2000). Phase I and pharmacokinetic study of farnesyl protein transferase inhibitor R115777 in advanced cancer. *Journal of Clinical Oncology* 18(4):927-941.

Zutic H. (1999). [Bronchial carcinoma—An overview]. *Med Arh* 53(3 Suppl 1):27-31.

Zwilling BS, Brown D, Pearl D. (1992). Induction of major histocompatibility complex class II glycoproteins by interferon-gamma: Attenuation of the effects of restraint stress. *Journal of Neuroimmunology* 37(1-2):115-122.

Index

Order a copy of this book with this form or online at:
http://www.haworthpress.com/store/product.asp?sku=5064

MEDICAL ETIOLOGY, ASSESSMENT, AND TREATMENT OF CHRONIC FATIGUE AND MALAISE
Clinical Differentiation and Intervention

_____in hardbound at $89.95 (ISBN: 0-7890-2195-1)
_____in softbound at $49.95 (ISBN: 0-7890-2196-X)

Or order online and use special offer code HEC25 in the shopping cart.

COST OF BOOKS_____

POSTAGE & HANDLING_____
(US: $4.00 for first book & $1.50
for each additional book)
(Outside US: $5.00 for first book
& $2.00 for each additional book)

SUBTOTAL_____

IN CANADA: ADD 7% GST_____

STATE TAX_____
(NJ, NY, OH, MN, CA, IL, IN, & SD residents,
add appropriate local sales tax)

FINAL TOTAL_____
(If paying in Canadian funds,
convert using the current
exchange rate, UNESCO
coupons welcome)

☐ **BILL ME LATER:** (Bill-me option is good on
US/Canada/Mexico orders only; not good to
jobbers, wholesalers, or subscription agencies.)
☐ Check here if billing address is different from
shipping address and attach purchase order and
billing address information.

Signature_____

☐ **PAYMENT ENCLOSED: $**_____

☐ **PLEASE CHARGE TO MY CREDIT CARD.**

☐ Visa ☐ MasterCard ☐ AmEx ☐ Discover
☐ Diner's Club ☐ Eurocard ☐ JCB

Account #_____

Exp. Date_____

Signature_____

Prices in US dollars and subject to change without notice.

NAME_____

INSTITUTION_____

ADDRESS_____

CITY_____

STATE/ZIP_____

COUNTRY_____ COUNTY (NY residents only)_____

TEL_____ FAX_____

E-MAIL_____

May we use your e-mail address for confirmations and other types of information? ☐ Yes ☐ No
We appreciate receiving your e-mail address and fax number. Haworth would like to e-mail or fax special
discount offers to you, as a preferred customer. **We will never share, rent, or exchange your e-mail address
or fax number.** We regard such actions as an invasion of your privacy.

Order From Your Local Bookstore or Directly From
The Haworth Press, Inc.
10 Alice Street, Binghamton, New York 13904-1580 • USA
TELEPHONE: 1-800-HAWORTH (1-800-429-6784) / Outside US/Canada: (607) 722-5857
FAX: 1-800-895-0582 / Outside US/Canada: (607) 771-0012
E-mailto: orders@haworthpress.com

For orders outside US and Canada, you may wish to order through your local
sales representative, distributor, or bookseller.
For information, see http://haworthpress.com/distributors

(Discounts are available for individual orders in US and Canada only, not booksellers/distributors.)
PLEASE PHOTOCOPY THIS FORM FOR YOUR PERSONAL USE.
http://www.HaworthPress.com   BOF04